MANAGEMENT AND LEADERSHIP FOR NURSE ADMINISTRATORS

FIFTH EDITION

Edited by

Linda Roussel, DSN, RN, NEA, BC
Professor/Executive Nurse Program
University of South Alabama
College of Nursing
Mobile, Alabama

with

Russell C. Swansburg, PhD, RN
Consultant in Nursing and Hospital Administration
San Antonio, Texas

JONES AND BARTLETT PUBLISHERS
Sudbury, Massachusetts
BOSTON   TORONTO   LONDON   SINGAPORE

World Headquarters

Jones and Bartlett Publishers
40 Tall Pine Drive
Sudbury, MA 01776
978-443-5000
info@jbpub.com
www.jbpub.com

Jones and Bartlett Publishers
Canada
6339 Ormindale Way
Mississauga, Ontario L5V 1J2
Canada

Jones and Bartlett Publishers
International
Barb House, Barb Mews
London W6 7PA
United Kingdom

Jones and Bartlett's books and products are available through most bookstores and online booksellers. To contact Jones and Bartlett Publishers directly, call 800-832-0034, fax 978-443-8000, or visit our website, www.jbpub.com.

Substantial discounts on bulk quantities of Jones and Bartlett's publications are available to corporations, professional associations, and other qualified organizations. For details and specific discount information, contact the special sales department at Jones and Bartlett via the above contact information or send an email to specialsales@jbpub.com.

The authors, editor, and publisher have made every effort to provide accurate information. However, they are not responsible for errors, omissions, or for any outcomes related to the use of the contents of this book and take no responsibility for the use of the products and procedures described. Treatments and side effects described in this book may not be applicable to all people; likewise, some people may require a dose or experience a side effect that is not described herein. Drugs and medical devices are discussed that may have limited availability controlled by the Food and Drug Administration (FDA) for use only in a research study or clinical trial. Research, clinical practice, and government regulations often change the accepted standard in this field. When consideration is being given to use of any drug in the clinical setting, the health care provider or reader is responsible for determining FDA status of the drug, reading the package insert, and reviewing prescribing information for the most up-to-date recommendations on dose, precautions, and contraindications, and determining the appropriate usage for the product. This is especially important in the case of drugs that are new or seldom used.

Production Credits
Publisher: Kevin Sullivan
Aquisitions Editor: Emily Ekle
Aquisitions Editor: Amy Sibley
Associate Editor: Patricia Donnelly
Editorial Assistant: Rachel Shuster
Associate Production Editor: Amanda Clerkin
Associate Marketing Manager: Rebecca Wasley
Manufacturing and Inventory Control Supervisor: Amy Bacus
Composition: Auburn Associates, Inc.
Cover Design: Kristin E. Ohlin
Cover Image Credit/Chapter Opener Image: © marivlada/ShutterStock, Inc.
Printing and Binding: Malloy, Inc.
Cover Printing: Malloy, Inc.

Library of Congress Cataloging-in-Publication Data
Management and leadership for nurse administrators/edited by Linda Roussel ; with Russell C. Swansburg.—5th ed.
    p. ; cm.
  Includes bibliographical references and index.
  ISBN-13: 978-0-7637-5714-4 (alk. paper)
  ISBN-10: 0-7637-5714-4 (alk. paper)
  1. Nursing services—Administration. 2. Nurse administrators. 3. Leadership. I. Roussel, Linda. II. Swansburg, Russell C.
    [DNLM: 1. Nursing, Supervisory. 2. Administrative Personnel. 3. Nurse Administrators. WY 105 M2655 2009]
  RT89.S885 2009
  362.17′3068—dc22

            2008027267

6048

Printed in the United States of America
12 11 10 09   10 9 8 7 6 5 4 3 2

To my contributors and their staff, patients, families, and students:
Thank you for your passion, tireless work, and dedication to improving quality for our consumers and creating healthy work environments for those entrusted to our care.

To Russell and Laurel Clark Swansburg:
Thank you for this opportunity and for your mentorship throughout my career.

CONTENTS

Preface. vii
Contributors. ix

Part I: Leading in Times of Complexity and Rapid Cycle Change. 1
Chapter 1:   Trends Shaping Nursing Leadership: Implications for
             Education and Practice. 2
Chapter 2:   Concepts and Theories Guiding Professional Practice 18
Chapter 3:   Emotionally Intelligent Leadership in Nursing and Healthcare
             Organizations 50
Chapter 4:   Ethical Nurse Leadership 74
Chapter 5:   Change, Complexity, and Creativity 102
Chapter 6:   Collaborative Decision Making and Communication: Skills and
             Practices 136

Part II: Leading the Business of Health Care: Processes and Principles 183
Chapter 7:   Organizational Structure and Analysis 184
Chapter 8:   Human Resource Development: Recruitment, Retention,
             and Managing Conflict. 260
Chapter 9:   Strategic Planning and Management 288
Chapter 10: Staffing and Scheduling 334
Chapter 11: Budgeting Principles for Nurse Managers 368
Chapter 12: Managing the Process of Care Delivery 406
Chapter 13: Information Management and Technology 428

**Part III: Leading to Improve the Future Quality and Safety of Healthcare
         Delivery Systems. 453**
Chapter 14: Health Policy, Laws, and Regulatory Issues 454
Chapter 15: Risk Management and Legal Issues. 470
Chapter 16: Tools for Evaluating Operations and Care Delivery Systems 494
Chapter 17: Quality Management 522
Chapter 18: Performance Appraisal 548
Chapter 19: The Professional Nursing Staff Educator 592
Chapter 20: Building a Portfolio for Academic and Clinical Partnership 608
Chapter 21: Transformational Leadership and Evidence-Based Management in
             a Changing World. 618
Chapter 22: Creating a Culture of Magnetism 642
Chapter 23: Managing a Culturally Diverse Workforce. 664

Index 681

PREFACE

The conventional definition of management is getting work done through people, but real management is developing people through work.
—Agha Hasan Abedi

This book is organized around the *Scope and Standards for Nurse Administrators*, American Organization of Nurse Executive competencies, the American Nurses Credentialing Center's "Forces of Magnetism", and current trends in healthcare management and leadership. *Management and Leadership for Nurse Administrators, Fifth Edition*, is suitable as an introductory course in nursing administration graduate programs. This book can also be used in upper level baccalaureate programs where traditional students and registered nurses (RNs) back to obtain a bachelors degree will find a basic course in management essentials. Staff development nurse managers in the service setting will also find this reference important in the mentoring and development of staff, specifically from a quality improvement and evidence-based practice perspective. This reference can also serve as an important resource to the advanced generalist role of the clinical nurse leader (CNL) which considers change, microsystems, complexity, systems thinking, collaboration, and leadership as core work in their program of study. The theory and principles of *Management and Leadership for Nurse Administrators, Fifth Edition*, apply to the entire spectrum of healthcare institutions and settings.

Management and Leadership for Nurse Administrators, Fifth Edition, provides theoretical and practical knowledge that will aid professional nurses in meeting the demands of constantly changing patient care services managed within complex adaptive systems. Because the demand for nurses in some specialties and geographical areas exceeds supply, it is essential that management processes create a culture of innovation, creativity, productivity, and greatness. Financial considerations and technology have increasingly dominated the healthcare industry, making the job of managing costly human and material resources urgent. Time is of the essence.

Healthcare institutions have been restructured, demassed, and decentralized along with other business and industrial institutions. This book has been revised to provide the best management concepts and theory of management available from the fields of generic management as well as nursing and management sources.

Chapters have been updated and streamlined. New chapters have been written to reflect changing markets and trends and to better address the critical need to collaborate and work with our clinical and academic partners. Chapters on trends, portfolio development, risk management, and a culture of magnetism have been added to this new edition.

The need for a diverse workforce as well as shortages of students in generic nursing programs and graduate nurses in practice require application of sound leadership and management principles to recruit and retain nurses in these areas.

CONTRIBUTORS

Chapter 3: Emotionally Intelligent Leadership in Nursing and Health Care Organizations
Susan H. Taft, PhD, RN, MSN
Associate Professor and Director, MSN in Nursing & Healthcare Management
MSN-MBA/MPA, Dual Degree Programs, College of Nursing
Kent State University
Kent, Ohio

Chapter 5: Change, Complexity, and Creativity
Anne Longo, MBA, BSN, RN-BC
Sr. Director, Center for Professional Excellence/Education
Cincinnati Children's, ML3020
Cincinnati, Ohio

Chapter 7: Organizational Structure and Analysis
Denise Danna, RN, DNS, NEA, BC, FACHE
Louisiana State University Health Sciences Center
School of Nursing
New Orleans, Louisiana

Chapter 8: Human Resource Development: Recruitment, Retention, and Managing Conflict
Elizabeth Thomas, MSN, RN
Clinical Associate Professor
The Loewenberg School of Nursing
University of Memphis
Memphis, Tennessee

Kathy S. Thompson, MSN, RN
Clinical Associate Professor
Loewenberg School of Nursing
University of Memphis
Memphis, Tennessee

Robert W. Koch, DNS, RN
Associate Dean
Loewenberg School of Nursing
University of Memphis
Memphis, Tennessee

Chapter 9: Strategic Planning and Management
Sandra Smith Pennington, PhD, RN
Dean, Graduate DNSc Nursing Program
Rocky Mountain University of Healthcare Professions
Provo, Utah

Elizabeth Simms, RN, MSN
Nurse Manager
New Orleans, Louisiana

Chapter 10: Staffing and Scheduling
Elizabeth Anderson, RN, MSN
Chief Executive Officer/Chief Nursing Officer
University of South Alabama Medical Center
Mobile, Alabama
Elizabeth Simms, RN, MSN
Nurse Manager
New Orleans, Louisiana

Chapter 11: Budgeting Principles for Nurse Managers
Beth Anderson, RN, MSN
Chief Executive Officer/Chief Nursing Officer
University of South Alabama Medical Center
Mobile, Alabama

Denise Danna, RN, DNS, NEA, BC, FACHE
Louisiana State University Health Sciences Center
School of Nursing
New Orleans, Louisiana

Chapter 12: Managing the Process of Care Delivery
Robert W. Koch, DNS, RN
Associate Dean
Loewenberg School of Nursing
University of Memphis
Memphis, Tennessee

Marylane Wade Koch, RN, MSN, CNA
Instructor
Loewenberg School of Nursing
University of Memphis
Memphis, Tennessee

Chapter 13: Information Management and Technology
Donna Faye McHaney, DNP, BSCS, RN, ARNP-C
Family Nurse Practitioner/Faculty
University of Alabama
Birmingham, Alabama

Chapter 14: Health Policy, Laws, and Regulatory Issues
Valorie Dearmon, RN, MSN, CNAA, BC
University of South Alabama College of Nursing
Mobile, Alabama

Chapter 15: Risk Management and Legal Issues
Valorie Dearmon, RN, MSN, NEA, BC
Instructor
University of South Alabama College of Nursing
Mobile, Alabama

Chapter 16: Tools for Evaluating Operations and Care Delivery Processes
Amy Bearden, RN, MSN, NEA, BC
Director of Patient Care Services
St. Luke's Magic Valley Regional Medical Center
Twin Falls, Idaho

Chapter 17: Quality Management
Beverly Blain Wright, RN, MSN, CNA
Mobile, Alabama

Marylane Wade Koch, RN, MSN, CNA
Instructor
Loewenberg School of Nursing
University of Memphis
Memphis, Tennessee

Chapter 18: Performance Appraisal
Amy Bearden, RN, MSN, NEA, BC
Director of Patient Care Services
St. Luke's Magic Valley Regional Medical Center
Twin Falls, Idaho

Chapter 19: The Professional Nursing Staff Educator
Debbie Faulk, PhD, RN
Associate Professor of Nursing
Auburn Montgomery School of Nursing
Montgomery, Alabama

Arlene H. Morris, EdD, RN
Distinguished Teaching Assistant Professor of Nursing
Auburn Montgomery School of Nursing
Montgomery, Alabama

Chapter 20: Building a Portfolio for Academic and Clinical Partnership
James L. Harris, DSN, APRN-BC, MBA, CNL

Sandra E. Walters, MSN, RN
Associate Chief Nurse
VA Tennessee Valley Healthcare System
Nashville, Tennessee

Chapter 22: Creating a Culture of Magnetism
Anita J. K. Langston, MSN, RN, ANP-BC, CCNS, CCRN
Clinical Assistant Professor
Loewenberg School of Nursing
University of Memphis
Memphis, Tennessee

Robert W. Koch, DNS, RN
Associate Dean
Loewenberg School of Nursing
University of Memphis
Memphis, Tennessee

Chapter 23: Managing a Culturally Diverse Workforce
Dr. Francine Mancuso Parker, RN, MSN, EdD
Associate Professor
Auburn University
School of Nursing
Montgomery, Alabama

Jeanne-Marie Tapke, RN, MSN, SPHR
President
Tapke Solutions
Ft. Mitchell, Kentucky

PART I

LEADING IN TIMES OF COMPLEXITY AND RAPID CYCLE CHANGE

1

TRENDS SHAPING NURSING LEADERSHIP:
Implications for Education and Practice

Linda Roussel, DSN, RN, NEA, BC

LEARNING OBJECTIVES AND ACTIVITIES

- Consider personal, organizational, and systems changes needed to effect greatness.
- Describe current trends in the business of health care and its impact on nurse administration.
- Discuss major influences, particularly of the Institute of Medicine, Agency for Healthcare Research and Quality, Institute for Healthcare Improvement, and other major players in the health system.
- Describe the impact of evidence-based practice in promoting safety and quality patient and healthy work environments.

CONCEPTS

Complexity, complex adaptive systems, chaos, change, innovation safety, quality, healthy work environments, health promotion, competency, diversity, strategic thinking, globalization, lifelong learning

---

QUOTE

There comes a special moment in everyone's life, a moment for which that person was born. That special opportunity, when he seizes it, will fulfill his mission—a mission for which he is uniquely qualified. In that moment, he finds greatness. It is his finest hour.

—Winston Churchill

NURSE MANAGER BEHAVIORS

Outcome management, lifelong learner, professional, role model

NURSE EXECUTIVE BEHAVIORS

Visionary, change agent, influencer, servant leader, mentor, systems analyzer, professional, advocate, communicator

Introduction

In the past decade, health care has witnessed dramatic swings, including a change in social demographics, advancements in medical technologies, heightened consumer awareness, and greater demand for high-quality, cost-effective care. This consumer-driven, competitive environment heralds in transformation that all healthcare organizations must embrace to be successful. Quality improvement, evidence-based practice, and systems thinking are essential to maintaining one's competitive edge. The traditional hierarchical, bureaucratic, and insulated organizational models no longer work in this new business of health care. An emerging model needs to be flat, innovative, nimble, and responsive to change. If a healthcare organization is to survive in today's frenetic pace, greater flexibility and the ability to deal with ambiguity are essential.[1]

Being great or going from good to great takes the courage of one's conviction, vision, and energy. We are charged with keeping up with trends that impact short- and long-term planning. Collins contends that visionary companies have better management development and succession planning than comparison companies, thereby ensuring greater continuity in leadership talent grown from within. Level five leadership does matter.[2]

Visioning and futuristic thinking do embrace an openness to change. Leaving the 20th century workplace, driven by innovation and technological transformation, new knowledge, skills, and abilities are demanded from everyone. New roles to address the demands are critical. High trust, encouraging the heart, authentic leadership, and relationship-based care are important in balancing quality, safe health care, efficiency, and cost constraints. There is a different emphasis and skill set for nurse administrators today than from those that dominated the past century. Logic, predictability, and linear reasoning were the order of the day and did give some measure of success in a stable environment. These skills are not enough and alone no longer serve us well.

ORGANIZATIONAL SYSTEM: CONTEXT FOR TRENDS AND CHANGE

Considering trends in light of organizations and systems propels the nurse administrator to consider different, innovative ways to structure and redesign processes and outcomes necessary to transform care delivery. Moving from an organization dominated by an over-rationalistic thinking "machine" focused on predictability, theorists of complexity and chaos show us that the natural world does not operate this way. Stacey purports that this revelation of the role of "creative disorder" in the universe needs to be taken to heart by managers. The consequences, as Stacey summarizes, turns management practices upside down. Considering complexity theory and organizations as complex adaptive systems (CAS), Stacey postulates the following points[3]:

- Analysis loses its primacy.
- Contingency (cause and effect) loses its meaning.
- Long-term planning becomes impossible.
- Visions become illusions.
- Consensus and strong cultures become dangerous.
- Statistical relationships become dubious.

The list goes on. An organization seeking stable relationships within an unpredictable environment is a recipe for failure. Organizations expecting predictable outcomes by focusing on its strengths, continuing what it does best, and making limited adjustments will likely be left in the dust by its innovative rivals. Successful strategies, in the long run, do not come by fixing organizational intention and circling around it; they emerge from complex and continuing interactions between people. According to Stacey, the dominant 1980s approach to strategy, which distanced itself from the strategic planning paradigm of preceding decades, still managed to maintain the aim of strategic management as its intent. "Management complexity theorists emphasize, rather, the importance of openness to accident, coincidence, serendipity. Strategy is the emerging resultant."[4]

Management in times of chaos requires a new way of thinking and being in the world. Managing in light of intense demands for greater quality, efficiency, and effectiveness of patient care necessitates consideration of alternatives to business as usual. The unusual becomes the usual; the ordinary becomes the extraordinary. Both have a place in managing and leading organizations.

Stacey distinguishes ordinary from extraordinary management. Ordinary management considers a logical analytic process to the day-to-day operations, using data analysis, goal setting, evaluating available options against goals, rationality, implementation, and evaluation, generally through hierarchical monitoring. Control is at the center of ordinary management. Cost-effective performance is often the yardstick by which effective and efficient systems are judged.[5]

According to Stacey, extraordinary management is also essential if the organization is to transform itself in situations of open-ended change. "Extraordinary management requires the activation of the tacit knowledge and creativity available within the organization. This necessitates the encouragement of informal structures—for example, workshops around particular issues or processes, with membership drawn from different business units, functions, and levels."[5]

Establishing informal groups requires spontaneity within the organization, often stimulated by paradoxes, inconsistencies, and conflicts occurring in the process of ordinary management. Informal groups need to be self-organizing systems, capable of redefining or extending their purpose versus being bound by fixed terms of reference. Such conditions enhance group learning, and its results are influenced as arguments to the broader management view. Stacey proposes that "in the necessary absence of hard evidence, arguments in favor of new assumptions and directions will be analogical and intuitive, and the process of decision making will be political as champions attempt to persuade others to their point of view."[6]

It is within this frame of references that the nurse executive can truly be innovative, moving the organization to think differently, try out new ideas, fail, start over again and again, and embrace the willingness to deal with ambiguity and uncertainty.

COMPLEX SYSTEMS

Healthcare systems are complex. The emerging field of complexity science offers alternative leadership and management strategies for the chaotic, complex, health care environment. A survey revealed that healthcare leaders intuitively support principles of complexity science. Leadership that uses complexity principles offers opportunities in the chaotic health care environment to focus less on prediction and control and more on fostering relationships and creating conditions in which CAS can evolve to produce creative outcomes.[7]

Zimmerman, Lindberg, and Plsek, in their work with CAS, note that this theory has much in common with general systems thinking, the learning organization, total quality, empowerment, gestalt theory, organizational development, and other approaches. Conceptualizing CAS purports an understanding of how things work in the real world. The authors provide the following principles in their work with CAS[8]:

1. View your system through the lens of complexity.
2. Build a good-enough vision.
3. When life is far from certain, lead with clockware and swarmware in tandem.
4. Tune your place to the edge.
5. Uncover and work with paradox and tension.
6. Go for multiple actions at the fringes, and let direction arise.
7. Listen to the shadow system.
8. Grow complex systems by chunking.
9. Mix cooperation with competition.

Working through these principles affords the nurse executive the opportunity to consider work from a number of different angles. For example, in principle 5, the authors suggest one balance data and intuition, planning and acting, safety and risk, giving due credit to each. "Clockware," coined by Kelly, describes the management processes that involve operating the core production processes of the organization in a manner which is rational, planned, standardized, repeatable, controlled, and measured. In contrast, "swarmware," also coined by Kelly, refers to management processes that discover new possibilities through experimentation, trials, autonomy, freedom, intuition, and working at the edge of knowledge and experience. Good-enough vision, minimum specifications, and metaphor are examples of swarmware. This process provides just enough of an idea, concept, or paints a landscape that leads individuals in CAS to become more participatory in trying whatever might work.[9]

Another example when working on principle 4 (tune your place to the edge) could be interpreted as placing the group at the edge of chaos, which increases the likelihood that creative approaches would emerge. The authors put forth the following paradoxical questions to consider:

- How can we give direction without giving directives?
- How can we lead by serving?
- How can we maintain authority without having control?

- How can we set direction when we don't know the future?
- How can we oppose change by accepting it? How can we accept change by opposing it?
- How can a large organization be small? How can a small one be large?
- How can we be both a system and many independent parts?
- What other questions might be relevant to the context of your work environment?[10]

The chaos manager must recognize these "forks in the road" and create a context supporting the new line of development by finding interventions that transcend the paradoxes or make them irrelevant.... The task hinges on finding new understandings or new actions that can reframe the paradox in a way that unleashes system energies in favor of the new line of development.

–Gareth Morgan

Furthering the need to understand macro-, micro-, and mesosystems as CAS, Plsek notes CAS as a "collection of individual agents who have the freedom to act in ways that are not always predictable, and whose actions are interconnected such that one agent's actions change the context for other agents."[11] By studying natural and human systems properties we can better understand the overall environment. These properties are described as follows[12]:

- Relationships as central to the system
- Structures, processes, and patterns
- Actions based on internalized simple rules and mental models
- Attractor patterns
- Constant adaptation
- Experimentation and pruning
- Inherent nonlinearity
- Systems embedded within other systems that coevolve

Using these properties, Plsek describes specific ways that such properties can be considered in adopting healthcare innovation within a complexity framework. Actions based on internalized simple rules and mental models would consider how individuals respond to their environment using internalized rules that drive action. For example, in a biochemical system, the "rules" are a series of chemical reactions. According to Plsek,[13]

> At a human level, the rules can be expressed as instincts, constructs and mental models. "First, do no harm" is an example of an internalized rule that might be behind an individual's reluctance to embrace the risk of an innovative change. These mental models need not be shared, explicit, or even logical when viewed by others, but they nonetheless contribute to the patterns in the complex system.

Plsek notes that mental models often are so ingrained in one's thinking that it is difficult (without reflection and examination) to embrace other perspectives and view points. Without this much needed work, it is likely that "fads and gimmicks" will be touted without real change, thus sustainability of new ways of doing business are unlikely to last and spread throughout the organization.

Zimmerman, Lindberg, and Plsek pose the question of how complexity science might improve management and the health of organizations. They put forth the following questions to ponder[14]:

- How does coevolution impact the role of a leader? If everything is changing and I am part of that change, how do I plan?
- If a CAS self-organizes, what is the job of manager or leader of a CAS?
- Can we use ideas of self-organization to unleash the full potential of our staff?
- Can we create the conditions for emergence as two or more organizations are coming together in a merger?

- What do we have to change to improve the quality of our services and reduce costs? Can complexity science provide us with any insights to this question?
- If an organization is a CAS, what does this imply about strategic planning?
- Can we use insights from complexity to improve the health of communities?
- If the edge of chaos is the area of greatest innovation, how do we stay on the edge of chaos? What are the risks of staying on the edge?
- What organizational structures, designs, processes etc. are consistent with a complexity science perspective? How would implementing these "complex" ideas improve organizations and the services they offer?
- How can we ensure complexity science enhances and complements proven management approaches? Where and when does complexity science add most value? Where are "traditional" approaches more appropriate?

Such foundational work in rethinking, questioning, and reflecting one's organization, its core business, and its relationship often provides a first step to developing policies and procedures within the system.

WORKING IN COMPLEX ADAPTIVE SYSTEMS

Nurses continue to top Gallup's annual survey of honesty and ethics among professions. We are in a strategic position to make a difference in managing and sustaining positive healthcare outcomes. Our hope is that our citizens count on nurses to bring about real change that ensures safe patient care by setting a path toward greatness and that we make good on our promises.[15]

Conceptualizing organizations as CAS provides a more useful framework for today's chaotic organizations. The content and context of leadership and management affect what nurse leaders do and how they must now behave in fundamentally altered work environments.

In 1996 the Institute of Medicine took on healthcare improvement to resolve unsafe care by ambitiously moving toward quality initiatives. The Institute of Medicine's seminal works, *To Err Is Human: Building a Safer Health System*[16] (1991) and *Crossing the Quality Chasm*[17] (2001), underscore the failings of the current healthcare system in which an estimated 98,000 hospitalized patients die annually in this country as a result of medical error. These well-documented sources of evidence also provide a vision for healthcare reform required for transformation and to bridge the gap between the current state of healthcare delivery and the ideal state. Small fixes are not enough to repair a broken system. Because of its strategic positioning in the healthcare arena as well as its strength in numbers, nursing must take up the challenge (it is there for the taking!), focusing on safe patient outcomes within healthy work environments. *Keeping Patients Safe*[18] provides well-grounded evidence, practices, and models in which care delivery lead by nurses can make the difference. The American Organization for Nurse Executives, the American Association of Critical Care Nurses, and other major nursing organizations have provided models to work with in making these changes.[19,20] Understanding complexity, complex adaptive system, and change are all a part of this drive to not only improve care but also to strive for greatness. Transforming the workplace by translation are skills and competencies that can be learned and embraced in this new world of health care work. Authentic leadership can make the difference in translating evidence into practice.

CREATING HEALTHY WORK ENVIRONMENTS

Creating and sustaining healthy work environments must be taken on by nurse leaders. Unhealthy work environments contribute to medical errors, outdated care delivery systems, and stress among health care providers. Our workplaces cannot allow unsafe conditions that demoralize the workforce. Unhealthy work environments often tolerate lateral and horizontal violence; thus basic civility, respect, and courtesy are not a part of the organization's culture. Healthy work environments support meaningful work and are a joyful place to be, charged with energy and vitality. The American Organization of Nurse Executives identify six critical factors to improve workplace initiatives, extracted from their study of workplace improvement and innovation[21]:

1. Leadership development and effectiveness
2. Empowered collaborative decision making
3. Work design and service delivery innovation
4. Values-driven organizational culture
5. Recognition and rewards systems
6. Professional growth and accountability

Using the above as a framework and an agenda for change, nurse executives are poised to initiate innovations and sustain healthy workplaces in the midst of persistent health care provider shortages, shrinking Medicare and Medicaid reimbursement, increasing health care costs and double-digit health premium increases, an aging population, and increased chronic illness management. To address such demands requires a major overhaul of our thinking and an unearthing of our mental models as we engage our workforce and carry out our business mission and professional responsibility. Professional nursing organizations are making strides to improve care delivery within a healthy work environment.

PROFESSIONAL ORGANIZATIONS FOR CHANGE TO IMPROVE CARE DELIVERY

A number of professional organizations have at their core mission patient safety and patient-centered care. For example, the American Association of Critical Care Nurses, in their Standards for Establishing and Sustaining Healthy Work Environments, reports that successful outcomes can only be supported by key elements: skilled communication, true collaboration, effective decision making, appropriate staffing, meaningful recognition, and authentic leadership.[22]

In the same vein, the American Organization of Nurse Executives also offers strategies and tools for addressing this critical work of sustaining healthy work places. American Organization of Nurse Executives has partnered with the Robert Wood Johnson Foundation in the support of Transforming Care at the Bedside (TCAB). The intent of this initiative is the advancing and informing with evidence of healthy workplace strategies for patients and staff to make a difference. TCAB provides a framework and direction to managers and staff as they move forward in taking these bold moves: safe and reliable care, vitality and teamwork, patient-centered care, and value-added care processes.[23] Working with the TCAB initiative, Martin et al. combine these moves and add six core values of work redesign, called the test of change. These work redesign strategies include an emphasis on the nursing staff, creating systems where work happens and, as it happens, improving efforts centering around patients' and employees' needs, executive leadership support, testing small samples to learn and spread to a larger scope, teaching along the way, and making it happen now.[24] Lessons learned in this journey focus on the importance of getting things started, with local spread moving to system spread. The concern was that this may have been considered a "flavor of the month" initiative, thus having a delay in the progression and sustainability of the change. Guidance by evidence, with the continuation of outcomes management and measurement, has offered further support for the importance of this work.

Other examples include the Registered Nurse Ontario Association, which provides guidelines and tools for developing healthy work environments. These evidence-based guidelines include such attention to professionalism, staffing, teamwork, ethics, and lifelong learning and development. These evidence-based guidelines and other tools equip the nurse executive with important resources for implementing, measuring, and evaluating change. Translating evidence into practice requires that the nurse executive has a working knowledge of how to find, use, and evaluate the evidence to support best practices.[24]

EVIDENCE-BASED PRACTICE

Evidence-based practice and organizational transformation requires that we be intentional and focused. Paying attention necessitates strategies to speed the rate of diffusing innovation. This is critical when innovation improves the quality of care. The evidence continues to grow; however, being slow to move is a barrier to best practice. The Institute of Medicine report, *Crossing the Quality Chasm*,[17] identified two barriers in particular that today are impeding health quality improvement: suboptimal investment in information technology and a reimbursement system that fails to provide coverage for innovative technologies in a timely manner. Understanding evidence-based practice underscores the need to be conversant with the drivers and barriers of diffusion, a major challenge today.

Nurse executives have a number of evidence-based practice models at their disposal, along with tools for appraising the evidence and best practice guidelines. For example, the University of Iowa, Johns Hopkins Medical Center, Academic Center for Evidence-Based Practice, and the Stetler Model of evidence-based practice offer exemplars for infusing evidence into professional nursing practice.[25–28] It is important that the nurse executive use these tools to inform clinical practice as well as create an evidence-based–rich environment with a culture that supports curiosity and inquisitiveness.

Competent nurse leaders must push on the drivers and reduce or eliminate barriers, when appropriate. If nurse executives have no systematic way of identifying breakthrough innovations early in their development, they are not able to give them the drive they need. Identifying innovations alone is not enough. Nurse executives must overcome resistance to change and embrace new information, knowledge, and skills in this aspect of the change process. In *Accelerating Quality Improvement in Health Care: Strategies to Speed the Diffusion of Evidence-Based Innovations*, examples are given to illustrate the need for thoughtful, rapid response. For example, when contemplating hospital redesign, consideration for optimum clinical care flow not only should take into account patient comfort but also ease of access to facilities and ease of movement for patients and their families. This would take into account infection control and other patient safety issues, allowing both integration of today's latest technology and technological upgrades over time. Along with clinical care concerns, creating a physical and working environment that would attract and retain the best medical, nursing, and administrative staff is also essential to this holistic approach.[29]

TRENDS AND TRANSFORMATION:
A FOCUS ON SAFETY, QUALITY, AND EDUCATION

The viability of our organizations depends on a successful transformation from traditional hierarchies to models of shared accountability that capitalize on the organizations' collective talent. Structures, processes, and outcomes are created and implemented to improve the quality of how we deliver health care. Patient safety is at the center of quality and is critical to what we do.

Integrating patient safety into nursing practice requires a change in the organizational culture. At most health care institutions, senior leadership identifies patient safety and quality as a strategic imperative within the organization. For example, the University of North Carolina Health Care System created a patient safety plan that emphasizes a focus on processes and systems rather than on the individual performance of a hospital staff member. Nurse managers on the University of North Carolina's inpatient units were challenged to identify areas for improvement, develop practice strategies to address these areas, and then work with staff to implement and evaluate the newly redesigned practice.[30]

The nurse manager's role has evolved into a highly complex pivotal position within health care organizations. This role is cornerstone to quality patient care, financial success, and patient and family satisfaction. At this level of leadership, strategic goals and objectives are translated and operationalized at the unit/departmental level. Through this evolutional process, traditional undergraduate nursing programs do not adequately prepare nurses for these complex middle management roles. Possessing advanced knowledge, skills, and abilities are no longer for the selected few! Based on the needs and complexity of our health care business, formal graduate-level education is critical for the development of the nurse manager. Graduate degrees in nursing administration or a combined advanced nursing degree with a master's in business administration can equip the new nurse manager with the fundamental tools and knowledge needed for development. The nurse executive, in leading the organization, can facilitate this by creating innovative programs for bridging this gap. Programs that might be included are partnerships with universities that grant the required degrees, special tuition reimbursement policies that accelerate completion of the degree, and flexible scheduling focusing on time management. A supportive and facilitative environment can do much to lay the groundwork for doctoral education for those nurse managers who ultimately move on to senior leadership roles. There must be evidence of organizational commitment for advancing the nurse manager's education.[31]

Evidence-Based Practice 1-1

A qualitative study described six themes critical to the work of chief nurse executive that included communication, continuous learning, quality health care, partnerships, relationship, and future orientation.[32]

Furthering this emphasis, Scoble and Russell developed a list of 130 competencies desired of nurse administrators. From this list, 13 key competency categories were ranked in order, with the top 6 identified as leadership behaviors and skills, financial acumen and budgeting, business acumen, management skills, communication skills, and human resource and labor relations. As the chief nurse executive considered priorities and challenges, five critical areas were enumerated and included: quality, patient safety and compliance, financial performance, leadership, and patient care delivery. These skill sets and competencies are underscored by current quality initiatives requiring interdisciplinary interventions often spearheaded by nursing.[33]

NURSING-SENSITIVE INDICATORS, SAFETY STANDARDS, AND QUALITY INDICATORS

Maas, Johnson, and Morehead proposed the phrase "nursing-sensitive indicators" to reflect patient outcomes influenced by nursing practice.[34] Needleman et al. noted that "nursing-sensitive indicators" may be a more comprehensive term focusing on the relationship of nursing with negative—or adverse—patient outcomes, such as medication errors, patient falls, and nosocomial infections. These authors note that there is less evidence that examines the relationship of nursing and positive patient outcomes, attributing the use of negative outcomes to the fact that adverse patient outcomes are more readily available in medical records and existing administrative data sets.[35]

Needleman et al. used the phrase "outcomes potentially sensitive to nursing" to recognize nursing contributions in the clinical care delivery process; however, the reluctance here points to the struggle in determining attribution when care delivery processes are interwoven.[35]

This is changing, however, with the National Database of Nursing Quality Indicators (NDNQI) translating data into quality care. The American Nurses Association pushed through efforts to collect and evaluate nursing-sensitive indicators in the early 1990s, providing ongoing support for database development activities through the National Center for Nursing Quality. University of Kansas School of Nursing, which ranks among the top nursing schools in the nation in National Institutes of Health funding for nursing research, continues to provide ongoing nursing-sensitive indicator consultation and research-based expertise to the NDNQI. This School of Nursing primarily conducts research on clinical and health policy topics in two areas: health care effectiveness and health behavior. The NDNQI continues to grow and is a powerful tool available to nurse executives. This national database program has two primary goals[36]:

- First, to provide comparative information to health care facilities for use in quality improvement activities
- Second, to develop national data on the relationship between nurse staffing and patient outcomes

According to the ANA, the database is growing and contains hundreds of participating health care facilities along with various kinds of data being collected. For example, patient outcome and nurse staffing data are being collected on critical care, step down, medical, surgical, medical/surgical, pediatric, psychiatric, and rehabilitation units. Nurse satisfaction data are being collected from a wide variety of nursing units. The data are collected according to strict standards; collaboration has been a key component in the growth of NDNQI. Participants can be part of the development process if they so choose.

NDNQI provides the capacity to trend data. NDNQI provides participants with quarter-by-quarter and unit-by-unit comparisons of nursing care, thus eliminating isolated and perhaps misleading snapshots of performance. The NDNQI data allow the nurse executive to mark progress, understand and improve the care of patients and the work environment of nurses, avoid costly complications, and assist in marketing the quality of nursing leadership's efforts. The NDNQI can also serve as a valuable tool for retention of nursing staff and recruitment of potential employees.[37]

In a similar vein, reports from the Institute of Medicine's Quality Initiative brought public attention to the urgent need for understanding, measuring, improving, and ensuring the quality of health care in the United States. Focused on important aspects of health care quality, such as revealing serious health care systems errors and patient safety concerns, these quality initiatives recommended taxonomy of quality attributes for the health care system. Recommendations are further proposed to enhance quality initiatives to coordinate quality-related efforts in six government programs, offering strategies for interdisciplinary education in the health professions and identifying changes needed in the work environment for nurses to improve patient safety. These major initiative reports represent a systematic effort to focus on quality and patient safety concerns in health care and to advance critical health care quality efforts in the United States.[16–18]

Additionally, although putting forth recommendations from these reports into practice is challenging, macro-level quality initiatives in the public and private sectors are ongoing. For example, within the federal government the Quality Interagency Coordination Task Force was formed, bringing together independent initiatives within various governmental agencies relating to or impacting health care quality.[38] Another example includes the National Healthcare Quality Report, developed by the Agency for Healthcare Research and Quality (AHRQ), which presented data on the quality of services for seven clinical conditions and includes a set of performance measures that serve as a baseline for the quality of health care.[39]

Private groups, such as the Leapfrog Group,[40] the National Quality Forum,[41] the Joint Commission,[42] and the Institute for Healthcare Quality,[43] are also proposing efforts and recommendations for improving and ensuring quality health care. Many of these initiatives attempt to move closer to the point of care delivery. As reported, professional organizations and provider groups, such as the American Nurses Association,[44] the American Medical Association,[45] and the Veterans Health Administration,[46] also proposed quality surveillance activities aimed at identifying and capturing provider- and profession-specific clinical quality indicators. Public reporting of health care quality data can drive quality improvement, expanding the potential value of quality indicators.

Another example comes from the AHRQ, which identifies quality indicators to measure health care quality by using available hospital inpatient administrative data. Patient safety indicators are tools to help health system leaders identify potential adverse events occurring during hospitalization.[47]

The AHRQ quality indicators expanded the original Healthcare Cost and Utilization Project quality indicators. The prevention quality indicators, the first set of AHRQ quality indicators, were released in November 2001. The second set, the inpatient quality indicators, were released in May 2002 and in March 2003. In February 2006 the fourth quality indicator module, the pediatric quality indicators, was added as the pediatric population was removed from the other modules.[48]

AHRQ is making the patient safety indicators software available without charge to hospitals and other users as SAS® and SPSS® programs with software documentation and a user guide that provides a synopsis of the evidence taken from the *Measures of Patient Safety Based on Hospital Administrative Data*. According to AHRQ, patient safety indicators[49]

- Can be used to help hospitals identify potential adverse events that might need further study
- Provide the opportunity to assess the incidence of adverse events and in hospital complications using administrative data found in the typical discharge record
- Include 20 indicators for complications occurring in hospital that may represent patient safety events
- Include six indicators with area level analogs designed to detect patient safety events on a regional level
- Are free and publicly available
- Can be downloaded

Evidence-Based Practice 1-2

Despite the Institute of Medicine reports calling for the creation of a standardized set of measures for monitoring the quality and effect of structural changes on the process and outcomes of nursing care, we did not observe a unified direction emerging in the literature. Reviews suggest that the following problems persist in efforts to examine profession-specific quality of care:

- Lack of standardized performance measure definitions
- Lack of consensus on a core set of evidence-based measures
- Limited availability of data at the unit and/or shift level

As such, controversy regarding the appropriate definition, number, and approach to indicator identification was found to persist.[50]

SUMMARY

We are in a new world of health care, and business is usual is the unusual order of the day. Understanding the organization through different lenses, such as CAS, may provide new tools for enhancing performance. Change, innovation, and infusion of evidence-based practice also contribute to greater efficacy and efficiency in leading. Armed with an understanding of evidence-based practice and quality indicators improves one's success in creating a safe environment for patients, their families, and the workforce. Without the authentic leadership that is transparent in its serving, there is little hope for real change that is sustained over time. The health of the patients and families entrusted to our care depends on our courage to be great and to continually strive for excellence. It is the hope of this author that increasing knowledge, skills, and abilities can serve this end.

APPLICATION EXERCISES

Exercise 1-1

Interview a nurse manager. Discuss nursing-sensitive indicators and how they are measured and evaluated. How are these data used to improve nursing care?

Exercise 1-2

Spend time on a nursing unit (department, service) that you have not been exposed to (work or field site). What do you observe in light of a complex adaptive system (CAS)? Write down what you are observing and compare and contrast to the principles of a CAS.

Notes

1. Malloch, K., & Porter-O'Grady, T. (2005). *The quantum leader: Applications for the new world of work.* Sudbury, MA: Jones and Bartlett.

2. Collins, J. C. (2001). *Good to great.* New York: HarperCollins.

3. Stacey, R. D. (1992). *Managing the unknowable: Strategic boundaries between order and chaos in organizations.* San Francisco: Jossey-Bass.

4. Stacey, R. D. (1993). *Strategic management and organizational dynamics.* London: Pitman.

5. Stacey, R. D. (1996). *Complexity and creativity in organizations.* San Francisco: Berrett-Koehler.

6. Ibid.

7. Ibid.

8. Zimmerman, B., Lindberg, C., & Plsek, P. (1998). Nine emerging and connected organizational leadership principles. In *Edgeware: Lessons for complexity science for health care leaders.* Dallas, TX: VHA, Inc.

9. Kelly, K. (1994). *Out of control: The new biology of machines, social systems and the economic world.* Reading, MA: Addison-Wesley.

10. Zimmerman et al., 1998.

11. Ibid.

12. Ibid.

13. Plsek, P. E. (1999). Innovative thinking for the improvement of medical systems. *Annals of Internal Medicine, 131,* 438–444.

14. Zimmerman et al., 1998.

15. Gallup Poll News Service. (2006). *Occupational outlook handbook: Registered nurses.* U.S. Department of Labor's Bureau of Labor Statistics.

16. Kohn, L. T., Corrigan, J. M., & Donaldson, M. S. (Eds). (1999). *To err is human: Building a safer health system.* Committee on Quality of Health Care in America, Institute of Medicine. Washington, DC: The National Academies Press.

17. Institute of Medicine. (2001). *Crossing the quality chasm: A new health system for the 21st century.* Committee on Quality of Health Care in America, Institute of Medicine. Washington, DC: The National Academies Press.

18. Page, A. (Ed.). (2004). *Keeping patients safe: Transforming the work environment.* Committee on the Work Environment for Nurses and Patient Safety, Institute of Medicine. Washington, DC: The National Academies Press.

19. American Organization of Nurse Executives. (2003). *Healthy work environments: Striving for excellence.* Retrieved January 17, 2008, from http://www.aone.org/aone/docs/hwe_excellence_intro.pdf

20. American Association of Critical Care Nurses. (n.d.). *Standards for establishing and sustaining healthy work environments.* Retrieved January 17, 2008, from http://www.aacn.org/aacn/pubpolcy.nsf/vwdoc/workenv

21. American Organization of Nurse Executives, 2003.

22. American Association of Critical Care Nurses, n.d.

23. Robert Wood Johnson/American Organization of Nurse Executives. (2005). *Transforming care at the bedside.* Retrieved February 18, 2008, from http://www.rwjf.org/pr/product.jsp?id=21085&catid=18

24. Martin, S. C., Greenhouse, P. K., Merryman, T., Shovel, J., Liberi, C. A., & Konzier, J. (2007). Transforming care at the bedside: Implementation and spread model for single hospital and multihospital systems. *Journal of Nursing Administration, 37,* 444–451.

25. Academic Center for Evidence-Based Practices. (2004). *ACE: Learn about EBP.* Retrieved February 1, 2008, from http://www.acestar.uthscsa.edu/Leran_model.htm

26. Melnyk, B., & Fineout-Overholt, E. (2005). *Evidence-based practice in nursing and healthcare: A guide to best practice.* Philadelphia: Lippincott Williams & Williams.

27. Stetler, C., Brunell, M., Giuliano, K., Morsi, D., Prince, L., & Newell-Stokes, V. (1998). Evidence-based practice and the role of nursing leadership. *Journal of Nursing Administration, 28,* 45–53.

28. *Conduct and utilization of research in nursing model.* Retrieved February 17, 2008, from http://www.medicalcityhospital.com/CustomPage.asp?guidCustomContentID={ABD30A7E-3A16-424C-A44F-51CCC1B1ED9B}

29. Accelerating quality improvement in health care: Strategies to speed the diffusion of evidence-based innovations (2003). The National Institute for Health Care Management (NIHCM) Research and Educational

Foundation and the National Committee for Quality Health Care (NCQHC), conference proceedings, January 27–28, Washington, DC.

30. University of North Carolina Health Care System. *Patient safety initiative.* Retrieved February 17, 2008, from http://www.unchealthcare.org/site.

31. Thomas, J. D., & Herrin, D. (2008). Executive Master of Science in Nursing Program: Incorporating the 14 forces of magnetism. *Journal of Nursing Administration, 38,* 64–67.

32. Scott, E. (2007). Nursing administration graduate programs in the United States. *Journal of Nursing Administration, 97,* 517–522.

33. Scoble, K., & Russell, G. (2003). Vision 2020, part 1. *Journal of Nursing Administration, 33,* 324–330.

34. Maas, M., Johnson, M., & Moorehead, S. (1996). Classifying nursing-sensitive patient outcomes. *Journal of Nursing Scholarship, 28,* 295–301.

35. Needleman, J., Buerhaus, P. I., Mattke, S., et al. (2001). *Nurse staffing and patient outcomes in hospitals* (contract no. 230-99-0021). Final report for Health Resources and Services Administration. Department of Health Policy and Management, Harvard School of Public Health, Boston, Mass 02115, USA. needlema@hsph.harvard. edu

36. American Nurses Association. (2004). *NDNQI: Transforming data into quality care.* Retrieved February 17, 2008, from http://nursingworld.org/MainMenuCategories/ThePracticeofProfessionalNursing/PatientSafety Quality/NDNQI/NDNQI_1/NDNQIBrochure.aspx

37. Ibid.

38. Quality Interagency Coordination Task Force. *Informing consumers about health care quality: New directions for research and action.* Retrieved February 17, 2008, from http://www.quic.gov/consumer/conference/summary/ index.html

39. Agency for Healthcare Research and Quality. (2005). *National healthcare quality report.* Retrieved February 17, 2008, from http://www.ahrq.gov/qual/nhqr05/fullreport/Index.htm

40. Leapfrog Group. (2008). Leapfrog hospital quality and safety survey and Leapfrog hospital rewards program. Retrieved February 17, 2008, from http://www.leapfroggroup.org/66445/hospital_contact. *Journal of Nursing Administration, 97.*

41. National Quality Forum. (2008). *Standardizing a patient safety taxonomy.* Retrieved February 17, 2008, from http://216.122.138.39/projects/completed/taxonomy.asp

42. Joint Commission. (2008). *National patient safety goals.* Retrieved February 17, 2008, from http://www. jointcommission.org/PatientSafety/NationalPatientSafetyGoals/

43. Institute for Healthcare Improvement. (2008). *Patient safety and the reliability of healthcare systems.* Retrieved February 17, 2008, from http://www.ihi.org/IHI/Topics/PatientSafety/MedicationSystems/Literature/Patient safetyandthereliabilityofhealthcaresystems.htm

44. American Nurses Association. (2008). *ANA statement for the Institute of Medicine's Committee on Work Environment for Nurses and Patient Safety.* Retrieved February 17, 2008, from http://nursingworld.org/ FunctionalMenuCategories/MediaResources/PressReleases/ 2006_1/ ANAonWorkEnvironment.aspx

45. American Medical Association. (2008). Quality of care campaign for patient safety. Retrieved February 17, 2008, from http://www.ama-assn.org/ama/pub/category/14785.html

46. U.S. Department of Veterans Affairs, Veterans Health Administration. (2008). *VA Interprofessional Fellowship Program in patient safety.* Retrieved February 17, 2008, from http://www.va.gov/oaa/specialfellows/programs/ SF_patient_safety.asp?p=17

47. Hussey, P. S., Mattke, S., Morse, L., & Ridgely, M. S. (2006). *Evaluation of the use of AHRQ and other quality indicators.* Agency for Healthcare Research and Quality. Retrieved February 17, 2008, from http://www.ahrq.gov/ about/evaluations/qualityindicators/qualityindicators.pdf

48. Agency for Healthcare Research and Quality. (2008). *Healthcare Cost & Utilization Project (HCUP).* Retrieved February 17, 2008, from http://www.ahrq.gov/data/hcup/

49. Agency for Healthcare Research and Quality. (2002). *Measures of patient safety based on hospital administrative data: The patient safety indicators.* Retrieved February 17, 2008, from http://www.ahrq.gov/downloads/pub/evidence/pdf/psi/psi.pdf

50. Eden, J., Wheatley, B., McNeil, B., & Sox, H. (Eds.). (2008). *Knowing what works in health care: A roadmap for the nation. Journal of Nursing Administration, 97.* Committee on Reviewing Evidence to Identify Highly Effective Clinical Services, Institute of Medicine. Washington, DC: National Academies Press.

References

American Nurses Association. (2004). *Scope and standards for nurse administrators* (2nd ed.). Washington, DC: American Nurses Publishing.

American Nurses Credentialing Center. *List of all magnet-designated facilities.* Retrieved February 17, 2008, from http://www.nursecredentialing.org/ANCC/magnet/getall.cfm

American Nurses Credentialing Center. (2007). *Overview of the ANCC magnet recognition program.* Silver Spring, MD: Author.

American Organization of Nurse Executives. *AONE nurse executive competencies.* Retrieved February 17, 2008, from http://www.aone.org

Christensen, C. M. (1997). *The innovator's dilemma.* Boston: Harvard Business School Press.

Collins, J. (2005). *Good to great and the social sectors.* New York: HarperCollins.

Collins, J. C., & Porras, J. I. (1997). *Built to last.* New York: HarperCollins.

Gladwell, M. (2002). *The tipping point.* New York: Little, Brown and Company.

Haig, K., Sutton, S., & Whittington, J. (2006). SBAR: A shared mental model for improving communication between clinicians. *Joint Commission Journal on Quality and Patient Safety, 32,* 167–175.

Hohenhaus, S., Powell, S., & Hohenhaus, J. (2006). Enhancing patient safety during hands-off. *American Journal of Nursing, 106,* 72A–72C.

Kerfoot, K. M., & Lavandero, R. (2005). *Healthy work environments: Enroute to excellence.* Retrieved January 17, 2008, from http://ccn.aacnjournals.org/cgi/content/full/25/3/72

Malloch, K., & Porter-O'Grady, T. (2006). *Introduction to evidence-based practice in nursing and health care.* Sudbury, MA: Jones and Bartlett.

Massoud, M. R., Nielsen, G. A., Nolan, K., Nolan, T., Schall, M. W., & Seven, C. (2006). *TCAB spread phase 2: a framework for spread: from local improvements to system-wide change.* IHI innovation series white paper. Cambridge, MA: Institute for Healthcare Improvement. Retrieved February 17, 2008, from http://www.ihi.org/IHI/Results/WhitePapers/AFrameworkforSpreadWhitePaper.htm

McClure, M., Hinshaw, A. S. (Eds.). (2002). *Magnet hospitals revisited: Attraction and retention of professional nurses.* Washington, DC: American Nurses Publishing.

Nurse Week. *The 14 forces of magnetism.* Retrieved May 22, 2007, from http://www.nurseweek.com/news/features/02-10/magnetism.asp

Oman, K. S., Duran, C., & Fink, R. (2008). Evidence-based policy and procedures: An algorithm for success. *Journal of Nursing Administration, 38,* 47–51.

Plsek, P. E. (1997). *Creativity, innovation, and quality.* Milwaukee, WI: ASQ Quality Press.

Plsek, P. E. (1998). Bringing creativity to reengineering efforts. In P. Lenz (Ed.), *Reengineering health care: A practical guide.* Tampa, FL: American College of Physician Executives.

Plsek, P. E. (1999). No special gift needed: Generating creative ideas for health care organizations. *Health Forum Journal,* March/April, 24–28.

Plsek, P. E. (1999). Quality improvement methods in clinical medicine. *Pediatrics, 103,* 203–214.

Plsek, P. E. (2001). Redesigning health care with insights from the science of complex adaptive systems. In IOM Committee on Quality of Health Care in America, *Crossing the quality chasm: A new health system for the 21st century.* Washington, DC: National Academy Press.

Plsek, P. E., & Greenhalgh, T. (2001). The challenge of complexity in health care. *British Medical Journal, 323,* 625–628.

Plsek, P. E., & Kilo, C. M. (1999). From resistance to attraction: A different approach to change. *Physician Executive, 25,* 40–46.

Porter-O'Grady, T., & Malloch, K. (2003). *Quantum leadership: A textbook of new leadership.* Sudbury, MA: Jones and Bartlett.

Quinn, R. E. (2000). *Change the world.* San Francisco: John Wiley & Sons.

Rodgers, K. (2007). Using the SBAR communication technique to improve nurse-physician phone communication. *American Academy of Ambulatory Care Nursing,* March/April.

Rogers, E. M. (2003). *Diffusion of innovations* (5th ed). New York: Free Press.

Sandlin, D. (2007). Improving patient safety by implementing a standardized and consistent approach to hand-off communication. *Journal of Perianesthesia Nursing, 22,* 289–292.

Senge, P. M. (2006). *The fifth discipline.* New York: Currency Doubleday.

Senge, P. M., Kleiner, A., Roberts, C., Ross, R. B., & Smith, B. J. (1994). *The fifth discipline fieldbook.* New York: Currency Doubleday.

Serling, R. J. (1992). *Legend and legacy.* New York: St. Martin's Press.

Shalizi, C. (2006). Methods and techniques of complex systems science: An overview. In T. Diesboeck & J. Kresh (Eds.), *Complex systems science in biomedicine* (pp. 33–95). Singapore: Springer.

Shortell, S. M., Bennett, C. L., & Byck, G. R. (1998). Assessing the impact of continuous quality improvement on clinical practice: What will it take to accelerate progress? *Millbank Quarterly, 76,* 593–624.

Transforming Care at the Bedside: microsystem level. Retrieved February 16, 2008, from http://www.ihi.org/IHI/Programs/TransformingCareAtTheBedside/TransformingCareAtTheBedside.htm?TabId=1

Watson, T. J., & Petre, P. (2001). *Father, son & co.* New York: Bantam.

Wheatley, M. J. (2005). *Finding our way.* San Francisco: Berrett-Koehle. *Journal of Nursing Administration, 97.*

Zimmerman, B., Lindburg, C., & Plsek, P. (1998). Edgeware (p. 263). Irving, TX: VHA Inc.

SELECTED WEB SITES

Agency for Healthcare Research and Quality

www.ahrq.gov

AHRQ funds, conducts, and disseminates research to improve the quality, safety, efficiency, and effectiveness of health care. The information gathered from this work and made available on the website assists all key stakeholders—patients, families, clinicians, leaders, purchasers, and policymakers—to make informed decisions about health care.

American Association of Critical Care Nurses

www.aacn.org

American Association of Critical Care Nurses provides leadership and resources to their members to improve health care for critically ill patients and their families. Core concepts of patient- and family-centered health care are integrated throughout their practice guidelines.

American Hospital Association

www.aha.org

The AHA is the premier membership organization for U.S. hospitals and provides leadership and advocacy for member hospitals to improve care for patients and their families. IFCC collaborated with AHA to develop the toolkit, *Strategies for Leadership: Patient- and Family-Centered Care,* available for download at http://www.aha.org/aha/key_issues/patient_safety/resources/patientcenteredcare.html

Center for Health Design

www.healthdesign.org

The Center for Health Design is a nonprofit research and advocacy organization of health care and design professionals *Journal of Nursing Administration, 97,* who are leading the effort to improve health quality through architecture and design. *Journal of Nursing Administration, 97.*

Center for Medical Home Improvement www.medicalhomeimprovement.org

2 CONCEPTS AND THEORIES GUIDING PROFESSIONAL PRACTICE

Linda Roussel, RN, DSN, NEA, BC

LEARNING OBJECTIVES AND ACTIVITIES

- Describe the importance of having a theory for professional nursing practice.
- Identify the scope and standards for nurse administrators as a framework for practice.
- Discuss the linkages of theory, evidence-based nursing, and practice.
- Discuss the guiding principles and competencies for nurse administrative practice and how they crosswalk to the scope and standards of nurse administrators.
- Define the terms *executive, manager, managing, management*, and *nursing management.*
- Identify five essential management practices that promote patient safety.
- Differentiate among concepts, principles, and theory.
- Describe critical theory.
- Discuss general systems theory.
- Illustrate selected principles of nursing management.
- Describe roles for nurse managers and nurse executives, differentiating among levels.
- Distinguish between two cognitive styles: intuitive thinking and rational thinking.
- Discuss the use of nursing theory in managing a clinical practice.
- Discuss the responsibility of the nurse administrator for managing a clinical discipline.

CONCEPTS

Aim of health care, scope of practice, standards of practice for nurse administrators, management theory, nursing management theory, critical theory, general systems theory, nursing management, management principles, management development, nursing management roles, role development, cognitive styles, intuitive thinking, rational thinking, management levels, modalities of nursing

NURSE MANAGER BEHAVIORS	NURSE EXECUTIVE BEHAVIORS
Applies postmodern management theory to organizational operations; assesses the impact of various influences from ethnic, political, social, financial, economic, and ethical issues perspectives; networks with state, regional, national, and global peers to share ideas and conduct mutual problem solving; demonstrates a commitment to lifelong learning and ongoing professional development through such activities as certification and participation in professional organizations	Examines the application of a nursing and management theory by creating a business plan that incorporates a pilot study; works with representatives of the professional nursing staff to develop and test the pilot study; leads initiatives in innovative programs and new implementation alternatives; pursues continuing education, certification, professional development, and networking; seeks experiences to advance one's skills and knowledge base in areas of responsibilities, including the art and science of nursing, changes in health care systems, application of emerging technologies, and administrative practices

Introduction

Patient safety and quality initiatives as well as magnet status continue to mandate that nurses practice from a framework of professionalism. A sound evidence-based management practice advances the overall practice of nursing administration. Nurse leaders guided by a conceptualized practice have an opportunity to transform health care. In 1999 the Institute of Medicine released *To Err Is Human: Building a Safer Health System*, a disturbing report that brought significant public attention to the crisis of patient safety in the United States. *Crossing the Quality Chasm: A New Health System for the 21st Century* followed in 2002, which was a more detailed reporting of the widening gap between how good health care is defined and how health care is actually provided. The latter report calls the divide not just a gap but a chasm, and the difference between those two metaphors is quantitative as well as qualitative. Not only is the current health care system lagging behind the ideal in large and numerous ways, but the system is fundamentally and incurably unable to reach the ideal. To begin achieving real improvement in health care, the whole system has to change.

Looking at the other side of the chasm, the 2002 report outlined an ideal health care with six "aims for improvement":

1. *Health care must be safe.* This means much more than the ancient maxim "First, do no harm," which makes it the individual caregiver's responsibility to somehow try extra hard to be more careful (a requirement modern human factors theory has shown to be unproductive). Instead, the aim means that safety must be a property of the system. No one should ever be harmed by health care again.

2. *Health care must be effective.* It should match science, with neither underuse nor overuse of the best available techniques—every elderly heart patient who would benefit from beta-blockers should get them, and no child with a simple ear infection should get advanced antibiotics.

3. *Health care should be patient centered.* The individual patient's culture, social context, and specific needs deserve respect, and the patient should play an active role in making decisions about her or his own care. That concept is especially vital today, as more people require chronic rather than acute care.

4. *Health care should be timely.* Unintended waiting that doesn't provide information or time to heal is a system defect. Prompt attention benefits both the patient and the caregiver.

5. *The health care system should be efficient,* constantly seeking to reduce the waste—and hence the cost—of supplies, equipment, space, capital, ideas, time, and opportunities.

6. *Health care should be equitable.* Race, ethnicity, gender, and income should not prevent anyone in the world from receiving high-quality care. We need advances in health care delivery to match the advances in medical science so the benefits of that science may reach everyone equally.

However, we cannot hope to cross the chasm and achieve these aims until we make fundamental changes to the whole health care system. All levels require dramatic improvement, from the patient's experience—probably the most important level of all—up to the vast environment of policy, payment, regulation, accreditation, litigation, and professional training that ultimately shapes the behavior, interests, and opportunities of health care. In between are the microsystems that bring the care to the patients, the small caregiving teams and their procedures and work environments as well as all the hospitals, clinics, and other organizations that house those microsystems. "We're trying to suggest actions for actors, whether you're a congressman or the president or whether you're a governor or a commissioner of public health, or whether you're a hospital CEO or director of nursing in a clinic or chairman of medicine," says Donald M. Berwick, MD, MPP, President and Chief Executive Officer of the Institute for Healthcare Improvement and one of the Chasm report's architects. "No matter where you are, you can look at this list of aims and say that at the level of the system you house, the level you're responsible for, you can organize improvements around those directions."

A framework for nursing administrative practice necessitates a redesigning of the various functions, roles, and responsibilities of a nurse administrator. Changes in the landscape of health care, such as new technology, increased diversity in the workplace, greater accountability for practice, and a new spiritual focus on the mind and body connection, require creativity, innovative leadership, and management models. A roadmap, with its definitive lines of direction, is not enough. A more appropriate analogy is that of using a compass to find true north in this new age of health care delivery systems and nursing practice models. Productivity and cost concerns remain important; however, there is an equal if not greater focus on safety, quality relationships, and healing environments. Sound nursing and management theories, along with evidence-based management practices, equip the nurse administrator with the tools to foster a culture of collaborative decision making and positive patient and staff outcomes. Core competencies identified by the Institute of Medicine in its work on educating health care professionals further underscore the work that needs to be done[1]:

1. Provide patient-centered care.
2. Work in interdisciplinary teams.
3. Use evidence-based practice.
4. Apply quality improvement.
5. Utilize informatics.

Core competencies apply to all health care professionals and emphasize greater integration of disciplines, creating a culture focused on improving safety outcomes in health care. Transformational leadership and evidence-based management are necessary for redesigning our current health care system. Creating a professional practice model of nursing can serve to strengthen this agenda and advance a safe, quality health care system.

PROFESSIONAL PRACTICE MODEL OF NURSING

If nursing is truly to be a professional practice, an environment supporting professional practice must be created. Models of care delivery by professional nurses further advance this important work. The impact of increasing demand and decreasing supply of registered nurses and rapid aging of the nursing workforce means that by the year 2020 there will be a 20% shortage in the number of nurses needed in the U.S. health care system. This translates into an unprecedented shortage of more than 400,000 registered nurses.[2] Given the anticipated shortage as well as the increased demand for nursing as a professional practice, the American Nurses Association (ANA) notes work environments that support professional practice to enhance positive staff and patient outcomes[3]:

1. Magnet hospital recognition
2. Preceptorships and residencies
3. Differentiated nursing practice
4. Interdisciplinary collaboration

Magnet Recognition Programs

The foundation for the magnet nursing services program is the *Scope and Standards for Nurse Administrators*.[4] The program provides a framework to recognize excellence in

1. Nursing services management, philosophy, and practices
2. Adherence to standards for improving the quality of patient care
3. Leadership of the chief nurse executive and competence of nursing staff
4. Attention to the cultural and ethnic diversity of patients, their significant others, and the care providers in the health care system

Nurse scientists continue to evaluate magnet hospitals. There have been substantial improvements in patient outcomes in organizational environments that support professional nursing practice. The magnet nursing services designation remains a valid marker of nursing care excellence.[5]

Preceptorships and Residencies

Clinical experiences facilitating students and graduates to make the transition to the work setting with more realistic expectations and maximal preparation are necessary.[6] Academic and clinical partnerships are essential, taking such forms as summer internships, externships, and senior capstone preceptored experiences. These partnerships offer opportunities for role socialization and for increasing clinical skills, knowledge, competence, and confidence.[7–9] Extended preceptorships serve as well-thought-out recruitment strategies to decrease costly, lengthy orientation programs and potentially reduce turnover rates.[10,11]

Along with socializing students and new nursing graduates, postgraduate residencies or internships are innovative ways to transition new graduates into practice. The National League for Nursing defines residencies as formal contracts between the employer and the new graduate that outline clinical activities performed by the new nurse in exchange for additional educational offerings and experiences.[12] In a survey of chief nursing officers, 85% of responding chief nursing officers reported having an extended program of orientation for new graduates.[13]

Differentiated Nursing Practice

Differentiated practice models are clinical nursing practice models defined or differentiated by level of education, expected clinical skills or competencies, job descriptions, pay scales, and participation in decision making.[14–16] Differentiated models of practice support clinical "ladders" or defined steps for advancement within the organization. These steps or "rungs" on the ladder are based on experience, additional education, specialty certification, or other indicators of professional excellence. Evidence supports differentiated practice models that foster positive patient and nursing staff outcomes.[17–20]

Interdisciplinary Collaboration

Interdisciplinary practice or collaboration is described as a joint decision-making and communication process among health care providers that is patient centered, focusing on the unique needs of the patient and the specialized abilities of those providing care. Characteristics of interdisciplinary collaboration include mutual respect, trust, good communication, cooperation, coordination, shared responsibility, and knowledge.[21]

Interdisciplinary practice emphasizes teamwork, conflict resolution, and the use of informatics, facilitating collaboration in patient care planning and implementation.[22] Best integrated health delivery systems evolve toward a model of care in which complex patients are managed by interdisciplinary providers. The Pew Health Professions Commission study supports collaboration among physicians, nurses, and allied health professionals. There is evidence of improved outcomes for both acutely and chronically ill patients when cared for by interdisciplinary teams.[23]

Professional nursing practice must be supported by an environment of professionalism, with exemplars of magnet recognition, preceptorships, residencies, differentiated practice, and interdisciplinary collaboration providing evidence that such an environment makes a difference. Using this as a backdrop, the ANA outlines components of a professional nursing practice environment[24]:

1. Manifests a philosophy of clinical care emphasizing quality, safety, interdisciplinary collaboration, continuity of care, and professional accountability, in that nursing staff assume responsibility and accountability for their own practice and nurse staffing patterns have an adequate number of qualified nurses to meet patients' needs, considering patient care complexity.
2. Recognizes contributions of nurses' knowledge and expertise to clinical care quality and patient outcomes, in that the organization has a comprehensive reward system that recognizes role distinctions among staff nurses and other expert nurses based on clinical expertise, reflective practice, education, or advanced credentialing. Nurses are encouraged to be mentors to less experienced colleagues and to share their enthusiasm about professional nursing within the organization and the community.
3. Promotes executive level nursing leadership, in that the nurse executive participates on the governing body and has the authority and accountability for all nursing or patient care delivery, financial resources, and personnel.
4. Empowers nurses' participation in clinical decision making and organization of clinical care systems, in that decentralized, unit-based programs or team organizational structure is used for decision making and review systems for nursing analysis and correction of clinical care errors and patient safety concerns are used.
5. Maintains clinical advancement programs based on education, certification, and advanced preparation, in that peer review, patient, collegial, and managerial input is available for performance evaluation on annual or routine basis and financial rewards are available for clinical advancement and education.
6. Demonstrates professional development support for nurses, in that professional continuing education opportunities are available and supported and long-term career support programs tar-

get specific populations of nurses, such as older individuals, home care or operating room nurses, or nurses from diverse ethnic backgrounds.
7. Creates collaborative relationships among members of the health care provider team, in that professional nurses, physicians, and other health care professionals practice collaboratively and participate in standing organizational committees, bioethics committees, the governing structure, and the institutional review processes.
8. Uses technological advances in clinical care and information systems, in that documentation is supported through appropriate application of technology to the patient care process and resource requirements are quantified and monitored to ensure appropriate resource allocation.

Professional nurse administrative practice considers the scope and standards for nurse administrators, providing a template for excellence in health care management.

SCOPE AND STANDARDS FOR NURSE ADMINISTRATORS: FRAMEWORK FOR PRACTICE

In a joint position statement on nursing administration education, the American Association of Colleges of Nursing and the American Nurses Association (ANA) outline core abilities necessary for nurses in administrative roles. These include the abilities to use management skills that enhance collaborative relationships and team-based learning to advocate for patients and community partners, to embrace change and innovation, to manage resources effectively, to negotiate and resolve conflict, and to communicate effectively using information technology. Content for specialty education in nursing administration includes such concepts and constructs as strategic management, policy development, financial management/cost analysis, leadership, organizational development and business planning, and interdisciplinary relationships. Being mentored by expert executive nurses, engaging in research, and enacting evidence-based management (such as the tracking of effectiveness of care, cost of care, and patient outcomes) are also critical to the education of nurse administrators.

The *Scope and Standards for Nurse Administrators* provides a conceptual model for educating and developing nurses in the professional practice of administrative nursing and health care. This document serves as a framework for this book, which focuses on the levels of nursing administration practice, the standards of practice, and the standards of professional performance for nurse administrators. Consideration of the scope and standards, the role of certification, magnet recognition, and best practice are also included from this frame of reference.[25] Management and leadership theory serves to further reinforce the concepts required for nursing administrative practice. Such concepts are essential to managing a clinical practice discipline.

THE NURSE ADMINISTRATOR

The nurse administrator has been described as a "registered nurse whose primary responsibility is the management of health care delivery services and who represents nursing service."[26] Nurse administrators can be found in a wide variety of settings, with entrepreneurial opportunities available throughout the health care arena. In addition to hospitals, home health care, and skilled care, nurse administrators can also serve in such settings as assisted living, community health services, residential care, and adult day care. In these settings, the nurse administrator must be adequately prepared to face challenges in diverse fields such as information management, evidence-based care and management, legal and regulatory oversight, and ethical practices.

Level of Nursing Administrative Practice

The ANA conceptually divides nursing administration practice into two levels, nurse executive and nurse manager, each with a particular focus that makes a unique contribution to the management of health care systems. The nurse executive's scope includes overall management of nursing practice, nursing education and professional development, nursing research, nursing administration, and nursing services. "The nurse executive holds the accountability to manage within the context of the organization as a whole, and to transform organizational values into daily operations yielding an efficient, effective, and caring organization."[27] Particular functions of the nurse executive include leadership, development, implementation, and evaluation of protocols, programs, and services that are evidence-based and congruent with professional standards.

Nurse managers are responsible to a nurse executive and have more defined areas of nursing service. Advocating and allocating for available resources to facilitate effective, efficient, safe, and compassionate care based on standards of practice are the cornerstone roles of the nurse manager. A nurse manager performs these management functions to deliver health care to patients. Nurse managers or administrators work at all levels to put into practice the concepts, principles, and theories of nursing management. They manage the organizational environment to provide a climate optimal to the provision of nursing care by clinical nurses and ancillary staff.

Management knowledge is universal; so is nursing management knowledge. It uses a systematic body of knowledge that includes concepts, principles, and theories applicable to all nursing management situations. A nurse manager who has applied this knowledge successfully in one situation can be expected to do so in new situations. Nursing management occurs at unit and executive levels. At the executive level, it is frequently termed administration; however, the theories, principles, and concepts remain the same.

With decentralization and participatory management, the supervisor, or middle management, level has been largely eliminated. Nurse managers of clinical units are being educated in management theory and skills at the master's level. Clinical nurses are being educated in management skills that empower them to take action in managing groups of employees as well as clients and families. Clinical nurse managers perform more of the coordinating duties among units, departments, and services. "Nurse managers are accountable for the environment in which clinical nursing is practiced."[28] Both the nurse executive and nurse manager use the standards of practice and standards of professional performance as priorities for nurse administrative practice.

The standards of practice (as framework for this edition) include the following[29]:

- Standard 1: Assessment. Considers data collection systems and processes. Analyzes workflow in relation to effectiveness and efficiency of assessment processes. Evaluates assessment practices.
- Standard 2: Problems/diagnosis. Considers the identification and procurement of adequate resources for decision analysis. Promotes interdisciplinary collaboration. Promotes an organizational climate that supports the validation of problems and formulation of a diagnosis of the organization's environment, culture, and values that direct and support care delivery.
- Standard 3: Identification of outcomes. Considers the interdisciplinary identification of outcomes and the development and utilization of databases that include nursing measures. Promotes continuous improvement of outcome-related clinical guidelines that foster continuity of care.
- Standard 4: Planning. Considers development, maintenance, and evaluation of organizational systems that facilitate planning for care delivery. Creativity and innovation that promote organizational processes for desired patient-defined and cost-effective outcomes are also included in this standard. Collaborates and advocates for staff involvement in all levels of organizational planning and decision making.
- Standard 5: Implementation. Considers the appropriate personnel to implement the design and improvement of systems and processes that assure interventions. Considers the efficient documentation of interventions and patient responses.
- Standard 6: Evaluation. Considers support of participative decision making. Develops policies, procedures, and guidelines based on research findings and institutional measurement of quality

outcomes. Evaluation includes the integration of clinical, human resource, and financial data to adequately plan nursing and patient care.

Standards of professional performance such as quality of care and administrative practice, performance appraisal, professional knowledge, professional environment, ethics, collaboration, research, and resource utilization are also integrated in the framework of this edition. These standards are woven within the chapters and provide continuity of processes and systems of nursing administration (Figure 2-1).

Magnet Recognition Program and Scope and Standards for Nurse Administrators

The American Nurses Credentialing Center provides guidelines for the magnet recognition program. This program's purpose is to recognize health care organizations that have demonstrated the very best in nursing care and professional nursing practice. Such programs have been recognized for having the best practices in nursing, and they also serve to attract and retain quality employees. A key objective of the program is to promote positive patient outcomes. This program also offers a vehicle for communicating best practices and strategies among nursing systems. "Magnet designation helps consumers locate health care organizations that have a proven level of nursing care."[30] Quality indicators and standards of nursing practice as identified by the ANA's Scope and Standards for Nurse Administrators are cornerstone to the magnet recognition program. Qualitative and quantitative factors in nursing are also included in the appraisal process. Certification of nurse administrators is also endorsed through the magnet recognition program.

Qualifications of Nurse Administrators

Attaining the license, education, and experience required for levels of nursing administrative practice is paramount to success in the role as well as to the organizational responsibilities accepted. The nurse

---

FIGURE 2-1	ANA SCOPE AND STANDARDS FOR NURSE ADMINISTRATORS

Standards of Practice	Standards of Professional Performance
Assessment	Quality of Care and Administrative Practice
Problem/diagnosis	Performance Appraisal
Appraisal	Identification of *Journal of Nursing Administration, 97, Journal of Nursing Administration, 97,* outcomes
Professional	Knowledge
Planning	
Professional	Environment
Implementation	Ethics
Evaluation	
Collaboration	
Research	
Resource	Utilization

manager and nurse executive must hold an active registered nurse license and meet the requirements in the state in which they practice. The nurse executive should hold a bachelor's degree and master's degree (or higher) with a major in nursing.

In the nurse manager's role, preparation should be a minimum of a bachelor's degree with a major in nursing. A master's degree with a focus in nursing is recommended along with nationally recognized certification in nursing administration with an appropriate specialty. "The experience backgrounds of professional nurses who serve as nurse administrators must include clinical and administrative practice, which enables these registered nurses to consistently fulfill the responsibilities inherent in their respective administrative roles."[31]

Certification of Nursing Administration

The American Nurses Credentialing Center offers two levels for nursing administration, including an advanced level. Both certification examinations include the following domains: organization and structure, economics, human resources, ethics, and legal and regulatory issues. The domain of organization and structure accounts for the highest percentage of questions for the advanced level. For the nurse manager level, the domain of human resources ranks highest. Both certification examinations include 175 questions with 150 questions scored. Review and resource materials for certification are available and can provide continuing education units for the certification examination.

Using management theory as an underlying framework supports the work of the nurse administrator through the Scope and Standards for Nurse Administrators.

MANAGEMENT: HISTORICAL PERSPECTIVES

Consideration of premodern, modern, and postmodern eras provides a broader perspective on management. The premodern era includes the concepts of work as craft, apprenticeship, journeyman artisan, fraternal organization of professions, and tradition. The modern management era considers pyramids, hierarchy, and systems of money, materials, manpower, inspection, distribution, and production in specialized cells that minimize interaction. The postmodern era includes networks, network stakeholders, and team planning.

Mary Parker Follett is credited with being the "mother of modern management." Taylor, Fayol, and Weber have had considerable influence on modern management and are called the "fathers of modern management." Scientific management (efficiency) provided information on standards, time/motion studies, task analysis, job simplification, and productivity incentives.

Modern management theory evolved from the work of Henri Fayol, who identified the activities or functions of the administrator as planning, organizing, coordinating, and controlling.[32] His work has been called "process management." Fayol defined management in these words:

> To manage is to forecast and plan, to organize, to command, to coordinate, and to control. To foresee and provide means [of] examining the future and drawing up the plan of action. To organize means building up the dual structure, material and human, of the undertaking. To command means binding together, unifying and harmonizing all activity and effort. To control means seeing that everything occurs in conformity with established rule and expressed demand.[33]

Although some persons believed these were technical functions that could be learned only on the job, Fayol believed that they could be taught in an educational setting if a theory of administration could be formulated.[34] He also stated that the need for managerial ability increases in relative importance as an individual advances in the chain of command. The principles of management described by Fayol are listed in Figure 2-2.[35]

FIGURE 2-2	FAYOL'S PRINCIPLES OF MANAGEMENT

1. Division of work
2. Authority
3. Discipline
4. Unity of command
5. Unity of direction
6. Subordination of individual interests to the general interests
7. Remuneration
8. Centralization
9. Scalar chain (line of authority)
10. Order
11. Equity
12. Stability or tenure of personnel
13. Initiative
14. Esprit de corps

Human relations management and behavioral science and management are also integrated into the modern management paradigm. The Hawthorne studies validated the influence of working conditions on employee efficiency and productivity. Labor and management relationships, communication, and democratization of the workplace are key aspects of human relations management. Maslow, Hertberg, MacGregor, Argyris, and Likert have been instrumental in developing behavioral science management theory. Additionally, Blake, Mouton, Fiedler, Hersey, and Blanchard are also noted for their work in this aspect of the modern era. Building on the work of human relations management, the behaviorists paid particular attention to leadership, participative management, personal motivation and hygiene factors, and hierarchy of workers' needs. During the modern management era, there was noted stability in the workforce, limited diversity in the workplace, and a better educated workforce.

Throughout management literature, the original functions of planning, organizing, directing (command and coordination), and controlling as defined by Fayol and others have been accepted as the principal functions of managers. Although linear structures, bureaucracy, rationality, and control define the modern area, the postmodern era considers a new universe of pattern, purpose, and process. Postmodern organizations are described as loosely coupled, fluid, organic, and "adhocratic." Organic, continuum-based, and living systems are inherent to this era. Wilson and Porter-O'Grady contrast linear integration with meta-integration, which focuses on long-term service orientation, systems design, and population/person-driven, continuum-based, and outcome-driven systems. According to the authors, the postmodern manager's role is accountability based, resource oriented, and service driven. The term "service driven" highlights the manager's role as facilitator, integrator, and coordinator.[36]

Peter Drucker first applied the term *postmodern* to organization in 1957, identifying a shift from the Cartesian universe of mechanical cause and effect (subject/object duality) to this new order of pattern, purpose, and process. Knowledge workers were also included in this discussion with greater emphasis on providing management processes and systems that supported decision making at the point of service by those knowledgeable about the processes. Evidence-based management is viewed as critical to transforming work environments and providing safe and quality care.[37]

Evidence-based management has particular significance in health care, because the work environment experiences greater turbulence, chaos, and instability than do those of other disciplines. Dated and untested management practices are no longer useful and may be detrimental to providing safe care. In *Keeping Patients Safe: Transforming the Work Environment of Nurses*, the importance of sound, evidence-based management practices are underscored. Using an evidence-based frame of reference, managers, like their clinical counterparts, are accountable for searching for, appraising, and applying empirical evidence from management research in their practices. Additionally, thoughtful reflection, decision making, and actions by managers should be systematically recorded and evaluated in ways that further add to the evidence base of effective management practice. The Committee identified five essential management practices.[38] These five practices have not been consistently applied, adding further evidence to their importance in today's health care environment:

1. *Balancing the tension between efficiency and effectiveness.* Best practices in this domain include putting redundancy into work design, which has proven effective in the air traffic control industry. Consideration of production efficiency, balance and alignment of organizational goals, accountability processes, rewards, incentives, and compensation are aspects of this practice, which can improve patient outcomes.

2. *Creating and sustaining trust.* Trust and honest, open communication are critical to successful organizational change. When there is openness and trust, individuals are more willing to make contributions to the organization without immediate payoffs. Trust in an organization's leaders and management practices has been linked to positive business outcomes such as increased productivity and greater profitability, whereas distrust has been linked to increased absenteeism, turnover, and risk aversion.

3. *Actively managing the process of change.* This management practice is related to human resource management and includes practices such as ongoing communication; training; designing mechanisms for feedback, measurement, and redesign; sustained attention; and worker involvement. The concept of investment in change as being good for the organization and individual is illuminated in this practice.

4. *Involving workers in work design and workflow decision making.* Hierarchically structured and highly controlled organizations lack the flexibility to respond to situations that are highly variable and associated with reduced safety. The concepts of shared governance, nursing empowerment, control over nursing practice, and clinical autonomy have been noted to improve patient outcomes as well as worker satisfaction. The key element in this practice is nurses' control over their practice. This influences care of the individual patient as well as organizational policies and practices carried out within nursing units, the effects of the health care organization as a whole on nursing care, and the control of resources in care provision. Magnet hospitals support these aspects of nurses' involvement. Studies reveal that both autonomy and control over nursing practice are consistent magnet characteristics. Additionally, nurses' autonomy and control over practice are positively related to trust in management.[39]

5. *Creating a learning organization.* Learning organizations constantly manage the learning process and consider all sources of knowledge, the use of systematic experimentation to generate new knowledge within the organization, and the quick and efficient transfer of knowledge within the organization. Understanding the existing knowledge culture within the organization is important to the work of creating a learning organization with enough time to think, learn, and train. Incentives and reward systems must be aligned and must facilitate knowledge management practices in the creation of a learning environment.[40]

These five essential management practices in nurses' work environment and health care at large are inconsistent at best and create barriers to positive patient outcomes. An understanding of management theory and practices provides a foundation for best practice.

Managing means accomplishing the goals of the group through effective and efficient use of resources. Specifically, project management is considered a core competency for nurses and managers. Some organizations have adopted project management as their main management approach (management-by-project); other organizations superimpose project management on their current organizational structure and management practices. The manager creates and maintains an internal environment in an enterprise in which individuals work together as a group. Managing is the art of doing, and management is the body of organized knowledge underlying the art. In modern management, staffing is frequently separated from the planning function, directing is labeled leading, and controlling is used interchangeably with evaluating. The ANA's standards for nursing administration are based on these principles, which support the science of nursing administration.[41]

THEORY, CONCEPTS, AND PRINCIPLES

The knowledge base of management science includes theory, which in turn includes concepts, methods, and principles. The principles are related and can be observed and verified to some degree when they are translated into the art or practice of management. Concepts are thoughts, ideas, and general notions about a class of objects that form a basis for action or discussion. Concepts tend to be true but are not always true. Principles are fundamental truths, laws, or doctrines on which other notions are based. Principles provide guidance to concepts and to thought or action in a situation.[42]

White explores a viewpoint on nursing theories in which she addresses prescriptive theories. She notes that their use as practice guidelines must be broad enough to provide a wide range of practice situations but not so broad as to be meaningless. A theory of decision making might be as beneficial in practice as a theory of nursing. If nursing is going to base its theory on laws, nurses need to validate principles through research—a difficult task, as theorists in the social sciences have discovered. It is not easy to reduce human behavior to laws. Nurses deal with human behavior in all roles but particularly in nursing management. Nurses believe that for nursing to be a real profession, it should have a scientific and theoretical base. Nursing is thus a practice profession based on the physical and social sciences.[43]

Nurse managers learn to merge the disciplines of human relations, labor relations, personnel management, and industrial engineering into a unified force for effective management. Nurse managers would add the theory of nursing to this list. A successful synthesis of these disciplines can promote employee commitment, increased productivity, enhanced competency, good labor relations, and competitiveness in health care. The workforce is poorly managed when these goals are not achieved.

Critical Theory versus Critical Thinking

Steffy and Grimes note that a strict natural science approach to social science is naive, because subjective or qualitative analysis is important to quantitative research. This holds true for management and consequently for nursing management. Health care organizational models are not objective and value free. Steffy and Grimes suggest using a critical theory approach to organizational science rather than a phenomenological or hermeneutic approach.

A phenomenological approach uses second-order constructs, or "interpretations of interpretations." This approach requires researchers to become participants in the organization and to suspend all judgments and preconceived ideas about possible meanings. The nurse manager interprets the meaning of nursing management experiences or observations and arrives at a nursing management theory from the aggregate of meanings.

Hermeneutics is the art of textual interpretation. In this approach, the nurse manager as researcher views self as a historically produced entity and recognizes personal biases in doing research. He or she considers the specific context and historic dimensions of data collected and reflect on the relationship between theory and history.[44]

Critical theory is an empirical philosophy of social institutions. Decision makers, such as nurse managers, translate theories into practice. Theories in use are behavioral technologies that include organizational development, management by objectives or results, strategic planning, planned change, performance appraisal, and other practice-oriented activities performed by managers. Critical theory aims to do the following:

1. Critique the ideology of scientism, the institutionalized form of reasoning that accepts the idea that the meaning of knowledge is defined by what the sciences do and thus can be adequately explicated through analysis of scientific procedures
2. Develop an organizational science capable of changing organizational processes

These aims are compatible with a theory of nursing management. Nurses use science to legitimize the practice of clinical nursing and nursing management.[45]

General Systems Theory

General systems theory is an organic approach to the study of the general relationships of the empirical universe of an organization and human thought. The theory comes from the field of biology and poses an analogy between an organism and a social organization. General systems concepts form the theoretical underpinnings for other leadership and management theories. Boulding describes nine levels of a general systems theory,[46] which are given here with nursing management applications:

1. *A static structure: the framework.* Nursing is a discipline with an aggregate population of registered nurses educated at several levels (including those with hospital diplomas and those with degrees from associate through doctoral levels), licensed practical nurses, and unlicensed assistive personnel (e.g., aides, orderlies, attendants, nursing assistants, and clerks). This population functions within a dynamic and flattening structure that may change frequently. Superior/subordinate relationships are giving way to decentralized, participatory, and transformational management at the practice level. Flat organizations usually have a top administrator, first-line managers, and practitioners. These nursing persons usually function in an environment in which the focus of attention is the client. One approach to a framework in nursing is that nursing persons apply the nursing process in giving care to patients. Many similarities exist between the nursing process and nursing management.
2. *A moving level of necessary predetermined motions: the clockwork.* Nurse managers process the knowledge and skills of management—planning, organizing, leading, and evaluating—to produce nursing care. The function of nursing management is the use of personnel, supplies, equipment, clinical knowledge, and skills to give nursing care to clients within varying environments. The nurse manager may also have other ancillary personnel to manage, such as therapists, housekeepers, and social workers, adding to the complexity of providing overall quality services for client care. One such environment is the hospital physical plant. Nursing planning + nursing organizing + nursing leading + nursing evaluating = nursing management. To this we may add that nursing management + nursing practice = nursing care of clients. The move is toward equilibrium of all forces that go into the nursing management equation.
3. *A control mechanism: the thermostat.* In nursing administration this thermostat could be the top administrator or any first-line manager. This person maintains a management information system that transmits and interprets information and communication to and from employees. Production of nursing care of satisfactory quality and quantity depends on the manager maintaining an environment satisfactory to employees.
4. *An open system or self-maintaining structure: the cell.* Nursing management will survive and maintain the nursing organization by being open to new ideas, new management techniques,

---

FIGURE 2-3   **AN OPEN SYSTEM**

External Environment

Transformation process

INPUT

Nursing personnel
Supplies
Equipment
Physical plant
Clients
Knowledge, values,
ethics, skills, and beliefs

Management of nursing
care of clients by nursing
personnel
Critical thinking
Application of nursing
theory in management
and clinical care

OUTPUT

Resolution of nursing
problems of clients
Outcome: client
improvement; client
health care goals met,
healing, peaceful death

Feedback

---

and the input of human and material resources to produce the nursing care needed by clients. An open system reproduces itself by keeping up to date and by developing replacements. Keep up to date by adding nursing education: nursing management + nursing planning + nursing evaluation = nursing care of clients (see Figure 2-3).

5. *The genetic–societal level.* There is a division of labor even within nursing management but especially among nursing personnel who produce the nursing care of patients. Further integrating multiple skill-level personnel into the mix offers more comprehensive complimentary care in meeting clients' health care needs. The raw materials—that is, the human and material resources—are input. These resources are processed as put through by a group of nursing personnel with varying knowledge and skills using a theory-based nursing care delivery system. The output is resolution of the nursing needs and problems of clients, with their improvement, accomplishment of health care goals, and healing, or their succumbing to a peaceful death.

6. *The "animal" level.* This level has increased mobility, teleological (designing or purposeful) behavior, and self-awareness. Some evidence indicates that nursing management is reaching this level. As nurse managers learn the knowledge and skills of the business and industrial world, they adapt these skills to the management of health care services. This gives nursing management and

nursing practice a more scientific basis, the result of which may be that nurses will be able to demonstrate empirically and theoretically that what they do affects client outcomes.

7. *The "human" level.* The nurse manager develops an increased awareness and knows that he or she can process the knowledge and skills of management to produce specific results.

8. *The level of social organization.* Nurse managers at this level distinguish themselves from other groups of managers. Nurse managers operate within complex roles; their functions are made effective by communication, relationships, and other interpersonal processes.

9. *Transcendental systems.* At this level nurse managers ask questions for which there are as yet no answers. Theoretical models of nursing management extend to level 4 (the cell), the level of application of most other models. Empirical knowledge is deficient at nearly all levels. Descriptive models are needed to catalogue events in nursing. The movement toward decentralization and participatory and service-line management, although still a very simple system, is growing each year as nurse scientists develop and apply new nursing administration models and theories of nursing. General systems theory is the skeleton of a science. Adding nursing research gives: nursing management + nursing planning + nursing evaluation + nursing research = nursing care of clients.

Disciplines and sciences have bodies of knowledge that grow with meaningful information. The empirical universe provides general phenomena relevant to many different disciplines; these phenomena can be built into theoretical models, including one for nursing management. Nursing as a discipline has varied populations (phenomena) that interact dynamically among themselves. These include professional nurses, technical nurses, practical nurses, and unlicensed assistive nursing personnel as well as professional nursing teachers, researchers, and managers. Individuals within the discipline interact with the environment (another phenomenon). Through knowledge and experience they grow. The media for growth are information, interpersonal processing, relationships, and communication, which are themselves phenomena.[47]

With the emerging changes in health care systems, nurse leaders need to accelerate changes in nursing organizations. The goal may be nursing modules centered on closely related operations, such as differentiated practice delivery models matched with intensity of care or specialized services. Standardization and flexibility can be melded to develop systems based on a requirement for a theory of nursing practice as a foundation for all modules, but with different theories being used in different modules chosen by professional clinical nurses.[48]

Full realization of systems theory is as far in the future for nursing as it is for manufacturing. Nursing is a "head, heart, and hands" discipline. Nursing management and practice tie the parts of the health care system together. Transformational nurse leaders will be fully knowledgeable about the work being done by their constituents because they will be coaches, mentors, and facilitators. Followers of the systems concept will also have to implement the integration of people, materials, machines, and time.[49]

ROLES AND NURSING MANAGEMENT

Role Development

The nurse manager draws from the best and most applicable theories of management to create an individual management style and performance.[50] This requires knowledge and the skills to use it. The nurse manager continues to acquire and use management knowledge to solve managerial problems, which require a contingency approach because no single approach works for all situations.[51] The nurse manager acts with the assumption that clinical nurses and other health care providers want to be competent and that with managerial support they will be motivated to achieve competence and greater levels of productivity. With achievement of competence and productivity goals, higher goals are set. Clinical nurses will seek out the organization that fits their needs.[52]

Adding to the nurse manager's ever-expanding role is the need to increase knowledge of and sensitivity to other health care individuals providing clinical services. These services are integrated into the client's overall experience of health care, of which nursing is a critical component.

McClure points out that nurse managers manage a clinical discipline performed by professional nurses. Because most nurses are women, conflicts may arise between their professional and personal lives. The nurse manager devises strategies to deal with these conflicts. Some blue-collar nurses lack knowledge of nursing research and do not read to keep up to date; they want nurse managers to do everything. White-collar nurses often want to be treated differently; they want job enrichment, with primary nursing duties and professional autonomy, and they want to be organized like the medical staff, with staff appointments and peer review. The nurse manager manages these two groups differently.[53]

Management Levels

Nurse managers perform at several levels in the health care organization. These include first-line patient care management at the unit level, middle management at the department level, and top management at the executive level. In some organizations decentralization has displaced the middle management level and redistributed department-level functions to staff functions under a matrix or another organizational structure. The middle management role is often reconsidered in work redesign effort, particularly as leadership moves further away from clinical care. The roles of managers are developmental, building on knowledge and skills as the scope of the nurse manager's role increases in breadth and depth. Middle nurse manager roles are frequently eliminated, and clinical nurses become empowered through management education.[54]

First-Line Nurse Managers

The following are some of the knowledge and skills needed by nurses in first-line management roles:

- Financial management knowledge and skills to prepare and defend a budget for expenses of unit personnel, supplies, and capital equipment and for revenues to meet expenses; the ability to manage scarce and expensive resources for performance
- The ability to match moral and ethical choices with respect to human needs, moral principles for behavior, and individual feelings in making decisions
- Recognition of and advocacy for patients' rights
- Active and assertive effort to share power within the organization, including shared power for nursing's practitioners. This includes nursing autonomy, which is threatened by authoritarian management. In turn, practicing nurses are involved in solving managerial problems.
- The ability to communicate and to promote effective communication and interpersonal relationships among nursing staff and others; presentation skills
- Knowledge of internal factors related to purpose, tasks, people, technology, and structure
- Knowledge of external factors related to economy, political pressures, legal aspects, sociocultural characteristics, and technology
- The ability to study situations and use management concepts and techniques, analyze the situations correctly, make diagnoses of problems, and tie the processes together to arrive at decisions
- The ability to provide for staff development
- The ability to provide a climate in which nurses clearly perceive that they are pursuing meaningful and worthwhile goals through their individual efforts
- Knowledge of organizational culture and its impact on productivity and problem solving
- Ability to effect change through an orderly process
- Commitment to maintain self-development by reading and attending workshops and other educational programs

- Knowledge of how to empower clinical nurses through committee assignments, quality circles, primary nursing, and even assigning titles
- Knowledge of recruitment and retention strategies to promote and retain valued nursing and health care personnel

To these could be added staffing and scheduling, management reports, hiring, performance appraisal, job productivity and satisfaction, constructive discipline dealing with stress and conflict, personnel management, diversity, and awareness of culture, values, norms, and ways of doing things.[55] Although these skills and this knowledge may be obtained through staff development, master's level management preparation is essential.

In no way are these lists complete. They are a beginning, however, and are built on in succeeding chapters.

The Nurse Executive

Executive nurse managers increase their knowledge and skills by building on what they learned as lower level managers. Executive nurse managers should be able to do the following:

- Apply financial management principles to costing and pricing nursing care and convey this knowledge to the nurses providing care
- Coordinate the division budget
- Empower lower level nurse managers
- Undertake corporate self-analysis of what nursing can do (skills, capabilities, weaknesses, the work of nursing) and its assumptions about itself, its environment, and its beliefs and convey results to employees
- Specify, weigh, interrelate, and simultaneously accomplish multiple goals
- Abandon obsolete principles of standardization, centralization, specialization, and concentration
- Decentralize and share authority and power through participatory management and transformational leadership, shared governance, professional nursing models, employee involvement, and programs on the quality of work life
- Establish a matrix organization using task forces and project teams with project leaders
- Set the stage for clinical nursing practice. This does not necessarily require that the nurse executive be clinically competent.
- Promote application of a theory of nursing within a nursing care delivery system
- Advise nursing educators on content of nursing administration programs
- Set depth and breadth of nursing research programs
- Anticipate the future of health care and of nursing
- Manage strategic planning
- Serve as mentor, role model, and preceptor to lower level managers, graduate students, and others
- Recognize and use authority and the potential for power

Evidence from research indicates that executive nurses prepared at the doctoral level need courses in ethical and accountable decision making, including missions and goals, policies, human resources, financial and material resources, databases, and communication management. These courses would be organized into organizational structure and governance, resources, and information management.[56]

With major changes in business practices, lessons learned from Japan offer meaningful strategies to American business, including the business of health care. For example, the Japanese have found that less variety is best when it comes to cutting costs and saving time. Consensus decision making does not always work. With the help of high-tech information systems, lone decisions based on multiple data sources and data points may be the best decisions.[57] The understanding of theories, roles and responsibilities, and evidence-based management provides the foundational work for the nurse administrator to manage a clinical practice.

MANAGING A CLINICAL PRACTICE

Nursing is a clinical practice discipline. Professional nurses want autonomy and control of their practice. They want to apply their nursing knowledge and skills without interference from nurse managers, physicians, or persons in other disciplines. The effective nurse manager trusts the professional nurse to apply knowledge and skills correctly in caring for a group of patients. In turn, the clinical nurse trusts the nurse manager to coordinate supplies, equipment, and support systems with personnel in other departments. Clinical nurses trust a human relations management in which they participate rather than one in which they have rules and regulations imposed on them. They use the body of nursing knowledge (theory) gained in nursing school and maintained through continuing education and staff development to practice nursing as they determine it should be practiced. In doing so, they adhere to management policies regarding such issues as documentation or quality improvement, because these requirements are also part of clinical nursing practice.

Use of Nursing Theory in Professional Practice

In developing nursing as a professional scientific discipline, nursing educators and researchers have developed theoretical frameworks for the clinical practice of nursing that are used by clinical nurses as models for testing and validating applications of nursing knowledge and skills. The results are added to the body of knowledge commonly called the theory of nursing. Theory gives practicing nurses a professional identity. It is based on scientific inquiry: nursing research. Each result of nursing research adds tested facts to nursing theory that can be learned by nursing students and active practitioners.

Watson's Theory of Caring

Caring is central to nursing, and most persons choosing nursing as a profession do so because they desire to care for others. Caring as a science has been defined by Jean Watson. She describes science of caring as one that encompasses a humanitarian, human science orientation, human caring processes, phenomena, and experiences. Watson outlines caring from a science perspective, grounded in a relational ontology of being-in-relation and a world view of unity and connectedness. Transpersonal caring, as Watson notes, acknowledges unity of life and connections that move in concentric circles of caring—from individual, to others, to community, to world, and to the universe. Caring science embraces inquiry that is reflective, subjective, and interpretative as well as objective-empirical. Caring science inquiry includes ontological, philosophical, ethical, historical inquiry, and studies.[58]

An example of how Watson's theory of caring can serve as a framework is illustrated in the Attending Nursing Caring Model (ANCM). ANCM is an exemplar for advancing and transforming nursing practice within a reflective, theoretical, and evidence-based context. The ANCM serves as a program for stimulating the profession and its professional practices of caring–healing arts and science, when nursing is experiencing decline, shortages, and crises in care, safety, and hospital and health reform. With the ANCM, Watson's theory of human caring is used as a guide for integrating theory, evidence, and advanced therapeutics in the area of children's pain. The ANCM raises contemporary nursing's caring values, relationships, therapeutics, and responsibilities to a higher level of caring science and professionalism, interacting with other professions, while sustaining the finest of its heritage and traditions of healing.[59]

Orem's Theory

Orem's theory of self-care is composed of three related theories: the theory of self-care, the theory of self-care deficit, and the theory of nursing systems. She viewed each person as a self-care agent who possesses capabilities, termed *self-care agency*, essential to performing self-care actions. Deliberate action is taken to meet the therapeutic self-care demand arising out of known needs for care. Self-care needs and demands vary throughout the lifespan. If the demand is not met, a self-care deficit exists, which creates the need for nursing. In the nurse–patient experience, a joint decision is made between the nurse and the patient. The role of the nurse is to facilitate and increase the self-care abilities of the individual. Self-care is not instinctive or reflexive but is performed rationally in response to a known need, which is learned through the individual's interpersonal relations and communication. Self-care agency is the power to engage in action. This is a complex developed capability that enables adults and maturing adolescents to recognize and understand factors that must be controlled and managed to regulate functioning and developing as well as the capability to decide about and perform proper care measures. This capability is dependent on lifelong experiences and values related to culture. This is aided by intellectual curiosity and by instruction and supervision from other persons.[60]

Parissopoulos and Kotzabassaki describe Orem's self-care theory in the management of elderly rehabilitation. Orem's theory provides common language in self-care leading to improved communication and enhances consistency in care delivery and building consensus of goals and outcomes of nursing. Nurses are in key positions to facilitate the achievement of self-care that requires sophisticated communication skills, teaching skills, specialized knowledge, and an awareness of the multiple factors affecting nurse–patient relationships during the provision of care.[61]

Roy's Theory

Roy advocates adaptation level theory to nursing intervention. She notes that a person adapts to the environment through four modes: physiologic needs and processes, self-concept (beliefs and feelings about oneself), role mastery (behavior among people who occupy different positions within society), and interdependence (giving and receiving nurturance).[62] Just as the individual patient adapts to changes in the environment, so does the nursing worker.

According to Roy, the goal of nursing is to assist the patient to adapt to illness so as to be able to respond to other stimuli. The patient is assessed for positive or negative behavior in the four adaptive modes. Once the assessment is made at the necessary (first or second) level, intervention is established by a nursing care plan of goals and approaches. The approach is selected to match the goal.[63] According to Mastal and Hammond, Roy's views are "that the developing body of nursing knowledge now contains verifiable theories and general laws related to: (1) persons as holistic beings, and (2) the role of nursing in promoting the person's maximum potential health and harmonious interaction with the environment."[64]

Frederickson illustrates application of the Roy adaptation model to the nursing diagnosis of anxiety. He describes or defines anxiety from the nursing perspective as exhibited by "poor nutritional status, reduction in usual physical activity, and lowered self-esteem, in addition to concern for job security." The nurse diagnoses the symptoms of anxiety through assessment of the four modes and then designs and implements an intervention that promotes client adaptation.[65]

Evaluation criteria for empirical testing of nursing theory were developed by Silva and expanded by others. Theory testing includes processes of verifying whether what was purported or experienced is true or solves problems in one's discipline or practice. Silva and Sorrell define nursing theory as "a tentative body of diverse but purposeful, creative, and logically interrelated perspectives that help nurses to redefine nursing and to understand, explain, raise questions about, and seek clarification of nursing phenomena in their research and practice."[66] They list three alternative approaches of testing to verify nursing theory:

1. Through critical reasoning
2. Through description of personal experiences
3. Through application to nursing practice (This concept has been applied at the National Hospital for Orthopedics and Rehabilitation, Arlington, Virginia, where the Roy adaptation model has been implemented throughout the hospital.)

Newman's Theory

Margaret Newman's theory of health as expanding consciousness emphasizes the whole pattern of the person in interaction with the environment and the process of nursing practice as the content of nursing research.[67] Newman's theory is grounded in Martha Rogers' science of unitary human beings and is consistent with the unitary transformative paradigm of nursing. Newman describes her model as the process of nursing intervention from the unitary–transformative paradigm. The outline of this intervention process can be applied to research and takes into account the following steps:

Step 1: Determining the mutuality of the process of inquiry

Step 2: Zeroing in during the interview on the most meaningful persons and events in the participant's life

Step 3: Sharing the researcher's depiction of the participant's life pattern, which has been translated from the interview data into a diagram as sequential patterns over time

Step 4: Determining evidence of pattern recognition and concomitant insight into the meanings of the client's life pattern

According to Newman, this process is the unitary–transformative nursing intervention via pattern recognition. It is the dynamic flow of patterning through the researcher and the researched interaction within the larger dynamic context. Newman's theory has been used in working with cancer patients and provides a conceptualization of intervening in a meaningful way.

Johnson's Theory

Johnson incorporated the nursing process (assessment, diagnosis planning, intervention, and evaluation) into a general systems model. Rawls applied this model to care of a patient for the purpose of testing, evaluating, and determining its utility for predicting the effect of nursing care on a patient. Rawls indicates that the model has disadvantages but is a tool that can be used "to accurately predict the results of nursing interventions prior to care, formulate standards of care, and most importantly, administer truly holistic empathic nursing care."[68]

Derdiarian sampled 223 cancer patients to verify the relationship among the eight subsystems of Johnson's behavioral system model. These eight subsystems (achievement, affiliative, aggressive/protective, dependence, eliminative, ingestive, sexual, and restorative) function through behavior to meet a person's demands. Illness disrupts and changes behavior sustained in the subsystems, resulting in negative effects on the behavioral systems. Changes in one subsystem initiate changes in others. Findings of this research indicated "fairly large, statistically significant (P < .001) direct relationships between the aggressive/protective subsystems and each of the other subsystems." The research presents a model for continued research of Johnson's behavioral system model with "implications for comprehensive assessment, early intervention, prevention of patients' potential problems, and ultimately for efficient care."[69]

Peplau's Theory

Peplau's theory defines nursing as a "significant, therapeutic, interpersonal process."[70] Peplau's theory involves such concepts as communication techniques, assessment, definition of problems and goals, direction, and role clarification.

Peplau states that four components make up the main elements of the nurse–patient relationship: nurse, patient, professional expertise, and client need. The nurse–patient relationship has three phases: the orientation phase, the working phase, and the resolution phase. During encounters with patients, the nurse observes, interprets what he or she observes, and then decides what needs to be done.

Interpersonal relations use the theoretical constructs of concepts, processes, and patterns:

- A concept is a small, circumscribed set of behaviors pertaining to a particular phenomenon such as conflict.
- A process is more complicated, more comprehensive, and longer lasting.
- A pattern is made up of separate acts that may have variations but share a common theme, aim, or intention.

Interpersonal theory is especially useful in psychiatric nursing and is useful in relation to psychosocial problems and nurse–patient relationships in all clinical areas of nursing. The joint effort of the nurse–patient relationship "includes identification of the presenting problems, understanding the problems and their variation in pattern, and appreciating, applying, and testing remedial measures in order to produce beneficial outcomes for patients."[71]

Case Management: An Example of a Nursing Practice Modality

Case management is more than a modality of nursing. It has been described as all of the following: clinical system that focuses on the accountability of an identified individual or group for conditioning care for a patient or a group of patients across a continuum of care; ensuring and facilitating the achievement of quality and clinical and cost outcomes; negotiating, procuring, and coordinating services and resources needed by the patient or family; intervening at busy points (and/or when significant variance occurs) for individual patients; addressing and resolving patterns in aggregate variances that have a negative quality/cost impact; and creating opportunities and systems to enhance outcomes.[72] Simply stated, case management is a process of coordinating services, and the case manager is the person who does the coordinating.[73]

The Center for Case Management's model of case management was designed as a clinical one. The model's underlying assumption was that caregivers of each discipline needed to have management skills, better patient care management tools, and more responsible administrative support to create quality clinical outcomes within a new cost-conscious milieu. The organizational structure is flat, with attending-level physician and "selected primary care nurses expanded into case managers to produce the integration of processes, aided by critical paths."[74] Critical paths have been integrated into CareMaps®. The CareMap® is used as the nursing care plan and for documentation.

A collaborative team approach is used when integration of care occurs across geographical care units such as the emergency room, the coronary care unit, the step-down unit, and the ambulatory clinic. Primary nurses from these units who have undergone formal orientation join the team.[75]

Personnel at the Center for Case Management believe that 100% of patients need their care managed by a CareMap®. The CareMaps® provide the documented standards for specific patient populations and disease states. With this infrastructure of care delivery, only 20% believe that patients need a case manager in addition to a CareMap® system.[76]

Quality improvement is an integral part of the case management system. Quality management is operationalized by the use of critical paths, CareMaps®, and case management, all of which provide the tools for accomplishing the nursing process.[77] CareMaps® present problems by defining quality as a product.[78] When interventions and goals are recorded that are different from those planned, they are termed *variances*. A variance indicates deviations from a norm or standard. Variance indicates intervention that works or does not work. Variances alter discharge dates, expected costs, and expected outcomes.

Variances show how the CareMap® and reality differ both positively and negatively. Variance that shows negative outcomes requires action to improve quality. Variance data are collected, totaled, analyzed, and reported; they then result in decisions that revise CareMaps® critical paths, procedures, and other elements of the plan–do–check–act cycle.[79] Because CareMaps® can be used to document nursing care, are outcome based, and have been found to be effective and efficient, nurses may want to use a computerized version for documentation.

Other Models of Case Management

University of Kentucky Hospital Model The University of Kentucky Hospital model of case management uses a problem-solving process. Case managers are master's-prepared nurses to whom cases are referred by quality-monitoring groups. Case managers verify problems, design strategies to fix them, and evaluate outcomes.

The priority in this model is efficient movement through the health care system. Case managers consult with finance personnel, administrators, and health care providers; they collaborate with physicians, primary nurses, and other health care providers; and they establish therapeutic relationships with patients and families. A case management advisory board meeting takes place quarterly. Members perform prospective or retrospective surveys for clinical problems. Case managers follow up with diagnoses and procedure codes specific to the cases with verified problems. Sample problems of outcomes include poor continuity in patient's care, inadequate discharge planning, inadequate patient teaching, extended preoperative and postoperative stays, and poor nutritional status of patients.

Among the results were the following:

- Reduced glucose levels in diabetic, adult, open-heart surgery patients (which resulted in a savings of $11,585 in room charges during a 6-month period)
- Decreased arterial blood gas charges in cardiovascular patients
- Intensive care newborn patients home 218 days earlier than comparable patients during the previous year (a savings of $82,731 for Medicaid patients alone)

Management will pay for performance when hiring case managers in the future.[80]

Carondelet/St. Mary's Hospital and Health Center Model Another model of case management is the Carondelet/St. Mary's Hospital and Health Center in Tucson, Arizona. In this model, nurse case managers work in partnership with high-risk individuals in the hospital (30%) and in the community (70%). Reports of applications of this model of nursing case management indicate that it results in financial savings and liability defenses. It is case management in which the nurse manages and coordinates the entire spectrum of a patient's care in all settings, hospital and community. Effective case management wins the confidence of all team members, including social workers and physicians. Nursing case management supports the highest use of clinical nursing skills. Rogers, Riordan, and Swindle report that case management reduced total admissions, mean admissions per patient, mean length of stay per patient, and net reimbursement. The authors recommend mandating Bachelor of Science in nursing qualifications for case managers and 5 years of clinical experience. They worked out comparable arrangements with social workers.[81]

Other Factors Related to Case Management

Bower reported that case managers at Hennepin County Medical Center in Minneapolis were responsible for the following[82]:

- Over $1 million in direct cost savings
- Readmission rates for patients having major bowel procedures reduced from 67% to 26%

- Readmission rates for patients with cerebrovascular disorders (except transitory ischemic attacks) reduced from 43% to 31%
- Compliance with antibiotic protocols in patients having hip and femur procedures increased from 38% to 89%

Nurses have been at the forefront of case management as it relates to moving patients through the hospital efficiently. There may be conflicts between nurse case managers and other providers within the community. Professional nurses should become educated about case management programs, interagency groups, use of interdisciplinary teams, and legal issues and should keep respect for clients' wishes and rights continually in mind.[84]

Strong indicates that clinical nurse specialists have the expert clinical and management skills to enhance planning, clinical decision making, and evaluation of resource use. The case management system has been applied to promote cost-effective, long-term wellness in migrant children by addressing cultural, nutritional, and dental care needs and by using available resources. This has also been done with homeless families. Case management identifies the clients' needs and makes and implements plans to meet those needs efficiently and effectively. Case management may be performed by a group practice of primary nurses.[85]

Discussing clients with learning disabilities, Thomas describes case management applied to clients in their local communities as managing a team of field workers who assess clients' needs and make action plans with them.[86] These plans address assessment, action planning, package development, and financial management. Case managers draw up contracts for clients' services.

These packages include an estimate of hours required for 1 month's care and residential versus home care costs, and they break down costs into those for such workers as community care assistant, respite care home outreach worker, physiotherapist, and occupational therapist and for transportation. Contracts involving groups of clients may obtain discounts. Third-party payers usually approve contracts. Thomas states that caseworkers are frequently social workers, and case management may develop into a new autonomous profession.

Dowling states that nursing case management makes the patient's nurse the central decision hub for the entire spectrum of patient care requirements and services.[87] He calls this matrix management. The common results of nursing case management fall into five primary areas:

1. Early, or appropriate, patient discharges
2. Expected, or standardized, clinical outcomes
3. Promotion of collaborative practice, coordinated patient care, and true continuity of care
4. Promotion of nurses' professional development and job satisfaction
5. Use of appropriate, or reduced, resources

The model is the critical path forecasting physician intervention, diagnostic testing, ancillary department patient care, support department input, and supply and equipment requirements. The individual critical path is a communication tool for all care given. It is a production schedule. The critical path provides the hospital material manager with a dynamic distribution of patient care supplies and equipment needed in advance of any requests. Hospital information supplements provide the information needed for supplies and equipment planning to be case specific. Just-in-time programs can provide patient-specific supplies for multiple supply-retention locations on a nursing unit.

Research indicates that using the critical path technique for assessing the postoperative recovery of coronary artery bypass graph patients prevents complications, reduces lengths of stay, and reduces hospital costs. Nursing interventions such as use of inspirometers, resumption of activity, and patient education support this finding. Critical paths may be used by nurses to identify appropriate nursing interventions and their costs.[88]

Case management is outcome based and supports evidence-based practices. The Medical Center of Central Georgia in Macon used outcome-based nursing practice. Researchers studied a population of stable cardiovascular patients receiving specialty infusions. By treating these patients on the telemetry unit rather than in the coronary care unit, the center realized cost avoidance of $46,121.83 in 1 year. Patient classification systems estimate caregiver time and caregiver costs. The weighted salary of caregivers was $14.34 per hour in the coronary care unit and $10.00 per hour in the telemetry unit. Cost per patient day was $102.45 versus $49.23, for a cost avoidance of $53.22 per patient day.[89]

Zander states that the complete results of case management must include length of stay statistics, readmission rates, and some tally of patient satisfaction.[90]

Bower catalogues the reasons for implementing case management[91]:

1. A client/family focus on the full spectrum of needs
2. Outcome orientation to care
3. Coordination of care by team collaboration
4. Cost management through facilitation through the health care system
5. Response to insurers and payers
6. A merger of clinical and financial interests, systems, and outcomes
7. Inclusion for marketing strategies

PATIENT OUTCOMES

Outcomes and their relation to productivity are a major concern in human relations management. At the University of Iowa College of Nursing, nurse researchers and practitioners have developed the nursing outcomes classification. At the College of Nursing, the nursing outcomes classification has been integrated with the nursing diagnoses classification, the nursing interventions classification, and the nursing management minimum data set.[92] Patient outcomes are the outcomes resulting from care of patients by nurses or an interdisciplinary care team. Patient outcomes include those related to patient satisfaction and health status, nosocomial infection control, and risk events and adverse outcomes. Activities related to patient outcomes are directed toward improving organizational performance continually over time.[93]

SUMMARY

The Scope and Standards for Nurse Administrators provides a conceptualization for practice. Levels of nursing administration further delineate the roles of nurse manager and nurse executive.

A theory of nursing management evolves from a general theory of management that governs effective use of human and material resources. The four major functions of management are planning, organizing, directing (or leading), and controlling (or evaluating). All management activities—cognitive, affective, and psychomotor—fall within one or more of these major functions, which operate simultaneously.

Nursing management focuses on human behavior. Nurse managers with knowledge and skills in human behavior manage professional nurses and nonprofessional assistive nursing workers to achieve the highest level of productivity of patient care services. To do this, nurse managers must become competent leaders to stimulate motivation through relationships and interpersonal processes and communication with the workforce.

The primary role of the nurse manager is that of managing a clinical practice discipline. To accomplish this requires numerous competencies supported by a theory of nursing management.

Nurse managers work with staff consisting of clinical practitioners. Educated in nursing management, they can assist these practitioners in their work according to the models of such theorists as Watson, Orem, Roy, Newman, Johnson, and Peplau.

Several modalities of nursing have evolved over the past 50 years. Functional nursing, the oldest nursing practice modality, is a method in which each staff member is assigned a particular nursing function, such as administering medications, admitting and discharging patients, and making beds and serving meals. Later, team nursing became the modality of choice for many hospital nursing services. Under the leadership of a professional nurse, a group of nurses works together to provide patient care. Team nursing rests on theoretical knowledge related to philosophy, planning, leadership, interpersonal relationships, and nursing process.

Since the 1970s the modality of total patient care through primary nursing has evolved. With primary nursing, the total care of a patient and a case load is the responsibility of one primary nurse. Joint or collaborative practice by a physician–nurse team has developed as a modality of nursing in a few hospitals. A more recent development is case management, a method of practicing nursing that incorporates any modality and in which the knowledgeable nurse becomes the case manager, making or facilitating all clinical nursing decisions about a case load of patients during an entire episode of illness.

As new technologies of patient treatment develop and the health care delivery system evolves around managed care, nurses need avenues to pursue the ensuing ethical dilemmas. Nursing practice is further complicated by the need for multicultural assessments as part of the nursing process and its outcomes.

Evidence-Based Practice 2-1

Professional nursing practice makes a difference in care delivery by empowering nurses. A study describing the experiences of work empowerment among nurses engaged in elderly care in southern Finland found that education and work experience related to behavioral empowerment. The data were collected with a questionnaire that included items on verbal, behavioral, and outcome empowerment. A response rate of 80.8% (252) was received with nurses experiencing strong verbal and behavioral empowerment. Nurses reported that they were less confident about outcome empowerment than in the two other fields of empowerment. "All fields of empowerment showed a statistically significant correlation with each other. Education and work experience were also related to behavioral empowerment. The results provide important clues for the development of elderly care."[94]

APPLICATION EXERCISES

Exercise 2-1
Define nursing management as it relates to your job. If you are a student, observe the work of a nurse manager and define management in terms of your observations.

Exercise 2-2
Describe a belief you have about nursing management in the organization in which you work or are doing clinical practice. Discuss your belief with your peers in clinical practice or students and with your nurse manager or instructor.

Summarize the conclusions. Is your belief valid? Totally? Partly? Not at all? Validity can be established by comparing your conclusions with viewpoints found in publications or by obtaining agreement from practicing nurse managers. You will codify selected theory of nursing management.

Exercise 2-3

Translate the management of time into nursing management theory with examples such as: "A nurse who practices good management will know how to use time effectively." The example may be one that applies to you as manager or to the observed behavior of another nurse manager. Keep a log for a day, making entries at 15-minute intervals on a separate sheet of paper. Use the following format:

Time   Activity   Delays and Bottlenecks

Analyze your log. How much of your day was productive? How much was unproductive? What can be done to increase productive time? Using the following format, make a management plan to make better use of your time.

Management Plan
   Goal:
   Actions   Target Dates   Assigned to   Accomplishments

Based on your observations from this exercise, write a theory statement that describes management as the effective use of time.

Exercise 2-4

The following functions originate from a theory of the institution or organization and the division of nursing:

Plans for accomplishing objectives are made.
Strategies for accomplishing objectives are formulated.
Activities are organized by priority.
Work is assigned.
Managerial jobs are designed.
An organizational structure evolves.

Describe how each of these activities is evident in your place of practice as a student or a practicing professional nurse.

Exercise 2-5

Write a short theory of nursing management based on information presented in this chapter. Remember that a theory of nursing management is an accumulation of concepts, methods, and principles that can be or have been observed and verified to some degree and translated into the art or practice of nursing management.

Exercise 2-6

Examine the periodicals listed for the last 12-month period:

The Journal of Nursing Administration
Nursing Administration Quarterly
Nursing Management
Nursing Research

Note the following:

- The number of articles on nursing theory versus nursing management theory.
- Theories of nursing that could be incorporated into a theory of nursing management. Did the research indicate that the theory fulfilled its claim? Explain.

- According to these periodicals, what theory of nursing management is being used in the organization in which you are gaining clinical experience as a student or in which you are employed?
- According to these periodicals, what theory of nursing management could be used in the organization in which you are gaining clinical experience as a student or in which you are employed? Consider the value the research has for meeting the goals of the organization, the division of nursing, and the nursing unit.
- Make a management plan for putting the research results into practice.

Exercise 2-7

Use your student group or form an ad-hoc committee of nurses to plan for needed implementation of nursing theory in a nursing unit. Make a management plan using the following format. To help make a decision, access the Internet and find applications of theories of Watson, Orem, Roy, Newman, Johnson, and Peplau.

Management Plan
    Problem:
    Objective:
    Actions   Target Dates   Assigned to   Accomplishments

Exercise 2-8

Evaluate case management as practiced in the agency in which you are employed or to which you are assigned as a student. Do this by gathering and analyzing data that do the following:

1. Describe the model of case management being used.
2. Identify the standards used to trigger the case management process.
3. Trace the continuum of case management from patient's entry through discharge.
4. Measure the achievement of stated outcomes.
5. Relate the nursing modality to case management.

Exercise 2-9

Consider the *Scope and Standards for Nurse Administration*. Interview a nurse executive to determine how this individual meets the standards.

Notes

1. Greiner, A. C., & Knebel, E. (Eds.). (2003). *Health professions education: A bridge to quality.* Washington, DC: The National Academies Press.
2. Buerhaus, P., Staiger, D., & Auerbach, D. (2000). Implications of an aging registered nurse workforce. *Journal of the American Medical Association, 283,* 2948–2954.
3. American Nurses Association (ANA). (2004). *Scope and standards for nurse administrators* (2nd ed.). Washington, DC: Author.
4. Ibid.
5. Aiken, L., Havens, D. S., & Sloane, D. M. (2000). The magnet nursing services recognition program: A comparison of two groups of magnet groups. *American Journal of Nursing, 100,* 26–36.
6. Mills, M. E., Jenkins, L. S., & Waltz, C. F. (2000). Emphasis courses: Preparing baccalaureate students for transition to the workforce. *Journal of Professional Nursing, 16,* 300–306.
7. Letizia, M., & Jennrich, J. (1998). A review of preceptorship in undergraduate nursing education: Implications for staff development. *The Journal of Continuing Education in Nursing, 29,* 211–216.
8. Mills et al., 2000.

9. Nordgren, J., Richardson, S. J., & Laurella, V. B. (1998). A collaborative preceptor model for clinical teaching of beginning nursing students. *Nurse Educator, 23,* 27–32.

10. Mills et al., 2000.

11. Woodtli, A., Hazzard, M. E., & Rusch, S. (1988). Senior internship: A strategy for recruitment, retention and collaboration. *Nursing Connections, 1,* 37–50.

12. National League for Nursing. (1983). *Internships for the new nurse graduate.* New York: Author.

13. University Health System Consortium. (2000). *Survey on professional recognition and nurse internship and residency programs.* Oak Brook, IL: Author.

14. American Nurses Credentialing Center. (2001). *Magnet nursing services recognition program.* Retrieved July 6, 2001, from http://www.ana.org/ancc/magnet.htm

15. American Organization of Nurse Executives. (2000). *Perspectives on the nursing shortage: A blueprint for action.* Chicago, IL: Author.

16. Bellack, J. P., & Loquist, R. S. (1999). Employer responses to differentiated nursing education. *Journal of Nursing Administration, 29,* 4–8, 32.

17. Anderko, L., Uscian, M., & Robertson, J. F. (1999). Improving client outcomes through differentiated practice: a rural nursing center model. *Public Health Nursing, 16,* 168–175.

18. Anderko, L., Robertson, J., & Lewis, P. (1999). Job satisfaction in a rural differentiated-practice setting. *Journal of Nursing Connections, 12,* 49–58.

19. Hutchens, G. C. (1994). Differentiated interdisciplinary practice. *Journal of Nursing Administration, 4,* 52–58.

20. Malloch, K. M., Milton, D. A., & Jobes, M. O. (1990). A model for differentiated nursing practice. *Journal of Nursing Administration, 20,* 20–26.

21. Arcangelo, V., Fitzgerald, M., Carroll, D., & David, J. (1996). Collaborative care between nurse practitioners and physicians. *Primary Care: Clinics in Office Practice, 23.*

22. Wakefield, M., & O'Grady, E. (2000). Putting patients first: Improving patient safety through collaborative education. In *Health Resources and Services Administration (HRSA), Collaborative Education to Ensure Patient Safety, Report to the Secretary of Health and Human Services and the Congress.* Joint Meeting, Council on Graduate Medical Education and National Advisory Council on Nurse Education and Practice. Washington, DC: Author.

23. Pew Health Professions Commission. (December, 1998). *Recreating health professional practice for a new century. The Fourth Report of the Pew Health Professions Commission.* University of California, San Francisco: Pew Health Professions Commission.

24. American Nurses Association (ANA). (2003a). *Nursing scope and standards of practice.* Washington, DC: American Nurses Publishing.

25. ANA, 2004.

26. ANA, 2004, p. 9.

27. ANA, 2004, p. 11.

28. ANA, 2004, p. 13.

29. ANA, 2004, p. 15.

30. ANA, 2004, p. 17.

31. ANA, 2004, pp. 9–10.

32. Fayol, H. (1949). *General and industrial management* (C. Storrs, Trans., p. 3). London: Pitman & Sons.

33. Ibid., pp. 5–6.

34. Hodgetts, R. M. (1990). *Management: Theory, process, and practice* (5th ed., p. 38). Orlando, FL: Harcourt Brace.

35. Fayol, 1949, pp. 8–9.

36. Wilson, C. K., & Porter-O'Grady, T. (1999). Leading the revolution in health care: Advancing systems, igniting performance. Gaithersburg, MD: Aspen Publishers.

37. Drucker, P. F. (1999). The emerging theory of manufacturing. *Harvard Business Review,* 94–98.

38. Page, A. (Ed.). (2004). *Keeping patients safe: Transforming the work environment of nurses.* Washington, DC: The National Academies Press.

39. Ibid., pp. 112–125.

40. Ibid., p. 122.

41. Ibid., p. 125.

42. Megginson, L. C., Mosley, D. C., & Pietri, P. H., Jr. (1996). *Management: Leadership in action* (5th ed., pp. 15–20). New York: Harper & Row.

43. White, V. (1984). Nursing theory: A viewpoint. *Journal of Nursing Administration, 6,* 15.

44. Steffy, B. D., & Grimes, A. J. (1986). A critical theory of organizational science. *Academy of Management Review, 11,* 322–336.

45. Ibid.

46. McKenzie, L. (1992). Critical thinking in health care supervision. *Health Care Supervisor, 2.*

47. Boulding, K. E. (1956). General systems theory: The skeleton of science. *Management Science,* 197–208.

48. Ibid.

49. Drucker, 1999.

50. Ibid.

51. Drucker, 1999, p. 96.

52. Huey, J. (1994). The leadership industry. *Fortune,* 54–56; Perry, N. J. (1994). How to mine human resources. *Fortune,* 96.

53. McClure, M. L. (1984a). Managing the professional nurse, part I: The organizational theories. *Journal of Nursing Administration,* 15–21; McClure, M. L. (1984b). Managing the professional nurse, part II: Applying management theory to the challenges. *Journal of Nursing Administration,* 11–17.

54. Ibid.

55. Rew, L. (1986). Intuition: Concept analysis of a group phenomenon. *Advances in Nursing Science,* 21–28.

56. Mathews, J. J. (1988). Designing a first line manager development program using organization-appropriate strategies. *Journal of Continuing Education in the Health Professions, 8,* 181–188.

57. Princeton, J. C. (1993). Education for executive nurse administrators: A databased curricular model for doctoral (PhD) programs. *Journal of Nursing Education,* 59–63.

58. Henkoff, R. (1995). New management secrets from Japan. *Fortune,* 135–146.

59. Watson, J., & Foster, R. (2003). The attending caring model: Integrating theory, evidence, and advanced caring-healing therapies for transforming professional practice. *Journal of Clinical Nursing, 12 ,* 360–365.

60. Orem, D. E. (1985). *Nursing: Concepts of practice* (3rd ed.). McGraw-Hill, New York.

61. Parissopoulos, S., & Kotzabassaki, S. (2004). Orem's self-care theory, Transactional analysis and the management of elderly rehabilitation. *Journal of ICUS, 17.*

62. Roy, C. (1971). Adaptation: A basis for nursing practice. *Nursing Outlook,* 254–257; Frederickson, K. (1993). Using a nursing model to manage symptoms: Anxiety and the Roy adaptation model. *Holistic Nursing Practice,* 36–43.

63. Ibid.

64. Mastal, M. F., & Hammond, H. (1980). Analysis and expansion of the Roy adaptation model: A contribution to holistic nursing. *Advances in Nursing Science,* 71–81.

65. Frederickson, 1993.

66. Silva, M. C., & Sorrell, J. M. (1992). Testing a nursing theory: Critique and philosophical expansion. *Advances in Nursing Science,* 12–23.

67. Newman, M. A. (1995). Recognizing a pattern of expanding consciousness in persons with cancer. In M. A. Newman (Ed.), *A developing discipline. Selected works of Margaret Newman* (pp. 159–171). New York: National League for Nursing.

68. Rawls, A. C. (1980). Evaluation of the Johnson behavioral system model in clinical practice. *Image,* 12–16.

69. Derdiarian, A. K. (1990). The relationships among the subsystems of Johnson's behavioral system model. *Image,* 219–225.

70. Thompson, L. (1986). Peplau's theory: An application to short-term individual therapy. *Journal of Psychosocial Nursing,* 26–31.

71. Peplau, H. E. (1992). Interpersonal relations: A theoretical framework for application in nursing practice. *Nursing Science Quarterly,* 13–18; Schafer, P. (1999). Working with Dave: Application of Peplau's interpersonal nursing theory in the correctional environment. *Journal of Psychosocial Nursing and Mental Health Services,* 18–24.

72. Herman, J., & Ziel, S. (1999). Collaborative practice agreements for advanced practice nurses: What you should know. *AACN Clinical Issues,* 337–342.

73. Center for Case Management. (1983). Toward a fully-integrated CareMap® and case management system. *The New Definition*, 1.

74. Center for Case Management. (1994). Part 1: Rationale for care-provider organizations. *The New Definition*, 1.

75. Ibid.

76. Ibid.

77. Center for Case Management. (1992). Quantifying, managing, and improving quality, part I: How CareMaps® link CQI to the patient. *The New Definition*, 1.

78. Ibid.

79. Center for Case Management. (1992). Quantifying, managing and improving quality, part III: Using variance concurrently. *The New Definition*, 1–2.

80. Brockopp, D. Y., Porter, M., Kinnaird, S., & Silberman, S. (1992). Fiscal and clinical evaluation of patient care. *Journal of Nursing Administration*, 23–27.

81. Rogers, M., Riordan, J., & Swindle, D. (1991). Community-based nursing case management pays off. *Nursing Management*, 30–34.

82. Bower, K. (1992). *Case management by nurses* (2nd ed., pp. 33–34). Washington, DC: American Nurses Publishing, 33–34.

83. Williams, R. (1992). Nurse case management: Working with the community. *Nursing Management*, 33–34.

84. Strong, A. G. (1992). Case management and the CNS. *Clinical Nurse Specialist*, 64.

85. Thomas, J. (1992, July 15). Package Deals. *Nursing Times*, pp. 48–49.

86. Dowling, G. F. (1991). Case management nursing: Indications for material management. *Hospital Material Management Quarterly*, 26–32.

87. Strong, A. G., & Sneed, N. V. (1991). Clinical evaluation of a critical path for coronary artery bypass surgery patients. *Progress in Cardiovascular Nursing*. 6(1): 29–37, Jan-Mar.

88. Servais, S. H. (1991). Nursing resource applications through outcome based nursing practice. *Nursing Economic*, 171–174, 179.

89. Zander, K., & McGill, R. (1994). Critical and anticipated recovery paths: Only the beginning. *Nurse Manager*, 25, 34–37, 40.

90. Bower, 1992, pp. 7–8.

91. The University of Iowa College of Nursing. (2000). *CHAOS*. Iowa City, IA: University of Iowa Press.

92. Titler, M. G., & McCloskey, J. M. (Eds.). (1999). On the scene: University of Iowa hospitals and clinics: Outcomes management. *Nursing Administration Quarterly*, 31–65.

93. Ibid.

94. Suominen, T., Savikko, N., Kiviniemi, K., Doran, D. K., & Leino-Kilpi, H. (2008). Work empowerment as experienced by nurses in elderly care. *Journal of Professional Nursing*, 24, 42–45.

References

Adams, A., & Bond, S. (2000). Hospital nurses' job satisfaction, individual and organizational characteristics. *Journal of Advanced Nursing*, 32, 536–543.

American Association of Colleges of Nursing. (2000). *Amid nursing shortages, schools employ strategies to boost enrollment*. Issue Bulletin. Washington, DC: Author.

American Association of Colleges of Nursing. (2000). *Position Statement: The baccalaureate degree in nursing as minimal preparation for professional practice*. Washington, DC: Author.

American Nurses Association. (2000). *Survey on nurses' working environment*. Washington, DC: American Nurses Publishing.

American Nurses Association/California. (2001). *Nurse staffing in California hospitals 1998–2000*. California Nursing Outcomes Coalition Database Project. Sacramento, CA: Author.

American Nurses Credentialing Center. (1999). *A role delineation survey of baccalaureate, diploma, and associate degree nurses*. Report of the Chauncey Group International to the American Nurses Credentialing Center, April, 1–17. Washington, DC: Author.

American Organization of Nurse Executives. (2000). *Nurse recruitment and retention study.* Chicago, IL: AONE Institute for Patient Care Research and Education.

American Organization of Nurse Executives. (2001). *Strategies to reverse the new nursing shortage: Tri-Council policy statement, January 31.* Washington, DC: Author.

Bednash, G. (2000). The decreasing supply of registered nurses: Inevitable future or call to action. *Journal of the American Medical Society, 283,* 1–8.

Brafman, O., & Beckstrom, R. A. (2006). *The starfish and the spider.* New York: Penguin Group.

Buiser, M. (2000). Surviving managed care: The effect on job satisfaction in hospital-based nursing. *Medical-Surgical Nursing, 9,* 129–134.

Cangelosi, J. D., Markham, F. S., & Bounds, W. T. (1998). Factors related to nurse retention and turnover: An updated study. *Health Marketing Quarterly,* 15, 25–42.

Caroselli, C. (2000). Scarce staff not your mother's nursing shortage. *Surgical Services Management, 6,* 23–25.

Caroselli, C. (2001). The first six months of practice: Strategies for success. *Imprint,* January 2001.

Center for Health Policy, Research and Ethics, George Mason University. (2001). *Hard numbers, hard choices: A report on the nation's nursing workforce.* Fairfax, VA: Author.

Coile, R. C. (1999). Magnet hospitals: Ten strategies to becoming a model nursing employer. *Russ Coile's Health Trends, 11,* 8–12.

College of Nurses of Ontario. (April 12, 2000). *News release: College of Nurses welcomes baccalaureate requirement for registered nurses.* Toronto, Ontario: Author.

Cotlier, S. N. (2000). *Allied health workforce 2000: Building a foundation for health care in the 21st century.* Baltimore, MD: Center for Health Policy and Workforce Research, Towson University.

Department of Veterans Affairs. (1999). *Nurse qualification standard. A guide for registered nurses.* Washington, DC: Author.

Department of Veterans Affairs, Nursing Strategic Health Care Group. (2000). RN education by grade, September 30. 1999. Washington, DC. (Unpublished data received August 1, 2000 from Author.)

Gosbee, J. (2005). *Using human factors engineering to improve patient safety.* Oakbrook Terrace, IL: Joint Commission Resources, Inc.

Gothberg, S. (2000). Retention of nurses: an organizational priority. *Medical-Surgical Nursing, 9,* 109, 143.

Havens, D. S. (2001). Comparing nursing infrastructure and outcomes: ANCC magnet and nonmagnet CNEs report. *Nursing Economics, 19,* 258–266.

Health Resources and Services Administration. (2000). *Collaborative education to ensure patient safety.* Report to the Secretary of Health and Human Services and the Congress. Joint Meeting, Council on Graduate Medical Education and National Advisory Council on Nurse Education and Practice. Washington DC: Author.

Health Resources and Services Administration. (2001). *National survey cites slowdown in number of registered nurses entering profession.* Washington, DC: Author.

Hendrickson, M. L. (1999). Nursing intern program eases new graduates into career. *Nursing Matters, 10,* 1, 9.

Hurson, T. (2008). *Think better.* New York: McGraw Hill.

Institute of Medicine. (2001). *Crossing the quality chasm: A new health system for the 21st century.* Washington, DC: National Academy Press.

Kangas, S., Kee, C., & McKee-Waddle, R. (1999). Organizational factors, nurses' job satisfaction and patient satisfaction with nursing care. *Journal of Nursing Administration,* 32–42.

Mahoney, J. (2000). The importance of job satisfaction in retaining nurses. *Home Healthcare Nurse Manager, 4,* 28–30.

McGilton, K. S., & Pringle, D. M. (1999). The effects of perceived and preferred control on nurses' job satisfaction in long-term care environments. *Research in Nursing and Health, 22,* 251–261.

McNeese-Smith, D. K. (1999). A content analysis of staff nurse descriptions of job satisfaction and dissatisfaction. *Journal of Advanced Nursing, 29,* 1332–1341.

Minnick, A. F. (2000). Retirement, the nursing workforce and the year 2005. *Nursing Outlook, 48,* 211–217.

Nelson, E. C., & Baralden, P. B. (2000). Knowledge for improvement: Improving quality in the micro-systems of care. In Goldfield, N. & Nash, D. B. (Eds.), *Managing quality of care in a cost-focused environment* (pp. 75–87). Tampa, FL: American College of Physician Executives.

Phelan, B. (1999). Yale-New Haven critical care nurse internship program. *Connecticut Nursing News, 72,* 27.

Prothero, M. M., Marshall, E. S., Fosbinder, D. M., & Hendrix, K. (2000). Personnel values and work satisfaction of registered nurses working in hospitals. *Journal of Nursing Scholarship, 32,* 81–82.

Scott, J. G., Sochalski, J., & Aiken, L. (1999). Review of magnet hospital research findings and implications for professional nursing practice. *Journal of Nursing Administration, 29,* 9–19.

Taylor, S., White, B., & Muncer, S. (1999). Nurses' cognitive structural models of work-based stress. *Journal of Advanced Nursing, 9,* 974–983.

Tovey, E. J., & Adams, A. E. (1999). The changing nature of nurses' job satisfaction: An exploration of sources of satisfaction in the 1990s. *Journal of Advanced Nursing, 30,* 150–158.

U.S. Department of Health & Human Services, Office of Disease Prevention & Health Promotion. (2000). *Healthy pPeople 2010* (2nd ed.). Washington, DC: Author.

Ventura, M. J. (1999). Staffing issues—Ethics on the job: A survey, part 4. *RN, 62,* 26–31.

3 EMOTIONALLY INTELLIGENT LEADERSHIP IN NURSING AND HEALTH CARE ORGANIZATIONS

Susan H. Taft, PhD, RN, MSN

LEARNING OBJECTIVES AND ACTIVITIES

- Define emotional intelligence.
- Distinguish between emotional intelligence and emotional competencies.
- Name the four emotional intelligence clusters.
- Identify the 18 emotional competencies discussed in the emotional intelligence clusters.
- Identify factors that may enhance or diminish one's innate emotional intelligence and learned emotional competencies.
- Describe the five core competencies and why they are considered crucial.
- Discuss why nursing settings are intensely emotional.
- Discuss the emotional competencies that may be most important to practicing nurses.
- Identify the emotional intelligence strengths and weaknesses of the nurses in these case studies: Figures 3-2, 3-3, and 3-6.
- Describe how to develop emotional competencies.
- Examine the characteristics of best and worst bosses you have known.
- Identify areas of research—from nursing and other disciplines—that support emotional competencies as predictors of leadership success.
- Describe how middle- and executive-level nurse leaders might use emotional competencies in different situations.
- Discuss how emotionally intelligent nurse leaders might improve nursing work environments.
- Identify the desirable characteristics and capabilities of middle- and executive-level nurse leaders and how to select for these qualities.
- Identify how emotional intelligence relates to national leadership standards.

CONCEPTS

Emotional intelligence, emotional competency, socioemotional leadership, effective and ineffective leaders, self-awareness, self-assessment, self-confidence, self-control, trust and trustworthiness, adaptability, achievement drive, initiative, optimism, empathy, influence, organizational politics, service orientation, developing others, inspirational leadership, change agent, conflict management, teamwork, collaboration, nurse manager, leader competencies

---

QUOTE

My continuing passion is to part a curtain, that invisible shadow that falls between people, the veil of indifference to each other's presence, each other's wonder, each other's human plight.

—Eudora Welty

NURSE MANAGER BEHAVIORS

Managing oneself successfully, relating effectively to others, leading change initiatives and other people, communicating effectively, managing relationships and diversity, sharing decision making, influencing, understanding and working with organizational politics, building trust, promoting teamwork and collaboration, and managing conflict are all strengthened with greater concentrations of emotional competencies.

NURSE EXECUTIVE BEHAVIORS

Executive-level leaders select and develop nurse middle managers, and middle managers select and develop members of their staff.

Introduction

Effective leadership in organizations requires numerous talents, skills, and types of knowledge, as the existence of this textbook demonstrates. At its core, leadership is about relationships with other people. Leaders' accomplishments are largely achieved through the individual and coordinated efforts of others. Without followers, there are no leaders.[1]

Leadership theories have developed since before the time of Machiavelli, but the most recent theories originated in the industrialized world of the 20th century. In the works of scholars, researchers, exemplary leaders, and undistinguished nonleaders alike, there are few topics in management about which more has been written. Since the 1950s, research has tended to focus on Western methods of leadership in traditional industries. More recently, leadership research has expanded our traditional understanding by focusing on leadership behaviors at different levels and within different functional areas of organizations, women's leadership styles, leader diversity as a competitive advantage to organizations, multicultural and global leadership,[2] the role of leaders in attaining quality outcomes, and an acknowledgment that "no one size fits all" practicing leaders. But consistently throughout time and across cultures, leadership has been recognized as a people-oriented business.

This chapter is devoted to exploring the people skills of good leaders—leaders who enable "their people" to be happy and productive workers and committed employees, who allow workers to grow and develop to their full potentials, and who themselves work successfully as committed organizational agents. As the standard bearers for high performance, effective leaders enable good performers but also counsel irretrievably poor employees to leave a setting where they perform poorly. The leadership framework discussed in this chapter is emotional intelligence,[3] a composite of 18 intra- and interpersonal competencies that predicts successful leadership at work.

WHAT IS EMOTIONAL INTELLIGENCE?

Emotional intelligence is defined as "the capacity for recognizing our own feelings and those of others, for motivating ourselves, and for managing emotions well in ourselves and in others."[4] Emotional intelligence includes capabilities distinct from, but complementary to, academic intelligence or the purely cognitive capacities measured by intelligence quotient. Emotional competencies are defined as "learned capabilities based on emotional intelligence that contribute to effective performance at work."[4] Based on extensive research conducted by Goleman and his associates and by the Hay Group of Boston, emotional competence has been found to matter twice as much as intelligence quotient and technical skill combined in producing superior managerial job performance.

Emotional intelligence develops in humans as a result of genetic inheritance and the socializing influences of childhood, adolescence, and adulthood; emotional competencies are a result of emotional intelligence plus opportunities we have to develop those competencies. They are capabilities we can learn and expand. Thus an individual born with average emotional intelligence might become exceptionally emotionally competent in adulthood if she had parents who, during her upbringing, tuned in well to her feelings, practiced leadership in college through her sorority, and worked with emotionally competent managers (positive role models) in her early work experiences. Similarly, it is possible to have life experiences that erode one's emotional intelligence. An individual born with high natural emotional intelligence could become limited in emotional competencies if she came from a home in which a parent was an alcoholic, suffered taunting or hazing in school, or had previous bosses who were abusive (negative role models).

The nursing profession requires a high degree of emotional labor—the ability of nurses to regulate their own emotions and the expression of emotions for the sake of their patients' needs. Nurses are expected to display emotions that convey caring, understanding, and compassion toward patients while regulating their own feelings. For newly graduated nurses, the added emotional burdens of coping with the transition from school to work are enormous.[5] The role of the nurse leader, then, becomes critical "in creating a supportive and positive work environment to help nurses cope with the stress of managing their own and others' emotions" concurrently.[6] Emotional intelligence provides a framework for understanding the ways in which leader behaviors are necessary for the creation of a positive emotion-intensive work environment.

Emotional Intelligence Framework

The emotional intelligence framework consists of two dimensions: the ability to understand and manage oneself and the ability to understand and relate well to others. These dimensions are further subdivided into self-awareness and self-management and social awareness and relationship management. In each dimension the ability to manage oneself or others is predicated on the awareness one has of self and others. Figure 3-1 shows the framework of the emotional intelligence dimensions.

Self-awareness can be considered the inner barometer, or rudder, people have to understand and direct the moment-to-moment and situation-to-situation variation in internal emotions. Humans are emotional, constantly reacting to internal and external stimuli. These stimuli may cause feelings that are positive or negative, uplifting or discouraging, threatening or pleasing, exciting or boring, and so on. An emotionally intelligent individual is aware of feelings as they emerge, understands them accurately, and has the self-confidence to continue activity in the world regardless of his or her emotions. Self-management extends one's emotional intelligence by allowing for self-control of emotions, maintenance of one's integrity, and adaptability to emerging situations. Individuals low in self-awareness or emotional self-management or both may "blurt" reactions in social situations, show rigidity or brittle-

---

FIGURE 3-1   **FRAMEWORK OF EMOTIONAL INTELLIGENCE**

Self	Others
Self-awareness	Social awareness
Self-management	Relationship management

---

ness when faced with differences of opinion, be defensive to criticism, act contrary to their espoused values, or project insecurity when around others (Figure 3-2).

Emotionally intelligent interactions with other people depend and build on an individual's strengths in self-awareness and self-management. Without a solid base of self-understanding, self-control, emotional security, trustworthiness, and adaptability, it is virtually impossible to be open to others and constructive in work relationships. Thus good leaders must know themselves well and be able to choose how they will respond in social situations. These strengths then provide the foundation for working well with others.

Good relationships with others are shown through social awareness and relationship management. They are considered "social radar"—the ability to understand others and work with them productively. Social awareness is founded, most directly, on the skills of empathy: sensing others' feelings, needs, and concerns and taking an active interest in them. Social awareness in work settings extends into the ability to use good political skills and an active, principled orientation to service toward customers or patients. To exhibit political astuteness at work and to serve patients with sensitivity, the nurse draws on his or her empathy for others, whether they are individuals or people who are part of groups. Relationship management includes areas frequently depicted in books and journal articles about leadership. Of all the emotional competencies, these are the most readily learned, either through study, reading, and practice or through leadership development programs. Relationship management encompasses capabilities in inspiring and influencing others, visioning, developing others, collaboration and teamwork, leading change initiatives, and managing conflict. The effective use of relationship management at work involves leadership that builds individual, group, and organizational engagement toward future accomplishments (see, for example, Figures 3-2 and 3-3).

FIGURE 3-2   **THE NEW NURSE MANAGER**

Tiffany worked in a large university medical center. She completed her BSN 3 years ago and in her first job as a staff nurse on a complex surgical unit rapidly proved herself to be a competent staff nurse. Because of her capabilities and positive attitude, she was promoted to charge nurse after 1 year. In her third year she was promoted to unit manager when the previous manager left to direct an ambulatory surgery center within the medical center system. Although a "quick study" in managing the logistics of her unit, she lost trust among the nurses in the unit when she reacted defensively and impatiently to criticisms and complaints from the staff, tended to give summary orders, and projected an "I'm too busy to talk to you now" response to staff concerns. For the first time since she started on the unit, Tiffany began to dread going to work. She believed that her former colleagues had turned against her and didn't appreciate how hard she worked for them. She often saw their concerns as petty and viewed them as not taking enough responsibility for their own roles on the unit. She talked to her nursing director regularly about the staff issues, but the director just laughed and told her that the "honeymoon was over" and that things would even out in time. After 6 months her relationship with her staff had deteriorated to the point that Tiffany, feeling betrayed, scapegoated, and disillusioned, left the medical center to work in a position with an insurance agency.

FIGURE 3-3	THE QUALITY MANAGER

Joe had worked as a staff nurse on medical floors at two different institutions for 6 and 5 years, respectively. When his first child was born, he decided to accept a job offer as the quality manager for a suburban community hospital so that he could enjoy regular hours and arrange his schedule to coordinate with the working hours of his wife. The position he accepted turned out to have more challenges than he anticipated: uneven patient quality outcomes on different nursing units, physicians angry with implied "report cards" on their medical practices, a new nurse executive who was trying to surmount the multiple demands of her position, a recently completed Joint Commission on Accreditation of Healthcare Organizations survey that enumerated more than a dozen deficiencies that needed correcting within 6 months, and declining patient satisfaction scores in many areas. His first meeting with the executive team of the hospital, in which his charge to "fix things" was laid out, was a demoralizing and overwhelming experience. For a day, Joe regretted having left the comfort of staff nursing, where he knew what to do and how to do it. As a staff nurse, problems could be addressed one patient at a time.

After talking with several nurse manager colleagues from his previous place of work and with a nurse educator at a local university where he had enrolled for master's study, Joe began to get a handle on how to approach his new responsibilities. He understood hospitals. He trusted his own ability to learn what he needed to learn and to move forward one step at a time, and he recognized that the amount he needed to accomplish required a systematic and comprehensive plan. Over the next week he talked to many different employees of the hospital and some of the physicians in leadership positions. Some of his meetings involved listening to people venting about the problems they faced in their work or the people they worked with; several included angry accusations about the perceived "quality agenda" of the chief executive officer. Joe made no attempt to counter the comments he heard, nor did he allow himself to get defensive and angry in return. Instead, he reiterated frequently that he was just trying to learn about the issues the hospital faced so that he could put together some ideas on how to move forward.

Emotional Competencies

Emotional competencies are developed from life experiences in combination with an individual's innate emotional intelligence. Humans tend to become increasingly emotionally competent with age as we accumulate experiences that help us understand ourselves and others better. We learn from positive as well as negative experiences. Who has not made political mistakes in a job early in a career? How many haven't suffered through a performance appraisal that found us less than perfect? Who has not failed to influence a peer group to do something we thought was an obvious "no-brainer?" To our benefit or detriment, we learned from these experiences. Similarly, almost everyone can identify a teacher who helped us come to know ourselves better and, in the process, improved us or a leader whom we would follow "anywhere." Parenting, socialization experiences, role models, and the practice of new behaviors all help or hinder us in developing emotional competence. The positive or negative influence on any individual depends on the quality of the experience and how it is processed by that person. The fields of child and adult development focus on how one's natural endowment, culture, and life experiences interact to create the unique mature individual.

Eighteen work competencies, depicted in Figure 3-4, constitute the emotional intelligence framework. Four clusters—self-awareness, self-management, social awareness, and relationship management— contain lists of the emotional competencies relevant to self and others. Though all competencies are considered important for leadership effectiveness, five are core competencies on which all the other competencies depend. For knowing and managing oneself, core competencies include emotional self-awareness, accurate self-assessment, self-confidence, emotional self-control, and, for working effectively with others, empathy. Without these core competencies, one cannot effectively exercise leadership. For example, one must be self-aware—in tune with one's own emotions—to practice emotional self-control. Emotional self-control is essential to collaborate with others, build teamwork, or manage

FIGURE 3-4	THE EMOTIONAL INTELLIGENCE FRAMEWORK & 18 COMPETENCIES[7]

Personal Competence	Social Competence
Self-awareness	Social awareness
Emotional self-awareness*	Empathy*
Accurate self-assessment*	Organizational awareness
Self-confidence*	Service orientation
Self-management	Relationship management
Emotional self-control*	Developing others
Transparency	Inspirational leadership
Adaptability	Change catalyst
Achievement orientation	Influence
Initiative	Conflict management
Optimism	Teamwork and collaboration

Note: *Core competencies, on which the remaining 13 competencies depend.
Source: Goleman, 1995, 1998a; Goleman et al., 2002; The Hay Group, 2004.

conflict. Empathy is required to develop others constructively, understand organizational politics, or respond proactively to customer needs.

In Figure 3-2 Tiffany's behavior as a new nurse manager reflects limitations in emotional self-awareness, self-control, adaptability, and self-confidence in how she understands and manages herself; in working with others, empathy, organizational awareness, developing others, inspirational leadership, conflict management, and teamwork and collaboration all appear to be weak. Although she has been a competent and effective staff nurse, Tiffany lacks the skills and emotional competencies to move effectively into a management role. It is common in all industries, including health care, for good workers to be promoted into management positions with little or no additional training or mentoring. Sometimes these promotions work well, but often they do not. It is a management myth that the best staff workers make the best leaders. Leading people requires skills and knowledge that even the most talented employees can lack.[8] Emotional intelligence is just one of many areas in management in which plans for human resource development are critical for leader success.

Because the core emotional competencies are essential leadership traits, they are the areas in which leadership development should, in the case of deficiencies, begin. Once integrated well into leadership behavior, the core competencies can be used to support or leverage further emotional competency development.

Figure 3-3 gives the scenario of Joe, the new quality manager at a community hospital. Like Tiffany, Joe came from a staff nurse position to a management role. Unlike Tiffany, Joe demonstrates a number of emotional competencies as he takes on a difficult work assignment: Although initially overwhelmed and discouraged by his new responsibilities, he is aware of his emotional reactions to those responsibilities. Rather than recede into self-doubt and make a choice to resign, he shows confidence in his own abilities to learn and move forward. He adapts to the magnitude of the job, seeks counsel from others (initiative and optimism), and sets out to gather information necessary for him to succeed (achievement orientation). His meetings with others in the organization are conducted with good political insight (organizational awareness) and empathy. He avoids responding emotionally to the comments he hears (emotional self-control). Joe recognizes that the job requires him to be a champion of change and that it takes collaboration and teamwork, plus development of others, to be effective. Within a reasonable period of time, Joe creates a vision for quality improvements at the hospital. In the near future, he stands a good chance of becoming an influential and inspirational leader for quality improvement.

Why was Joe so much more effective than Tiffany? We cannot say for sure, but some combination of innate emotional intelligence, socialization, positive role models, and age and experience probably provided him with the opportunities to develop his emotional competencies. In contrast, Tiffany came to her new position with serious limitations and, presumably, less positive prior growth opportunities relative to leadership. Nurse leaders who are responsible for selecting, hiring, and promoting personnel need to be aware of the great variation in emotional intelligence that exists among employees. Though Joe needed some coaching in his new position, which he obtained primarily from external sources, Tiffany required far greater in-house development to become a successful nurse manager. At a minimum, management classes and good mentoring would have provided Tiffany with some necessary initial support for her to face the challenges she encountered in her new position. In her organization, Tiffany's development needs were not identified, so she floundered and failed, carrying negative views of leadership with her to future jobs. Most likely, the harm done to her as a potential leader will need to be "unlearned" before she can develop leadership capabilities later in her career.

The 18 emotional competencies that constitute emotionally intelligent leadership are summarized in Figure 3-5. In the upper left cell are the competencies of self-awareness: emotional self-awareness, accurate self-assessment, and self-confidence. They are the foundation for effective leadership. Self-awareness gives an individual a constant internal monitoring system. It reports feelings and reactions to experiences in the present but also includes knowing and anticipating situations in which one is apt to feel stress, joy, anger, insecurity, defensiveness, impatience, and so on. Self-awareness is a prerequisite for the social competency of empathy. The individual who is emotionally self-aware or has accurate self-assessment knows his or her strengths and weaknesses and is comfortable "owning" them around other people. Comfort with one's own capabilities, values, and skills—both those that are strong and those that are limited—leads to self-confidence and the potential for behavioral integrity. The self-confident leader uses these competencies to support his or her self-assurance, self-efficacy, and often the courage to voice unpopular views in the workplace. Any leader in today's health care settings needs to have some toughness to survive; self-confidence is a core component of a good survival strategy.

The capacity for good self-management, shown in the lower left cell, includes the emotional competencies of emotional self-control, transparency, adaptability, the drive to achieve, initiative, and optimism. Emotional self-control prevents us from being hijacked by our feelings, but it does not imply that the expression of all emotions at work is undesirable. There are many experiences in the workplace that call for the appropriate expression of feelings, such as events that stimulate anger, sadness, frustration, humor, or happiness. The key to self-control is that the individual is aware of his or her feelings and makes a choice as to whether to express them or keep them submerged. Thus a nurse might choose to let a manager know when he or she is frustrated with an ongoing lack of supplies to care for patients but decide not to express indignation when a coworker makes a mistake with a patient, as the latter case may be more constructively dealt with through rational discussion.

The rules for emotional expression or emotional control vary greatly across ethnic groups, cultures, national origins, social class, organizations, and other contexts. Some organizations enable both staff and leaders to be frank and open in the expression of feelings, whereas others maintain codes of formality that tend to limit the sharing of feelings. Leaders need to understand the norms of their own workplaces and use these to guide how they manage their own feelings and those of others.

Transparency—being honest, open, trustworthy, and authentic—is the competency that most expresses an individual's integrity. Transparent leaders can be depended on and trusted. They model ethical behavior. When pressured to do something they believe to be wrong, transparent leaders demonstrate

| FIGURE 3-5 | EMOTIONAL COMPETENCIES CONSTITUTING EMOTIONALLY INTELLIGENT LEADERSHIP[9] |

Personal Competence	Social Competence
Self-awareness One's "inner barometer," rudder **Emotional self-awareness*** A fundamental and essential emotional competence Recognizing your own emotions and their effects Knowing where your "buttons" are **Accurate self-assessment*** Knowing your strengths & weaknesses Seeking out and "taking in" feedback from others **Self-confidence*** Sense of self-worth & capabilities that can sustain you during failures & defeats; having "presence"	**Social awareness** One's "social radar" **Empathy*** Sensing others' feelings, needs, concerns and perspectives and taking an active interest **Organizational awareness** Reading a group's emotional/political currents and power relationships, and acting on this awareness **Service orientation** Anticipating, recognizing, and meeting customers' needs, and the motivation
Self-management Enables one to resist the tyranny of emerging moods **Emotional self-control*** Being unfazed in stressful situations; influenced by biochemistry and neurological system **Transparency** Trustworthiness, credibility, accountability for self; others can count on you High integrity: acting consistently with your own values **Adaptability** Ability to let go of previous ways of doing things, willingness to try new ways **Achievement orientation** A drive to accomplish goals, stretch for high performance; sets apart high achievers Core for entrepreneurs **Initiative** Motivation; seeking out new ideas and methods; taking responsibility; readiness to act **Optimism** Persisting despite obstacles and setbacks; not fearing failure	**Relationship management** Enables one to act in the interests of others with out tripping over his or her own ego **Developing others** Sensing others' development needs and bolster ing the development of others' abilities **Giving timely feedback** **Inspirational leadership** Having vision; inspiring and guiding; communicating often and effectively **Change catalyst** Recognizing the need for change; removing barriers; communicating widely; modeling **Influence** Winning people over; indirectly building consensus and support; orchestrating effective tactics of persuasion; good communication Fine-tuning presentations/appeals to fit the audience **Conflict management** Understanding all perspectives and negotiating with these in mind; does not mean suppressing conflict **Teamwork and collaboration** Working toward shared goals using individual strengths and group synergy; nurturing relationships, building esprit de corps, sharing credit lavishly Includes managing meetings well

Note: *Core competencies.
Source: Goleman, 1995, 1998a; Goleman et al., 2002; The Hay Group, 2004.

courage by standing up against it, even when taking a stand may be personally risky. Almost everyone would like to have a transparent leader because he or she engenders trust. Such leaders live and model the behaviors they expect of others,[10] in the process enabling others to act with integrity. Trust in a leader gives rise to positive emotions in employees, and positive emotions are what attach people to their work.

The emotional competency of adaptability enables leaders to be flexible in changing situations or in overcoming obstacles to getting work done. It provides for emotional resiliency in the face of multiple demands, complex or ambiguous situations, shifting priorities, and painful realities. Though people who lack adaptability may be ruled by anxieties and fears about change, it is also true that an adaptive response to every challenge is not always desirable. There are values and principles to which leaders should adhere, and too much flexibility on these may be the wrong choice. Examples include nurse executives who hold to a floor of safe staffing rather than agree to cut budgets that could result in dangerously low nurse-to-patient ratios; an agency director who rejects requests for special treatment for family members of local politicians; or the medical department head who refuses gifts to his department offered by pharmaceutical representatives in exchange for promotion of specific brand-name drugs. Because health care organizations are complex, fast moving, and concerned with the health of humans, adaptability is important for any nurse leader, but equally important is knowing those areas in which existing practices should be maintained.

The ability to harness internal motivation, the readiness to take responsibility and to persist, and the drive to stretch for high performance, take risks, and accomplish goals typify leaders high in achievement orientation and initiative. High achievers are inwardly directed, holding challenging standards for themselves. They are proactive, love to learn, seek challenges, and are willing to bend rules. In the business world entrepreneurs tend to have these characteristics to an extreme degree, although they often lack some of the other important leadership competencies associated with social awareness and relationship management. In health care, high achievers/initiators operate in a constant state of readiness. They are frequently results oriented and focus on performance improvements by mobilizing themselves and others.

People at work take their emotional cues from their leader(s). Because positive or negative emotions from a leader powerfully penetrate the work climate, the presence of the former is clearly preferable to the latter. An optimistic leader is one who carries a "can do" attitude and who persists despite obstacles and setbacks. Optimism enables a leader and his or her employees to learn from mistakes and move forward. He or she is a carrier of hope.

Displayed in the upper right cell of Figure 3-5 are the competencies of social awareness: empathy, organizational awareness, and service orientation. As a core competency, empathy provides the foundation for the remaining two competencies in this cell as well as the ability to manage relationships (as shown in the lower right cell). Empathy is the "sine qua non of all social effectiveness in working life,"[11] a critical competency for working with a diverse group of people and those from different cultures. Every organization has an invisible nervous system of connection and influence.[12] Political astuteness, a part of the competency of organizational awareness, derives from being attuned to individuals, groups, and organizational power dynamics; detecting social networks and unspoken rules; and knowing how to use other people and processes to advance one's own interests. For middle managers, awareness of politics needs to include those above and below them. The politically aware leader tends to have an organizational, as opposed to subunit or departmental, perspective. Even for empathetic leaders, this perspective may be the most difficult of emotional competencies to learn. As an educator, I have found that the competency of organizational awareness is best learned by my graduate students through mentoring experiences with politically gifted leaders.

Service orientation, whether customers are patients or members of other departments, draws on the ability of the leader to grasp the customer's perspective and to create systems responsive to that perspective. He or she seeks ways to increase satisfaction and loyalty.[13]

The lower right cluster of Figure 3-5 lists the emotional competencies of relationship management: development of others, inspirational leadership, change catalyst, influence, conflict management, and teamwork and collaboration. These too are built on a foundation of the core competencies of emotional self-awareness, accurate self-assessment, self-control, self-confidence, and empathy.

Healthy organizations cultivate formal and informal leadership throughout the system by developing leaders. Nurse executives, for example, play a pivotal role in the development of nurse managers.[14] In performance-oriented cultures, all staff are considered worthy of development. This can be informally addressed through coaching and feedback—giving accurate, specific, timely, descriptive feedback that the receiver can use effectively and from which he or she can grow.[15] Such cultures disparage the singular use of "overly nice" feedback that excludes critical, but important, appraisal information.

To guide others, leaders must first have a clear sense of their own direction, values, and priorities. Inspiring leaders rely on core values to orient decisions; they are intentional and authentic,[16] leading by example, whether supporting people through day-to-day work challenges or episodes of difficult change. They value and nurture the relationship between leader and followers,[17] typically creating an empowered staff. Honest, authentic, frequent two-way communication[18] enables trust development and is the hallmark of the inspirational leader. It is an "emotional craft".[19] Some research has found that the intent of staff nurses to leave is negatively correlated with their leader's transformational leadership style[20]—that is, transformational leadership contributes to nurse retention.

Any leader in health care is a change agent: It comes with the job. Most health care leaders essentially lead change all the time. No longer is most change "planned"; it usually originates outside of health care organizations in the form of government regulations, alterations in reimbursement, technological innovation, shifts in the economy and demographics, and so on. More often than not, we respond to changes beyond our control. All changes in organizations evoke some resistance. The best change agents do not give ultimatums; they use the competencies of self-awareness and self-management, as well as empathy, politicking, influence, visionary leadership, conflict management, and teamwork and collaboration, to engage employees and lead successful change efforts. Because changes are always occurring, the skills and abilities of change management need to be fully integrated into the daily practices of managers.

The desire to exert influence can be directed at individuals or groups. Skills in influencing others in the workplace are not routinely taught in nursing school, nor do staff nurses typically learn to be influential through their work except in the area of patient care. Influence skills are built on self-awareness and empathy—being in touch with your own agenda and sensing how others are likely to respond and then fine-tuning your appeal to engage others. Nurses use these skills frequently to influence the medical and administrative staffs. The persuasive leader intentionally uses her or his emotions and body language to affect the emotions of others. This requires good communication skills,[21] a collaborative stance, trust, and both direct and indirect methods of influencing others. Indirect methods may be especially useful, as when one builds support for an idea before presenting it to the intended audience.

Managing conflict in organizations can include such actions as intervening in interpersonal or group frictions, confronting one's boss, addressing interdepartmental conflicts, facilitating a restructuring, and bargaining with labor unions.[22] Facility in handling difficult people and tense situations constructively is not a widely distributed skill in American society. It is one of the most demanding of emotional intelligence competencies, requiring all the competencies of self-awareness and self-management, as well as empathy, organizational awareness, the ability to develop others and exert influence, and collaboration. Although organizations rife with conflict are unhealthy work environments, it is often the organization in which differences are suppressed and conflicting views are disallowed that is the most dysfunctional. Differences of opinion and the emotions that accompany them can become toxic if not addressed. In most cases conflicting views can be expressed, acknowledged, and addressed in positive ways. Part of Victoria's difficulty in Figure 3-6 was that she never surfaced and addressed differences in perspectives

FIGURE 3-6	THE REMOTE NURSING AGENCY DIRECTOR

Victoria was the director of nursing for a large, multidisciplinary home health agency serving 12 acute care hospitals in a multicounty region. Her boss, the chief operating officer (COO), was a physician who worked offsite because of numerous other responsibilities with one of the medical centers. Victoria saw the COO about one or two times a month; otherwise, they communicated by telephone, e-mail, and fax. The COO was erratic in his oversight of the agency. Most of the time he let it "run itself," but at other times he would arrive unannounced and demand data and financial reports all at once, often grilling the directors about what he found. Victoria and the other directors of the agency didn't like the COO's style, but they were content because, most days, he didn't meddle with them. Although not yielding much profit, the agency nonetheless covered its costs, had reasonable patient and family satisfaction scores, and continued to have a steady flow of referrals.

As time went on, Victoria focused on her staff nurses and team leaders, patient care needs, interdisciplinary coordination, and referring hospitals. She attended to accreditation preparedness and compiled required reports in collaboration with her codirectors. Staff at the agency was reasonably content, although scheduling and salary complaints never seemed to go away. E-mails and faxes from the COO came frequently but were primarily concerned with issues of regulation, quality developments in health care, and cost-saving ideas. Victoria responded to these when she had something to share back with the COO, but mostly she filed or saved his communications for future reference. He knew little about home nursing care and was not much of a team player when he interacted with others, so she tended to avoid discussions with him when possible.

After 18 months in her position, Victoria came in on a Friday morning to find the COO and the director of human resources waiting for her. They took her into the conference room, where the COO informed her that she was being relieved of her duties. He had completed a performance review about her that stated he had found her resistant to direction, aloof, unwilling to innovate, and stuck in a "narrow nursing frame of mind." He indicated he had lost confidence in her. Shocked, Victoria responded as calmly as she could manage, noting that the agency's referrals, nursing statistics, cost per visit, patient satisfaction, profitability, turnover rates, and staff satisfaction ratings were all as good as, if not better than, those of similarly sized home health agencies. Since her departmental outcome measures were better than acceptable, how could he justify firing her? He told her the nursing department needed a change of leadership, so that's what he was doing. He then gestured to the director of human resources, who had said nothing to this point, and indicated that she and the director could work out her termination arrangements. After their meeting, the director walked Victoria to her office for her personal items and then to her car, collecting the agency's keys before she indicated that Victoria should leave and not return to the premises.

between the chief operating officer and herself. A politically savvy leader often anticipates where and when conflicts are likely to surface and prepares to address them. The insightful use of varying viewpoints can enable the leader to channel strong feelings into problem solving and creative solutions.

Across all types of industries, teamwork is one of the most consistently valued attributes of managers. Teamwork and collaboration are related to the emotional intelligence of groups[23] and are the means by which virtually all work is accomplished in health care organizations. Collaborative styles typically reflect an equal focus on task accomplishment and concern for relationships. Individuals able to function effectively as team players do so as a result of emotional intelligence, especially the competencies associated with self-awareness and self-management, plus empathy and service orientation. Cognitive intelligence, technical expertise, or ambition alone does not make people collaborative. Well-functioning teams consistently outperform the collective contributions of skilled individuals as a result of the synergy of "social intelligence." Combined talents and knowledge on a team interactively and unpredictably catalyze the best in everyone, leveraging the full capabilities of the team members.[24] Thus leaders who are good team builders and facilitators (i.e., running meetings well, building esprit de corps) greatly enhance work performance while generating an atmosphere of friendly collegiality. Group cohesion has been found to be partially predictive of nurse job satisfaction,[25] as has nurse–physician collaboration.[26]

It is important to note that all forms of interactions at work need to be considered relevant to emotionally intelligent behaviors. This means that e-mails, faxes, voice mails, and written memos or reports are subject to the same sensitivities that the emotional competencies address. An example of this is using empathy when sending an e-mail or writing a memo; the emotionally intelligent sender is aware of what the recipient knows and thinks before framing the message. Often, providing a sentence or two of background before stating a message or stating at the outset what the sender wants from the receiver helps the message reach the receiver. For example, as a nurse educator it is not unusual for me to get e-mails from my undergraduate students that contain no signature at the end of the message. If I don't recognize the e-mail address, I often have no idea who sent me the message. In these cases, clearly the student is focused entirely on his or her needs and not thinking about my ability to receive the message.

No leaders, good or bad, have equal strengths or equal weaknesses in all 18 emotional competencies. Leaders and managers have their own unique constellations of the components of emotional intelligence.

Best and Worst Bosses

In training individuals in emotional intelligence, I have worked with health care professionals from many different organizations. I often ask people to list the characteristics of their best and worst bosses and found that the results of this exercise are very consistent across settings. People tend to list variations of the behaviors shown in Figure 3-7.

FIGURE 3-7   CHARACTERISTICS OF MY "BEST" AND "WORST" BOSSES

Best Bosses	Worst Bosses
Understands my strengths and weaknesses	Poor listener
Always has an open-door policy	Micro-manager
Is available and accessible	Is too busy to help me
Is genuinely interested in others	Gives orders and expects them to be carried out without question
Works with me on difficult projects	Gives negative feedback but rarely says anything positive
Has a good sense of humor	
Admits to own mistakes; open to feedback	Gets angry easily; tends to "shoot the messenger"
Expects effort and conscientiousness but not perfection	Has no insight into him- or herself
Willing to change plans based on input from me and others in my workgroup	Gives unclear instructions and then blames others when it's done wrong
Gives an assignment and then lets us do it; doesn't meddle	Doesn't want to know my opinion
Is positive and upbeat	Prefers to fire off e-mails rather than sit down and talk
Often brings in bagels or fruit for us	Incompetent; can't acknowledge own weaknesses; is insecure
Is quick to give credit to others for good work	Wants to look good to his or her boss at all costs
Takes a lot of stress from upper management but never brings it back to us	Is unavailable, inaccessible, never "around"
Always has our department's best interests at heart	Is often in a bad mood
Really cares about how our patients are treated	Lazy; I have absolutely no idea what he or she does all day

(continues)

Will "handle" anyone who is abusive to one of us on the unit; won't back down or let us down	Is unethical
Works harder than anyone else	Will lie or misrepresent things rather than admit she or he made a mistake
Has high standards, sticks to values	Takes credit for the work that others do
"Walks the talk"	Is clueless about our feelings about things
Understands the "big picture;" is visionary	Can't deal with conflict, so avoids it
Always looks for new and better ways to do things; is open	Seems unhappy with in home life, and brings a lot of that into work
Knows a lot about what's going on in other organizations like ours and brings new ideas back to us	Changes direction all the time
Treats everyone fairly and equally	Is rigid and defensive
Gives feedback—all kinds—frequently; is collaborative	Is cold and distant
Encourages us to have different points of view and to express them; helps us find resolutions	Holds grudges
Will sit down with two people who are not working well together and get them to work it out	Doesn't advocate for us at higher levels or with other departments; "sells out"
Shares information; is upfront with us when something can't be changed	Doesn't tell me how he or she thinks I'm doing until I get slammed in my annual performance evaluation (which is usually months late)
Encourages us to come up with our own solutions to problems; will intervene if we're stuck	Listens to gossip (and selectively believes it)
Is creative; willing to take risks	Has "favorites" (who get special treatment)
Is very well liked and respected by people in other departments	Is not a team player
Makes us want to follow him or her	Doesn't deal well with office politics
	Doesn't address important issues, even when they go on for months or years
	Talks all the way through meetings without letting anyone else say anything
	Doesn't want to change anything—or the opposite: makes changes willy-nilly without thought
	Poor/no communication
	Has no vision, no charisma

Note that the characteristics of best and worst bosses tend to be opposites of each other: creative versus rigid, gives credit versus takes credit, shares information versus withholds information, advocates versus sells out, and so on. What people report seeing and valuing in a best boss includes the competencies associated with emotionally intelligent leadership.

Although we know that knowledge, skills, and capabilities in addition to those characteristics listed in Figure 3-7 are necessary for good leadership and management (e.g., the ability to secure and distribute resources for work tasks or the use of sound staffing and scheduling principles), it is noteworthy that how others evaluate their leaders rests disproportionately on the followers' perceived relationships with those leaders. This strikingly illustrates the basis for the importance of emotionally competent leaders.[27] Because nursing in all its forms is a people-oriented business, top-performing nursing work groups are powered by their leaders' abilities to manage themselves and work well with others.

RESEARCH AND PROFESSIONAL SUPPORT FOR EMOTIONALLY INTELLIGENT NURSING LEADERSHIP

The American Organization of Nurse Executives sets research and education priorities that address critical issues facing the profession.[28] The American Organization of Nurse Executives, which represents the perspective of nursing leaders across the United States, consistently calls for professional leadership and leadership development at all levels of nursing activity. Strong, effective executive leaders in nursing can be scarce commodities, but even where they exist their organizations frequently have inconsistent leadership strength throughout the ranks. American Organization of Nurse Executives executive leadership competencies call for strengths in communication and relationship building with all stakeholders and in leading change. At the nurse manager level, the critical art of leading others includes a cluster of relationship and diversity management, influence, human resource leadership, and shared decision-making competencies.[28]

The American Nurses Association publishes a booklet outlining the scope and standards for nurse administrators[29] that includes nurse executive and nurse manager levels. Both levels of nursing leadership call for knowledge and qualifications that, in part, fall within the domain of the emotional competencies framework: customer service; ethical conduct; effectiveness in communication; developing and fostering relationships; negotiation and conflict resolution abilities; organizational behavior and development; performance appraisal and improvement; strategic visioning; advocacy for patients and staff; collaboration with other disciplines and leaders; leadership in human resources management and development; facilitation of continuous quality improvement; change agency; innovation; accountability; empowerment of staff and nurse participation in decision making; maintenance of a healthy climate and culture; competence with diversity; supervision; recruitment, selection, and retention of staff; self-assessment and openness to constructive feedback; and transmission of values. The standards reflect the values and priorities of the profession, direct the leadership of professional nursing practice, and identify areas in which nurse leaders are accountable to the public.

A growing research base documents the relationship between nursing, environments of care, staffing ratios, and nurse education levels and patient outcomes.[30] Most of this research focuses on hospital nursing and appears in journals such as *Health Affairs*, the *Journal of Nursing Administration*, *Nursing Economics*, and *Policy, Politics, & Nursing Practice* as well as in specialty nursing journals. Additionally, national foundations, such as the Robert Wood Johnson Foundation, and government agencies, such as the Agency for Healthcare Research and Quality (part of the U.S. Department of Health and Human Services), periodically issue reports on patient safety and outcomes research they have funded.[31] The documented importance of nursing to quality care is evident throughout these studies and, with it, the necessity for effective nursing leadership at all levels of health care organizations.

Several areas of need for emotionally intelligent nursing leadership are especially prominent in the research literature: recruiting and retaining qualified staff and limiting stress, transfer, grievance, turnover attrition, and nurses leaving the profession,[32] promoting positive work climates[33]; promoting nurse participation in decision making and enhancing power and control[34]; improving nurse recognition, advancement opportunities, and lifelong learning[35]; enhancing management responsiveness to and communication with nurses; and providing better administrative support for nursing activities.[36] These areas of need are especially critical because of the shortage of nurses nationwide, the costs of turnover (replacement costs for a registered nurse are estimated to average $42,000–$64,000[37]), and the disruptions in organizational effectiveness and patient care quality associated with unstable staffing.

In spite of the common practice of promoting nonmanagement-prepared staff nurses into charge and leadership positions, the need for well-prepared managers is well established in the nursing literature.[38] Nurse leaders make a significant difference in how nurses perceive and perform in their jobs. Repeatedly, effective behaviors and practices of nurse leaders have been found to influence work environments in innumerable ways, resulting in greater levels of staff nurse job satisfaction and organizational commitment. Exceptional nurse executive leadership, with the proper infrastructural support,[39] positively influence the entire climate of nursing work in an organization. And because nurse middle managers can "make or break" the care delivery process, there is growing evidence that well-run nursing units provide higher levels of care quality.

Nurse executives in any health care setting establish standards, provide resources, buffer staff nurses from the effects of ongoing uncertainties in the health care industry, lead with high expectations, and negotiate with other professional groups for control over nursing practice. Additionally, top-level emotionally intelligent nursing leadership is necessary to support the effective selection and development of nurse middle managers. In turn, nurse executives need support from their executive colleagues to create work environments that enable professional practice by nurses. Nationally, the strongest nursing organizations have tended to be those in which the chief executive officer understands and values nursing and "gets it" in regard to what is needed to maintain a strong base of nursing practice. He or she trusts and grants full authority to the nurse executive to run the nursing operation (Figure 3-8).

FIGURE 3-8　EMOTIONAL INTELLIGENCE AT WORK

For nearly 30 years, until the managed care decade of the 1990s, the Beth Israel (BI) Hospital in Boston served as an icon for the empowerment of nursing. With its chief nurse executive, Joyce Clifford, working in a unique partnership with CEO physician Mitchell Rabkin, the BI helped to pioneer an innovative model of nursing care.... The hospital.... employed an almost all registered nurse staff, hired only RNs with bachelor's degrees, and was committed to enhancing the collaboration between nurses and physicians and giving nurses a greater voice in their institution.... [T]hose nurses received institutional support from the highest levels.... [N]ursing care does not depend on the personal kindness or the moral virtuousness of the nurse. Instead it depends on education and experience and on the institutional support that nurses receive from the hospital in which they are employed.... Nurses there were among the most satisfied in the nation.[40]

Historically, Beth Israel had been one of the best hospitals in the world in which to practice as a nurse. Organizational features that both enhanced nurses' work satisfaction and improved patient outcomes included support for nurses' stature and representation in the hospital, control over the resources required to perform their work, autonomy in decisions about how to care for their patients, and teamwork and collegiality with physicians.[41] This did not happen by chance—all of its great accomplishments were voluntary creations constructed over years[42] by the collaborative relationship between the chief executive officer and chief nursing operator.

I interviewed Dr. Rabkin in 1992 as part of Beth Israel's participation in the program Strengthening Hospital Nursing, a national initiative funded by the Robert Wood Johnson Foundation and the Pew Charitable Trusts. His support for nursing and nurses was both seriously and humorously relayed through the following comments:

> There are very few places, I think, where other than by some dictatorial policy, nursing is deemed to be co-equal with medicine, surgery, etc. My argument is that nursing is a clinical service just like medicine and surgery, OB/GYN, and so on.... Hospitals—not this place alone—are nursing institutions primarily, not doctoring institutions. Now if you don't have a truly professional nursing service, [empowering nurses] is not going to work. You need two things: one, you need nurses who are smart, because doctors don't tolerate people as colleagues who are not as smart as they are. You need to have smart nurses. The other thing is that they have to be true colleagues, and that comes about not only in nurses' education but also with their image of themselves, the capacity to understand what nursing really is, and I see that here [at Beth Israel].
>
> In fact, there was a marvelous incident a number of years ago, with a head nurse who couldn't have weighed more than 90 pounds, and this was with a new resident on the orthopaedic service; these kids [residents] rotate through all of the Harvard hospitals. This one had spent some 6 months at [another hospital], and literally within 30 minutes of his arrival at BI, he had some floor nurse in tears. The head nurse manager asked him to come into her office, and she said to him, 'You're new here, you've been [at the other hospital] for 6 months, and I've got to tell you that the way we do things around here is rather different, and what you've done is completely unacceptable. This is the way we work here [and she went on to explain the co-equal role of nurses at BI]. This is your first day and I realize it and we're certainly going to give you time to learn.' Then this pipsqueak put her finger on this guy's chest—he's about 6'2"—and she said, 'If you do not learn, we will send you back to the minor leagues where you came from.' The guy got beet red, stormed out, and then went to see the senior orthopaedic surgeon, who said, 'Well, maybe you've got something to learn.' About 3 or 4 days later he came back and asked to speak to the head nurse in private. 'I have to apologize,' he said, 'I had no idea that nurses were so good and so confident, and so capable, I really had no idea at all.' So they [new residents] learn. They also learn from role modeling by the other physicians. It's not only the nurses standing up for themselves; the nurses know that the administration backs them up.[43]

Rabkin's story suggests many aspects of the BI culture that support nursing practice, but it also illustrates an emotional intelligence characteristic of "best bosses"—"handling" anyone who is abusive to nurses.

HOW TO DEVELOP YOUR EMOTIONAL COMPETENCIES

All emotional competencies can be learned and developed. The core competencies—emotional self-awareness, accurate self-assessment, self-confidence, emotional self-control, and empathy—are the most important because they are fundamental. A leader deficient in the core competencies will encounter difficulty mastering any of the remaining 13 competencies. In Figure 3-6 Victoria appears to have the competencies associated with self-awareness and self-management. She knows that she doesn't like the chief operating officer and his leadership style, is able to maintain self-control in his presence, and is confident of her abilities to run the nursing component of the home health agency. Her crucial mistake, however, is her lack of empathy for the chief operating officer. She didn't really know what motivated him or what was important to him, nor did she have any idea how he might be viewing her performance. It is likely that the chief operating officer, though not often present, had expectations that his direct reports would demonstrate attention and responsiveness to his communications, regardless of how important (or irrelevant) his direct reports believed those communications were. When Victoria ignored or deflected a good number of his e-mails and faxes, the chief operating officer probably found her behavior disrespectful, perhaps even offensive. As a result, he interpreted her behavior as resistant, aloof, and not innovative. Had Victoria been more aware of the chief operating officer's expectations and what his unique leadership behaviors meant to him, she could have been more astute in managing the politics between her and her boss. The competency of organizational awareness, which concerns one's political savvy at work, cannot be developed without first having the ability to empathize with the needs and feelings of other individuals and groups. Victoria used her own frame of reference to determine what was important in her job, giving little thought to what her chief operating officer viewed as important. She also let his relatively infrequent appearances on-site lull her into a false sense of security.

Developing emotional competencies first requires an awareness of areas of strength and weakness and then an identification of what ideal behavior would be in a targeted area of weakness (Figure 3-9). The individual needs to assess honestly his or her motivation to change and willingness to practice new behaviors. From a feasibility standpoint, it is important to focus changes on just one or two competencies.

Behavior change is most effective when it connects to activities in the individual's work life that are most in need of and likely to show improvements. Many young and inexperienced nurses, for example, are uncomfortable approaching physicians with recommendations for changes in patient management. Reticence with physicians can be a good starting point for behavior change: More self-assertion leads to high payoffs for both the nurse and his or her patients. Self-development in such a situation might focus on self-awareness (exactly what is the staff nurse afraid of?) and self-confidence (with a peer, practice strategies for managing the conversation). Nurse managers who are uncomfortable standing up and addressing groups might choose to work on empathy (anticipate what the members of the group might be thinking and feeling) and self-confidence (plan the presentation thoroughly, rehearse with a peer, and actively seek responses from the group members during the presentation). Even minor successes in self-directed behavior change can be highly motivating for continuing development efforts.

Change in behaviors driven by emotional habits requires that as we practice new behaviors, we actively seek to unlearn the old behaviors. The old behaviors become a source of resistance and backsliding unless they are identified, acknowledged, and actively transformed. This kind of change depends on the ability to engage one's own emotions in order to change them. For example, use self-awareness to monitor how you are reacting emotionally to giving up an old habit (e.g., avoiding conflict) while trying a new one (asking conflicting parties to express their differences).

The engagement of an emotionally competent coach, mentor, or friend to aid self-development efforts is essential. We cannot change what we do not see or know, so external observation and feedback

FIGURE 3-9 | STEPS TO DEVELOPING EMOTIONAL COMPETENCIES[44]

1. Determine your behavioral goals.

   • Ground them in your assessment of your emotional strengths and weakness, and use feedback from others who know you well. Make sure you understand the gaps between your actual and your preferred "ideal" behavior.
   • Build on and engage your strengths.
   • Develop clear, manageable goals; have them reflect your personal vision for self-development.
   • Pick no more than one or two areas (competencies) at a time. Determine whether your plans for self-directed change will fit smoothly into your life: Are there day-to-day events that can be used as a learning laboratory?
   • Honestly assess your commitment to working on self-development.

2. Create a plan to reach your behavioral goals.

   • Select a coach and establish a verbal contract.
   • Identify and agree on the developmental priorities and behavioral indicators.
   • Identify how behavioral development will facilitate your career goals.
   • Identify opportunities for trials and action, using ways that fit your learning style.
   • Identify times and places for the coach (and any others you choose to involve) to observe you and provide feedback.
   • Identify role models you would like to emulate.
   • Understand that self-development will take time and sustained focus. It doesn't happen overnight!

3. Monitor your progress regularly.

   • Practice, practice, practice; use work and outside settings.
   • Tune in to behaviors you need to unlearn in order to learn new ones.
   • Meet and talk with your coach. Ask questions to help clarify issues.
   • Seek feedback from others as possible.
   • Identify in which situations it is easier or harder for you to improve.
   • Don't "slip" in other strength areas of emotional competency while you are focused on development in new areas; avoid relapses.
   • Do reading and thinking on your own behavior and developmental goals.
   • Keep a written record of thoughts, feedback, insights, difficulties, and successes.
   • Assess your continued commitment.

4. Celebrate successes.

   • Give yourself credit for evidence of developmental improvements; reinforce your growth.
   • Seek ways to further sharpen your developmental progress.
   • Assess your continued commitment to behavior change.

Source: Based on research conducted by Goleman, 1995, 1998a; Goleman et al., 2002; The Hay Group, 2004.

provides indispensable data. A coach also enables the individual to learn by talking over the situation, exploring alternatives, and reflecting on behavioral options. Importantly, the coach can also function as a motivator, encouraging and holding the person accountable for his or her self-development plan.

Behavior change requires practice, typically sustained over weeks and months—often up to 6 months—to develop a new competency. With extended practice, reflection, reinforcement, and success, mastery is possible. Supplementary activities can facilitate behavior change: reading and studying about leadership or emotional intelligence, self-reflection (journals, discussion, reflective learning groups),[45] experiential learning exercises,[46] and measurement feedback.[47] Like athletic performance, proficiency development requires ongoing cycles of practice–trial–feedback and correction.

Finally, even without intentional behavior change, there is evidence that humans intuitively develop emotional competencies with age and experience.[48]

> ## Evidence-Based Practice 3-1
>
> The researchers critically reviewed the conceptualization and empirical evidence in support of emotional intelligence and its stated role in the occupational environment. The researchers considered the objectives of emotional intelligence in occupational and career assessment, focusing on selection of personnel, job placement, job performance, and satisfaction. This review demonstrated current evidence to support important strides toward understanding the usefulness of emotional intelligence in the workplace. However, the ratio of "hype" to hard evidence is high, with over-reliance in the literature on expert opinion, anecdote, case studies, and unpublished proprietary surveys. The review does summarize a number of practical guidelines for the development and implementation of emotional intelligence measures within occupational settings.[49]

SUMMARY

Throughout life we observe leaders and learn about what makes them proficient. A complex phenomenon, leadership occurs in all work settings and is enacted through countless individual behaviors. In this chapter, I focused on those aspects of leadership that involve relationships between leaders and other people—the "people" skills of leaders. Using a framework of emotional intelligence, I address the relevance of 18 emotional competencies to the successful intra- and interpersonal work lives of nurse leaders. Evidence is presented that emotionally competent organizational leadership raises the level of performance for everyone and enhances the patient experience.

Notes

1. Kellerman, B. (2008). *Followership: How followers are changed and changing leaders.* Harvard Business Press.

2. Rotondo, D. M., Carlson, D. S., & Kincaid, J. F. (2003). "Coping with multiple dimensions of work-family conflict." *Personnel Review, 32*(3), 275–296; Shipper, F. M., Hoffman, R. C., & Rotondo, D. M. (2007). "Does the 360 feedback process create knowledge equally across cultures?" *Academy of Management Learning and Education, 6,* 1, 22–50; Rahim, M. A., Psenicka, C., Polychroniou, P. Zhao, J. H. (2002). A model of emotional intelligence and conflict management strategies: A study in seven countries. *International Journal of Organizational Analysis, 10*(4).

3. Goleman, D. P. (1995). *Emotional Intelligence: Why It Can Matter More Than IQ for Character, Health and Lifelong Achievement.* New York: Bantam Books; Goleman, D. (1998). Working with Emotional Intelligence. New York: Bantam Books; Goleman, D., Boyatzis, R., and McKee, A. (2002). The emotional reality of teams. *Journal of Organizational Excellence, 21(2),* 55–65.

4. Hay Group. (2004). Communication: The Foundation for Successful HR Program Implementation—Six Key Goals of a Strategic Communication Plan. Accessed on May 5, 2008: http://resources.bnet.com/topic/hay+ group.html

5. Duchscher, L. (2001). Experiences and learning during a graduate nurse program: An examination using a focus group approach. *Nurse Education in Practice, 4*(4), 258–263.

6. Vitello-Cicciu, L. M. (2002). Learning from success: Improving undergraduate education through understanding the capabilities of successful nurse graduates. *Nurse Education Today, 25*(3), 181–188.

7. Goleman, D. P. (1995). *Emotional Intelligence: Why It Can Matter More Than IQ for Character, Health and Lifelong Achievement.* New York: Bantam Books; Goleman, D. (1998). Working with Emotional Intelligence. New York: Bantam Books; Goleman, D., Boyatzis, R., and McKee, A. (2002). The emotional reality of teams. *Journal of Organizational Excellence, 21*(2), 55–65; Communication: The Foundation for Successful HR Program Implementation—Six Key Goals of a Strategic Communication Plan. Accessed on May 5, 2008: http://resources.bnet.com/topic/hay+group.html

8. Boyatzis, R. E., Smith, M., & Blaize, N. (2006). Developing sustainable leaders through coaching and compassion. *Academy of Management Journal on Learning and Education, 5*(1), 8–24.

9. Goleman, D. P. (1995). *Emotional Intelligence: Why It Can Matter More Than IQ for Character, Health and Lifelong Achievement.* New York: Bantam Books; Goleman, D. (1998). *Working with Emotional Intelligence.* New York: Bantam Books; Goleman, D., Boyatzis, R., and McKee, A. (2002). The emotional reality of teams. *Journal of Organizational Excellence, 21*(2), 55–65; *Communication: The Foundation for Successful HR Program Implementation—Six Key Goals of a Strategic Communication Plan.* Accessed on May 5, 2008: http://resources.bnet.com/topic/hay+group.html

10. Dickenson-Hazard, N. (2004). World health, global health: Issues and challenges. *Journal of Nursing Scholarship, 36*(1), 6–10.

11. Goleman, D., Boyatzis, R., & McKee, A. (2002). *Primal leadership: Realizing the power of emotional intelligence.* Harvard Business School Press, 50.

12. Goleman, D. (1998). *Working with emotional intelligence.* Bantam Press, 160.

13. Goleman, D. (1998). *Working with emotional intelligence.* Bantam Press.

14. Corning, P. A. (2002). The re-emergence of emergence: A venerable concept in search of a theory. *Complexity, 7*(6), 18–30.

15. Michaelsen, L. K., & Schultheiss, E. E. (1998–1989). Making feedback helpful. *Organizational Behavior Teaching Review, 13,* 109–113.

16. Dickenson-Hazard, N. (2004). World health, global health: Issues and challenges. *Journal of Nursing Scholarship, 36*(1), 6–10.

17. Institute of Medicine & Page, A. (2003). *Keeping patients safe: Transforming the work environment of nurses.* Washington, D.C.

18. Woolf, R. (2001). How to talk so people will listen. *Journal of Nursing Administration, 31,* 401–402.

19. Goleman, D. (1998a). *Working with emotional intelligence.* New York: Bantam Books, 197.

20. Larrabee, J. H., Janney, M. A., Ostrow, C. L., Withrow, M. L., Hobbs, G. R., & Burant, C. (2003). Predicting registered nurse job satisfaction and intent to leave. *Journal of Nursing Administration, 33*; Laschinger, H. K. S., Almost, J., & Tuer-Hodes, D. (2003). Workplace empowerment and magnet hospital characteristics. *Journal of Nursing Administration, 33,* 410–422.

21. Woolf, R. (2001). How to talk so people will listen. *Journal of Nursing Administration, 31,* 401–402; O'Connor, M. (2001). Reframing communication: Conversation in the workplace. *Journal of Nursing Administration, 31,* 403–405.

22. Forman, H., & Grimes, T. C. (2002). Living with a union contract. *Journal of Nursing Administration, 32,* 611–614.

23. Druskat, V. U., & Wolff, S. B. (2001). Building the emotional intelligence of groups. *Harvard Business Review, 79,* 81–90; Rapisarda, B. A. (2002). The impact of emotional intelligence on work team cohesiveness and performance. *International Journal of Organizational Analysis, 10,* 363–379.

24. Goleman, D. (1998a). *Working with emotional intelligence.* New York: Bantam Books, 205; Druskat, V. U., & Wolff, S. B. (2001). Building the emotional intelligence of groups. *Harvard Business Review, 79,* 81–90; Rapisarda, B. A. (2002). The impact of emotional intelligence on work team cohesiveness and performance. *International Journal of Organizational Analysis, 10,* 363–379.

25. Larrabee, J. H., Janney, M. A., Ostrow, C. L., Withrow, M. L., Hobbs, G. R., & Burant, C. (2003). Predicting registered nurse job satisfaction and intent to leave. *Journal of Nursing Administration, 33.*

26. Boyle, D. K., & Kochinda, C. (2004). Enhancing collaborative communication of nurse and physician leadership in two intensive care units. *Journal of Nursing Administration, 34,* 60–70.

27. Goleman, D. (1998b). What makes a leader? *Harvard Business Review, 76,* 93–102.

28. American Organization of Nurse Executives, 2002; American Organization of Nurse Executives, Retrieved July 19, 2007 at http://www.aone.org/aone/resource/NMLC/nmlcLEARNING.html; Ritter-Teitel, J. (2003). Nursing administrative research: The underpinning of decisive leadership. *Journal of Nursing Administration, 33,* 257–259.

29. American Nurses Association. (2004). *Scope and standards for nurse administrators* (2nd ed). Washington, DC: Author.

30. Aiken, L. H., Clarke, S. P., Sloane, D. M., Sochalski, J., & Silber, J. H. (2002). Hospital nurse staffing and patient mortality, nurse burnout, and job dissatisfaction. *Journal of the American Medical Association, 288,* 1987–1993; Aiken, L. H., Clarke, S. P., Sloane, D. M., Sochalski, J., Busse, R., Clarke, H. (2001). Nurses' reports on hospital care in five countries. *Health Affairs, 20,* 43–53; Blegen, M. A., Vaughn, T., & Goode, C. (2001). Nurse experience and education: Effect on quality of care. *Journal of Nursing Administration, 31*(1), 33–39; Blegen, M. A., Goode, C. J., & Reed, L. (1998). Nurse staffing and patient outcomes. *Nursing Research, 47,* 43–50; Institute of Medicine & Page, 2003; Mullan, 2001; Institute of Medicine & Page, A. (2003). *Keeping patients safe: Transforming the work environment of nurses.* Washington, DC: The National Academies Press.

31. Kaissi, A., Johnson, T., & Kirschbaum, M. S. (2003). Measuring teamwork and patient safety attitudes of high-risk areas. *Nursing Economics, 21,* 211–218.

32. Mark, B. A. (2002). What explains nurses' perceptions of staffing adequacy? *Journal of Nursing Administration, 32,* 234–242; McKinnon, C. (2002). You can do it too in 2002: Registry reduction. *Journal of Nursing Administration, 32,* 498–500; McNeese-Smith, D. (1995). Job satisfaction, productivity, and organizational commitment: The result of leadership. *Journal of Nursing Administration, 25,* 17–26; McNeese-Smith, D. K., & Crook, M. (2003). Nursing values and a changing nursing workforce. *Journal of Nursing Administration, 33,* 260–270.

33. American Nurses Association. (2004). *Scope and standards for nurse administrators* (2nd ed). Washington, DC: Author.

34. Larrabee, J. H., Janney, M. A., Ostrow, C. L., Withrow, M. L., Hobbs, G. R., & Burant, C. (2003). Predicting registered nurse job satisfaction and intent to leave. *Journal of Nursing Administration, 33,* 271–283; Laschinger, H. K. S. (2004). Hospital nurses' perceptions of respect and organizational justice. *Journal of Nursing Administration, 34,* 354–364; Laschinger, H. K. S., Almost, J., & Tuer-Hodes, D. (2003). Workplace empowerment and magnet hospital characteristics. *Journal of Nursing Administration, 33,* 410–422.

35. Carroll, T. L., & Austin, T. (2004). Career coaching: A hospital and a university link hands to retain nursing talent. *Reflections on Nursing Leadership, 30,* 30–31. Cathcart, D., Jeska, S., Karnas, J., Miller, S. E., Pechacek, J., & Rheault, L. (2004). Span of control matters. *Journal of Nursing Administration, 34,* 395–399.

36. Aiken, L. H., Clarke, S. P., Sloane, D. M., Sochalski, J., & Silber, J. H. (2002). Hospital nurse staffing and patient mortality, nurse burnout, and job dissatisfaction. *Journal of the American Medical Association, 288,* 1987–1993; Aiken, L. H., Clarke, S. P., Sloane, D. M., Sochalski, J., Busse, R., Clarke, H. (2001). Nurses' reports on hospital care in five countries. *Health Affairs, 20,* 43–53; Aiken, L. H., Smith, H. L., & Lake, E. T. (1994). Lower medicare mortality among a set of hospitals known for good nursing care. *Medical Care, 32,* 771–787.

37. Aiken, L. H., Clarke, S. P., Sloane, D. M., Sochalski, J., & Silber, J. H. (2002). Hospital nurse staffing and patient mortality, nurse burnout, and job dissatisfaction. *Journal of the American Medical Association, 288,* 1987–1993.

38. Corning, P. A. (2002). The re-emergence of emergence: A venerable concept in search of a theory. *Complexity, 7*(6), 18–30.

39. Cooper, R. W., Frank, G. L., Gouty, C. A., & Hansen, M. C. (2002). Key ethical issues encountered in healthcare organizations: Perceptions of nurse executives. *Journal of Nursing Administration, 32,* 331–337.

40. Weinberg, D. B. (2003). *Code green: Money-driven hospitals and the dismantling of nursing.* Ithaca, NY: Cornell University Press.

41. Ibid, p. 13.

42. Ibid, pp. 2 & xii.

43. Taft, S. (1992). Interview with Mitchell Rabkin, personal communication, Boston, MA, July.

44. Goleman, D. P. (1995). *Emotional Intelligence: Why It Can Matter More Than IQ for Character, Health and Lifelong Achievement.* New York: Bantam Books; Goleman, D. (1998). *Working with Emotional Intelligence.* New York: Bantam Books; Goleman, D., Boyatzis, R., and McKee, A. (2002). The emotional reality of teams. *Journal of Organizational Excellence, 21*(2), 55–65.

45. Brewer, J., & Cadman, C. (2000). Emotional intelligence: Enhancing student effectiveness and patient outcomes. *Nurse Educator, 25,* 264–266.

46. de Janasz, S. C., Dowd, K. O., & Schneider, B. Z. (2002). *Interpersonal skills in organizations.* Boston: McGraw Hill.

47. Hay Group. (2004). *Communication: The Foundation for Successful HR Program Implementation—Six Key Goals of a Strategic Communication Plan.* Accessed on May 5, 2008: http://resources.bnet.com/topic/hay+ group.html

48. Goleman, D. P. (1995). *Emotional Intelligence: Why It Can Matter More Than IQ for Character, Health and Lifelong Achievement.* New York: Bantam Books; Goleman, D. (1998). *Working with Emotional Intelligence.* New York: Bantam Books; Goleman, D., Boyatzis, R., and McKee, A. (2002). The emotional reality of teams. *Journal of Organizational Excellence, 21*(2), 55–65.

49. Zeidner, M., Matthews, G., & Roberts, R. D. (2004). Emotional intelligence in the workplace: A critical review. *Applied Psychology, 53,* 371–399.

References

Aiken, L. H., Clarke, S. P., Sloane, D. M., Sochalski, J., & Silber, J. H. (2002). Hospital nurse staffing and patient mortality, nurse burnout, and job dissatisfaction. *Journal of the American Medical Association, 288,* 1987–1993.

Aiken, L.H., Clarke, S. P., Sloane, D. M., Sochalski, J., Busse, R., Clarke, H. (2001). Nurses' reports on hospital care in five countries. *Health Affairs, 20,* 43–53.

Aiken, L. H., Smith, H. L., & Lake, E. T. (1994). Lower medicare mortality among a set of hospitals known for good nursing care. *Medical Care, 32,* 771–787.

American Nurses Association. (2004). *Scope and standards for nurse administrators* (2nd ed). Washington, DC: Author.

American Organization of Nurse Executives (AONE). (2002). AONE 2002 research and education priorities. *Journal of Nursing Administration, 32,* 228.

American Organization of Nurse Executives (AONE). Retrieved July 19, 2007, from http://www.aone.org/aone/resource/NMLC/nmlcLEARNING.html

Beecroft, P. C., Kunzman, L. A., Taylor, S., Devenis, E., & Guzak, F. (2004). Bridging the gap between school and workplace: Developing a new graduate nurse curriculum. *Journal of Nursing Administration, 34,* 338–345.

Benner, P., Sheets, V., Uris, P., Mallock, K., Schwed, K., & Jamison, D. (2002). Individual, practice, and system causes of errors in nursing. *Journal of Nursing Administration, 32,* 509–523.

Bingham, R. (2002). Leaving nursing. *Health Affairs, 21,* 211–217.

Blegen, M. A., Goode, C. J., & Reed, L. (1998). Nurse staffing and patient outcomes. *Nursing Research, 47,* 43–50.

Blegen, M. A., Vaughn, T., & Goode, C. (2001). Nurse experience and education: Effect on quality of care. *Journal of Nursing Administration, 31*(1), 33–39.

Boyle, D. K., & Kochinda, C. (2004). Enhancing collaborative communication of nurse and physician leadership in two intensive care units. *Journal of Nursing Administration, 34,* 60–70.

Brewer, J., & Cadman, C. (2000). Emotional intelligence: Enhancing student effectiveness and patient outcomes. *Nurse Educator, 25,* 264–266.

Brodeur, M. A., & Laraway, A. S. (2002). States respond to nursing shortage. *Policy, Politics, & Nursing Practice, 3,* 228–234.

Buerhaus, P. I., Needleman, J., Mattke, S., & Stewart, M. (2002). Strengthening hospital nursing. *Health Affairs, 21,* 123–132.

Carroll, T. L., & Austin, T. (2004). Career coaching: A hospital and a university link hands to retain nursing talent. *Reflections on Nursing Leadership, 30,* 30–31.

Cathcart, D., Jeska, S., Karnas, J., Miller, S. E., Pechacek, J., & Rheault, L. (2004). Span of control matters. *Journal of Nursing Administration, 34,* 395–399.

Cooper, R.W., Frank, G. L., Gouty, C. A., & Hansen, M. C. (2002). Key ethical issues encountered in healthcare organizations: Perceptions of nurse executives. *Journal of Nursing Administration, 32,* 331–337.

Corning, S. P. (2002). Profiling and developing nursing leaders. *Journal of Nursing Administration, 32,* 373–375.

Cowin, L. (2002). The effects of nurses' job satisfaction on retention: An Australian perspective. *Journal of Nursing Administration, 32,* 283–291.

de Janasz, S. C., Dowd, K. O., & Schneider, B. Z. (2002). *Interpersonal skills in organizations.* Boston: McGraw Hill.

de Ruiter, H.-P., & Saphiere, D. H. (2001). Nurse leaders as cultural bridges. *Journal of Nursing Administration, 31,* 418–423.

Dickenson-Hazard, N. (2004). Cultivating effective leadership skills for nurses: A commentary. *Policy, Politics, & Nursing Practice, 5,* 145–146.

Druskat, V. U., & Wolff, S. B. (2001). Building the emotional intelligence of groups. *Harvard Business Review, 79,* 81–90.

Duchscher, J. E. B. (2001). Out in the real world: Newly graduated nurses in acute-care speak out. *Journal of Nursing Administration, 31,* 426–439.

Duffield, C., Aitken, L., O'Brien-Pallas, L., & Wise, W. J. (2004). Nursing: A stepping stone to future careers. *Journal of Nursing Administration, 34,* 238–245.

Fletcher, C. E. (2001). Hospital RN's job satisfactions and dissatisfactions. *Journal of Nursing Administration, 31,* 324–331.

Foley, B. J., Kee, C. C., Minick, P., Harvey, S. S., & Jennings, B. M. (2002). Characteristics of nurses and hospital work environments that foster satisfaction and clinical expertise. *Journal of Nursing Administration, 32,* 273–282.

Forman, H., & Grimes, T. C. (2002). Living with a union contract. *Journal of Nursing Administration, 32,* 611–614.

Garrett, D. K., & McDaniel, A. M. (2001). A new look at nurse burnout: The effects of environmental uncertainty and social climate. *Journal of Nursing Administration, 31,* 91–96.

Goleman, D. (1995). *Emotional intelligence.* New York: Bantam Books.

Goleman, D. (1998a). *Working with emotional intelligence.* New York: Bantam Books.

Goleman, D. (1998b). What makes a leader? *Harvard Business Review, 76,* 93–102.

Goleman, D., Boyatzis, R., & McKee, A. (2002). *Primal leadership: Realizing the power of emotional intelligence.* Boston: Harvard Business School Press.

Goode, C. J., & Williams, C. A. (2004). Post-Baccalaureate nurse residency program. *Journal of Nursing Administration, 34,* 71–77.

The Hay Group. (2004). *Emotional intelligence services.* Retrieved November 30, 2004, from http://ei.haygroup.com/about_ei/

Hill, K. S. (2003). Development of leadership competencies as a team. *Journal of Nursing Administration, 33,* 639–642.

Holtom, B. C., & O'Neill, B. S. (2004). Job embeddedness: A theoretical foundation for developing a comprehensive nurse retention plan. *Journal of Nursing Administration, 34,* 216–227.

Horton-Deutsch, S. L., & Wellman, D. S. (2002). Christman's principles for effective management: Reflection and challenges for action. *Journal of Nursing Administration, 32,* 596–601.

HSM Group, Ltd. (2002). Acute care hospital survey of RN vacancy and turnover rates in 2000. *Journal of Nursing Administration, 32,* 437–439.

Ingersoll, G. L., Olsan, T., Drew-Cates, J., DeVinney, B. C., & Davies, J. (2002). Nurses' job satisfaction, organizational commitment, and career intent. *Journal of Nursing Administration, 32,* 250–263.

Institute of Medicine & Page, A. (2003). *Keeping patients safe: Transforming the work environment of nurses.* Washington, DC: The National Academies Press.

Irvine, D. M., & Evans, M. G. (1995). Job satisfaction and turnover among nurses: Integrating research findings across studies. *Nursing Research, 44,* 246–253.

Jeffries, E. (2002). Creating a great place to work: Strategies for retaining top talent. *Journal of Nursing Administration, 32,* 303–305.

Kahn, W. A. (1993). Caring for the caregivers: Patterns of organizational caregiving. *Administrative Science Quarterly, 38,* 539–563.

Kaissi, A., Johnson, T., & Kirschbaum, M. S. (2003). Measuring teamwork and patient safety attitudes of high-risk areas. *Nursing Economics, 21,* 211–218.

Kalisch, B. J. (2003). Recruiting nurses: The problem is the process. *Journal of Nursing Administration, 33,* 468–477.

Kalliath, T., & Morris, R. (2002). Job satisfaction among nurses: A predictor of burnout levels. *Journal of Nursing Administration, 32,* 648–654.

Kleinman, C. S. (2003). Leadership roles, competencies, and education: How prepared are our nurse managers? *Journal of Nursing Administration, 33,* 451–455.

Kleinman, C. S. (2004). Workforce issues: Leadership strategies in reducing staff nurse role conflict. *Journal of Nursing Administration, 34,* 322–324.

Krugman, M., & Smith, V. (2003). Charge nurse leadership development and education. *Journal of Nursing Administration, 33,* 284–292.

Kupperschmidt, B. R. (1998). Understanding Generation X employees. *Journal of Nursing Administration, 28,* 36–43.

Larrabee, J. H., Janney, M. A., Ostrow, C. L., Withrow, M. L., Hobbs, G. R., & Burant, C. (2003). Predicting registered nurse job satisfaction and intent to leave. *Journal of Nursing Administration, 33,* 271–283.

Laschinger, H. K. S. (2004). Hospital nurses' perceptions of respect and organizational justice. *Journal of Nursing Administration, 34,* 354–364.

Laschinger, H. K. S., Almost, J., & Tuer-Hodes, D. (2003). Workplace empowerment and magnet hospital characteristics. *Journal of Nursing Administration, 33,* 410–422.

Letvak, S. (2002). Retaining the older nurse. *Journal of Nursing Administration, 32,* 387–392.

Ma, C.-C., Samuels, M. E., & Alexander, J. W. (2003). Factors that influence nurses' job satisfaction. *Journal of Nursing Administration, 33,* 300–306.

MacPhee, M., & Scott, J. (2002). The role of social support networks for rural hospital nurses. *Journal of Nursing Administration, 32,* 264–272.

Manion, J. (2003). Joy at work! Creating a positive workplace. *Journal of Nursing Administration, 33,* 652–659.

Manojlovich, M., & Laschinger, H. K. S. (2002). The relationship of empowerment and selected personality characteristics to nursing job satisfaction. *Journal of Nursing Administration, 32,* 586–595.

Mark, B. A. (2002). What explains nurses' perceptions of staffing adequacy? *Journal of Nursing Administration, 32,* 234–242.

McKinnon, C. (2002). You can do it too in 2002: Registry reduction. *Journal of Nursing Administration, 32,* 498–500.

McNeese-Smith, D. (1995). Job satisfaction, productivity, and organizational commitment: The result of leadership. *Journal of Nursing Administration, 25,* 17–26.

McNeese-Smith, D. K., & Crook, M. (2003). Nursing values and a changing nursing workforce. *Journal of Nursing Administration, 33,* 260–270.

Michaelsen, L. K., & Schultheiss, E. E. (1998–1989). Making feedback helpful. *Organizational Behavior Teaching Review, 13,* 109–113.

Moore, S. C., & Hutchison, S. A. (2007). Developing leaders at every level: Accountability and empowerment actualized through shared governance. *Journal of Nursing Administration, 37,* 564–568.

Mullan, F. (2001). A founder of quality assessment encounters a troubled system firsthand. *Health Affairs, 29,* 137–141.

Navaie-Waliser, M., Lincoln, P., Karuturi, M., & Reisch, K. (2004). Increasing job satisfaction, quality care, and coordination in home health. *Journal of Nursing Administration, 34,* 88–92.

Neuhauser, P. C. (2002). Building a high-retention culture in healthcare. *Journal of Nursing Administration, 32,* 470–478.

Nierenberg, R. J. (2003). The use of a strategic interviewing technique to select the nurse manager. *Journal of Nursing Administration, 33,* 500–505.

Nikolaou, I., & Tsaousis, I. (2002). Emotional intelligence in the workplace: Exploring its effects on occupational stress and organizational commitment. *International Journal of Organizational Analysis, 10,* 327–342.

Noyes, B. J. (2002). Midlevel management education. *Journal of Nursing Administration, 32,* 25–26.

O'Brien-Pallas, L., Thomson, D., Alksnis, C., & Bruce, S. (2001). The economic impact of nurse staffing decisions: Time to turn down another road? *Hospital Quarterly, 4,* 42–50.

O'Connor, M. (2001). Reframing communication: Conversation in the workplace. *Journal of Nursing Administration, 31,* 403–405.

O'Hara, N. F., Duvanich, M., Foss, J., & Wells, N. (2003). The Vanderbilt Professional Nursing Practice Program, part 2: Integrating a professional advancement and performance evaluation system. *Journal of Nursing Administration, 33,* 512–521.

Ohio Nurses Association. (2004). Creating a compelling workplace. *Ohio Nurses Review, 79,* 6.

Rahim, M. A., & Psenicka, C. (2002). A model of emotional intelligence and conflict management strategies: A study in seven countries. *International Journal of Organizational Analysis, 10,* 302–326.

Rapisarda, B. A. (2002). The impact of emotional intelligence on work team cohesiveness and performance. *International Journal of Organizational Analysis, 10,* 363–379.

Ritter-Teitel, J. (2003). Nursing administrative research: The underpinning of decisive leadership. *Journal of Nursing Administration, 33,* 257–259.

Robert Wood Johnson Foundation, Kimball, B., & O'Neil, E. (2002). Health care's human crisis: The American nursing shortage. Retrieved September 30, 2004, from http://www.rwjf.org/publications/publicationspdfs/nursing_report.pdf

Roberts, B. J., Jones, C., & Lynn, M. (2004). Job satisfaction of new baccalaureate nurses. *Journal of Nursing Administration, 34,* 428–435.

Robinson, K., Eck, C., Keck, B., & Wells, N. (2003). The Vanderbilt Professional Nursing Practice Program, part 1: Growing and supporting professional nursing practice. *Journal of Nursing Administration, 33,* 441–450.

Russell, G., & Scoble, K. (2003). Vision 2020, part 2: Educational preparation for the future nurse manager. *Journal of Nursing Administration, 33,* 404–409.

Safire, W., & Safire, L. (1982). *Good advice.* New York: Wing Books.

Shipper, F., Rotondo, D. M., & Hoffman, R. C. IV. (2003, August). A cross-cultural study of linkage between emotional intelligence and managerial effectiveness. Paper presented at the Academy of Management, Seattle, Washington.

Smeltzer, C. H. (2002a). The benefits of executive coaching. *Journal of Nursing Administration, 32,* 501–502.

Smeltzer, C. H. (2002b). Succession planning. *Journal of Nursing Administration, 32,* 615.

Snow, J. L. (2001). Looking beyond nursing for clues to effective leadership. *Journal of Nursing Administration, 31,* 440–443.

Sochalski, J. (2002). Trends: Nursing shortage redux: Turning the corner on an enduring problem. *Health Affairs, 21,* 157–164.

Stevens, S. (2002). Nursing workforce retention: Challenging a bullying culture. *Health Affairs, 21,* 189–193.

Sullivan, J., Bretschneider, J., & McCausland, M. P. (2003). Designing a leadership development program for nurse managers: An evidence-driven approach. *Journal of Nursing Administration, 33,* 544–549.

Sullivan, T., Kerr, M., & Ibrahim, S. (1999). Job stress in health care workers: Highlights from the National Population Health Survey. *Hospital Quarterly, 2,* 34–40.

Tourangeau, A. E. (2003). Building nurse leader capacity. *Journal of Nursing Administration, 33,* 624–626.

Tzeng, H. M., & Ketefian, S. (2002). The relationships between nurses' job satisfaction and inpatient satisfaction: An exploratory study in a Taiwan teaching hospital. *Journal of Nursing Care Quality, 16,* 39–49.

Upenieks, V. V. (2002a). What constitutes successful nurse leadership? A qualitative approach utilizing Kanter's theory of organizational behavior. *Journal of Nursing Administration, 32,* 622–632.

Upenieks, V. V. (2002b). Assessing differences in job satisfaction of nurses in magnet and non-magnet hospitals. *Journal of Nursing Administration, 32,* 564–576.

Upenieks, V. V. (2003). What constitutes effective leadership? Perceptions of magnet and nonmagnet nurse leaders. *Journal of Nursing Administration, 33,* 456–467.

Vitellow-Cicciu, J. M. (2002). Exploring emotional intelligence: Implications for nursing leaders. *Journal of Nursing Administration, 32,* 208.

Wagner, C. M., & Huber, D. L. (2003). Catastrophe and nursing turnover: Nonlinear models. *Journal of Nursing Administration, 33,* 486–492.

Watson, C. A. (2002). Understanding the factors that influence nurses' job satisfaction. *Journal of Nursing Administration, 32,* 229–231.

Watson, C. A. (2004). Evidence-based management practices: The challenge for nursing. *Journal of Nursing Administration, 34,* 207–209.

Weinberg, D. B. (2003). *Code green: Money-driven hospitals and the dismantling of nursing.* Ithaca, NY: Cornell University Press.

Wellins, R., & Weaver, P. S. Jr. (2003). See-level leadership. *Training and Development* (September 2003), 58–65.

Woolf, R. (2001). How to talk so people will listen. *Journal of Nursing Administration, 31,* 401–402.

4 ETHICAL NURSE LEADERSHIP

Linda Roussel, DSN, RN, NEA, BC

LEARNING OBJECTIVES AND ACTIVITIES

- Identify core bioethic terms and basic ethical principles for the nurse administration in health care agencies.
- Describe professional ethics and a code of ethics for nursing.
- Define critical aspects of an ethics committee and the role of the nurse administrator.
- Identify major ethical dilemmas as they relate to managing health care services.
- Describe ethical issues related to collective bargaining.
- Describe traditional and nontraditional collective bargaining strategies to improve the patient care environment.
- Identify major reasons for greater unionization among professional nurses.
- Discuss the meaning of collective bargaining.
- Discuss the history of collective bargaining in nursing.
- Identify the characteristics of a profession and their relationship to collective bargaining.
- Identify and discuss the issues that lead to unions and collective bargaining.
- Describe the process of collective bargaining.
- Describe a grievance procedure and illustrate how it should work.
- Discuss the processes of arbitration and mediation.
- Discuss the benefits of collective bargaining.
- Discuss the ills of collective bargaining.

CONCEPTS

Bioethic terms, professional ethics, code of ethics, ethical dilemmas, ethical principles, ethics committee, managerial ethics, collective bargaining, professional employee, grievance, arbitration, supervisory influence, strike, organizational autonomy, mandatory overtime, unions

QUOTE

Sometimes leaders communicate by the most elegant and simple symbols—Gandhi nakedly facing his enemies, Churchill issuing a defiant sign for victory, Martin Luther King, Jr. standing resolutely behind bars.

—Howard Gardner

Maintains privacy and confidentiality of patients/consumers/staff and organizational data; advocates for nonjudgmental and nondiscriminatory behaviors in serving patients/consumers/staff in culturally diverse environments; designs human resource management policies to prevent possible union organizing activities; shares knowledge and skills with students, colleagues, and others, serves as a mentor and role model	Advocates for patients/consumers/personnel who are recipients of services; adheres to Code of Ethics with Interpretive Statements (American Nurses Association, 2001); complies with regulatory and professional standards as well as integrity of health care business practices; maintains processes to identify and address ethical issues and dilemmas; designs human resource management policies to make employment satisfying to employees and to facilitate open communication among employees and managers; establishes and facilitates a framework for professional nursing practice based on core ideology, which includes vision, mission, philosophy, core values, evidence-based nursing practice, and standards of practice

Introduction

Ethics is the discipline involved in the judgment of rightness or wrongness, unfairness or fairness, virtue or vice, ends, objects, or states of affairs. "Professions are defined in part by the ethics that govern their practice."[1] Morals and principles are incorporated into any discussion about ethics, ethical decision making, and ethical dilemmas. Collective bargaining also poses ethical issues for consideration in leading health care environments.

PROFESSIONAL ETHICS AND INTEGRITY

True professional status implies a code of ethics. Ethics has always been significant in professional nursing practice. This commitment has been further intensified with the establishment in 1990 of the Center for Ethics and Human Rights under the umbrella of the American Nurses Association (ANA). The Center's guiding mission is to address the complex ethical and human rights confronting nurses and to designate activities and programs that serve to increase ethical competence and human rights sensitivity of nurses.[2] Professional integrity reinforces the Code of Ethics for Nurses with Interpretive Statements and can be defined as strict adherence to a code of conduct.

Standard 11 in the Scope and Standards for Nurse Administrators describes the decisions and actions made by nurse administrators that are based on ethical principles. Measurement criteria are identified as follows[3]:

1. Advocates on behalf of recipients of services and personnel
2. Maintains privacy, confidentiality, and security of patient/client/resident, staff, and organization data
3. Adheres to the Code of Ethics for Nurses with Interpretive Statements[4]
4. Ensures confidentiality with regulatory and professional standards as well as integrity in business practices
5. Fosters a nondisciplinary climate in which care is delivered in a manner sensitive to sociocultural diversity
6. Ensures a process to identify and address ethical issues within nurses and the organization

This standard and the code of ethics provide a framework for decision making and managing health care systems.

Ethical Principles

Biomedical ethicists describe three primary principles—respect for persons, beneficence, and justice—that are sometimes stated as rules or obligations. Ethics addresses three types of moral problems: moral uncertainty (doubt about moral principles or rules that may apply or the nature of the ethical problem itself), moral dilemma (conflict of moral principles that support different courses of action), and moral distress (inability to take the action known to be right because of external constraints).[5]

The principle of respect for persons describes individuals' ability to take rational action and make moral choices. Autonomy, veracity (truth telling), confidentiality, and informed consent evolve from the principle of respect for persons.[6]

The principle of beneficence has two purposes: first, do no harm, and second, promote good. This principle is basic to those providing health care services and is often contradictory. For example, aggressive treatment causes pain and complications as it possibly promotes a positive outcome.[7]

The principle of justice involves fairness, rights, and obligation. The possible rationing of scarce resources may create ethical dilemmas and may be perceived as promoting or neglecting the principle of justice. For example, Mickey Mantle's liver transplant (given his history of alcoholism and later diagnosis of cancer) may have been perceived as preferential treatment and an unfair allocation of this limited resource.[8]

Ethical Theories

A number of ethical theories are foundational to health care and biomedical ethics. These theories provide principles and guidelines for ethical discussion and debates centered on ethical dilemmas. Using a theoretical framework when forming an ethics committee can further guide discussion and decision making. Useful theories include the utilitarianism theory of Jeremy Bentham (1748–1832) and John Stuart Mill (1806–1873), the natural rights theory of John Locke (1632–1704), and the contractarian theory of Thomas Hobbes (1588–1679). The consequentialist, or utilitarian, view purports that the consequences of our acts are of primary concern, that the means justify the ends, that one should consider the greatest good for the greatest number, and that the concepts of good and bad are personalized for each of us. John Locke's theory provided guidelines for the U.S. Declaration of Independence, which discusses our inalienable rights and the government's obligation to respect these rights. The contractarian theory states that morality involves a social contract, which provides the principles of what an individual can and cannot do.[9]

Other theoretical approaches, which are more traditional from a health care perspective, include the deontologic style (from the Greek root meaning "knowledge of that which is binding and proper") and teleologic style (from the Greek root meaning "knowledge of the end"). The deontologic approach assigns duty or obligation based on the intrinsic features of the act; the teleologic approach assigns duty or obligation based on the consequences of the act (its extrinsic nature).[10]

Holistic ethics has also been proposed as an ethical framework. "Holistic ethics is a philosophy that couples both reemerging and rapidly evolving concepts of holism and ethics."[11] Unity and integral wholeness of all people and of all nature is identified and sought out for unity and wholeness of self and within humanity. Dossey, Keegan, and Guzzetta further note that within this framework, "acts are not performed for the sake of law, precedent, or social norms; they are performed from a desire to do freely in order to witness, identify, and contribute to unity of the self and of the universe, of which the individual is a part."[12] Raising consciousness and being concerned about the effect of the act on an individual's larger self is the focus of holistic ethics. Decision making, problem solving, and the management of health care services can be guided by a holistic perspective, which considers all aspects within systems.

Ethical Terms

Ethical terms that are used in ethical discussions with health care providers provide a common language. Such terms may include the following[13]:

- *Autonomy:* One's actions are independent from the will of others. Moral autonomy denotes freedom to reach one's own values about what is right and wrong.
- *Beneficence:* Engaging in an act that is good or that brings about good effects
- *Competence:* Capacity to make decisions about the provision of medical care for oneself (decision-making capacity). Competence is also considered the legal capacity to make decisions.
- *Confidentiality:* Not divulging information that an individual considers secret
- *Consent:* One person voluntarily agrees to allow another to do something
- *Decision-making capacity:* One's ability to make decisions about the provision of medical care for oneself. This is a clinical determination that is specific to the decision at hand and, as such, may vary from time to time or from decision to decision (see Competence).
- *Euthanasia:* "Happy death" (Greek); has come to mean the deliberate ending of a human life. Active euthanasia refers to the direct killing of a patient. Passive euthanasia involves the withdrawal of medical technologies to allow the underlying disease to take its natural course. Voluntary euthanasia means that the act is undertaken at the behest of the patient and should be distinguished from nonvoluntary euthanasia, in which the patient has made no such request, and involuntary euthanasia, in which the action is performed against the patient's wishes.
- *Informed consent:* Generally, a formal written consent patients give to health care professionals expressing their complete understanding and agreement and allowing tests, procedures, or experimentation
- *Nonmaleficence:* Not performing actions that cause harm to patients
- *Obligations:* Responsibilities assumed by human beings toward one another by law, morality, custom, or tradition
- *Rights:* Justified claims upon others for actions or nonactions
- *Slippery slope argument:* If X is allowed, Y will follow, and Y is ethically unacceptable
- *Utilitarianism:* A normative ethical theory that advocates bringing about the greatest good for the greatest number of people; originally advocated by John Stuart Mill
- *Value:* Any object or quality that is found to be desirable or worthwhile

Other terms that may be useful to understand include the following:

- *Natural law:* Human good cannot be reduced to a mere function of what people desire; this theory considers the fulfillment of natural purpose, design, or essence.[14]
- *Feminist ethics:* An ethical framework that considers concepts that link relational autonomy, contextual reasoning, and indeterminate boundaries and that underscores caring[15]
- *Rights-based ethics:* An ethical theory that emphasizes the role of rights. One of the three kinds of

ethics developed by R. Dworkin; the others are goal-based ethics (utilitarianism) and duty-based ethics (Kantian ethics).[16]

- *Virtue-based ethics:* Recognizes the reality of the moral agent[17]

It is important to have a working knowledge of the above terms in discussing ethical concerns and issues. This serves as a foundation to working with ethics committees and provides some foundational information for this critical work.

DEVELOPING A HEALTH CARE ETHICS PROGRAM

A health care ethics program can be instrumental in developing ethical competence and creating a climate conducive to ethical practice. Clinical practice, research, and administration can reinforce ethical competence. "Competence in ethics requires moral sensibility, moral responsiveness, moral reasoning, and moral leadership."[18] A sound health care ethics program should support the mission, philosophy, strategic plans, and policies related to human resource management and patient care. The Joint Commission on Accreditation of Healthcare Organizations standards address ethical issues, specifically focusing on respect for patients, responding to patient values and preferences, and patient responsibilities.[19]

Elements of an ethics program include education, consultation, and policy development and review[20]:

1. *Education* includes classes and information on such topics as natural law, deontology, utilitarianism, emotionalism, feminist ethics, and others. Developing a glossary of terms useful to understanding the vocabulary of an ethics committee is also important and may include principles such as autonomy, justice, beneficence, nonmaleficence, veracity, and confidentiality. Discussing clinical topics related to services offered in the facility helps to make the information disseminated applicable to the management of ethical dilemmas within the organization.

2. *Consultation* requires individuals skilled in assessment, process, and interpersonal competencies. "Ethics consultation is often assigned to an individual or group with demonstrated competency and skill in ethics consultation."[21] The American Society for Bioethics and Humanities provides core competencies for successful ethics consultation.[22]

3. *Policy development* provides guidance to organizations in addressing ethical dilemmas. "Tasks that must be assigned are (a) reviewing existing policies from an ethical perspective; and (b) developing and writing policies on such topics as informed consent, withholding/withdrawing treatment, advance directives, surrogacy, DNR, medical futility, privacy, confidentiality, organ transplant, donation, and procurement, research, conflict of interest, impaired providers, conscientious objectors, and the use of reproductive and other technologies."[23]

Evidence-Based Practice 4-1

Jones found that offering ethics consultation reduces nonbeneficial life-sustaining treatments and that those patients receiving ethics consultation had fewer hospital, intensive care unit, and ventilation days than those who received usual care.[24]

Developing a health care ethics program gives support and a foundation to an organization's ethics committee, which responds to the many challenging dilemmas facing health care providers. Hospital ethics committees began to appear in the 1970s and gained a high profile in 1982, when two Kaiser Permanente physicians were charged with first-degree murder. The physicians were adhering to a family's wishes to remove intravenous feeding tubes from a comatose, severely brain-damaged patient. At the time of the investigation, the judge found no guidelines within the organization to handle these issues.[25] Ethics committees' responsibilities include the following[26]:

- Defuse existing fears within an institution.
- Educate caregivers on how ethics committees can be used for personal and professional benefit.
- Be knowledgeable and nonthreatening.
- Serve in an advisory role to aid and assist decision makers.
- Make available diverse values, knowledge, and experience.
- Not usurp authority from a primary physician.

Along with ethics committees, ethics networks and ethics centers are also important. Ethics quality indicators are particularly important to end-of-life care and caring for individuals who are seriously ill. Trinity Lutheran's medical staff put forth four performance improvement indicators related to end-of-life care[27]:

1. The patient's record contains physician documentation of the rationale for the patient's code status.
2. If the patient resuscitation category was changed during the patient's hospital stay, there is physician documentation by the physician about the reason for the change and patient/surrogate agreement.
3. If the patient has an advance directive, the wishes of the patient were followed.
4. For patients placed on life support, the record reflects
   a. That a meaningful discussion took place with the patient/surrogate.
   b. That the treatment decision supports the patient's known values and goals of life.

These guidelines and other types of protocols provide useful information in managing a clinical practice.

ETHICAL IMPLICATIONS FOR MANAGING A CLINICAL PRACTICE DISCIPLINE

Many ethical issues are directly related to the providing of patient care services. These have become more important since the 1990s because of several factors: the increased sophistication of medical science and technology; interprofessional relationships; organ donations and transplants; special concerns relating to patients with AIDS, the uninsured, the aged, and high-risk neonates; concern about practical limits on financial resources for health care; changes in society; and growing emphasis on the autonomy of the individual.[28]

Professional nurses implement the employer's policy concerning the moral responsibility of health care. Nurses have responsibility for supervising and reviewing patient care, meeting quality standards, making certain that decisions about patients are based on sound ethical principles, developing policies and mechanisms that address questions of human values, and responding to social problems and dilemmas that affect the need for health care services.[29]

To fulfill this responsibility, professional nurses support nurses confronted with ethical dilemmas and help them think through situations by open dialogue. Nurse managers establish the climate for this discussion. Davis recommends ethics rounds as a means of discussing ethical dilemmas. Such discussions can stem from hypothetical cases, case histories, or a case based on a current patient. Ethical reasoning requires participation by a knowledgeable person. Ongoing awareness and reinforcement of ethical principles and reasoning increases the organization's awareness of the nature of professional practice. Davis describes four ethical principles[30]:

1. *Autonomy.* Personal freedom of action is an ethical principle to be applied by nurse managers toward professional nurses, who in turn apply the principle in the care of their patients. The pro-

fessional nurse is given autonomy to deliberate about nursing actions and has the capacity to take nursing actions based on this deliberation. Hospitalized or ambulatory patients may have diminished autonomy, and the professional nurse becomes an advocate or autonomous agent for these patients' rights. The patient is responsible for making decisions about his or her care, and the family may be involved with the patient's consent.

2. *Nonmaleficence.* This ethical principle is defined as the avoidance of intentional harm or the risk of inflicting harm on someone. The use of restraints is an area that pits the principle of autonomy and self-determination against that of nonmaleficence. When risks outweigh costs, one must protect the patient. Side rails, safety vests, tranquilizers, and wrist restraints all have the potential for abuse. Discharge planning can prevent negative outcomes and potential errors. When errors occur, the nurse should acknowledge them to the patient or a surrogate, with full and immediate disclosure to the physician and the institution's administration. Nurses can protect patients from incompetent practitioners and protect their own rights at the same time.

3. *Beneficence.* Beneficence is the principle of viewing persons as autonomous, not harming them, and contributing to their health and welfare.

4. *Justice.* Justice involves giving people what is owed, deserved, or legitimately claimed.

The four ethical principles of autonomy, nonmaleficence, beneficence, and justice are being studied and debated in relation to nursing research and practice, to drug trials (including the use of placebo control subjects), and to cost-cutting in provider organizations.[31]

Many ethical issues relate to nursing and health care, including the issue of the right to health care. However, the United States does not provide health care as a matter of law. The following are some other ethical issues:

1. The rights of individuals and their surrogates versus the rights of the state or society. This issue creates confrontations between consumers and practitioners and may lead to management efforts to cut costs by cutting services (staff) or closing treatment centers. A survey of the Association of Community Cancer Centers indicated that 84% of these institutions staffed oncology units higher than other medical/surgical units.[32]

2. The rights of patients unable to make their own decisions weighed against the rights of patients' families and the rights of institutions

3. The rights of patients to forgo treatment versus the rights of society

4. Issues related to the following:
   a. Reproductive technology and preselection of desired physical characteristics of children; genetic screening
   b. Organ harvesting and transplants
   c. Research subjects
   d. Confidentiality
   e. Restraints
   f. Disclosure
   g. Informed consent
   h. Patient incapacity
   i. Court intervention

5. Reporting of ethical abuse of patients and staff

The ANA Committee on Ethics published several position statements and guidelines that seek to assist nurses in making ethical decisions in their practice. These guidelines are based on ethical theory and the ANA Code for Nurses, an expression of "nursing's moral concerns, goals, and values." They are designed to provide nurses with guidance on a range of ethical issues, including the withdrawing or withholding of food or fluid; risk versus responsibility in providing care; safeguarding client health and safety from illegal, incompetent, or unethical practices; nurses' participation in capital punishment; and nurses' participation and leadership in ethical review practices.[33]

Nurse managers need to know the legal framework for their actions. They should help clinical nurses to balance teaching, research, clinical investigation, and patient care. Practicing from an evidence-based framework provides a strong foundation for ethical work. All should work for social justice to ensure a desirable quality of life and health care services. Nurses may promote compassion and sensitivity through protest of public policies that reduce quality of or access to health care for the poor. Nurses should pursue human values, wholeness, and health values.[34] This does not mean that nurses must subsidize health care by working for lower salaries; rather, they should work to have the cost shared by all of society.

Evidence-Based Practice 4-2

A study of ethical issues and problems encountered by 52 nurses in their work in one hospital used a 32-item ethical-issues-in-nursing instrument. Results indicated that nurses encountered few ethical issues. The five most common issues were inadequate staffing patterns, the prolonging of life through heroic measures, inappropriate resource allocations, situations in which patients were being discussed inappropriately, and irresponsible activity of colleagues. Ethical issues were more frequent in critical care units than in medical or surgical units. The study group recommended institutional ethics committees and nursing ethics rounds to sensitize nurses to ethical issues.[35]

Evidence-Based Practice 4-3

A survey of institutions in the metropolitan New York area studied how nurses addressed ethical concerns in their practice. In this survey, 71 of 116 hospitals responded. Topics addressed by hospital ethics committees included allocation of resources, patients' rights, death and dying, abortion, prison health, and institutional issues. Formats used to address ethical issues included nursing meetings, in-service hospital committees, hospital ethics committees, and interdisciplinary rounds. All ethics committees had nursing representatives, mostly from administrative and management positions. It was concluded that most institutions do not adequately address nursing issues and concerns.[36]

Among the ethical dilemmas seldom addressed by nurse managers are ethical boundaries, particularly those involving sex. Nurse managers and administrators should provide continuing education to increase nurses' awareness of improper nurse–patient relationships, including accepting gifts and favors, doing business with patients and their families, being coerced or manipulated by patients, visiting patients at home while off duty, and making nontherapeutic disclosures. Risk environments include inpatient psychiatric services and chemical dependency treatment programs.[37]

Patients are sometimes denied pain relief by lazy or policy-focused providers, despite mandates for a patient's right to freedom from pain and pain management. Although letters to Ann Landers are not scientific, their anecdotes can be revealing. One writer wrote that a physician would not give her father pain medication the night before he died of terminal cancer because that physician would have had to walk to another unit for a small needle. In another letter, the wife of a terminal cancer patient requesting relief of intense pain was told by a nurse, "He has to wait another 30 minutes." The ethical and professional answer to such incidents is for assertive nurses to obtain adequate pain medication orders and implement them.[38]

One of the leading experts in nursing ethics, Leah Curtin, advocates creation of moral space for nurses to preserve their integrity. A nurse who believes an action to be wrong should not be forced to take that action. Curtin states that because ethics deals with values as well as with facts and interests, answers to ethical questions do not fall strictly within the bounds of any one discipline. Because ethical questions are complex, they are puzzling, even bewildering. Because any answer we frame touches many areas of concern, we cannot foresee all the consequences of the answers we choose. To solve an ethical problem, Curtin recommends that we do the following[39]:

1. Gather as much information as possible to understand precisely what the problem is.
2. Determine as many ways as possible to resolve the problem as they present themselves.
3. Consider the arguments for and against each alternative we can discover or imagine.

The nurse has an obligation to protect the welfare of patients and clients by virtue of his or her legal duties, the code for nurses, and nurses' social role. From a moral perspective, one must not knowingly harm another person. Any freely chosen human act is right insofar as it protects and promotes the human rights of individual nurses. Professionals have duties to guide their young colleagues, and nurses on all levels have mutual duties to support and guide one another.[40]

Values-based management stems from the actions of chief executive officers who set the stage for using a values credo of shared beliefs that govern the decisions and actions of top management. Two companies that do this are Levi Strauss & Company and Holt Companies. Their values include openness, teamwork, diversity, ethical behavior, and honest communication. Their priorities are ethics, human dignity, and self-fulfillment. The employees believe that they make important contributions to the company, customers, and the community. Such companies find that productivity and products increase as a result of this attention to ethics.[41]

Ethics committees should be established to prevent burnout. Their goals should include being a forum for expressing concerns, promoting awareness and education, participating in clinical decision making and policy and procedure development, developing professional identity, and communicating with other committees. Issues that are often reviewed by ethics committees are described in the following sections.[42]

Advance Directives

An advance directive is "a written instruction, such as a living will or a durable power of attorney for health care, recognized under state law (whether statutory or as recognized by the courts of the state) and relating to the provision of such care when the individual is incapacitated." Advance directives are mandated by the Patient Self-Determination Act (a provision of the Omnibus Budget Reconciliation Act of 1990).[43] Advance directives are considered necessary because people face choices about procedures to prolong life. Studies related to advance directives indicate the following[44]:

1. Use of proxies for persons with serious mental illness is neither meaningful nor beneficial.
2. Increased use of advance directives reduces use of health care services without affecting satisfaction or mortality of persons in nursing homes.
3. Elderly persons can use an interactive multimedia CD-ROM program to learn about advance directives.

The advance directive is a directive to physicians and other health care providers given in advance of incapacity with regard to a person's wishes about medical treatment. As an example, the Texas Natural Death Act gives a person the right to provide instructions about care when faced with a terminal condition. It covers such procedures as cardiopulmonary resuscitation, tube feeding, respirators, intravenous therapy, and kidney dialysis. A durable power of attorney for health care allows a person to name another person to make medical decisions for the incapacitated person.

A directive to physicians may be called a living will. The attending physician and another physician certify that a person has a terminal condition that will result in death in a relatively short time and that the person is comatose, incompetent, or otherwise unable to communicate.

An advance directive is a legal document. In Texas, for example, it does not have to be drawn up by a lawyer or notarized but does have to be witnessed. An oral statement suffices when made in the presence of two witnesses and the attending physician. Witnesses cannot be physicians, nurses, hospital personnel, fellow patients, or persons who will have claim against a person's estate.[45]

Under Texas law (Consent to Medical Treatment Act), the following people have the option to make medical decisions for an incompetent person: spouse, sole child who has written permission from all other children to act alone, majority of children, parents, a person whom the patient clearly identified before becoming ill, any living relative, or a member of the clergy (surrogate).[46]

Ethics in Business

Lee writes that all organizations should develop a policy on ethics. Business ethics helps people find the best way to satisfy the demands of competing interests. Ethics is part of corporate culture. Ethical organizations try to satisfy all of their stockholders, are dedicated to high purpose, are committed to learning, and try to be the best at whatever they do. Leaders of ethical organizations have the moral courage to change direction, hire brilliant subordinates, encourage innovation, stick to values, and persist over time. Polaroid established internal conferences on ethics in 1983 and 1984. These included philosophers, ethicists, and business professors who looked at the language and concepts of ethics. The conferences were broadened to include leadership and dilemma workshops to apply the knowledge to company cases.[47]

Nurse managers can explore similar modes of studying ethics. They can do so with clinical nursing staff to include looking at how business is done versus how it should be done. Such a study can set the organizational climate for ethical decision making. Ethics can be built into orientation, management development, participative management, and policies and procedures.

According to Beckstrand, "The aims of practice can be achieved using the knowledge of science and ethics alone."[48] To apply Beckstrand's theory to nursing management, nurse managers would apply their knowledge to change the nursing work environment to realize a greater good where and when needed.

Donley states that a health care system should be based on values that promote both the individual and the common good.[49] Limitations in nursing management knowledge can cause dilemmas for nurses. There could be a hierarchy of values in managing practice. Nurse managers need to determine how much decision-making power clinical nurses want and how much managers can delegate. A theory of ethics should be meshed with a theory of nursing management that is congruent with a theory of ethical conduct for clinical nurses.

Both clinical nurses and managers use scientific knowledge to determine whether conditions support change. The intrinsic value of the management actions should be given careful thought and should be debated by nurse managers who consciously attempt to practice management that realizes the highest good. The manager is more apt to be successful if scientific management knowledge is applied.

Ethics in management translated into nursing theory can be summed up as follows:

1. Nurse managers can influence the ethical behavior of nursing personnel by treating them ethically.
2. Nurse managers have a code of ethics on which peers have agreed. They enter into ethical dilemmas when they go against that code.
3. Nurse managers fall into moral dilemmas when they go against their internal values.
4. Although ethical and moral dilemmas differ, an ethical nurse manager is a moral nurse manager.

5. Ethical decisions can be clarified by three questions:
   a. Is it legal? This question resolves some dilemmas but not when questionable laws and policies are involved.
   b. Is it balanced? The nurse manager should aim for a win–win solution.
   c. How will it make me feel about myself? The nurse manager should consider the impact of each action on his or her self-respect.
6. Nurse managers with positive self-images usually have the internal strength to make the ethical decision.
7. An ethical leader is an effective leader.
8. Nurse managers should apply six principles of ethical power:
   a. The chief nurse executive promotes and ensures pursuit of the stated mission or purpose of the nursing division, because this statement reflects the vision of practicing nurses. Although the mission statement should be reviewed periodically, goals or objectives are set for yearly achievement.
   b. Nurse managers should build an organization to succeed, thereby building up employees through pride in their organization.
   c. Nurse managers should work to sustain patience and continuity through a long-term effect on the organization.
   d. Nurse managers should plan for persistence by spending more time following up on education and activities that build commitment of personnel.
   e. Nurse managers should promote perspective by giving their staff time to think. They should practice good management for the long term.
   f. Nursing service managers should consider developing an organization-specific code of ethics expressed in observable and measurable behaviors.[50]

A code of ethics should be ingrained in employees to create a strong sense of professionalism. Such a code should be the basis of a planned approach to all management functions of planning, organizing, leading, and evaluating. Nursing employees can help develop the code of ethics, help implement it, and determine its associated rewards and punishments. A code of ethics should be read and signed by employees and regularly reviewed and revised.

Contents of a code of ethics include definition of ethical and unethical practices, expected ethical behavior, enforcement of ethical practices, and rewards and punishments. To be objective, a code of ethics specifies rules of conduct. To be effective, it should be applied to all persons.[51]

ETHICS AND COLLECTIVE BARGAINING

Ethical decision making regarding work environment issues such as safety on the job and control over practice is important to professional practice. Transforming care at the bedside requires attention to the political as well as physical and emotional environment in the work site. Redesigning and negotiating for safe, healthy workplaces necessitates an understanding of collective bargaining, particularly in unionized work settings.

Improvement in wages, the primary purpose of collective bargaining in the past, is no longer the focal point of most negotiations. "Much more essential to nurses is assuring they have a safe practice environment free of mandatory overtime and other work issues, and a voice in the resource allocation decisions that affect their ability to achieve quality health outcomes for patients."[52] Control over practice, flexible scheduling, and a collegial environment are viewed as essential to a quality work life for professional nurses. Nurse activists note that finding processes, structures, and methods, such as collective bargaining, may offer nurses control over practice. This control is crucial to the survival of professional nursing in the face of an acute nursing shortage crisis.[53]

Research validates the importance of professional nurses having control of their practice; in fact, for many nurses this control is the deciding factor to remain in one's job and the profession. In 2001, Peter D. Hart Research Associates found that 21% of a sample of 700 nurses in current practice reported the desire to leave their positions due to stress and physical demands of work. Participants further reported that an improvement in staffing ratios would be a primary reason for remaining on the job and in the profession.[54] Nurses who had been in their positions longer than 5 years were asked why they remained. Satisfactory pay and benefits, collegial environment, and flexible scheduling were identified as the top reasons that nurses stayed longer than 5 years in their positions.[55] Additionally, research on shared governance models (which are prevalent in magnet hospitals) found positive patient outcomes; these models were also found to create nursing practice environments that attracted and retained professional nurses. Such structures were described as being conducive to autonomy and control over practice.[56] Recurrent themes are control over professional nursing practice, flexible schedules, and collegial respect.

These themes are also common subjects of collective bargaining agreements, which often cover the following issues[57]:

- Mandatory and voluntary overtime
- Acuity-based staffing systems
- Use of temporary nurses
- Protections from reassignments, work encroachment by non-nurses, and mandated non-nursing duties
- Provisions for work orientation and continuing education
- Whistle-blower protection
- Health and safety provisions, such as free hepatitis B vaccines
- "Just cause" language for discipline and termination
- Provisions for nursing and multidisciplinary practice committees

Collective Bargaining Defined

Collective bargaining is the "process by which organized employees participate with their employers in decisions about their rates of pay, hours of work, and other terms and conditions of employment."[58] Collective bargaining is the process through which the representatives of the employers and employees meet at reasonable times; confer in good faith about wages, hours, and other matters; and put into writing any agreements reached. The duty to bargain is required of both the employer and union.[59]

Collective bargaining is the means by which professional nurses can influence hospital nursing care delivery systems and labor–management relations through a united voice.[60] Collective bargaining is often viewed as a power relationship, either adversarial or cooperative.[61] Executives of firms have learned that employee empowerment and autonomy is good for business. As productivity increases, this knowledge has led to increased training of employees at the production level, elimination of middle management, decentralization of decision making with participatory management at the production level, and an upsurge in the success of the firm. This commitment to sharing power gives employees less reason to resort to collective bargaining.

The National Labor Relations Act of 1947 defines a professional employee as

> (a) any employee engaged in work (i) predominantly intellectual and varied in character as opposed to routine mental, manual, mechanical, or physical work; (ii) involving the consistent exercise of discretion and judgment in its performance; (iii) of such a character that the output produced or result accomplished cannot be standardized in relation to a given period of time; (iv) requiring knowledge of an advanced type in a field of science or learning customarily acquired by a prolonged course of specialized intellectual instruction and study in an institution of higher learning or a hospital, as dis-

tinguished from a general academic education or from an apprenticeship or from training in the performance of routine mental, manual, or physical processes; or (b) any employee who (i) has completed the courses of specialized intellectual instruction and study described in clause (iv) of paragraph (a), and (ii) is performing related work under the supervision of a professional person to qualify himself to become a professional employee as defined in paragraph (a).[62]

Strauss summarizes the characteristics of professional behavior[63]:

- Specialized education and expertise
- Autonomy
- Commitment
- Societal responsibility for maintenance of standards of work

Pavalko differentiates between professionals and other workers by stating that professionals have the following[64]:

- A systematic body of knowledge and theory as a basis for work and expertise
- Social ability in times of crisis; the professional is sought out by the public
- Specified training, including transmission of ideas, symbols, and skills
- Motivation for service to clients
- Autonomy, self-regulation, and control by individual practitioners
- A sense of long-term commitment
- A need for common identity and destiny, with shared values and norms
- A code of ethics

Professional nursing organizations have supported the development of nursing theory, the goal of self-regulation, and a code for nurses with interpretive statements. Such a code includes behaviors such as maintaining competency in nursing and participation in activities that contribute to the development of the profession's body of knowledge. When unable as individuals to attain their goals, professional nurses pursue them through collective bargaining.

Collective Bargaining Issues: Ethical Considerations

Issues that lead to petition for unions develop between employers and employees and usually occur because employers do not want to share power with employees. Historically, the chief executive officers of firms built bureaucratic organizations to retain power in the management structure. This has been costly for firms and has resulted in their restructuring to eliminate layers of management, empower employees with management knowledge and skills, and improve productivity and profits.

There are several major issues that lead to unions and collective bargaining[65]:

- Absence of procedures for reporting unsafe or poor patient care. Quality of patient care is the number one issue.
- Short staffing and improper skills mix to correspond to patient acuity
- Floating without orientation and training
- Use of temporary personnel and unlicensed assistive personnel
- Resistance of employers to accept joint decision making
- Adversarial relationships between nurses and management and exploitation of nurses by management
- Lack of respect for employees
- Lack of autonomy, that is, incursion by management into the scope of practice
- Lack of promotional opportunities
- Lack of professional practice committees

- Lack of staff development and continuing education opportunities
- Lack of child care and elder care
- Lack of involvement
- Poor differentials for shift work, education, and experience
- Low wages and limited benefits
- No pension portability
- Lack of employee assistance programs
- Poor on-call arrangements and lack of flexible schedules
- Overwork, mandatory overtime, and shift rotation
- Low morale
- Performance of non-nursing duties
- Poor management and poor communication
- No ability to take sufficient breaks
- Fair policies and practices for discipline and dismissal
- Assurance that patient classification systems have practicing nurse inputs
- Fair and consistent standards, policies, and practices
- Adequate health insurance
- Assurance that competence and qualification are considered with seniority
- Vacancy posting so that all nurses have an opportunity
- Lack of a system to apply peer review
- Lack of career ladders

The professional nurse works in an environment where human resources are not always valued but are viewed as a commodity. Professional nurses might get fired for such actions as questioning physician authority or refusing to work where they believe they are not qualified. Additionally, horizontal and lateral hostility in the workplace also increased risks to the health and safety for those in the workplace. Thus nurses often work in a climate of fear that results in poor morale, poor productivity, stifling of creativity, reluctance to take risks, ineffective communication, and reduced motivation.[66] Ultimately, these factors lead to an unbearable level of job stress, which culminates with a letter of resignation.

Process

Once nurses have decided to pursue collective bargaining because they believe they have no alternative, the general process is as follows:

1. An organization committee is formed. It should be broad-based in structure and representative of the major issues so as to represent all prospective members on all shifts and in all practice areas. Members should be well known and respected.
2. The major campaign issues are identified and discussed.
3. The organizing committee does research to obtain extensive knowledge of all facets of the institution, including history, structure, organization, finances, administration, and culture.
4. A timetable is prepared, delineating the specific organizing activities.
5. Possible employer tactics are identified and discussed, and specific strategies are developed to manage them.
6. A system is established for keeping in constant communication with nurses.
7. A structural plan is made, including adoption of a set of bylaws and election of officers.
8. Recognition occurs by the employer or National Labor Relations Board (NLRB) certification. Voluntary recognition requires authorization cards signed by a majority of nurses. If the employer does not recognize the action, NLRB certification requires that at least 30% of the nurses sign cards. A majority is best.[67]

9. An election is held in which nurses vote for or against a collective bargaining unit. The NLRB sets the election date by mutual agreement. Notices posted on employee bulletin boards include the date, hours, and places of election; payroll period for voter eligibility; description of the voting unit; a sample of the ballot; and general rules for conduct of the election. With a majority of voting nurses (50% plus 1) voting for it, the NLRB certifies the petitioners as the exclusive bargaining unit. If there is no majority, the NLRB will not accept another petition for 1 year.

10. A bargaining committee is elected by the nurses to negotiate a contract.[68]

11. A contract is negotiated. Members of the bargaining committee should survey the membership to gather data for contract proposals. At the first bargaining meeting proposals are made. The easiest ones should be settled first. Management strategy will be to try to set the tone of the sessions and to package proposals so that they can slip some past the nurses. Their strategies will include flattery, conciliation, anger, astonishment, and total silence. For this reason, nurse members should track all proposals using minutes of the meetings and make index cards listing the proposals of each side. Debriefings at the end of each session are helpful. The nurse team should respond to management with care, spirit, and no unconditional concessions.[69]

12. When all proposals have been fully discussed and agreed on, the contract is written.

13. The contract is then presented to union members who vote to ratify or reject it. If ratified, it is signed by both sides.

14. The contract is enforced through grievance and arbitration procedures. It is reviewed or amended on a regular basis.[70]

Grievance Procedures

A strong grievance procedure increases employee satisfaction, so it is a good human resource management tool, with or without a union. Potential trouble spots are identified early and may include claims for higher wages when jobs are modified. Grievance procedures must be perceived as fair. Their contents should be told to all employees, and managers should be trained to follow them. This training allays managers' fears.[71]

The grievance policy should be communicated as an employee benefit and included in the personnel handbook (Figure 4-1). Peer review should be used in employee appraisals involving grievances and final decisions. Some courts have equated peer review to due process. Peer review builds values of conflict resolution, teamwork, decision making at lower levels, employee empowerment, and ownership.[72]

Eldridge suggests the following points for effective settlement of grievances[73]:

1. Accurate definition of the problem: Does it violate the contract or the law? Is it timely? Documented?

2. Timely presentation: Follows the time limits and steps of the grievance procedure and for notifying appropriate persons.

3. Documentation: Facts; claim adjustment desired; form signed, dated, and given to appropriate persons.

4. All stops are performed with a businesslike attitude to facilitate objectivity and communication.

Nursing is difficult, complex, and requires specialized knowledge. All nurses should commit to a written employment agreement with a grievance procedure. This should be done whether they represent themselves or are represented by a union. When nurses use a labor organization, they should use one with a large membership and a long and successful history.[74] The ANA and some State Nurses Associations fall into this category.

FIGURE 4-1   SAMPLE EMPLOYEE GRIEVANCE PROCEDURE

GRIEVANCES AND DISCIPLINARY ACTIONS

4.1 GRIEVANCE AND APPEAL PROCESS

Metropolitan Medical Center provides a means for you, as a regular employee who has completed the probationary period, to appeal disciplinary actions, including dismissal, suspension, or demotion when used as a disciplinary action, that you believe are unjust or to submit a grievance for any working condition that results in inequities or other situations which have a negative effect on morale. The Medical Center, in its sole discretion, reserves the right to determine whether an action is a management right as outlined in Section 4.5 of this Handbook and, therefore, not subject to grievance and/or appeal. Layoffs and written warnings may not be appealed.

This process may be used in a situation where there are allegations that an individual has been discriminated against based on race, sex, religion, color, national origin, age, disability, disabled veteran, or Vietnam Era veteran status. In such an event, if the individual against whom such allegations have been made is either in the first or second step of the grievance and appeal process, the employee should contact the Department of Human Resources to institute a grievance. This process is available to an employee who alleges such discrimination is related to the issue of sexual harassment.

Employees in their probationary period may only appeal if they believe they have been discriminated against on the basis of race, sex, religion, color, national origin, age, disability, disabled veteran, or Vietnam Era veteran status. Additionally, this process is available to a probationary employee who alleges such discrimination is related to the issue of sexual harassment.

4.1.1 First Step

If you are considering initiating a grievance or appeal, you should first discuss the matter with your Department Head. You should state your case, in writing, to your Department Head and state the adjustment desired. This should be done within 10 working days of the occurrence.

4.1.2 Second Step

If your grievance is not settled to your satisfaction with your Department Head, you may appeal, in writing, to your Assistant Hospital Administrator within 10 working days of the response to step one.

4.1.3 Third Step

If your grievance is not handled to your satisfaction in step two, you may appeal, in writing, to your Division Head within 10 working days of the response to step two.

4.1.4 Final Step

If your grievance is not handled to your satisfaction in step three, you may request, in writing, the Assistant Vice President of Human Resources to schedule a hearing before the Staff Grievance and Appeal Committee.

A hearing before the committee is a nonadversarial proceeding, and attorneys are not allowed to participate on either side. You may select another university employee who is both willing and able to arrange his or her work schedule accordingly to represent you in the grievance/appeal hearing.

The committee's recommendations are presented to the Vice President for Financial Services for a final decision. The Assistant Vice President of Human Resources will advise the concerned parties of the decision and assist in any personnel action required.

4.2 Disciplinary Guidelines

Disciplinary guidelines have been established by the Metropolitan Medical Center so that you and other employees will be accorded a process of progressive discipline as set forth in these guidelines. The guidelines on the following pages show example violations and the degree of disciplinary action that may be required for each.

Your supervisor has the authority to determine an appropriate corrective measure through disciplinary action for any other violation of conduct not listed in the guidelines. The Medical Center reserves the right to change the particular type of discipline noted on the listed guidelines, due to the extent and severity of a particular offense. In some instances, even though previous violation of policy has not occurred, the severity of the offense may result in disciplinary action, up to and including dismissal.

So that the safety and productivity of all employees of the Medical Center is ensured, a progressive disciplinary program has been established. If you fail to observe the accepted norm of behavior, your super-

(continues)

visor may issue either a verbal or written warning. Written warnings will be made a part of your permanent personnel file. Oral and written warnings may not be appealed. A layoff may not be appealed as it is not a disciplinary action.

4.2.1 Felony Charges

If you, as a regular or temporary employee of the Medical Center, are charged with a felony offense, you shall be suspended without pay pending the outcome of your trial. A temporary or grant-funded employee who is charged with a felony offense shall be suspended without pay pending the outcome of the trial or the ending date of the employee's temporary appointment or grant funding, whichever is earlier. You are responsible for notifying your supervisor if you are charged with a felony offense.

If you are suspended without pay because of a felony charge and are otherwise eligible for benefits, you may continue to participate in the group medical and life insurance programs. You are responsible for making arrangements with the Payroll Office to pay the total monthly premium costs for these benefits. If you are convicted of a felony offense, you shall be immediately dismissed.

If you are found not guilty of the felony offense as charged, you shall be reinstated with back pay for the period during which you were suspended without pay pending outcome of your trial with no break in service and you shall retain accrued vacation and sick leave benefits. A temporary or grant funded employee shall be reinstated with back pay until the ending date of the employee's temporary appointment or grant funding, whichever is earlier.

Mediation

Mediation is assisted negotiation. When the negotiating parties cannot reach agreement on an issue during contract negotiations or during a labor dispute unresolved by grievance procedures, the issue is referred to a mediator trained to resolve such disputes. The mediator assists the parties in defining the issues, dissolving obstacles to communication, exploring alternatives, facilitating the negotiations, and reaching an agreement. In law cases, mediation works 80% of the time or more.[75]

Successful mediation involves good faith: All parties are present during the entire mediation session; there is adequate time; the mediator lays ground rules, describes the process, and answers questions; the session is private; the parties are separated into "caucuses" in which their conversations are private; and the mediator shuttles between parties until a settlement is reached. The parties negotiate the settlement.[76]

Arbitration

Whereas a mediator works with the parties in a dispute to get them to resolve their differences, an arbitrator examines the facts and makes a decision that is binding. Arbitration uses as the source of law the express provisions of the contract, past practices of the industry, and the shop (health care and nursing). Past practices must[77]

- Be unequivocal (clear, consistent, acceptable); be accepted by the people involved as the normal and proper response to the underlying circumstances presented
- Have longevity; have existed for a sufficient length of time to have developed a pattern
- Have mutuality; both parties regard the conduct as correct and customary in handling the situation

Practices that are long-standing and have been accepted by both parties are as binding as if written. Subjects not covered in the agreement are the residual rights of management, including the methods of operation and direction of the workforce. Union rights include areas of benefits, wages, and working conditions. Unchallenged customs and practices are considered accepted as part of the agreement by both parties. Arbitrators should effectuate the agreement and contain conflict.[78]

Supervisory Influence

With the power of unions generally declining, goals for unions of professional nurses are best met by multipurpose organizations that can respond and adapt to the particular concerns of nurses, such as "supervisory influence." Generally, employers raise these concerns with relation to who will represent professional nurses. Rank-and-file nurses may be concerned that nurse managers will dominate the bargaining unit through membership in the SNA. The bargaining unit needs some insulation from SNA members who are managers. The issue usually extends beyond legal characterizations to political overtones of power and control within the organization. The California Nurses Association established the legal standard on the issue of supervisory influence in the Sierra Vista case in 1979. This standard is best met by an integrated, multipurpose professional association as a bargaining agent.[79] This agent would include and meet the needs of clinical nurses of all specialties along with nurse managers, educators, and researchers who are members of the SNA.

Advantages of Unionization

Unions view the health care field as a potential pool for membership, which is a threat to hospital leaders. Concrete evidence shows "that collective bargaining, when used effectively, actually facilities delivery of the best care and services."[80]

Collective bargaining has contributed to the high standard of living for the working people of Western countries. Employee compensation levels are higher when they are determined at the bargaining table.[81]

Collective bargaining is viewed by employees as an enforceable way to secure justice in the workplace and a way for them to share power with employers. It provides fundamental protection against arbitrary or unfair treatment in the matter of promotions, remuneration, dismissal, and retirement. The bargaining agreement or contract balances management power with the combined might of all the employees. Protection under collective bargaining is greater than the contract itself. Unfair management authority can be challenged through a grievance system.[82] Contracts with nurses frequently include reference to the ANA code for nurses and standards of nursing practice.[83]

Research indicates that nurses have been reluctant to exercise collective power. Involvement peaks during organizing activity and in times of crisis or conflict. Nurses are more involved with committees related to the nursing product than with those related to bargaining unit affairs.[84]

The Michigan Nurses Association views its members as nurses who have combined the philosophies of professional nursing care and collective bargaining. The goal of this association is protection of patients through protection of nurses' professional and economic rights.[85]

Contracts give nurses input on nursing care standards, policies, and procedures. Unions improve working conditions related to shift rotation, floating, non-nursing duties, flexible staffing, meal breaks, rest periods, time away from work, continuing education, tuition reimbursement, educational leave, grievance and arbitration procedures, maternity/paternity leave, discipline, posting of vacancies, recall from layoffs, peer review, career ladders, joint committees to improve safety and quality of patient care, and adherence to the code for nurses.[86]

The success of unions depends on the quality of the work environment and the credibility and effectiveness of the organization as a bargaining agent and workplace advocate.[87] Outcomes of labor negotiations depend on employee and employer relationships, attitudes, and philosophies.[88] Evidence on unionization estimate that union members average salaries that are 6% higher than those of nonunion workers.[89]

Hannah and Shamian state that the foundation of modern nursing is a professional practice model of nursing. This model can be achieved through collective bargaining and nursing information. The following are the characteristics of a professional practice model of nursing[90]:

- Multidisciplinary and interdisciplinary collaboration
- Accountability
- Practice based on a sound and discipline-specific scholarly foundation (i.e., knowledge, theory, and inquiry)
- Autonomy rooted in a clear understanding of the scope and boundaries of the discipline of nursing
- Awareness of the sociopolitical context of practice

- Self-motivated professional development, including self and peer evaluation, aimed at maintaining currency of practice knowledge

The professional practice model of nursing care can be achieved through functional, team, primary, or case management methodologies. The best environment is a decentralized organizational structure using self-governance. Collective bargaining environments can be suitable for a professional practice model of nursing that provides for career mobility, advancement, and wage increases using criteria beyond mere seniority.[91]

The purposes of collective bargaining include "facilitating communication between the parties to the contract; establishing and maintaining mutually satisfactory salaries, hours of work, and working conditions; prompt disposition of differences of opinion or grievances; and resolution of disputes."[92] The goal is collaboration. A fully implemented nursing information system provides clinical data quickly; improves nurses' work; and coordinates management activities, physician-delegated tasks, and professional nursing practice. Decision-support systems are information systems designed to provide the information needed to make clinical decisions about patient care. Inputted data (such as history and test results) are processed against stored data to give decision outputs, such as differential nursing diagnosis and suggested therapeutic recommendations.

Source data entry should be conducted from bedside terminals or through two-way radio transmission. Patient discharge abstracts should be expanded to include nursing care delivery information. A nursing minimum data set is available. The collective bargaining unit can be a powerful ally to nursing management in integration of a professional practice model of nursing informatics.[93]

Disadvantages of Unionization

Unions cost money and create adversarial relationships. They focus on seniority rather than merit. Before joining a union, the nurse should study its experience or history and its track record. The nurse should talk to union members, tally the annual costs for dues and fees, and read the financial statement.[94]

Because they are elected as are politicians, union officials have a vested interest in maintaining a combative relationship with management. Unions may discourage hard work and personal ambition while encouraging dependence.[95]

Once nurses gain collective bargaining status they exhibit low participation in related activities. A survey of 261 registered nurses employed in voluntary hospitals in New York State and represented by the New York State Nurses Association for collective bargaining produced the following results[96]:

1. Few nurses attended union meetings regularly, although more did than do blue-collar workers.
2. Only 10.3% of respondents attended union conventions. Excuses included family responsibilities, location, expense, time off, and lack of interest.
3. Members read literature from the bargaining agent.
4. Few nurses submit bargaining demands.
5. Of respondents, 45% voted in local bargaining unit elections and 35% in statewide elections.
6. About two-thirds read the bargaining agreement.
7. Few file formal grievances. Of those who did file, 65% filed for professional concerns and 37.5% for economic concerns. One-third knew little about the grievance procedure. They handled grievances informally first.
8. Nurses do not appear to be prepared to assume leadership roles in bargaining units.
9. College-educated nurses were more aggressive about work stoppages and picketing.

The writer concluded that "nurses who have adopted collective bargaining and who fail to exercise their responsibilities are responsible for the abridgement of their own rights and the success or failure of collective bargaining in their institutions."[97]

Strikes

Strikes are usually a last resort. Striking nurses are frequently portrayed in a negative way by the media. A content analysis of 893 U.S. newspaper articles presented a more negative image of the nurse than did newspaper articles on other nursing subjects. There were more negative headlines, criticism of nurses, and negative relationships reported in the articles about strikes. A desire for higher salaries was the major strike issue reported by newspapers, conveying the message that nurses were more interested in personal economic gain than in quality of patient care.[98]

Causal factors may contribute to a strike vote[99]:

1. Perceived lack of responsiveness by nurse administrators in solving everyday problems experienced by nursing staff
2. Fear of change experienced by nursing staff
3. Resistance by nurses to the national trend of using unlicensed, assistive personnel to reduce operating costs
4. Perceived reduction in benefits for the nursing staff
5. Environmental and workplace health and safety concerns
6. Perceived inequities in salaries between the nursing staff and senior executives

Firing striking workers is illegal, but it is standard management strategy for companies to threaten to hire permanent replacements. Companies are then obligated to hire former strikers only as future openings occur. Approximately 21,000 workers in U.S. companies lost their jobs through permanent replacement policies. Organized labor has been unable to obtain federal legislation banning replacement of employees who strike. In 1938 the Supreme Court ruled that permanent replacements are legal.[100]

Vulnerability

There has been increased interest in collective bargaining among health care workers since the 1991 Supreme Court decision. The long-term goal of the ANA is to "enable the country's two million nurses to achieve control over their own practice and work environment."[101] If nurse administrators wish to avoid dealing with collective bargaining units, they should create the conditions under which nurses have equivalent control.

The signs and symptoms of increased vulnerability to collective bargaining activity are those of an unhealthy environment[102]:

1. Increased nursing staff turnover
2. Increased employee-generated incidents
3. Increased grievances filed
4. Breakdown in communication
5. Sudden changes in staff behavior
6. Increased inquiries about personnel policies and practices
7. Changes in behavior of "problem children"
8. Pro-union, collective bargaining, or professional organization literature, posters, or graffiti
9. Organization of and invitation to off-site meetings for staff members only
10. Formation and submission of petitions
11. Managers' "gut" feelings

Nurse administrators should do a formal assessment of collective bargaining and make a plan for action that prevents it. Some of the activities to consider in this plan of action are training of front-line management in communications, counseling, mentoring, participatory management, shared governance, and addressing quality-of-care issues immediately.[103] Other actions to take include the following:

- Make the nurses feel like stakeholders. This is especially important with advanced, technically trained nurse specialists.
- Make nurses feel connected and invested in their work so they can be creative and productive.
- Prepare nurses to increase their role functions as members of interdisciplinary teams.
- Examine the possibility of new partnership models with nurses: shared ownership, gain sharing, bonuses, pay for performance, outcome pay, per diem contracting, caseload payment structures, benefit smorgasbords, increased autonomy of work, participation, and self-managed teams.
- Work can be redesigned as a result of union leadership and management partnership, with mutually formed mission, goals, and planning for the future.[104]

Collective bargaining is unnecessary when nurses and management communicate well and participate in decision making. It is unnecessary when nurses receive adequate support and appropriate recognition. Nurses should be provided with a voice in decision making, resources to do the job, safeguarding of standards of nursing practice, protection of employment rights, and attractive terms and conditions of employment.[105] These are all aspects of a model of Human Resource Management that works and that keeps nurse employees happy.

One of the most important benefits of collective bargaining is increased job security. Nurses can be fired for economic reasons and for incompetence, but management should be sure terminations are done only for good and just causes. Laws prevent discrimination on the basis of sex, race, religion, national origin, age, handicap, and for some types of whistle-blowing. The NLRA prevents discrimination on the basis of union activity. Termination should never be related to acts violating public policy or for refusal to perform an illegal practice.[106]

The employer is considered to have the absolute right to determine staffing patterns, ratios, and other personnel requirements. Employers should consider input from nurses in formulating standards of nursing practice; providing education benefits; and ridding nurses of non-nursing work; and for hiring, promotions, and transfers.[107]

ETHICS AND GOOD WORK IN NURSING

Gardner and colleagues proposed a tool kit reflective of their Good Work Project which strives for excellence, ethics, and engagement in the professions. According to Gardner,[108]

> The Good Work® Project is a large scale effort to identify individuals and institutions that exemplify good work—work that is excellent in quality, socially responsible, and meaningful to its practitioners—and to determine how best to increase the incidence of good work in our society.

The Good Work Project provides a variety of references and resources, along with courses, a tool kit, and traveling curriculum to help increase ethical, professional work. Miller, through her work with the Good Work Community of Interest through Sigma Theta Tau International, use these resources to better define Good Work in Nursing.[109]

Evidence-Based Practice 4-4

Paolillo and Vitell conducted an exploratory study of ethical decision making by individuals in organizations. The researchers found that moral intensity, as defined by Jones (1991), significantly influences ethical decision-making intentions of managers. According to the researchers, moral intensity explained 37% and 53% of the variance in ethical decision making in two decision-making scenarios. The research, in part, supports the need for a theoretical understanding of ethical/unethical decision making and serves as a foundation for future research.[110]

SUMMARY

The ANA's *Scope and Standards for Nurse Administrators* identifies ethics and ethical principles as critical to the nurse administrator's decisions and actions. This includes adherence to the Code of Ethics for Nurses with Interpretive Statements as well as compliance with regulatory and professional standards. Integrity in business practices requires checks and balances to decisions and actions taken within health care systems. Ethics committees, ethics networks, and ethics centers heighten awareness of patients' rights and consumer protection. Understanding ethical theories and principles guides thinking and decision making. Developing a health care ethics program requires education, consultation, and policy review. Identifying ethics quality indicators further advances a health care ethics program and increases the competency of those involved in analyzing ethical dilemmas. As technologies of patient treatment develop and the health care delivery system evolves around managed care, nurses need avenues to pursue the ensuring ethical dilemmas.

Collective bargaining through unionization is a process whereby employees join together to gain collective power that somewhat neutralizes the power of management. Ethical consideration should also be given to the collective bargaining process. Collective bargaining has been used in the nursing profession for over 50 years. In 1991 the U.S. Supreme Court affirmed the ruling of the NLRB that professional nurses could form a distinctly separate bargaining unit within hospitals.

Issues related to collective bargaining include pay, benefits, and conditions of work related to provision of quality care to patients. Many professional nurses are reluctant to use the process of collective bargaining. Those who do put the safety of patients above their own concerns.

Implementing the theory of human resource management that puts trust in employees by training them to manage themselves is the best management strategy to deter collective bargaining. Nursing and health care leaders who work collaboratively with practicing clinical nurses through decentralization and participatory management prevent collective bargaining. It has been proven time and again that people who manage their own work and who make professional decisions about their practice increase the productivity and profitability of the firm.

APPLICATION EXERCISES

Exercise 4-1

Form a group of six to eight peers. Each group member identifies and describes, orally or in writing, an ethical dilemma. Discuss each dilemma from the viewpoints of care for the patient and support for the caregiver. What are the implications for interpersonal relationships among caregivers and care recipients?

Exercise 4-2

Set up two teams to debate the following issue:

Professional nurses should intervene in instances in which they observe unethical conduct or illegal or unprofessional activities

   Versus

Professional nurses should not intervene in instances in which they observe unethical conduct or illegal or unprofessional activities.

Select a moderator. Decide on rules for selection and then decide on rules of procedure. For example, each speaker from each side may be allowed to speak to a question for 3 minutes.

   Consider the following questions:

1. What is the individual responsibility of the professional nurse employee in instances where he or she observes unethical conduct or illegal or unprofessional activities by the employer?

2. What is the responsibility of professional nursing organizations once they are made aware of such instances?
3. What is the responsibility of community organizations if they are made aware of such instances?

Consider the following issues:

- Accreditation action
- Government action (Medicare)
- Publicity (media)
- Prevention

Exercise 4-3

Examine organizational policies related to patients' rights as well as statements made by nursing associations and hospital associations and articles in professional journals. What authority or source would lead one to believe that the patient has a right to know his or her nursing diagnosis, the goals of care related to that diagnosis, and the nursing actions prescribed to meet those goals? What authority or source would lead one to believe that the patient has a right to assist in the planning of his or her nursing care? What authority or source would lead one to believe that the patient has a right to know what to expect as a result of his or her nursing care?

Exercise 4-4

Interview a professional nurse who is a member of a union. Determine his or her perceptions of the benefits of collective bargaining. What does he or she perceive as the weaknesses of collective bargaining?

Exercise 4-5

Prepare a plan to evaluate the vulnerability of a health care organization to collective bargaining. Use it to assess the organization. Prepare a list of recommendations for decreasing the vulnerability of the organization to collective bargaining. Present the results to the nurse administrator. This exercise may be done by a small group of nurse managers or students.

Notes

1. Baker, L., & Marquis, B. (Eds). (2003). *Nursing administration review and resources manual* (p. 67). Washington, DC: Institute for Research, Education, and Consultation at the American Nurses Credentialing Center.
2. Ibid.
3. American Nurses Association. (2004). *Scope and standards for nurse administrators* (2nd ed.). Washington, DC: Author.
4. Ibid., p. 27.
5. Dossey, B. M., Keegan, L., & Guzzetta, C. E. (2005). *Holistic nursing: A handbook for practice* (4th ed., p. 94). Sudbury, MA: Jones and Bartlett.
6. Veatch, R. M. (Ed.). (2002). *Medical ethics.* Upper Saddle River, NJ: Prentice Hall.
7. Orentlicher, D. (2001). *Matters of life and death: Making moral theory work in medicine and the law.* Princeton, NJ: Princeton University Press.
8. Fowler, M. (1989). Ethical decision making in clinical practice. *Nursing Clinics of North America, 24,* 955–965.
9. Milner, S. (1993). An ethical practice model. *Journal of Nursing Administration, 23,* 22–25.
10. Ibid.
11. Dossey et al., 2005, p. 96.
12. Ibid.

13. Ibid.
14. Kantor, J. E. (1989). *Medical ethics for physicians-in-training*. New York: Plenum Medical Book Company.
15. Wolf, S. (1996). Introduction: Gender and feminism in bioethics. In S. Wolf (Ed.), *Feminism and bioethics: Beyond reproduction* (pp. 3–45). New York: Oxford University Press.
16. Bandman, E., & Bandman, B. (2002). Nursing ethics through the life span (4th ed., p. 294). Upper Saddle River, NJ: Prentice Hall.
17. Veatch, 2002.
18. Turner, M. (2003). A toolbox for healthcare ethics program development. *Journal for Nurses in Staff Development, 19,* 9–15.
19. Joint Commission on Accreditation of Healthcare Organizations. (1996). *Comprehensive accreditation manual for hospitals.* Oakbrook Terrace, IL: Author.
20. Turner, 2003.
21. Ibid.
22. Worthley, J. A. (1999). *Organizational ethics in the compliance context.* Chicago, IL: Health Administration Press.
23. Pellegrino, E. D. (2000). Interview with Edmund D. Pellegrino, M.D. In M. Boylan (Ed.), *Medical ethics* (pp. 25–36). Upper Saddle River, NJ: Prentice Hall.
24. Jones, T. (2004). Ethics consultations reduced hospital, ICU, and ventilation days in patients who died before hospital discharge in the ICU. *Evidence-Based Nursing, 7,* 53.
25. Eckberg, E. (1993). The continuing ethical dilemma of the do-not-resuscitate order. *The Association of Perioperative Registered Nurses, 67,* 784.
26. Ibid.
27. Christopher, M. (2001). Role of ethics committees, ethics networks, and ethics centers in improving end-of-life care. *Pain Medicine, 2,* 162.
28. Special Committee on Biomedical Ethics. (1985). *Values in conflict: Resolving ethical issues in hospital care.* Chicago, IL: American Hospital Association.
29. Ibid.
30. Davis, A. J. (1982). Helping your staff address ethical dilemmas. *Journal of Nursing Administration, 29*(6), 9–13.
31. Flaherty, M. (1999, August 30). Search for answers: Drug trials create ethical balancing act. *HealthWeek, 1,* 10; Noble-Adams, R. (1999). Ethics and nursing research, 1: Development, theories and principles. *British Journal of Nursing,* 888–892; Dwyer, M. L. (1998). Genetic research and ethical challenges: Implication for nursing practice. *AACN Clinical Issues,* 600–605; Kawas, C. H., Clark, C. M., Farlow, M. R., Knopman, D. S., Marson, D., Morris, J. C., et al. (1999). Clinical trials in Alzheimer disease: Debate on the use of placebo controls. *Alzheimer Disease & Associated Disorders, 19,* 124–129; Brommels, M. (1999). Sliced down to the moral backbone? Ethical issues of structural reforms in healthcare organizations. *Acta Oncology, 38,* 63–69.
32. Mortenson, L. E. (1984). Are oncology nurses too expensive? *Oncology Nursing Forum,* 14–15; Committee on Ethics, American Nurses Association. (1988). *Ethics in nursing: Position statements and guidelines.* Kansas City, MO: Author.
33. American Nurses' Association. (1988). *Ethics in nursing: Position statements and guidelines.* Kansas City, MO: Author.
34. Sauer, J. E. (1985). Ethical problems facing the healthcare industry. *Hospital & Health Services Administration,* 44–53.
35. Berger, M. C., Seversen, A., & Chvatal, R. (1991). Ethical issues in nursing. *Western Journal of Nursing Research,* 514–521.
36. Scanlon, T. M., & Fleming, C. (1990). Confronting ethical issues: A nursing survey. *Nursing Management, 5,* 63–65.
37. Pennington, S., Gafner, G., Schilit, R., & Bechtel, B. (1993). Addressing ethical boundaries among nurses. *Nursing Management, 7,* 36–39.
38. Landers, A. (1994, June 17). Pain-free death is a right worth defending. *San Antonio Express-News,* p. 5J.
39. Curtin, L. L. (1993). Creating moral space for nurses. *Nursing Management,* 18–19.
40. Curtin, L. L. (1992). When the system fails. *Nursing Management,* 21–25.

41. Konstam, P. (1992, December 12). Values-based system focuses on ethics. *San Antonio Light,* p. D1.

42. Buchanan, S., & Cook, L. (1992). Nursing ethics committees: The time is now. *Nursing Management,* 40–41.

43. U.S. Cong. House. 101st Congress, 2nd Session. S. 4206, Medicare provider agreements assuring the implementation of the patients right to participate in and direct health care delivery affecting the patient [introduced in the U.S. House; 26 October 1990]. 101st Congress. Congressional Record-House, H12456–H12457.

44. Murphy, C. P., Sweeney, M. A., & Chiriboga, D. (2000). An educational intervention for advance directives. *Journal of Professional Nursing,* 21–30; Molloy, D. W., et al. (2000). Systematic implementation of an advance directive program in nursing homes: A randomized controlled trial. *JAMA,* 1437–1444; Geller, J. L. (2000). The use of advance directives by persons with serious mental illness for psychiatric treatment. *Psychiatric Quarterly,* 1–13; Burt, J. G. (1999). Compliance with advance directives: A legal view. *Critical Care Nursing Quarterly,* 72–74.

45. Bexar County Hospital District. (1991). *Understanding advance directives: Your rights as a patient.* San Antonio, Texas: Author.

46. Premack, P. (1993, July 23). Medical OK law has a key change. *San Antonio Express-News,* p. 11D.

47. Lee, C. (1986). Ethics training: Facing the tough questions. *Training,* 30–33, 38–41.

48. Beckstrand, J. (1978). The need for a practice theory as indicated by the knowledge used in the conduct of practice. *Research in Nursing and Health,* 175–179.

49. Donley, R. (1993). Ethics in the age of health care reform. *Nursing Economics,* 19–23.

50. Fernicola, K. C. (1988). Take the high road . . . to ethical management: An interview with Kenneth Blanchard. *Association Management,* 60–66.

51. Mizock, M. (1986). Ethics: The guiding light of professionalism. *Data Management,* 16–18, 29.

52. Budd, K. W., Warino, L. S., & Patton, M. E. (2004). Traditional and non-traditional collective bargaining: Strategies to improve the patient care environment. *Online Journal of Issues in Nursing.* Retrieved July 24, 2005, from http://www.nursingworld.org/ojin/topic23/tpc23_5.htm

53. Goodin, H. J. (2003). Collective bargaining. *Journal of Advanced Nursing, 43,* 335–350; McClure, M. L., Poulin, M. A., Sovie, M. D., & Wandelt, M. A. (2002). Magnet hospitals: Attraction and retention of professional nurses (the original study). In M. L. McClure, & A. S. Hinshaw (Eds.), *Magnet hospitals revisited: Attraction and retention of professional nurses.* Washington, DC: American Nurses Publishing.

54. Peter D. Hart Research Associates. (2003). *The nurse shortage: Perspectives from current direct care nurses and former direct care nurses.* Retrieved December 1, 2003, from http://www.aft.org/healthcare/downloadfiles/Hart_Report.pdf

55. Lacey, L. M. (2003). Called into question: What nurses want. *Nursing Management, 34,* 15–17; Lacey, L. M., & Shaver, K. (2004). Retaining staff nurses in North Carolina. *North Carolina Center for Nursing.* Retrieved January 17, 2004, from http://www.nursenc.org/research/retain_staff.pdf

56. Aiken, L. H. (2002). Superior outcomes for magnet hospitals: The evidence base. In M. L. McClure & A. S. Hinshaw (Eds.), *Magnet hospitals revisited: Attraction and retention of professional nurses.* Washington, DC: American Nurses Publishing.

57. Budd et al., 2004, pp. 1–20.

58. White, B. (1984). An introduction to collective bargaining. *Oregon Nurse, 23,* 27.

59. Common questions about union organizing and representation. (1985). *Michigan Nurse,* 3; Fulmer, W. E. (1982). *Union organizing: Management and labor conflicts.* New York: Praeger.

60. Hannah, K. J., & Shamian, J. (1992). Integrating a nursing professional model and nursing informatics in a collective bargaining environment. *Nursing Clinics of North America,* 31–45.

61. Beletz, E. E. (1982). Nurses' participation in bargaining units. *Nursing Management,* 48–50, 52–53, 56–58.

62. Project of the ABIM Foundation, ACP–ASIM Foundation, and European Federation of Internal Medicine (2002). *Medical Professionalism in the New Millennium: A Physician Charter, 136*(3), 243–246.

63. Strauss, G. (1968). Professionalism and occupational associations. *Industrial Relations, 2,* 7–31.

64. Pavalko, R. (1971). *Sociology of occupations and professions.* Itasca, IL: Peacock.

65. Fenner, K. M. (1991). Unionization: Boon or bane? *Journal of Nursing Administration,* 7–8; Benton, T. (1992). Union negotiating. *Nursing Management, 23,* 70, 72; Krasnansky, J. A. (1992). Time to stop the debate. *RN,* 116; Holmsted, L. (1991). E & GW annual business meeting. *The Maine Nurse,* 5.

66. Wheaton, D. (1991). Collective bargaining: Confronting the conflicts. *The Maine Nurse,* 10.

67. Kleingartner, A. (1969). Professional association: An alternative to unions? In R. Woodworth & R. Peterson (Eds.), *Collective negotiations for public and professional employees* (pp. 241–245). Glenview, IL: Scott, Foresman.

68. ChangHwan, K., & Sakamoto, A. (2008). Does inequality increase productivity? *Work and Occupations, 35*(1), 85–114.

69. Friedheim, M. K. (1982). Negotiating a union contract. *Medical Laboratory Observer,* 58–63.

70. Kleingartner, A. (1969). Professional association: An alternative to unions? In R. Woodworth & R. Peterson (Eds.), *Collective negotiations for public and professional employees* (pp. 241–245). Glenview, IL: Scott, Foresman.

71. Eubanks, P. (1990). Employee grievance policy: Don't discourage complaints. *Hospitals,* 36–37.

72. Ibid.

73. Eldridge, I. (1986). Some techniques and strategies of collective bargaining. *Washington Nurse,* 13.

74. Krasnansky, D. (1992). Professional and collective bargaining. Retrieved on July 4, 2008 from http://www.lotsofessays.com/viewpaper/1687107.html.

75. Brutsche, S. (1990). Mediation cross-examined. *Texas Bar Journal,* 584.

76. Ibid.

77. Dvorak, J. M. (1983). Past practice concepts in collective bargaining. *Michigan Nurse,* 5–7.

78. Ibid.

79. McLachlan, L. D. (1990). Meeting the challenges of collective bargaining. *California Nurse, 1,* 4–5.

80. Flanagan, R. (1999). Macroeconomic performance and collective bargaining: An international perspective, in *Journal of Economic Literature,* Vol. XXXVII (Sept. 1999), pp. 1150–1175.

81. Aidt, T., & Tzannatos, S. (2002). *Unions and collective bargaining: Economic effects in a global environment,* Washington, DC: World Bank.

82. Freeman, R., & Medoff, J. (1984). *What do unions do?* New York, Basic Books.

83. Layard, R., Nickell, S., & Jackman, R. (1991). *Unemployment: Macroeconomic performance and the labour market*, Oxford University Press, Oxford.

84. ChangHwan, K., & Sakamoto, A. (2008). Does inequality increase productivity? *Work and Occupations, 35*(1), 85–114.

85. Michigan Nurses Association. (2008). Access on May 5, 2008: http://www.minurses.org/Labor/benefits.shtml

86. Ibid.; Aidt, T., & Tzannatos, S. (2002). *Unions and collective bargaining: Economic effects in a global environment.* Washington, DC: World Bank.

87. Hoeven, van der, R. (2000). *Labour markets and income inequality. What are the new insights after the Washington Consensus?* UN/WIDER Working Papers 209. United Nations University, World Institute for Development Economics Research (UN/WIDER).

88. Aidt, T., & Tzannatos, S. (2002). *Unions and collective bargaining: Economic effects in a global environment.* Washington, DC: World Bank.

89. Hepner, J. O., & Zinner, S. E. (1991). Nurses and the new NLRB rules: Implications for healthcare management. *Health Progress, 72*(8), 20–2.

90. Hannah, K. J., & Shamian, J. (1992). Integrating a nursing professional practice model and nursing informatics in a collective bargaining environment. *Nursing Clinics of North America, 27*(1), 31–45.

91. Ibid.

92. Ibid.

93. Ibid.

94. Leipert, B. (1998). The use of professional nursing practice standards in nursing labour arbitrations in British Columbia, 1987–1994. *Journal of Advanced Nursing, 27*(3), 622–632.

95. Worsler, R. (1993, September 27). Still fighting yesterday's battle. *Newsweek,* 12.

96. ChangHwan, K., & Sakamoto, A. (2008). Does inequality increase productivity? *Work and Occupations, 35*(1), 85–114.

97. Ibid.

98. Kalisch, P. A., & Kalisch, B. J. (1985). Policy and perspectives on newspaper reports of nurse strikes. *Research in Nursing and Health,* 243–251.

99. Pointe, P. R., Fay, M. S., Brown, P., Doyle, M., Perron, J., Zizzi, L., et al. (1998). Factors leading to a strike vote and strategies for reestablishing relationships. *Journal of Nursing Administration,* 35–43.

100. Levinson, M., & Chideya, F. (1993, July 19). One for the rank and file. *Newsweek,* 38–39.

101. American Nurses Association. (2003). *Nursing's social policy statement* (2nd ed.). Washington, DC: American Nurses Association.

102. MacLeod, M., Browne, A. J., & Leipert, B. (1998). Issues for nurses in rural and remote Canada. *Australian Journal of Rural Health*, 6: 72–78.

103. Ibid.

104. Porter-O'Grady, T. (1992). Transformational leadership in an age of chaos. *Nursing Administration Quarterly, 17*(1), 17–24.

105. Hannah, K. J., & Shamian, J. (1992). Integrating a nursing professional practice model and nursing informatics in a collective bargaining environment. *Nursing Clinics of North America, 27*(1), 31–45.

106. Goodin, H. J. (2003). Collective bargaining. *Journal of Advanced Nursing, 43*, 335–350.

107. Cohen, A. (1989). The management rights clause in collective bargaining. *Nursing Management*, 24–26, 28.

108. Gardner, H. (2007). Good Work Project. *Excellence, ethics and engagement in the professions.* Retrieved February 28, 2008, from http://www.goodworkproject.org/

109. Miller, J. (2006). Opportunities and obstacles for Good Work in Nursing. *Nursing Ethics, 13*, 471–487.

110. Paolillo, J. P., & Vitell, S. J. (2002). An empirical investigation of the influence of selected personal, organizational and moral intensity factors on ethical decision making. *Journal of Business Ethics, 35*, 65–74.

References

Apfer, J., Zabava Ford, W. S., & Fox, D. H. (2003). Predicting nurses' organizational and professional identification: The effect of nursing roles, professional autonomy, and supportive communication. *Nursing Economics, 21*, 226–232.

Arras, J. D., & Steinbock, B. (1999). *Ethical issues in modern medicine* (5th ed.). Mountain View, CA: Mayfield.

Beauchamp, T. L., & Childress, J. F. (2001). Principles of biomedical ethics (5th ed.). New York: Oxford University Press.

Bell, S. E. (2003). Ethical climate in managed care organizations. *Nursing Administration Quarterly, 27*, 133–139.

Forman, H., & Davis, G. A. (2002). The rising tide of healthcare labor unions in nursing. *Journal of Nursing Administration, 32*, 376–378.

Malpas, P., & Schaffner, M. (2000). Managerial ethics: Arriving at decisions we can live with. *Gastroenterology Nursing, 23*, 239–240.

Szcepanski, A. (2003a). Just cause: Security for your job. *Michigan Nurse, 76*, 11, 13.

Szcepanski, A. (2003b). Mandatory subjects of bargaining. *Michigan Nurse, 76*, 7.

5 CHANGE, COMPLEXITY, AND CREATIVITY

Anne Longo, MBA, BSN, RN-BC

LEARNING OBJECTIVES AND ACTIVITIES

- Define and differentiate between creativity and innovation.
- Develop plans for recognizing and increasing the creativity, critical thinking skills, and innovation of clinical nurses.
- Identify methods of critical thinking.
- Perform a concept analysis of critical thinking.
- Identify reasons or need for change in nursing practice and management.
- Identify and differentiate between theories of planned change: Reddin, Lewin, Rogers, Havelock, Lippitt, Spradley, and Gladwell.
- Identify reasons for resistance to change; develop strategies to overcome that resistance.
- Describe change within complex adaptive systems.
- Describe the sound evidence and best practices in a service setting; develop a plan for an evidence-based project within that setting.

CONCEPTS

Creativity, innovation, critical thinking, change theory, scholarly inquiry, complexity science, complex adaptive systems

```
Q U O T E
```

Nursing is an art, and if it is to be made an art, it requires as exclusive a devotion, as hard a preparation, as any painter's or sculptor's work.

—Florence Nightingale

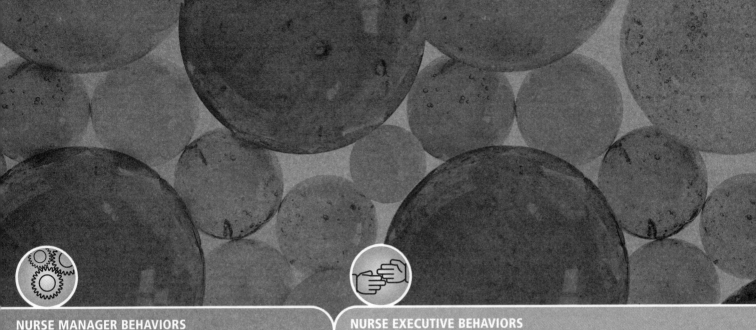

NURSE MANAGER BEHAVIORS	NURSE EXECUTIVE BEHAVIORS
The manager promotes an environment in which creativity, innovation, and critical thinking are recognized and rewarded. He or she considers change the domain of executive nursing and initiates all efforts for planned change accordingly.	A leader encourages all nursing employees to think freely, considers creative ideas critically, and recommends innovations in the practice of nursing and in the environment in which nursing is practiced. He or she involves nurses in implementing planned change and encourages nurses to be involved in the change process, scholarly inquiry, and evidence-based practice within the framework of a healthy work environment.

Introduction

In a climate of chaos and change within the healthcare industry, the trends at the forefront of the competitive market are based on the creativity and innovations of organizations. "Today's most sought-after talent is the ability to originate."[1] The creative process is not limited; it encompasses a range from organizations reaching out to develop new market strategies to bedside clinicians searching for new and better ways to provide care. Critical thinking skills must be applied to creative ideas, with successful innovations as the outcome, accomplished through planned change within an organization's stated policies and procedures. Changing organizations for excellence must afford opportunities and must change the ways people think and interact to create workplaces and systems that are purposeful and aligned with evidence-based results. Whether the nurse leader is involved in research, education, or administration, the use of change theories as a means of creating a healthy work environment is paramount to ensuring the intended goals of the Institute of Medicine as well as the environment in which the nurse leader seeks to make change.

The American Organization of Nurse Executives competencies include change management as part of a leadership skill set.[2] The responsibilities of the nurse leader in using change management are as follows:

1. Use change theory to plan for the implementation of organizational changes.
2. Serve as a change agent, assisting others in understanding the importance, necessity, impact, and process of change.
3. Support staff during times of difficult transitions.
4. Recognize one's own reaction to change and strive to remain open to new ideas and approaches.
5. Adapt leadership style to situational needs.

Using the change management theories addressed in this chapter provides the nurse leader with guidance in how to creatively think while problem-solving on a day-to-day basis.

CREATIVITY AND INNOVATION

Creativity and Innovation Defined

Creativity is defined in *Webster's New Twentieth Century Dictionary*, Unabridged (2nd edition) as "artistic or intellectual inventiveness." Innovation is defined as "the introduction of something new." These definitions suggest that the terms are interchangeable. Creativity is the mental work or action involved in bringing something new into existence, whereas innovation is the result of that effort.[3] To differentiate between the two, one might say that a nurse can create or invent a new nursing product, process, or procedure (creativity) and then can effect change by putting a new product, process, or procedure into use (innovation). Creativity is a way of using the mind.[4] Creativity is a special talent and an important tool for survival in the 21st century. Research indicates that creativity is separate from intelligence.[5]

Why Creativity?

A constant flow of new ideas is needed to feed the mandate for change in every aspect of our lives. Business leaders argue that creativity yields profits. With creativity, new products can be developed and a company can compete. New methods (innovations) are the fruits of that creativity. For many years nurses have tended to think of selling their services like a product as mercenary or unethical; this thinking has changed as nurses have acquired a higher level of education and have become more autonomous, with professional nurses becoming entrepreneurs in establishing businesses of their own. Sister Reinkemeyer predicted this development as early as 1968 when she wrote, "university programs try to produce independent personalities and thinkers capable of facing some of the modern scientific and psychosocial changes in nursing."[6]

Innovation is key to the survival and growth of both health care and nursing. Entrepreneurs create the new and different; entrepreneurial nurses create new businesses with new products and services, from which both the nurse and the organization benefit. The nurse gains personal satisfaction, rewards, and recognition, whereas the organization survives, thrives, and prospers.[7]

Establishing a Climate for Creativity

For creativity to prosper, the organization must provide an intellectual environment that gives employees recognition, prestige, and an opportunity to participate. Employees gain a sense of ownership and commitment by being involved in planning their work and making decisions. Nurse managers promote creativity through sensitivity, giving people the attention they want and treating them as distinct individuals. Competent managers inspire creativity by taking risks and by showing confidence, giving praise and support, being nourishing, using tact, and having patience.[8] Implementing the American Nurses Credentialing Center's 14 forces of magnetism as part of change management provides the nurse leader with a framework from within a climate of creativity can flourish. Critically thinking of how these forces impact each desired change allows the nurse leader to ensure the staff adopts and incorporates the changes necessary to improve the health care system at a local level.

The goals of the magnet program are to promote quality in a setting that supports professional practice, identifying excellence in the delivery of nursing services to patients/residents, and disseminate "best practices" in nursing services.[9]

Creative thinking can be developed with the intent of increasing the creative capacity and/or behavior of individuals or groups. Techniques of creativity training can include brainstorming, synectics, morphological analysis, forced fit, forced relationships, brainwriting, visualization, cueing, lateral thinking, and divergent thinking.[10] These techniques can be used when nurse leaders encourage free thinking and allow nurses to express their ideas openly.

Other motivators of creativity in nursing include the following:[11]

- Providing assistance to develop new ideas
- Encouraging risk taking while buffering resistant forces
- Providing time for individual effort
- Providing opportunities for professional growth and development
- Encouraging interaction with others outside the group
- Promoting constructive intragroup and intergroup competition
- Recognizing the value of worthy ideas
- Exhibiting confidence in workers

With motivators in place, leadership is able to allow the creative process to evolve. The following are actions that facilitate the production of goal-oriented ideas:[12]

1. Assemble the separate elements that will be creatively combined to produce a product or a new procedure. The problem must be identified in terms of usefulness of this product or process. If a known element is missing, what is available to replace it?
2. Use the available and assembled elements in combinations that produce original ideas.
3. Remove inhibitions to creativity such as excess motivation, anxiety, fear of taking risks, dependence on authority, and habitual modes of thinking and speaking. Creativity is not confined to a small, exclusive set of gifted people. Language contains the potential for creative thought, and everyone has this potential.
4. Study techniques of creativity so that the elements can be used.

Metamanagement

Metamanagement describes a cooperative effort of entrepreneurial or creative managers, strategic planners, and top management. It is a planning framework that cuts across organizational boundaries and facilitates strategic decision making about current practices and future directions. It is a flexible and creative planning process that stimulates in-house entrepreneurial thinking and behavior, and it is a consistent and accepted value system that reinforces management's commitment to the organization's strategy. Metamanagement stresses teamwork, organizational flexibility, open communication, innovation, risk taking, high morale, and trust.[13]

Nurse managers practicing metamanagement plan the organizational structure and its dynamics, nature, and position. They perform as an innovative, committed, enlightened, and disciplined group willing and able to restructure thinking and organizations and to generate and execute successful plans for a profitable nursing business. They stimulate the input of the clinical staff, thereby generating direction for the nursing organization and occupation.

The following task-related actions by nurse managers will help to develop and maintain a creative climate:[14]

1. Providing freedom to experiment without fear of reprimand
2. Maintaining a moderate amount of work pressure
3. Providing challenging yet realistic work goals
4. Emphasizing a low level of supervision in performance tasks
5. Delegating responsibilities
6. Encouraging participation in decision making and goal setting
7. Encouraging use of a creative problem-solving process to solve unstructured problems

8. Providing immediate and timely feedback on task performance
9. Providing the resources and support needed to get the job done

An example of action research that can be used in metamanagement is appreciative inquiry.[15] Appreciative inquiry, as interpreted by Cooperrider of Case Western Reserve University's Weatherhead School of Management, is a specific method for using metamanagement (represented as a four-dimensional cycle) and is guided by the following principles:

- The *constructive principle* focuses on understanding, reading, and analyzing organizations as living, human constructions.
- *Simultaneity* is the principle recognizing that inquiry and change are not truly separate but are simultaneous; inquiry is intervention.
- The *anticipatory principle* refers to our collective imagination and discourse about the future; bringing the future powerfully into the present as a mobilizing agent. This principle visualizes positive images of the future led by action.
- The *poetic principle* represents a metaphor that human organizations are much more like an open book than a machine; the organization's story is constantly being written and re-written and is a source of learning, inspiration and interpretation.
- The *positive principle* purports that for building and for sustaining change momentum large amounts of positive affect and social bonding are necessary.[16,17]

Creative Problem Solving

Creative problem solving starts by using vague or ill-defined problems as challenges. Problems can be attacked intuitively to generate as many ideas as possible. Solutions may create new challenges and new cycles of creative problem solving. The creative and innovative approaches to situations involve literacy and an exchange of ideas, perhaps more familiar to "right-brained" thinkers; in analytical thinking, an almost mathematical twist guides the process, stemming from "left-brain" thinking. Research indicates that both the right and left cerebral hemispheres contribute to the maintenance of multiple word meanings in highly creative persons.[18]

There are several theories of creative problem solving. Lattimer and Winitsky suggest the following:[19]

1. *Thinking:* Identifying factors to be used in solving an issue or developing a strategic plan; the choice is between a risk-free alternative and an alternative that involves risk
2. *Decomposing:* Breaking the situation into components—alternatives, uncertainties, outcomes, and consequences—and working with each component and combining the results for a decision
3. *Simplifying:* Determining the important components and concentrating the most crucial factors and the most essential relationships, then making intuitive judgments
4. *Specifying:* Establishing the value of key factors, the probabilities for the uncertainties, and the preferences for the outcomes
5. *Rethinking:* Examining the original analysis regarding omissions, inclusions, order, and emphasis

Godfrey recommends an alternative theory of creativity with the following five steps:[20]

1. *Perception:* Realizing there is a problem
2. *Preparation:* Research, data collection, and arrangement of information to define the problem
3. *Ideation:* Analysis and structure of a variety of formats that stimulate analogies and images; brainstorming
4. *Incubation:* Withdraw and relax when the flow of ideas ends. The unconscious takes off and forms images of possible solutions.
5. *Validation:* Test a solution

Drucker indicates that every corporation needs a strategy for innovation. He suggests four strategies:[21]

1. *The first with the most:* Be first in the market and first to improve a product or cut its price. This discourages prospective competitors.
2. *The second with the most:* Let someone else establish the market. Satisfy markets with narrow needs and specific capabilities. Provide excellent products for big purchasers with narrow needs. Offer new features. This strategy can be seen in the competitive healthcare market, in which certain corporations have specialized in psychiatric services, rehabilitation services, or drug-dependency services.
3. *The niche strategy:* Corner a finite market, making it unprofitable for others. When the niche becomes a mass market, change the strategy to remain profitable.
4. *Making the product your carrier; one product carries another:* This strategy is used by medical supply companies whose electronic thermometers are the basis for sales of disposable covers and intravenous pumps, which are in turn the basis for sales of fluid administration sets.

Creativity in the Workplace

Creative people, including nurses, have a broad background of knowledge. They have the mental skills of curiosity, openness, sensitivity to problems, flexibility, ability to think in images, and capability of analysis and synthesis.[22] Creative nurses use their knowledge to stimulate their sensory perceptions. In addition to solving problems, they identify new problems to solve by formulating questions about the hows and whys of established practices. Creative people are sometimes considered different from other people. This difference has been described by Levinson (1965) purporting that creativity is not so strangely mysterious and incomprehensible, however, does involve innovativeness, the ability to abstractly think and at time eccentric.[23] An individual may appear to be gifted with a brilliant intellect. During childhood this individual may have been the curious type who searched for books to read and tasks to do that satisfied his or her curiosity. Searching for the approval and encouragement of parents, friends, or teachers but not receiving it, he or she may have become something of a loner.

Creative individuals value the work and association of other creative individuals; they stimulate each other to think and perhaps even to be competitively creative. They can tolerate ambiguity; they have self-confidence, the ability to toy with ideas, and persistence.[24]

Nursing leaders possess the attributes of teamwork, global thinking, multitasking, creativity, and flexibility that are so important to the healthcare marketplace. They have integrated clinical and business principles and are a source of knowledge and skills to make their organizations prosper.[25] To foster independence and creative talents, nurse managers should assume that creative nurses are not odd or eccentric. As a consequence, barriers are not erected among peer groups. Nurse managers should communicate and cooperate with clinical nurses to set new goals or new practices for achieving goals.[26] Performance appraisals of creative employees should reward unconventional, intelligent efforts toward innovation, even if those efforts have failed. Evaluation must keep pace with human judgments resulting from complexity, uncertainty, theory, change, and control.[27]

Managing creativity can be challenging. Nurse managers must build an environment in which interpersonal relationships and trust are established to allow for the maximal creative effort among staff. With a willingness to listen and a spirit of cooperation, staff will accept differing behaviors and ideas without defensiveness or fear of losing control. Nurse managers can plan to nourish creativity in nursing personnel by doing the following:

1. Noting the creative abilities of those who develop new methods and techniques and enhancing employees' self-esteem

2. Providing time and opportunity for creative work, to be planned during performance appraisals and included in scheduling
3. Permitting time for educational offerings
4. Recognizing expertise in clinical practice, teaching, research efforts, and management skills
5. Encouraging nursing personnel to become involved in progress in the workplace, in community endeavors, and in professional organizations
6. Encouraging calculated risk taking and acceptance of personal responsibility, allowing for the freedom to fail

To encourage creativity, hire creative people. Frequently, they are the ones who have taken time off to learn and explore; sometimes considered "off-the-wall," they bring fresh viewpoints to their chosen profession. Weed out the complacent. Support generous sabbaticals. Model, measure, and teach curiosity; seek out curious work. Change the pace, and make it fun![28]

Developing a model of shared governance is one example of bringing creativity to the workplace whereby the decisions of care are made by staff working at the bedside. An example of shared governance in action is the innovative collaboration between Robert Wood Johnson Foundation and the Institute for Healthcare Improvement's Transforming Care at the Bedside initiative. Begun in 2003, the focus is on safe, reliable care, vitality and teamwork, patient-centered care, and value-added care processes.[29] It is at the bedside that the use of standardized measurements used rigorously will assist in evaluating successful change assisting the nurse leader to drive diverse healthcare systems to common evidence-based goals.[30]

This change project impacts the nurse leader seeking to implement change in her or his area of practice because it is an example of forced change that must be incorporated into practice by means of planned change requiring a great deal of critical thinking.

Social Intelligence

Planning for creativity in the workplace must take into account both emotional intelligence as outlined in Chapter 3 and social intelligence as described by Dr. Karl Albrecht. Social intelligence is the ability to get along well with others and to get them to cooperate with you. Why? Because the biggest obstacle to learning something new, in this case implementing change, is that you already believe you know it. There are three principles of perception related to change:

1. *Recognition:* We relate the change with something we already know. For example, cover the face of your cell phone and then try to describe it.
2. *Interpretation:* Misinformation about the change comes from misinterpretation. The brain converts incoming data into what we believe it should be.
3. *Expectation:* This controls much of our perception; it is how we organize our thoughts about the change that can often be a self-fulfilling prophecy.

Leaders who are creating a healthy work environment where change can flourish must ask if they and their staff are exhibiting nourishing behaviors or toxic behaviors regarding change:

1. Toxic behavior is a consistent problem of behavior that makes others feel devalued, inadequate, angry, frustrated, or guilty.
2. Nourishing behavior is a consistent pattern of behavior that makes others feel valued, loved, respected, capable, and appreciated, which are all behaviors required for change to be adopted and consequently successful.

Dr. Albrecht's model of social intelligence uses the mnemonic SPACE for the required skills a leader must use when interacting with staff:

- S = Situational awareness: This dimension is a kind of "social radar" or the ability to read situations and to interpret the behavior of people in change situations. What are their possible intentions, emotional states, and proclivity to interact?
- P = Presence: This incorporates a range of verbal and nonverbal patterns such as one's appearance, posture, voice quality, and subtle movements. In other words, presence is a whole collection of signals that others process into an evaluative impression of a person.
- A = Authenticity: Staff and others have a kind of "social radar" that enables them to pick up various signals from our behavior to judge whether we are honest, open, ethical, trustworthy, and well intentioned or inauthentic.
- C = Clarity: This is the ability to explain ourselves, illuminate ideas, pass data of action, and enable leaders to get others to cooperate.
- E = Empathy: The shared feelings between two people or a state of connectedness with another staff member creates the basis for positive interaction and cooperation.[31]

CRITICAL THINKING

The term *critical thinking* has been prominent in the field of education since the early 1980s. Although some believe the term is applicable across all genres, others believe the term is best defined as discipline specific.[33] This idea is particularly pertinent to nursing because the discipline is continuously concerned with purposeful, goal-directed thinking toward making judgments on evidence-based practice rather than on conjecture.[34] On a daily basis, nurses are required to assimilate an abundance of data and information to make decisions within their practice for which there are frequently no absolute or singly correct responses.[35]

The ideal critical thinker is habitually inquisitive, well informed, trustful of reason, open minded, flexible, fair minded in evaluation, honest in facing personal biases, prudent in making judgments, willing to reconsider, clear about issues, orderly in complex matters, diligent in seeking relevant information, reasonable in the selection of criteria, focused in inquiry, and persistent in seeking results which are as precise as the subject and circumstances of inquiry permit.

—P. A. Facione[32]

Nurses use critical thinking for several purposes, including applying professional and technical knowledge and skills in caring for clients. In these applications, critical thinking is the best guarantee that nurses will have successful outcomes. In the 10th edition of their book, entitled *Argumentation and Debate,* Freeley and Steinberg claim that competence in critical thinking is necessary for developing one's ability to participate effectively in human affairs, pursue higher education, and succeed in the highly competitive world of business and the professions. These authors also indicate that the ability to reach successful decisions is based on accurate evidence and valid reasoning.[36] Behaviors based on critical thinking are essential to a nurse's role as clinician, manager, researcher, or teacher.

Freeley and Steinberg identify seven methods of critical thinking:

1. *Debate:* Debate involves inquiry, advocacy, and reasoned judgment on a proposition. A person or group may debate or argue the pros and cons of a proposition in coming to a reasoned judgment. A debate usually entails opposing positions and specific rules.
2. *Individual decisions:* An individual may debate a proposition in his or her mind using problem-solving or decision-making processes. When consent or cooperation of others is needed, the individual may use group discussion, persuasion, propaganda, coercion, or a combination of these methods.
3. *Group discussion:* Five conditions for reaching decisions through group discussion are that "the group members (1) agree that a problem exists, (2) have comparable standards of value, (3) have compatible purposes, (4) are willing to accept the consensus of the group, and (5) are relatively few in number."[37]

4. *Persuasion:* Persuasion is communication to influence the acts, beliefs, attitudes, and values of others by reasoning, urging, or inducement. Debate and advertising are two forms of communication whose intent is to persuade.

5. *Propaganda:* Propaganda can be good or bad; it is multiple media communication designed to persuade or influence a mass audience. Propagandists may debate and argue. Their tactics need to be subjected to critical analysis.

6. *Coercion:* Threat or use of force is coercion. An extreme example is brainwashing, in which subjects are completely controlled physically for an indefinite period of time.

7. *Combination of methods:* Some situations require a combination of the foregoing communication techniques to reach a decision.[38]

A consensus is emerging that critical thinking should underlie the nursing process within nursing education programs. Critical thinking generally is regarded by academics as essential to the educated mind and superordinate to problem solving in the nursing process.[39]

❝*The rudiments of critical thinking are recalling facts, principles, theories, and abstractions to make deductions, interpretations, and evaluations in solving problems, making decisions, and implementing changes.* **❞**

Critical Thinking and Clinical Reasoning

What is the nurse leader's role in accountability for critical thinking as it relates to clinical reasoning and ultimately clinical judgment? Initially, it is nurturing the climate by

- Fostering an attitude of inquiry
- Encouraging staff to challenge assumptions
- Role modeling critical thinking strategies and skills by using the Socratic method of questioning out loud in front of others, thus making the process explicit for others
- Expecting colleagues at all levels to think critically and enforcing that expectation via rewards and consequences
- Modeling and expecting effective collaboration[40]

Thinking out loud by developing questions related to the domains of learning (affective, psychomotor, and cognitive) in relation to the specific desired change will assist staff in learning the expected behaviors required of the change. The nurse leader works with the educator to develop questions based in Bloom's taxonomy. For example, the taxonomy of cognitive verbs is knowledge, comprehension, application, analysis, synthesis, and evaluation.[41] What does the staff need to know about the planned change that can be addressed by developing questions related to each one of these areas with the ultimate goal of staff being able to assist with the evaluation of the desired change? Using the evidence to provide the initial knowledge and what facts need to be absorbed to understand the rationale for the change will then lead to valuing the change so that it is applied. Application of the desired change leads to critically thinking (analysis) and synthesis of how the change can be incorporated into the current work. Evaluation to ensure the change has the intended outcome leads to trusting the process in a creative healthy work environment.

Complex Adaptive Systems

The use of the various types of intelligence as part of managing change is critical to the leader working in a complex adaptive system. A complex adaptive system is often characterized by dynamic relationships among many agents, influences, and forces. The concept of complex adaptive systems comes from a body of literature known as complexity science, chaos theory, or network science. According to Dr. Cynthia Olney, the key traits of complex adaptive systems are as follows:[42]

- An entangled web of relationships among any agents and forces, both internal and external. These influences cause constant change, adaptation, and evolution of the system in an unpredictable, nonlinear manner.
- Self-organizing
- Chaotic and do not move predictably toward an end goal
- Communication laden, which are heaviest at the boundaries of a system
- Observable systemwide patterns of behaviors
- Feedback loops as the mechanisms for change in a system
- Repeated patterns of behavior themselves at different levels of a system and across systems

Plsek and Greenhalgh add the additional concepts of

- Tension and paradox are natural phenomena, not necessarily to be resolved.
- Inherent pattern of the system
- Attractor behaviors, which are patterns that provide comparatively simple understanding of what first seems to be extremely complex behavior

A great deal of nurse leaders and managers work within a complex adaptive system. Possessing the knowledge of your own areas of influence and how they integrate into the system as a whole increases the likelihood of sustainable change throughout the entire change process.[43]

Applications of Critical Thinking

Concept analysis is frequently advocated as a strategy for promoting critical thinking.[44] Concept analysis uses critical thinking to advance the knowledge base of nursing management and nursing practice.

A class of master's-level nursing students at Louisiana State University developed a method of concept analysis in their nursing management course using critical thinking. The students did literature searches before each class in preparation for concept analysis. In their first session, they developed the following format for concept analysis:

1. Identify and clarify the concept, including the philosophy and content analysis.
2. List the characteristics and attributes of the concept—for example, concrete/abstract, quality, and quantity.
3. Obtain perceptions, that is, what people believe or their interpretations about selling, marketing, and customers (determine whom the concept affects and what is perceived as needed).
4. Identify the use or application and the policies, procedures, practices (skills), and knowledge required.
5. Perform a researchable and synergistic evaluation to promote change, create energy, and validate theory.[45]

This format was used to study and analyze concepts such as organizational climate, legal and ethical nursing practices, nursing care delivery systems, theory of nursing management, standards of nursing practice, evaluation of patient care, and research in nursing administration.

Application of critical thinking theory to nursing management requires that the nurse manager have knowledge of the theory. Nursing staff development faculty also must have knowledge of the theory and the teaching skills that stimulate critical thinking and test it at the highest cognitive, affective, and psychomotor domains, not only in process but also in outcomes. Lectures are the least effective method for teaching critical thinking. Teaching methods to develop and test the higher level of the cog-

---

| **FIGURE 5-1** | **ACTIVITIES AND STRATEGIES FOR PROMOTING CRITICAL THINKING** |

Activities and strategies for promoting critical thinking include problem solving, decision making, clinical judgment, reflective thinking, questioning, dialogue, dialectical thinking, concept mapping, concept analysis, inquiry-based learning, script theory, two-way talks, case studies, clinical pathways, research findings, clinical rounds, peer review, shift reports, information processing, skills acquisition theory, conferences, context-dependent test items, and cognitive apprenticeship.

Models for studying critical thinking include the following:

- Loving's competence validation model.[49]
- The cognitive apprenticeship model.[50]

Source: Author.

---

nitive domain and competencies of the affective and psychomotor domains should be a part of the staff development process.[46] Critical thinking skills can be developed through the study of logic, problem-solving observation, analytic reading of books and articles about nursing and management, and group discussion[47] (Figure 5-1).

Critical thinking is consistent with the nursing process and should be evident in higher level learning objectives in the cognitive, affective, and psychomotor domains.

Futurist John Naisbitt describes high tech as technology that embodies both good and bad consequences. "High touch is embracing the primeval forces of life and death. High touch is embracing that which acknowledges all that is greater than we."[48] Professional nurses are high-tech, high-touch people whose work requires the cognitive abilities of synthesis and analysis; professional nurses are critical thinkers.

NEED FOR CHANGE

Four general reasons for designing orderly change have been defined by Williams:[51]

1. To improve the means of satisfying economic wants
2. To increase profitability
3. To promote human work for human beings
4. To contribute to individual satisfaction and social well-being

To these reasons one must add the concerns of the new millennium: the structures of healthcare organizations will continue to change, as will the structures of other industries. These changes encompass higher standards and superior performance, constant innovation in technology and corporate structure, the accomplishment of doing more for less, teamwork, customer preference, employee versus employer loyalties, industry regulations, corporate ownership, increased opportunities, shrinking resources, increased competition, and increasing complexity.[52] The need for organizational change may involve not only the whole system but also each of its units. This change will require management of the political dynamics and transition as well as motivation of constructive behavior.[53]

Change can help achieve organizational objectives as well as individual ones. The status quo of nursing will change with new models of patient care. Nurses are certainly aware of changes in relationships with those who hold authority and power, changes in responsibility and status, and changes in organizational, departmental, and unit objectives. Increased mobility within society at large has given rise to the creation of highly profitable travel nurses' agencies, creating increased staffing turnover as nurses leave to travel and as travel nurses are temporarily employed. Some employees resist change, but others welcome it as an opportunity to make adjustments in existing work situations, alter their relationships with their associates, and achieve personal growth and goals.

Structural change will greatly affect central staffers; these changes will include those in human resource development as well as those in nursing staff development. Central staffers will need to become project creators and network builders for the primary business units—the direct patient care units and the product sales units. As consultants to these units, central staffers can help develop the expertise necessary for success. If not involved in consulting for the existing structure, they can develop independent service centers, selling their services to the business units within the organization and to outside markets.[54] All this change is needed because of increasing competition, technological advancements, and human resource concerns.[55]

The end of the 20th century saw significant changes in the nature of healthcare organizations, the demands placed on nurse managers, and the needs and motivations of nursing personnel. Successful nurse managers have learned to manage change and have publicly related the role of nursing to being an involved and concerned member of society. They recognize the growing complexity of the health care organization, particularly in the division of nursing, and they recognize the changing values of nurses within the profession.

Nurses want opportunities for advancement or promotion, recognition for their work, and more help from their peers and supervisors to improve their job skills. One dramatic change for nurses has been the impetus to develop their professional standards to higher levels by raising their credentials, particularly with regard to education. Nurses have also recognized the need for continuing education to deliver up-to-date services. Evidence suggests that technological innovation can cause scientists' and engineers' knowledge to become obsolete in 10 years or fewer if they do not pursue further education; parallel evidence could be developed to support the same conclusion about nursing. A glance at the plethora of nursing journals shows nurses' awareness of society's current problems and their increasing involvement with them. These include problems of health, environmental pollution, poverty, ethnic equality, education, civil rights, religion, and advances in genetics.

Today's nurses are more committed to task, job, and profession than they are loyal to an organization; they are no longer bound by threat or ritual. Younger nurses, like other younger professionals, are mobile and have salable skills. They want to use all their skills and to be collaborative and democratic.[56] They look at the kind of services provided (short term, critical, or chronic), management's philosophy (participative vs. authoritarian), experimental outlook, and physical and geographical location. Nurses are willing to work hard; they desire an environment in which there is humor and the opportunity to use imagination and in which they can exert some control.

Nurse managers must change their behavior to suit the profile of this new breed of worker; they must be constantly aware of cues for the need for change. They must become more flexible and individualized in dealing with employees, and they must be candid, confronting conflict by allowing nurses to express their feelings, thoughts, and reactions. Management styles change, as do policies, procedures, relationships with subordinates, and employment and compensation practices. Individual needs and group motivations should be considered. The changes in nursing management aim to promote the ideas of all people, to encourage attentive listening, and to reward people for becoming personally involved and committed to their work. Nurse managers see themselves as agents of change functioning within a profession that draws its basic support from society. ". . . [T]he nurse manager will have to act as change agent in moving the organization forward, utilizing human-intensive skills to mobilize the resources available to her and her professional nursing peers. All of this effort will serve to define, implement, and evaluate the strategies and processes that will meet the healthcare needs of the future."[57]

What framework should the nurse leader use to answer the need for change? Incorporating the standards of the American Association of Critical Care Nurses *Healthy Work Environments* as part of the framework can guide the nurse leader to answer the call for change. The six standards with corresponding elements were developed in response to the Institute of Medicine's 1996 report, *Crossing the Quality Chasm*:

- *Standard 1—**Skilled Communication:*** Nurses must be as proficient in communication skills as they are in clinical skills.
- *Standard 2—**True Collaboration:*** Nurses must be relentless in pursuing and fostering true collaboration.
- *Standard 3—**Effective Decision Making:*** Nurses must be valued and committed partners in making policy, directing and evaluating clinical care, and leading organizational operations.
- *Standard 4—**Appropriate Staff:*** Staffing must ensure the effective match between patient needs and nurse competencies.
- *Standard 5—**Meaningful Recognition:*** Nurses must be recognized and must recognize others for the value each brings to the work of the organization.
- *Standard 6—**Authentic Leadership:*** Nurse leaders must fully embrace the imperative of a healthy work environment, authentically live it, and engage others in its achievement.[58]

Adaptation to change has always been a job requirement for nursing. Change is the key to progress and to the future; often that change begins with a focus on technology, without consideration for human relationships and political sensitivities. It is the task of nursing management to develop complimentary nursing systems that encompass new technology, improve patient care, and ultimately give greater satisfaction to nursing workers.

Change Theory

Some widely used change theories are those of Reddin, Lewin, Rogers, Havelock, Lippitt, and Spradley.

Reddin's Theory

Reddin developed a planned change model that can be used by nurses. He suggested seven techniques by which change can be accomplished:

1. Diagnosis
2. Mutual setting of objectives
3. Group emphasis
4. Maximum information
5. Discussion of implementation
6. Use of ceremony and ritual
7. Resistance interpretation

The first three techniques are designed to give those affected by the change an opportunity to influence its direction, nature, rate, and method of introduction. These individuals are then able to have some control over the change, to become involved in it, to express their ideas more directly, and to propose useful modifications.

Diagnosis (the first technique) is scientific problem solving. Those affected by the change meet and identify problems and the probable outcomes. Mutual objective setting (technique number 2) ensures that the goals of both groups, those instituting the change and those affected by it, are brought into line. It may be necessary for groups to bargain and compromise. Group emphasis (number 3) is sometimes referred to as team emphasis. Change is more successful when supported by a team rather than by a single person. "Groups develop powerful standards for conformity and the means of enforcing them."[59]

Maximum information (number 4) is important to the success of change. Discussion of implementation (number 5) by the use of ceremony and ritual (number 6) considers the culture of the organization, particularly the use of rewards to reinforce the change. Interpretation of any resistance to change (number 7) takes into account the processes and systems in place which may require a revisiting of the group's work and objectives set for implementation (numbers 3, 4, and 5). Management should make at least four announcements with regard to a proposed change:[60]

1. That a change will be made
2. What the decision is and why it was made
3. How the decision will be implemented
4. How implementation is progressing

Lewin's Theory

One of the most widely used change theories is that of Kurt Lewin, which involves three stages:

1. *The unfreezing stage:* The nurse manager or other change agent is motivated by the need to create change. Affected nurses are made aware of this need. The problem is identified or diagnosed, and the best solution is selected. One of three possible mechanisms provides input to the initial change: (a) individual expectations are not being met (lack of confirmation), (b) the individual feels uncomfortable about some action or lack of action (guilt anxiety), or (c) a former obstacle to change no longer exists (psychological safety). The unfreezing stage occurs when disequilibrium is introduced into the system, creating a need for change.[61]
2. *The moving stage:* The nurse manager gathers information. A knowledgeable, respected, or powerful person influences the change agent in solving the problems (identification). A variety of sources give a variety of solutions (scanning), and a detailed plan is made. People examine, accept, and try out the innovation.[62]
3. *The refreezing stage:* Changes are integrated and stabilized as part of the value system. Forces are at work to facilitate the change (driving forces). Other forces are at work to impede change (restraining forces). The change agent identifies and deals with these forces, and change is established with homeostasis and equilibrium.[63]

Rogers' Theory

Everett Rogers modified Lewin's change theory. Antecedents included the background of the change agent and the change environment. Rogers' theory has five phases:

- Phase 1: Awareness, which corresponds to Lewin's unfreezing phase
- Phase 2: Interest
- Phase 3: Evaluation
- Phase 4: Trial, which corresponds to Lewin's moving phase
- Phase 5: Adoption, which corresponds to Lewin's refreezing phase. In the adoption phase the change is accepted or rejected. If accepted, it requires interest and commitment.[64]

Rogers' theory depends on five factors for success:[65]

1. The change must have the relative advantage of being better than existing methods.
2. It must be compatible with existing values.
3. It must have complexity—more complex ideas persist even though simple ones get implemented more easily.

4. It must have divisibility—change is introduced on a small scale.
5. It must have communicability—the easier the change is to describe, the more likely it is to spread.

Havelock's Theory

Havelock's theory is another modification of Lewin's theory, expanded to six elements. The first three correspond to unfreezing, the next two to moving, and the sixth to refreezing:[66]

1. Building a relationship
2. Diagnosing the problem
3. Acquiring the relevant resources
4. Choosing the solution
5. Gaining acceptance
6. Stabilization and self-renewal

Lippitt's Theory

Lippitt added a seventh phase to Lewin's original theory. The seven phases of his theory of the change process are as follows:[67]

- Phase 1: Diagnosing the problem. The nurse as change agent looks at all possible ramifications and involves those who will be affected. Group meetings are held to win the commitment of others. To ensure success, key people in top management and policymaking roles are involved.
- Phase 2: Assessing the motivation and capacity for change. Possible solutions are determined, and the pros and cons of each are forecast. Consideration is given to implementation methods, roadblocks, factors motivating people, driving forces, and facility forces. Assessment considers financial aspects, organizational aspects, structure, rules and regulations, organizational culture, personalities, power, authority, and the nature of the organization. During this phase the change agent coordinates activities among a number of small groups.
- Phase 3: Assessing the change agent's motivation and resources. The change agent can be external or internal to the organization or division. An external change agent may have fewer bases but must have expert credentials. An internal change agent, however, knows the people. The process could involve both. The change agent must have a genuine desire to improve the situation, knowledge of interpersonal and organizational approaches, experience, dedication, and a personality to suit the situation. The change agent should be objective, flexible, and accepted by all.
- Phase 4: Selecting progressive change objectives. The change process is defined, a detailed plan is made, timetables and deadlines are set, and responsibility is assigned. The change is implemented for a trial period and evaluated.
- Phase 5: Choosing the appropriate role of the change agent. The change agent will be active in the change process, particularly in handling personnel and facilitating the change. The change agent will deal with conflict and confrontation.
- Phase 6: Maintaining the change. During this phase emphasis is on communication, with feedback on progress. The change is extended in time. A large change may require a new power structure.
- Phase 7: Terminating the helping relationship. The change agent withdraws at a specified date after setting a written procedure or policy to perpetuate the change. The agent remains available for advice and reinforcement.

Figure 5-2 compares these theories.

It should be noted that all five theories are similar to the problem-solving process itself, indicating that the latter could be used to implement planned change. The nurse manager should select the the-

FIGURE 5-2 COMPARISON OF CHANGE THEORIES

REDDIN	LEWIN	ROGERS	HAVELOCK	LIPPITT
1. Diagnosis	1. Unfreezing	1. Awareness	1. Building a relationship	1. Diagnosing the problem
2. Mutual objective setting	2. Moving	2. Interest	2. Diagnosing the problem	2. Assessing motivation and capacity for change
3. Group emphasis	3. Refreezing	3. Evaluation	3. Acquiring the relevant resources	3. Assessing change agent's motivation and resources
4. Maximum information		4. Trial	4. Choosing the solution	4. Selecting progressive change objective
5. Discussion of implementation		5. Adoption	5. Gaining acceptance	5. Choosing the appropriate role of the change agent
6. Use of ceremony and ritual			6. Stabilization and self-renewal	6. Maintaining change
7. Resistance interpretation				7. Terminating the helping relationship

Note: Author.

ory he or she feels most comfortable with after identifying the change to be made. A management plan is then made to cover the phases of making the change. The planning phase requires gathering data to support a decision for change. To set objectives, the nurse manager works with the nursing staff who will be affected by the change. Thus, the entire group becomes aware of and interested in the need for change. A relationship is built between the nurse manager and nursing employees. The plan can then become an opportunity made cooperatively, implemented by an enthusiastic group, and evaluated and maintained by the group. Decision making is implemented by planned change.

Spradley's Model

Spradley developed an eight-step model based on Lewin's theory. She indicates that planned change must be constantly monitored to develop a fruitful relationship between the change agent and the change system. Following are the eight basic steps of the Spradley model:[68]

1. *Recognize the symptoms:* There is evidence that something needs changing.
2. *Diagnose the problem:* Gather and analyze data to discuss the cause. Consult with the staff. Read appropriate materials.
3. *Analyze alternative solutions:* Brainstorm. Assess the risks and the benefits. Set a time, plan resources, and look for obstacles.
4. *Select the change:* Choose the option most likely to succeed that is affordable. Identify the driving and opposing forces, using challenges that include assimilation of the opposition.

5. *Plan the change:* This includes specific, measurable objectives, actions, a timetable, resources, budget, an evaluation method such as the program evaluation review technique, and a plan for resistance management and stabilization.

6. *Implement the change:* Plot the strategy. Prepare, involve, train, assist, and support those who will be affected by the change.

7. *Evaluate the change:* Analyze achievement of objectives and audit.

8. *Stabilize the change:* Refreeze; monitor until stable.

In a study of a nursing center for the community elderly, results showed that the use of change theory could determine a client's readiness to change health behaviors.[69]

Tipping Point

"The biography of an idea and the idea is very simple" is from the book, *The Tipping Point*, which the nurse leader can also choose to use as a framework for change.[70] The tipping point, or "the one dramatic moment in an epidemic when everything can change all at once," is exactly the moment the nurse leader seeks during the implementation phase of change.[71] Seeking out the few staff members who will support the change and are seen as informal leaders is an example of what Gladwell calls the law of the few. Change becomes an epidemic because of a few who are social, energetic, knowledgeable, and influential among their peers.

Stickiness is the second law in causing a tipping point. "Stickiness means that a message makes an impact. You can't get it out of your head."[72] To the nurse leader, this is the time when all staff applies the required change. The third law, the power of context, says "that human beings are a lot more sensitive to their environment than they may seem." It is the nurse leader's responsibility to assess the environment where the change is to occur in order to know the context in which the change will take place.

New Management Theory

Dunphy and Stace describe a differentiated contingency model for organizational change. It includes two contrasting theories of change (incremental and transformational) and two contrasting methods of change (participation and coercion).

Incremental change assumes that the effective manager moves the organization forward in small, logical steps. The long time frame plus the sharing of information increases confidence among employees and reduces the organization's dependence on outsiders to provide the impetus and momentum for change. The incremental model is similar to the systems approach to change and organizational development. It is used when the organization is ready for predicted future environmental conditions, but adjustments are needed in mission, strategy, structure, and/or internal processes.[73]

An organization may require transformational change on a large scale when there is environmental "creep," organizational "creep," diversification, acquisition, merger, shutdowns, industry reorganization, or major technological breakthroughs. Transformational strategies embody large-scale adjustments in strategy, structure, and process requirements.

Participative methods of change are used to overcome workforce resistance. Coercive methods are authoritarian and use force. The contingency model uses a mixture of methods as dictated by conditions.[74]

The new theory of management is one of transformation or change. Today, the fundamental sources of wealth are knowledge and communication, not natural resources and physical labor. Change means opportunity and danger. Information technology and the computer are the enablers of productivity. Customers have much more power; computers have replaced middle managers. Success requires quick responses to changing circumstances. Organizational design should be reconfigurable on an annual, monthly, weekly, daily, or hourly basis. Organizations should be able to develop new products rapidly, have flexible production systems, and use team-based incentives. Big companies are outsourcing many functions and paying for intellectual labor. Intellectual assets—networks and databases—have replaced physical assets. The most valuable devices will help people cope with change.[75]

Management theory is going through a massive transformation, referred to in management literature as a revolution. The new theory of change process has three steps:

1. *Awakening:* This is when the need for change is realized. During step 1 the leadership articulates why the change is necessary.
2. *Envisioning:* This is a group effort that addresses technical, political, and cultural resistance. During step 2, resistance is dealt with. There will be technical resistance, political resistance related to resource allocation and powerful coalitions, and cultural resistance related to the chain of command, media, and training.
3. *Rearchitecting:* This eliminates boundaries and compartments. To get rid of boundaries or ceilings, the hierarchy is de-layered, perks for executives are reduced, and gain-sharing incentive systems are broadened. To get rid of horizontal boundaries or internal walls, cross-functional teams, project teams, and partnership are used. To get rid of external boundaries, alliances are created, customer satisfaction is measured, and teams are built with customers and suppliers.

Leadership skills for the change include the following:[76]

1. Identify changes in the environment that will affect the business.
2. Lead others to overcome fear and uncertainty in making change.
3. Visualize the business through the eyes of the customer.
4. Have a clear vision of the future of the business.
5. Assume responsibility for own mistakes.
6. Build coalition and network across organizational lines to achieve important goals.
7. Lead the change.

Transformation is the process of reinventing an organization. Leaders create an atmosphere of continual change. Evaluation is done by peers, superiors, and subordinates. Transformed organizations have no boundaries; employees work up and down the hierarchy, across functions and geography, and with suppliers and customers. Goals center on numbers, total quality, and unity. Celebration is crucial, with emphasis on teamwork and using people's brains, imagination, and dedication. Let the team map the work to do it better and faster. The transformational manager views any process as susceptible to improvement. Reorganization focuses on customer segments and needs.[77]

In this transformation, leadership requires courage, judgment, and visibility. It requires a burning desire to change as healthcare organizations move to meet a world standard of quality. Managers need to motivate, empower, and educate employees. Managers may practice seven steps to being the best:[78]

1. Determine the world standard in every part of the process of providing care.
2. Use process mapping for the system's parts. Redesign to get rid of inefficiencies. Survey customers.
3. Communicate with your employees as though your life depended on it.
4. Distinguish what needs to be done from how hard it is to do it.
5. Set stretch targets. Let people decide how to reach them. Do not punish.
6. Never stop.
7. Pay attention to your inner self.

Change Agent

As one studies change theory, one notes that its application tends to mimic the problem-solving process. The nurse, operating as a change agent, uses change theory to identify and solve problems. This nurse learns to anticipate impending change, including that arising from interdependent systems, responds to change, and takes action to direct its course.

Nurses can compete successfully in the world of health care by doing things a new way. Professional nurses are expected to have the vision to change things and to be change agents.[79]

Examples of the Application of Change Theory

Retrenchments involving layoffs do not always use appropriate change theory. As a consequence, considerable unnecessary pressures, including unfavorable publicity, are placed on nurses. The organizational climate becomes tense and disruptive and gives personnel a sense of loss of security. Nurse executives feel tired and drained.

Causes of such problems include policies and plans that are developed after the fact, with few policies developed to deal with employees remaining with the organization. The media can be used to inform the public of changes in the healthcare system that necessitated the layoff.

The following are among the positive responses that minimize resistance to the change of retrenchment:[80]

1. Have a strong orientation toward reality, preparedness, knowledge of human behavior, stress management, and openness and honesty in dealing with employees.
2. Develop organization-wide retrenchment plans and policies with the advice of the personnel or human resource management department and legal counsel.
3. Consider the use of consultants.
4. Evaluate the criteria for layoffs: seniority, performance appraisal, and job categories. The principle of last hired, first fired should be weighed against the principle of keeping the most qualified employees.
5. Have the public relations department (or a consultant) handle publicity.
6. Deal positively with rumors through newsletters, informal discussions, and open meetings.
7. Reassure remaining employees by being visible and available. Make frequent rounds.
8. Do team building with chaplains, psychiatric specialists, and human resource specialists.
9. Form a nurse manager support group that includes families, friends, colleagues, and non-nursing professional peers.
10. Be fair and honest and handle people with dignity and care.

Transformational change brings radical change to the mission, structure, and culture of an organization. This change may be managed with consultation and employee participation. The nurse manager should keep training personnel abreast of organizational changes. Empowerment is a key factor in managing change, because empowered employees become change agents. Some coping strategies are problem focused, whereas some are emotion focused.

Employees need time to adjust to change, sometimes as long as several years. They can use this time to learn new skills and should become well trained. If they are to leave the organization, they need time to prepare resumes and perform a job search. All employees should be treated with respect and concern. Whenever possible, change should give employees choices.[81]

Resistance to Change

Resistance to change, or attempting to maintain the status quo when efforts are being made to alter it, is a common response. Change evokes stress that in turn evokes resistance.

Resistance is often based on a threat to the security of the individual, because change upsets an established pattern of behavior. If the problem-solving approach is used, answers should be provided to questions about the impact of the change, including the following:

- Will the change affect the work standard and subsequent employment, promotion, and raises?
- Will it mean an increased work load at an accelerated pace?
- Do employees visualize how they will fit into the picture if this change occurs?

In-service education and continuing education may help provide the answers.

Factors that stimulate resistance to change include habits, complacency, fear of disorganization, set patterns of response to change, conservatism, perceived loss of power, ego involvement, insecurity, perceived loss of current or meaningful personal relationships, and perceived lack of rewards.[82]

People are afraid of change because of lack of knowledge, prejudices resulting from a lifetime of personal experience and exposure to others, and fear of the need for greater effort or a higher degree of difficulty.

People have developed fears, biases, and social inhibitions from the cultural environment in which they live. Because they cannot be separated from these cultural factors, it is necessary to find ways of managing them within a system.

Barriers to change include a perception of implied criticism. "You are changing the system because you don't like the way I do it." Employees perceive that machines and systems are replacing them or making their jobs less interesting. For example, a programmed system could be used by patients to take their own nursing histories.

Change may demand the investment of a great deal of time and effort in relearning. If nurses are to be independent practitioners, what happens to those who are not prepared? "Probably the greatest single personal barrier is that individuals do not understand or refuse to accept the reasons for the change or the need for it. Unfortunately, it is not always easy to equate the reasons and the needs and to communicate them in meaningful and compelling language."[83]

People are members of a social system in a community and will resist change if it affects that social system. Social changes that threaten social customs, values, self-esteem, and security are resisted more than technical changes. One member of the social system may influence others even if that person is unaffected by the change.

Other causes of resistance to change include time and pace; different generations of nurses have different rates of change.

Values and Beliefs

Cognitive frameworks are based on values and beliefs about the effective means of achieving these values. Nurse managers who value the chain of command, policies, and procedures and who believe their management experience does not need input from clinical nurses may not look for problems needing change. As long as they are successful, these nurse managers are strengthened by success that builds their self-respect. This success fosters resistance to any change that threatens the integrity of the framework. People resist discarding their own ideas. Accepting another's idea reduces their self-esteem. They may consider a good idea a unique event to be preserved. Ideas should have life cycles. They shine and then dim and need to be replaced. Ideas need to be considered a depreciable.[84]

Change is affected by the crucial differences among geographical regions. Some regions are more open to fast change, whereas others accept slow changes. Cultural changes are affected by religious or political beliefs. People hold fast to meaningful beliefs.[85]

Evidence-Based Practice 5-1

Gillen claims that change stimulates increased levels of energy, which is called hyperenergy and is not stress. Hyperenergy is the heightened drive a person feels in response to a perceived challenge or threat. If not managed, hyperenergy is used by employees to think of surreptitious ways of preventing change. Hyperenergy can be pooled for collective resistance to change. It distracts employees, causing errors and accidents.[86] Skilled nurse leaders bring employees into the change process so the employees do not view the change as a threat. Employees' hyperenergy is then channeled into involvement in the change process.

One reason for resistance to change is that hierarchical, bureaucratic frameworks with rules achieve stability. It should be kept in mind that both individuals and organizations need such stability through continuity in policies and procedures so that recurring needs can be dealt with routinely and problems do not have to be resolved anew each time they appear.

The major symptoms of resistance to change are refusal, confrontation, and covert resistance such as no preparation for meetings or misunderstandings of the place or time, incomplete reports, refusal to accept responsibility, uncooperative employees, passive aggressiveness, absenteeism, and tardiness.[87]

Strategies for Overcoming Obstacles to Change

According to Drucker, "One cannot manage change. One can only be ahead of it."[88] Drucker suggests that the manager lead change and view it as an opportunity. Change can be led with nurse managers acting as change agents. One of the strategies a nurse manager can use is to hire a consultant to make the diagnosis and recommend programs that will improve the productivity of nurse personnel while giving them job satisfaction. Such measures can include educational programs to improve the areas in which problems exist.

Effectively led change leads to improvement of patient care services, raised morale, increased productivity, and meeting of patient and staff needs. Change is an art, the mastery of which can be exhilarating, refreshing, challenging, and exciting, because it represents opportunity. Change is facilitated when nurse employees are assigned to adapt to changing job requirements.

Collection and Development of Data

Nurse managers need to gather data about work so that it can be discussed, analyzed, and used to effect change when indicated. Personnel, particularly managers, can be educated to make and manage change. They will learn about labor power planning and utilization rather than leaving this entirely to the human resources department. They will learn about financial management rather than depend on the accounting office personnel to take care of it. These are areas in which effective strategies can be developed to foster external cooperative efforts among chief nurse executives of similar institutions and organizations within a community. Such concepts can be expanded to clinical services. If a division of nursing cannot afford to use such specialists as a full-time mental health nurse practitioner, several organizations can collectively contract for the services of one. Thus change becomes a cooperative venture.

Integration of computers and automated equipment is essential to the change process, particularly when managers are competing for professional nurses as well as for healthcare dollars. Within this domain, nurse educators can elicit the advice and skills of nursing management system personnel as impartial third-party critics of the change being effected. These personnel will give nurse educators effective feedback while providing management information support systems.

Adding the Evidence

Nurse leaders who use evidence as part of change management can facilitate innovation. Evidence-based decision making is not just for use by the bedside clinician. Communication, shared decision making, and quality improvement are all pieces of transformational leadership that promotes change in the diverse healthcare system. There are many evidence-based frameworks from which the nurse leader can choose to determine which evidence to use. For example, the five steps of evidence-based decision making below are based on Melnyk and Fineout-Overholt and are reframed from a management perspective:[89]

1. Ask the burning management question in the format that yields the most relevant and best evidence.
2. Collect the most relevant and best evidence to answer the question.

3. Critically appraise the evidence for its validity, relevance, and applicability.
4. Integrate all evidence with one's management expertise, preferences, and organizational values in making a management decision or change.
5. Evaluate the management decision or change from implementing the evidence.

Another framework is Kathleen Stevens ACE star model:

- *Discovery:* This is a knowledge-generating stage. In this stage, new knowledge is discovered through the traditional research methodologies and scientific inquiry. Research results are generated through the conduct of a single study. This may be called a *primary research study,* and research designs range from descriptive to correlational to causal and from randomized control trials to qualitative. This stage builds the corpus of research about clinical actions.
- *Evidence summary:* This is the first unique step in evidence-based practice—the task is to synthesize the corpus of research knowledge into a single, meaningful statement of the state of the science. The most advanced evidence-based practice methods to date are those used to develop evidence summaries (i.e., evidence synthesis, systematic reviews, e.g., the systematic review methods outlined in the *Cochrane Handbook*) from randomized control trials. Some evidence summaries use more rigorous methods than others, yielding more credible and reproducible results. The rigorous evidence summary step distinguishes evidence-based practice from the old paradigm of research utilization. Largely due to the work of the Cochrane Collaboration, rigorous methods for systematic reviews have been greatly advanced, using meta-analytic techniques and developing other statistical summary strategies, such as number needed to treat.
- *Translation:* The transformation of evidence summaries into actual practice requires two stages: *translation* of evidence into practice recommendations and *integration* into practice. The aim of translation is to provide a useful and relevant package of summarized evidence to clinicians and clients in a form that suits the time, cost, and care standard. Recommendations are generically termed *clinical practice guidelines* and may be represented or embedded in care standards, clinical pathways, protocols, and algorithms.
- *Integration:* Integration is perhaps the most familiar stage in health care because of society's longstanding expectation that health care be based on most current knowledge, thus requiring implementation of innovations. This step involves changing both individual and organizational practices through formal and informal channels. Major aspects addressed in this stage are factors that affect individual and organizational rate of adoption of innovation and factors that affect integration of the change into sustainable systems.
- *Evaluation:* The final stage in knowledge transformation is evaluation. In evidence-based practice, a broad array of endpoints and outcomes are evaluated. These include evaluation of the impact of evidence-based practice on patient health outcomes, provider and patient satisfaction, efficacy, efficiency, economic analysis, and health status impact. As new knowledge is transformed through the five stages, the final outcome is evidence-based quality improvement of health care.[90]

Planning helps overcome many obstacles to change. Planning keeps interpersonal relationships from being disrupted if persons with common frames of reference are brought together. The planner can assist people to meet their goals while minimizing their fear and anxiety. Fear is stimulated by the external threat of change. Anxiety, which is self-induced dread, is internally stimulated. Planning helps people accept change without fear or anxiety.

In making changes, nurse managers should plan to help people unlearn the old (unfreeze) and use the new (refreeze). Implementation and updating of nursing management information systems can refine much of the unfreezing and refreezing. Often, nurse managers help their staff learn the new without having them unlearn the old. This is a major problem in nursing because of the changing role of nurses.

To prepare a plan carefully, the nurse manager should share information and decision making, work for common perception and understanding, and support and reinforce the nursing staff's effort to effect change. Clear statements of philosophy, goals, and objectives are needed in preparing for change.

Beyers recommends that nurse executives be involved in the following elements of strategy planning:[91]

- Product/market planning
- Business unit planning
- Shared resource planning
- Shared concern planning
- Corporate-level planning

Nursing in all areas, both clinical and managerial, must consider competition. The patient will go where there is higher quality nursing care, which results from effectively planned and managed change. Nurse educators should perform market surveys to determine the nursing products and services that consumers want.[92] This activity itself constitutes change and results in changes.

Looking at the theory of the business of the healthcare organization and of nursing, what needs to be abandoned? This may include products, services, markets, distribution channels, and every end user who does not fit the theory of the business. End users do not need many organizations to get information; they use the Internet to obtain information on providers and services. Nursing's goal is to improve this information and these services in the interest of survival and progress. The opportunity is with maintaining physical and mental functioning of individuals and populations. Drucker suggests that managers look at windows of opportunity:[93]

- The organization's own unexpected successes and failures as well as the unexpected successes and failures of the organization's competitors
- Incongruities, especially incongruities in the process, whether of production or distribution, and incongruities in customer behavior
- Process needs
- Changes in industry and market structures
- Changes in demographics
- Changes in meaning and perception
- New knowledge

Plans list every person on whom the change depends and the level of involvement of each. Who will oppose and who will support the change? The dominant coalition in the organization and the forces that stimulate change should be identified and their support enlisted. Appropriate current events should be noted through reading and meetings; those that enhance the mission of the organization and for which the clinical nurses claim or share ownership should be highlighted.[94] This activity brings new ideas and new knowledge to stimulate and justify the need for change.

Planning also requires thinking in multiple time frames: changes to be effected in 6 months, 1 year, and so on. The nurse manager should identify the trade-offs between nursing and other departments, between clinical and management staffs, and within the change process itself, and he or she should list ways to enlist support.[95]

Nurse managers need to be careful not to overplan. They should leave some room for the people who implement the change to exercise intelligent initiative. They need to be sure that the rewards or benefits to individuals and to the group are carefully communicated. If people want a change to work, they will make it happen. Change leads to real innovation and, although it creates uncertainty and discomfort, requires nurse leaders to have the knowledge and skills to manage it.[96]

Training and Education

The frequency of training and education should match the frequency of change. Nursing personnel require constant staff development programs to keep from depreciating in knowledge and competence. From initial hiring and orientation, change should be portrayed as an integral part of the nurse's job.[91] Nurse managers should inform employees of the pressures that make change necessary.

Using the steps of the nursing process or the American Society of Training and Development's Analysis, Design, Develop, Implement and Evaluate model as a means of instructional design theory and process provides a path for determining the status of the education of the planned change.[97]

Critical Thinking

Nurse leaders need critical thinkers during the change process from start to finish. This is the individual who is an independent thinker. They base decisions on sound reasoning. Critical thinkers are observant and able to organize and prioritize data. The critical thinker does not hesitate to question yet functions as a good role model and educator. Critical thinking in the world of nursing is based on the nursing process, and in planning change the nursing leader must allow the staff who is impacted by the change time to critically reflect on how the change process is affecting their practice.

Rewards

Rewards for old behavior patterns should be removed after the individuals have been helped to see the reasons for the proposed change. Employees need to see the necessity for the new behaviors and should be given real incentives, financial or nonfinancial. Here is where job standards come in. The job standards should incorporate the new methods or skills and phase out the old ones. To provide an incentive, performance appraisal can be based on the new standards. Time must be allowed and opportunity provided for retraining. Nonfinancial rewards include enriching jobs and encouraging self-development. Such activities can satisfy individual needs.

Using Groups as Change Agents

Groups in themselves are often effective change agents. When the group appears to work in harmony and to have well-understood goals, it may be used to institute the change. If the idea can be planned in the group, it will be implemented more successfully. A group is more willing to assume risks than most individuals are. Planning should make clear the need for change and provide an environment in which group members identify with such need. Objectives should be stated in clear, concise, and qualitative terms. Administrative policy should contain broad guidelines with understandable procedures for achieving the objectives, and these guidelines and procedures should be communicated to the group.

As agents of change, nurse managers need to use staff talents by using temporary work teams to solve specific problems and effect change. They need to participate on interdisciplinary task forces and prepare people for job mobility through experiences planned to facilitate it. Third-party critics may help diagnose and solve problems.

The informal group can promote and support change. It can be formed by enlisting the help of a strong leader and by forming a strong group that will communicate its perception of needed change to nurse managers and educators.[98]

Communications

Too often change is announced by rumor when it should be clearly introduced. Because changes split teams and kill friendships, causing productivity to drop, employees should be told about upcoming changes before they become rumors.[99] Announcements should be factual and comprehensive and should state objectives, nature, methods, benefits, and drawbacks of the change. An announcement made face-to-face will be better received.

Discussion of implementation should give people maximum information. The discussion should cover the rate and method of implementation, including the first steps that will be taken and the sequence and people involved in each element.

Ceremonies may be effective in various aspects of the change. They are useful for retirement; promotion; introduction of a new coworker, superior, or subordinate; a move to a new job; start of a new system; and reorganization. When used well, ceremonies focus on the importance of the ongoing institution and underline the importance of individual loyalty to that institution and its positions. They convey that the organization and the employees are both needed.

As change agent, the nurse manager discusses with people reasons for resisting change. When people understand the real reasons for the change, they are not as resistant to it. They should be encouraged to sound off.

Planned change needs to be successfully communicated to all employees, even those who are not directly or immediately involved. Verbal announcements can be followed up with written ones and progress reports. Change occurs smoothly in direct proportion to the positive and democratic behavior that demonstrates management's philosophy and practice at all levels from the top down. Communication includes body language and tone of voice as well as words.[100]

Organizational Environment

Nurse managers could be more successful if they paid attention to the organizational environment into which change is introduced and the manner in which it is done. Managers need to be committed to a change and to support it by actions that express their attitudes. When the nurse leader attempts to impose change in an authoritarian manner, people often resist it. Concern for employees is as important as concern for patients. Managers can establish an environment for change by doing the following:

1. Emphasizing relationships with and between groups
2. Bringing out mutual trust and confidence
3. Emphasizing interdependence and shared responsibility
4. Containing group membership and responsibility by preventing individuals from belonging to too many groups and ensuring that the same responsibilities are not given to several groups
5. Having a wide sharing of control and responsibility
6. Resolving conflict through bargaining or problem-solving discussions[101]
7. Permitting job movement to facilitate careers
8. Anticipating and rewarding change, thus institutionalizing it[102]
9. Modifying the nursing organizational structure to accommodate changes that provide growth and development
10. Promoting a can-do attitude
11. Providing predictability and stability by maintaining job security, sharing bad news early, and shifting concern to teamwork and process improvement[103]

When the organizational climate changes, employees change behaviors. A desired organizational climate fosters high-quality patient care.[104]

Anticipating Potential Failures

Although preparation is the key to successful change, it should include anticipation of potential failure. Three questions need to be answered before actions for change begin. First, nurse leaders should determine what the risks are and how much they are willing to expend in terms of resources. Second, they should decide who would do the work. Third, they should have a flexible agenda and plan what will be done when it goes wrong.

Mistakes happen. The importance of the change determines how much risk the nurse leader is prepared to take. For example, one might risk a great deal and reorganize an entire unit to achieve the goal of having professional nurses perform as case managers. Changes can be introduced in one unit, evaluated, and modified before being extended to other units.

The positive aspect of resistance to change is that it pushes the change agent to plan more carefully, listen with sympathetic understanding, and reexamine goals, functions, priorities, and values. When properly addressed, resistance uses less of people's energy. Other effective responses to resistance are showing respect for honest questions and differences of opinion, altering strategy and tactics, altering composition of groups, and proceeding in an objective, firm, assertive, and nonjudgmental manner.[105]

Implementation Science

As the nurse leader determines what to change, when to change, and how to change, she or he must also consider how the staff behaves as they accept the change. One method of decreasing potential failures is to review the work of Sladek, Phillips, and Bond, who believe there are parallel dual processing models that need to be taken into account to assist staff in adopting behavior change. This is an example of implementation science: identifying and understanding behavior, barriers to changing behavior, and effective methods for changing behavior.

One mode of reasoning has been described as experiential, unconscious, fast, associative, heuristic, tacit, quick, intuitive, recognition primed, implicit, and automatic and acquired via biology or exposure. The other mode has been described as rational, conscious, deliberate, slow, rule-based, analytic, explicit, controlled, and acquired by cultural and formal tuition. Sladek et al. believe reasoning can be either-or and that experiential processing is chosen when a judgment is considered relatively unimportant, whereas rational processing is chosen when the stakes are high. The nurse leader needs to implement change taking into account this parallel dual-processing model as she or he outlines the specific components of the change that staff will be responsible for knowing.[106]

Managing Creativity

The nurse manager can encourage creativity through interpersonal relationships that establish trust. This requires acceptance of differing behaviors and ideas and a willingness to listen. It requires friendliness and a spirit of cooperation. It also requires respect for the feelings of others and a lack of defensiveness.[107]

Creative nurses produce a lot. They are unconventional and individualistic. Their critical skills are problem awareness and specification, skills that lead to problem resolution.[108]

Nurse managers can plan to nourish creativity in nursing personnel by doing the following:

1. Noting the creative abilities of those who develop new methods and techniques
2. Providing time and opportunity for people to do creative work. This can be planned during the performance appraisal process.
3. Recognizing those who are masters or experts in nursing work in clinical practice, teaching, research, and management
4. Encouraging nursing personnel to become involved in new nursing endeavors at work, in the community, and in professional organizations, as well as undertaking other activities that increase knowledge and skills
5. Encouraging risk taking and acceptance of personal responsibility

Successful companies hire and keep creative employees who create and market new products. They keep people by knowing how to manage, motivate, and reward them. Venture teams composed of persons with diverse expertise and experiences usually accomplish more than individuals alone. Human resources planning includes recruitment of employees with this expertise and experience. Venture teams are used by such firms as Motorola and the 3M Company.

Creative venture team members include those with technical skills and people skills. They have members who are practical problem solvers and team players. They include artists, scientists, and businesspersons. They must be decisive.

Successful companies do extensive interviewing before hiring. They then do extensive training. They seek people who are genuine in their desire to create new products and serve the customer. Performance appraisal rewards risk taking and intelligent effort that may result in failure.

Innovation results in profitability. Successful companies reward generation of new ideas from within and adoption from without. Performance evaluation should help marginal performers do better. Six-month evaluations are recommended. Peer evaluation and feedback are effective.

Innovative companies do technical audits of individual units to rate them on technical factors, business factors, and overall viability. Reward systems include freedom for creative individual research; freedom to fail; fellowships; in-house grants; autonomy; choice of own venture team; pay raises based on performance, not on seniority; three-track career systems—scientific, managerial, and research; in-house promotions; peer recognition awards; banquets; plaques; and letters of appreciation. Reward teams to foster cooperation. Research confirms results. Reward individuals when someone has "gone the extra mile" to encourage the newcomer, to thank someone who is leaving, when someone's contribution has been ignored by the team, to stir up the team from group-think, and when members differ greatly in their choice of rewards.

Encourage careers through empowerment to raise self-esteem, leading by example, continuing education, and sabbaticals. Motorola spent $60 million on training and $60 million on lost work time to reeducate its employees in 1989.[109]

Evidence-Based Practice 5-2

Kalisch and Curley describe a case study in which an organization identified its strengths, weaknesses, opportunities, and threats through an analysis process. A transformation process was illustrated that included five phases: (1) setting the stage for change, (2) management training, (3) strategic planning, (4) developing and implementing changes at the organizational level, and (5) developing and implementing changes at the unit level. Lessons learned included the following: support from the top, adequate resources, willingness to face the brutal facts, early attention to sustainability, infusion into the grassroots, unrelenting communication, emphasis on building and maintaining trust, ensuring early wins, not declaring success too soon, and recognizing that you cannot fully know how. The need for change and appreciating the ongoing challenge and continuing efforts to transform were underscored in this case study.[110]

SUMMARY

Ability to manage planned change is a necessary competency of all nurses, as it represents viability of the nursing organization. Because planned change is a necessity, nurse managers create the climate for its receptivity by nursing personnel. Change, the key to innovation and the future, has its basis in change theory.

Lewin's change theory is widely used by nurses and involves three stages: unfreezing, moving, and refreezing. In the unfreezing stage, employees are made aware of needed changes. A plan for change is made and tested in the moving stage. During the refreezing stage, the change becomes a part of the system, establishing homeostasis and equilibrium.

Rogers, Havelock, and Lippitt each modified Lewin's original change theory. Reddin's theory has many similarities, and all have common elements of problem solving and decision making.

Resistance to change is evoked by stress from threatened security of affected employees. It can be overcome by planning that involves those who will be affected, particularly if they can see a benefit. Established values and beliefs, imprinting, time perspectives, and hyperenergy all stiffen resistance to change.

The nurse as change agent is the manager of change and thus requires knowledge of the theory of change. Education and training are necessary for nursing personnel who will be affected. Intrinsic and extrinsic rewards are another management tool. Using groups to effect change will help absorb the risks of change; risks are part of the process.

Creativity and innovation are important aspects of nursing that lead to better practice as new knowledge and skills are applied. The result is change that leads to maintenance of a competitive share of the healthcare market, thus ensuring the position of nursing.

In essence, change is all about critical thinking as the nurse leader and nurse manager must think through all aspects of planning the change by answering the following:

- What is the desired outcome, is there evidence to support the change and how will it be measured, via research, performance improvement process or evidence-based practice project?
- Who are the stakeholders and how will they be involved?
- What change theory will be used?
- Has a baseline needs assessment been performed?
- How/where does this planned change fit into strategic initiatives such as implementation of the American Association of Critical Care Nurses's *Healthy Work Environments*?
- Will there be variations among the implementation plans depending on location?
- What is the level of understanding (dual processing) and commitment (social/emotional intelligence) of staff?
- Who needs to be involved in the design of the change process?
- Have the complex adaptive system issues been taken into consideration during the implementation?

Change involves nursing managers in many functions of nursing. It requires planning. The organization is adapted to accommodate the changes. The nurse manager uses communication, leadership, and motivation theory to overcome resistance and gain support in making the change work. The implemented change is continually evaluated to keep it working and effective.

APPLICATION EXERCISES

Exercise 5-1

In your own words, write a definition of critical thinking. Relate it to your use of the nursing process in caring for clients.

Exercise 5-2

We all make personal decisions daily that relate to work, home, family, community, or other aspects of our lives. State a personal problem facing you. Identify the outcome that you want. Determine the means available to achieve this outcome. List the pros and cons of each means, and decide which you will use. Do it!

Exercise 5-3

Refer to your daily newspaper. Identify an issue being discussed related to local (city or county) government.

- What are the arguments involved?
- Which do you support?
- What can you do about them?

Debate the issue. Form a group of your peers and do the following:

1. Determine the pros and cons of the issue.
2. Elect a team captain for each side of the issue.
3. Identify the members of each team.
4. Set rules for the debate: decide on a monitor, determine the speaking sequence and length of time each team member may speak, decide whether the team captains will give summaries, determine who will judge the debate, and decide when and where the debate will take place.
5. Evaluate the debate.

Note: If you wish to do a more formal debate, refer to the Freeley and Steinberg book of note 36, particularly pages 310–311.

Exercise 5-4

Select a change that needs to be made in managing nursing personnel or in nursing care of patients. The needed change may originate from the results of research or from a notable problem. Decide which change theory or theories to use and make a plan for the change.

Exercise 5-5

Ascertain whether your unit of employment has a business plan. If not, develop one with your peers. If there is a business plan, note whether it needs updating, and, if so, update it. Will this process result in any changes within the unit?

Exercise 5-6

Organize a group of professional nurses to do the following:
- Explore the theory of the nursing business within an organization (hospital, nursing home, home health care, professional organization).
- Identify products and activities to be abandoned.
- Identify products or activities to be developed. Select one for a pilot test.

Exercise 5-7

You may complete the following exercise as an individual or as a group.

Scenario: It was obvious to the entire nursing staff of a community hospital that the work load was decreasing. There were empty beds on every unit. Deliveries on the obstetrical unit were down to an average of one per day, and the daily census of the postpartum unit and newborn nursery was four to six patients. Work load and patient census on the pediatric unit were low as well. Rumors were rampant. One was that the pediatric and obstetrical units would be combined. Another was that they would both be closed and their patients would be combined with medical-surgical patients on other units. A third rumor was that the other community hospital was having similar problems and that negotiations were under way to combine several specialty services between the two institutions. It was even rumored that one would become an extended-care facility and that the management of both hospitals would be combined. Worries of nursing staff gave way to gossip among various groups in corridors, at coffee breaks, in the dining room, and everywhere employees chanced to meet, including areas to which patients were transported, such as the x-ray lab, the physical therapy room, and the medical laboratory. Employees were concerned most about job security and institutional stability—whether there would be jobs for all of them and whether the job benefits would be the same if they worked at either hospital. At a clinical nurse managers' meeting, the director of nursing was asked if any of the rumors were true. She stated that the administrator would make an announcement at the appropriate time and that until then the staff should continue with its work. That afternoon the local newspaper announced a merger of the two hospitals, describing in detail the missions and services each would provide to the community. No reference was made to the plans for employees.

Prepare a business plan (management plan) that embodies application of change theory that would be best under the preceding scenario.

Exercise 5-8

Scan the previous year's issues of 10 different nursing journals and answer the following.
How many articles report research in
Management or administration?
Teaching?
Practice?

Exercise 5-9

Form a group of your peers and have each member identify something that can be improved in nursing. This may be a policy or a procedure; a change in a form to make its use more effective; an interdepartmental protocol, such as how tests are scheduled or patients transported or handled; or a change in clinical practice. Using change theory, each person makes a plan for improvement and discusses it with the peer group. When the group decides the plan merits implementation, present it to nursing administration where you work or are assigned as a student.

Exercise 5-10

Explore the idea of creating a nursing research/evidence-based practice council, or think outside the box and call it a council of professional inquiry. Consider its mission, philosophy, and objectives. If there is enough interest among the nurses in the organization in which you work, make a management plan to launch the council as an organizational entity.

Exercise 5-11

Use the Internet to look at some of the practices of highly profitable companies. What business practices do they use that could be used in the health care industry? Pay particular attention to practices related to creativity, innovation, and research. Is there evidence of the application of change theory?

Exercise 5-12

Take time with subordinates and review a recently implemented change. Have subordinates identify how/if each of the 14 forces were impacted. Note areas not involved and determine if this would have made a difference in the adoption of the change and/or its sustainability.

Notes

1. Wynett, C., Fogarty, T., & Kadish, R. (2002). Inspiring innovation. *Harvard Business Review, 80*(8), 39–49.
2. American Organization of Nurse Executives. (2005). AONE nurse executive competencies. *Nurse Leader,* February, p. 51.
3. Newcomb, D. P., & Swansburg, R. C. (1971). *The team plan: A manual for nursing service administrators* (2nd ed., pp. 136–172). New York: Putnam.
4. Lattimer, R. L., & Winitsky, M. L. (1984). Unleashing creativity. *Management World,* 22–24.
5. Gilmartin, J. (1999). Creativity: The fuel of innovation. *Nursing Administration Quarterly, 23*(2), 1–8.
6. Reinkemeyer, M. H. (1968). A nursing paradox. *Nursing Research, 8,* 26–34.
7. Manion, J. (1991). Nurse entrepreneurs: The heroes of health care's future. *Nursing Outlook, 39*(1), 18–21.

8. Godfrey, R. R. (1986). Tapping employees' creativity. *Supervisory Management, 16–20.*

9. American Nurses Credentialing Center. (2005). *Magnet recognition program.* Silver Spring, MD: American Nurses Credentialing Center. Retrieved July 6, 2008 from http://www.nursecredentialing.org

10. Gordon, J., & Zemke, R. (1986). Making them more creative. *Training, 23,* 30–34.

11. Van Gundy, A. G. (1984). How to establish a creative climate in the work group. *Management Review,* 24–25, 28, 37–38.

12. Glucksberg, S. (1968). Some ways to turn on new ideas. *Think,* 24–28.

13. Munhall, P. (2007). *Nursing research: A qualitative perspective* (4th ed.). Boston: Jones and Bartlett.

14. Stefaniak, K. (2007). Discovering nursing excellence through appreciative inquiry. *Nurse Leader, 5*(2), April, 42–46.

15. Troxel, J. (2002). *Appreciative inquiry: An action research method for organizational transformation and its implications to the practice of group process facilitation.* Retrieved January 19, 2007, from http://www.consultmillennia.com/document/Appreciative%20Inquiry.pdf

16. Lattimer & Winitsky, 1984.

17. Van Gundy, 1984.

18. Atchley, R. A., Keeney, M., & Burgess, C. (1999). Cerebral hemispheric mechanisms linking ambiguous word meaning retrieval and creativity. *Brain Cognition,* 479–499.

19. Lattimer & Winitsky, 1984.

20. Godfrey, 1986.

21. Drucker, P. F. (1985). Creating strategies of innovation. *Planning Review,* 8–11, 45.

22. Godfrey, 1986.

23. Levinson, H. (1965). What an executive should know about scientists. *Notes & Quotes.* Hartford, CT: Connecticut General Life Insurance Company, 1.

24. Godfrey, 1986.

25. Kleinman, C. S. (1999). Nurse executives: New roles, new opportunities. *Journal of Health Administration Education, 8*(6), 15–26.

26. Newcomb & Swansburg, 1971.

27. Southon, G. (1999). IT, change and evaluation: An overview of the role of evaluation in health services. *International Journal of Medical Information, 4*(1),125–133.

28. Peters, T. (1990, August 11). Lack of curiosity may kill business. *San Antonio Light,* p. B2.

29. Rutherford, P., Lee, B., & Greiner, A. (2004). *Transforming care at the bedside.* IHI Innovation series white paper. Boston: Institute for Healthcare Improvement.

30. Newhouse, R. (2007). Accelerating improvement. *Journal of Nursing Administration, 37,* 264–268.

31. Albrecht, K. (2005). Social intelligence: A different kind of "smart." The American Society of Training and Development 2005 annual conference, concurrent session, Orlando, FL.

32. Facione, P. A. (1990). *The Delphi Report. Critical thinking: A statement of expert consensus for purposes of educational assessment and instruction* (p. 2). (Executive Summary). Milbrae, CA: The California Academic Press.

33. Scheffer, B. K., & Rubenfeld, M. G. (2000). A consensus statement on critical thinking. *Journal of Nursing Education,* 352–359.

34. Simpson, E., & Courtney, M. (2000). Critical thinking in nursing education: Literature review. *International Journal of Nursing Practice, 8,* 89–98.

35. Ibid.

36. Freeley, A. J., & Steinberg, D. L. (1999). *Argumentation and debate* (10th ed., pp. 1–3). Belmont, CA: Wadsworth.

37. Ibid., p. 8.

38. Ibid., pp. 9–12.

39. Jones, S. A., & Brown, L. N. (1993). Alternative views on defining critical thinking through the nursing process. *Holistic Nurse Practitioner,* 71–76.

40. Jackson, M., Ignatavicius, D., & Case, B. (2006). *Conversations in critical thinking and clinical judgment.* American Association of Critical Care Nurses. Boston: Jones and Bartlett.

41. Bloom, B. (1956). *Taxonomy of educational objectives—handbook 1.* New York: David McKay Company, Inc.

42. Olney, C. (2005). Using evaluation to adapt health information outreach to the complex environments of community-based organizations. *Journal of Medical Library Association, 93*(Suppl.), S57–S67.

43. Plsek, P., & Greenhalgh, T. (2001). The challenge of complexity in healthcare. *British Medical Journal, 323,* 625–628.

44. Kemp, V. H. (1985). Concept analysis as a strategy for promoting critical thinking. *Journal of Nursing Education,* 382–384.

45. Graduate students in the master's program in nursing management at Louisiana State University School of Nursing, New Orleans, LA, Fall 1993.

46. Woods, J. H. (1993). Affective learning: One door to critical thinking. *Holistic Nurse Practitioner,* 64–70.

47. McKenzie, L. (1992). Critical thinking in health care supervision. *Health Care Supervisor,* 2.

48. Naisbitt, J. (1999). *High tech high touch* (pp. 24–26). New York: Broadway Books.

49. Bos, S. (1998). Perceived benefits of peer leadership as described by junior baccalaureate nursing students. *Journal of Nursing Education,* 189–191.

50. Taylor, K. L., & Care, W. D. (1999). Nursing education as cognitive apprenticeship: A framework for clinical education. *Nurse Educator,* 31–36.

51. Williams, E. G. (1969). Changing systems and behavior. *Business Horizons,* 53–58.

52. Kanter, R. M. (1989). *When giants learn to dance* (pp. 9–26). New York: Simon & Schuster.

53. Nadler, D. A., & Tushman, M. L. (1989). Organizational frame bending: Principles for managing reorganization. *Executive,* 194–204.

54. Peters, T. (1991, November 19). Winds of change hit central staffs. *San Antonio Light,* p. E3.

55. Covin, T. J., & Kilmann, R. H. (1990). Participant perceptions of positive and negative influences on large-scale change. *Group & Organizational Studies,* 233–248.

56. Brynildsen, R. D., & Wickes, T. A. (1970). Agents of changes. *Automation, 17,* 36–40.

57. Porter-O'Grady, T. (1986). *Creative nursing administration: Participative management in the 21st century* (p. 109). Norcross, GA: Affiliated Dynamics.

58. Barden, C. E. (2005). *AACN standards for establishing and sustaining healthy work environments.* Aliso Viejo, CA: American Association of Critical-Care Nurses.

59. Reddin, W. J. (1969). Confessions of an organizational change agent. *Group and Organizational Management, 2*(1), 33–41.

60. Ibid.

61. Spradley, James. 1980. *Participant Observation.* United States: Holt Rinehart and Winston. Welch, L. B. (1979). Planned change in nursing: The theory. *Nursing Clinics of North America, 14*(2), 307–321.

62. Ibid.

63. Ibid.

64. Welch, 1979.

65. Ibid.

66. Ibid.; Oates, K. (1997). Models of planned change and research utilization applied to product evaluation. *Clinical Nurse Specialist,* 270–273.

67. Welch, 1979.

68. Spradley, 1980.

69. Kreidler, C. M., Campbell, J., Lanik, G., Gray, V. R., & Conrad, M. A. (1994). Community elderly: A nursing center's use of change theory as a model. *Journal of Gerontological Nursing,* 25–30.

70. Gladwell, M. (2000). *The tipping point: How little things can make a big difference.* Boston: Little, Brown and Company.

71. Ibid.

72. Ibid.

73. Dunphy, D. C., & Stace, D. A. (1988). Transformational and coercive strategies for planned organizational change: Beyond the O. D. model. *Organizational Studies, 9,* 317–334.

74. Ibid.

75. Stewart, T. A. (1993). Welcome to the revolution. *Fortune, 128,* 66–80.

76. Tichy, N. M. (1993). Revolutionize your company. *Fortune, 128,* 114–118.

77. Welch, J. A master class in radical change. (1993). *Fortune, 128,* 82–96.

78. Ibid.

79. Roach, J. V. (1988, April 4). U.S. business: Time to seize the day. *Newsweek,* p. 10; Beyers, M. (1984). Getting on top of organizational change: Part 1, process and development. *Journal of Nursing Administration,* 32–39; Freed, D. H. (1998). Please don't shoot me: I'm only the change agent. *Health Care Supervision,* 56–61.

80. Feldman, J., & Daly-Gawenda, D. (1985). Retrenchment: How nurse executives cope. *Journal of Nursing Administration,* 31–37.

81. Rosenberg, D. (1993). Eliminating resistance to change. *Security Management,* 20–21.

82. Williams, 1969.

83. Ward, M. J., & Moran, S. G. (1984). Resistance to change: Recognize, respond, overcome. *Nursing Management,* 30–33.

84. Hunt, R. E., & Rigby, M. K. (1984). Easing the pain of change. *Management Review,* 41–45.

85. Ibid.

86. Gillen, D. J. (1986). Harvesting the energy from change anxiety. *Supervisory Management,* 40–43.

87. Ward & Moran, 1984.

88. Drucker, P. F. (1999). *Management challenges for the 21st century* (p. 73). New York: HarperCollins.

89. Melnyk, B., & Fineout-Overholt, E. (2005). *Evidence-based practice in nursing and healthcare* (p. 8). Philadelphia: Lippincott Williams & Wilkins.

90. Stevens, K. R. (2004). *ACE star model of EBP: Knowledge transformation.* Academic Center for Evidence-based Practice. The University of Texas Health Science Center at San Antonio. Retrieved July 6, 2008 from http://www.acestar.uthscsa.edu

91. Beyers, M. (1984). Getting on top of organizational change. Part 2. Trends in nursing service. *Journal of Nursing Administration, 14,* 31–37.

92. Ibid.

93. Drucker, 1999.

94. Beyers, 1984; Gillen, 1986.

95. Gillen, 1986.

96. McPhail, G. (1997). Management of change: An essential skill for nursing in the 1990s. *Journal of Nursing Management,* 199–205.

97. Hunt & Rigby, 1984.

98. Ward & Moran, 1984.

99. Report on Victor E. Dowling's change theory, "How to wage the war on change." (1990). *Electrical World,* 38–39.

100. Levick, D. (1996). How do you communicate? Managing the change process. *Physician Executive,* 26–29.

101. Endres, R. E. (1972). Successful management of change. *Notes & Quotes.*

102. Hunt & Rigby, 1984.

103. Report on Victor E. Dowling's change theory, 1990.

104. Beyers, 1984.

105. Ward & Moran, 1984.
106. Sladek, R., Phillips, P., & Bond, M. (2006). Implementation science: A role for parallel dual processing models of reasoning? *Implementation Science, 1,* 1–8.
107. Van Gundy, 1984.
108. Gordon & Zemke, 1986.
109. Gupta, A. K., & Singhal, A. (1993). Managing human resources for innovation and creativity. *Resource Technology Management, 36,* 41–48.
110. Kalisch, B., & Curley, M. (2008). Transforming a nursing organization: A case study. *Journal of Nursing Administration, 38,* 76–83.

References

Barry-Walker, J. (2000). The impact of systems redesign on staff, patient, and financial outcomes. *Journal of Nursing Administration, 30*(2), 77–89.

Beasley, P. (2000, May 7). Ways to boost creativity in the workplace. *The Knoxville News Sentinel,* p. J1.

Bradshaw, M. J. (1999). Clinical pathways: A tool to evaluate clinical learning. *Journal of the Society of Pediatric Nurses,* 37–40.

Buckley, D. S. (1999). A practitioner's view on managing change. *Frontier Health Service Management,* 38–43, 49–50.

Greenwood, J. (2000). Critical thinking and nursing scripts: The case for the development of both. *Journal of Advanced Nursing,* 428–436.

Ingersoll, G. L., Kirsch, J. C., Merk, S. E., & Lightfoot, J. (2000). Relationship of organizational culture and readiness for change to employee commitment to the organization. *Journal of Nursing Administration,* 11–20.

Jones, D. C., & Sheridan, M. E. (1999). A case study approach: Developing critical thinking skills in novice pediatric nurses. *Journal of Continuing Education in Nursing,* 75–78.

Keenan, J. (1999). A concept analysis of autonomy. *Journal of Advanced Nursing,* 556–562.

Lyth, G. M. (2000). Clinical supervision: A concept analysis. *Journal of Advanced Nursing,* 722–729.

Muir, N. (2004). Clinical decision-making: Theory and practice. *Nursing Standard, 18,* 47–52, 54–55.

Oermann, M. H. (1998). How to assess critical thinking in clinical practice. *Dimensions of Critical Care Nursing,* 322–327.

Platzer, H., Blake, D., & Ashford, D. (2000). An evaluation of process and outcomes from learning through reflective practice groups on a post-registration nursing course. *Journal of Advanced Nursing,* 689–695.

Redfern, S., Christian, S., & Norman, I. (2003). Evaluating change in healthcare practice: Lessons from three studies. *Journal of Evaluation in Clinical Practice, 9,* 239–249.

Rodger, M. A., & King, L. (2000). Drawing up and administering intramuscular injections: A review of the literature. *Journal of Advanced Nursing,* 574–582.

Whitley, G. G. (1999). Processes and methodologies for research validation of nursing diagnosis. *Nursing Diagnosis,* 5–14.

6 COLLABORATIVE DECISION MAKING AND COMMUNICATION:
Skills and Practices

Linda Roussel, DSN, RN, NEA, BC
Russell C. Swansburg, PhD, RN

LEARNING OBJECTIVES AND ACTIVITIES

- Describe collaborative decision making.
- Define decision making.
- Distinguish among different models of decision making.
- Describe the steps in the decision-making process.
- Apply the decision-making process.
- Identify ways to make decision making more effective.
- Describe the place of intuition in the decision-making process.
- Describe the steps in the problem-solving process.
- Describe group problem-solving techniques.
- Illustrate the components of communication as it relates to decision making and problem solving.
- Interpret the elements of communication, evaluating the climate for effective communication.
- Distinguish between communication as perception and communication as information.
- Compare communication with feedback to communication without feedback.
- Distinguish among causes of listening habits and techniques to improve listening.
- Distinguish among media of communication.
- Contrast future impacts on communication on decision making and problem solving.

CONCEPTS

Collaborative decision making, decision making, normative model, decision-tree model, descriptive model, strategic model, cost–benefit analysis, intuition, organizational decision, personal decision, problem solving, communication, elements of communication, communication climate, perception, feedback, information, listening, media of communication, questions, oral communication, written communication, interviews, human capital

---

QUOTE

Imagination is the beginning of creation: you imagine that you desire, you will what you imagine, and at last you create what you will.

—George Bernard Shaw

A manager applies decision-making theory and the problem-solving process in achieving the mission of the nursing agency, supports the notion that all communication takes place within the principle of channel of communication, facilitates staff participation in decision making, considers the development and implementation of organizational systems, and specifies resources necessary to implement the plan.

A leader coaches and involves team members and associates when applying decision-making theory and the problem-solving process to achieve the mission of the nursing agency and collaborates in the design and improvement of systems and processes that ensure interventions and implemented by appropriate staff member.

Introduction

Collaborative decision making is important to decentralized problem solving. Communicating at the unit level provides a greater opportunity to make a difference in staff integration of outcomes. When staff is engaged and productive, greater creativity can be expected. Collaborative decision making can enhance transparency because there is greater openness to all involved and improved accountability and commitment, equity, and efficiency as information is shared and redundancy is avoided. These strategies incorporate staff members' feedback and involvement in the organization and its work. Collaborative decision making and problem solving are often praised as the best management practices in successful organization.[1] Research in magnet hospitals on attracting and retaining nurses as well as maintaining positive patient and organizational outcomes further advances this notion, identifying excellent communication, collaborative relationships, and participation in decision making as assets.[2–4] Keeping patients safe by transforming the work environment for nurses, a major initiative, underscores the critical nature of communication, collaborative decision making, and problem solving.[5] *Nursing's Agenda for the Future: A Call to the Nation* further strengthens these directives.[6] The nurse administrator's ability to meet these challenges requires an understanding of decision making, problem solving, and communication.

Complex decision making is a part of any level of nursing. Functioning successfully, the nurse must demonstrate problem-solving skills in uncertain and changing situations in which indecisiveness or poor decisions are costly. The ability to foster organizational decision making and problem solving is an essential personal skill for nurses. This chapter deals with models and strategies that nurses can use to strengthen personal skills and further develop the decision-making and problem-solving abilities of staff members. The theory of decision making, a required competency for professionals, is an essential component of the nursing and management process. Good decisions require internal and external information on how other people view the world of nursing and make decisions.

DECISION-MAKING PROCESS

Definition

Everyone at some time makes decisions, and it may be assumed that innate abilities, past experience, and intuition form the basis for making successful decisions. Decisions are often made by choosing among known alternatives. But what about unknown alternatives? Making a choice is not the only element of decision making. The process, which usually involves a systematic approach of sequenced steps, should be adaptable to the environment in which it is used. Lancaster and Lancaster define decision making as a systematic, sequential process of choosing among alternatives and putting the choice into action. This definition acknowledges natural and learned abilities while providing order and continuity to the process of decision making.[7]

Empirical evidence shows that timely decision makers are needed in today's environment. Such decision makers consider more alternatives, more batches of options, at one time. They are experienced mentors, or they rely on older, experienced mentors. Speedy decision makers thoughtfully integrate strategies and tactics. They juggle budgets, schedules, and organizational options simultaneously. They constitute the winning culture in decision making.[8]

Wah describes four predominate decision-making models: the rational model, incremental model, satisfying model, and garbage can model. The rational model is the most frequently used by managers because it is objective, logical, and systematic. Wah identifies eight common pitfalls in making good decisions:[9]

1. *Complexity of problem:* When one is only able to comprehend or handle seven pieces of information at any point of time, there is limited cognitive capability and information-processing capacity. This often results in managers being unable to fully comprehend the issue or problem. Given this predisposition, managers tend to reduce a problem's complexity to more manageable levels, often oversimplifying a problem. Teams can help to reduce such issues. Group decision making helps better diagnose and define the problem.

2. *Unclear problem:* Managers may not probe deep enough to get to the real cause or root of the problem; thus the problem may be defined too broadly or too narrowly. Symptoms may be confused with the problems. When a problem is not well defined, the solutions address the symptom and not the actual problem.

3. *Mental blocks:* Mental blocks may occur at the cultural, perceptual, emotional, or intellectual levels. "Perceptual blocks, also called biases, can distort problem identification, which in turn results in focusing on certain types of alternatives and not others. Similarly, cultural blocks prevent thinking out of the box and instead promote remaining in one's own comfort zone. Creating a multicultural team by bringing together members from different cultural backgrounds may help to reduce such a barrier."[10] Developing teams may take time, particularly if the organization's culture does not support innovative, diverse groups working together.

4. *Available information:* Decisions may be made with available, accessible information rather than quality, "fresh" alternatives. Quick fixes may be necessary; however, not all problems are urgent and thus require more time and more information, particularly if they are complex and far reaching.

5. *Uncertain evaluation criteria:* Deciding on the best, most useful criteria is an important step in the decision-making process. It is important to determine criteria as well as the weight, or ranking, of the outcome. Agreeing on the evaluation criteria is never an easy task. If the criteria are

not clearly defined, this will pose a difficulty in evaluating and choosing the right alternatives. Outcomes should be relevant and measurable.

6. *Choosing the best decision:* The organization's structure and culture are to be considered in choosing the best option in solving the problem. Individual self-interest or preference should be avoided. Discussions should be open and presented fairly and equitably. Teamwork and team spirit can reduce power struggles and are important in sustaining good decisions and change.

7. *Constraint in resources:* Decisions are interrelated, and a conceptual and holistic view is important to the process. A constraint on time, costs, and human resources limits the choice of the best alternative. The objective is to know how to use limited resources to achieve unlimited outcomes.

8. *Management involvement:* It is important that the right decisions be carefully considered. Implementation is the next step, often a more challenging task given the need for a motivated, committed workforce. A less than perfect alternative with good execution may likely bring about better results than a good alternative with poor execution.

In a holistic decision-making process, getting the "right" people involved in the process will not only increase acceptance of the alternative but will also enhance successful implementation and sustainability.

Clinical Decision Making

In the clinical decision-making arena, clinical nurses manage patients' histories and physical data, nursing diagnoses, nursing interventions, and nursing outcomes data to affect therapeutic results.[11] Many decision support systems are available in the medical treatment of patients. Evidence shows that most patients prefer to leave decision making to their healthcare providers. This is, however, changing with the widespread use of the Internet, informing patients of their illness and healthcare and treatment options. Evidence-based practices have also influenced patients' decision-making ability, giving sound information on which to base decisions.[12]

Patients' decision-making activity decreases with age and severe illnesses and increases with education.[10] Evidence on decision making related to individual protocols abounds. This literature includes decision making about cancer treatments, cardiovascular disease, growth hormone therapy, triage practices, and computer systems related to clinical decision-making models in general.[13] Nurse practitioners use these decision support systems while developing additional ones. Such nurse practitioner support systems are being studied in relation to general practice.[14]

A review of the literature yields a number of decision-making models. Four models are covered in this chapter.

Normative Model

This model is at least 200 years old. It is assumed to maximize satisfaction and fulfills the "perfect knowledge assumption" that in any given situation calling for a decision, all possible choices and the consequences and potential outcome of each are known.[15] Seven steps are identified in this analytically precise model:

1. Define and analyze the problem.
2. Identify all available alternatives.
3. Evaluate the pros and cons of each alternative.
4. Rank the alternatives.
5. Select the alternative that maximizes satisfaction.
6. Implement.
7. Follow up.

The normative model for decision making is unrealistic because it assumes that there are clear-cut choices between identified alternatives.

Decision-Tree Model

Various adaptations of decision-tree analysis are found in the literature; the essential elements described in the 1960s are standard. All factors considered important to a decision can be represented on a decision tree. Vroom arranged answers to seven diagnostic questions in the form of a decision tree to identify types of leadership style used in management decision-making models. The questions focus on protecting the quality and acceptance of the decision and deal with adequacy of information, goal congruence, structure of the problem, acceptance by subordinates, conflict, fairness, and priority for implementation.[16] Magee and Brown depict decision trees as starting with a basic problem and using branches to represent event forks and action forks. The number of branches at each fork corresponds to the number of identified alternatives. Every path through the tree corresponds to a possible sequence of actions and events, each with its own distinct consequences. Probabilities of both positive and negative consequences of each action and event are estimated and recorded on the appropriate branch. Additional options (e.g., delaying the decision) and consequences of each action–event sequence can be depicted on the decision tree. Computer simulations of decision trees are now available and can be adapted to a limited number or a highly complex network of branches involved in the decision-making process. Normal analysis of the tree is conducted by computing predicted consequences of all event forks (the right-hand edge of the tree), substituting that value for the actual event fork and its consequences, and selecting the action fork with the best expected consequences. Both the optimal strategy and its expected consequences are determined. Quantitative analysis in the form of decision trees can be used for any type of problem but may be unnecessary in simple problems involving limited consequences.[17]

Descriptive Model

Simon developed the descriptive model based on the assumption that the decision maker is a rational person looking for acceptable solutions based on known information. This model allows for the fact that many decisions are made with incomplete information because of time, money, or personnel limitations; it also allows for the fact that people do not always make the best choices. Simon wrote that few decisions would ever be made if people always sought optimal solutions. Instead, he contended, people identify acceptable alternatives. The following are the steps in the descriptive model:[18]

1. Establish an acceptable goal.
2. Define subjective perceptions of the problem.
3. Identify acceptable alternatives.
4. Evaluate each alternative.
5. Select an alternative.
6. Implement a decision.
7. Follow up.

The descriptive model may lend itself well to nurses faced with daily decisions that must be made rapidly and that have significant consequences. Steps in the model are not unlike those in the familiar nursing process, although the sequencing is different. Readers may readily identify conditions in their own environments similar to those described by Simon and see immediate application of this model.[19] Lancaster and Lancaster illustrated the use of this model for nursing administrators.[20]

Figure 6-1 was developed by Swansburg (one of this chapter's authors) after many years of experience using the descriptive model.

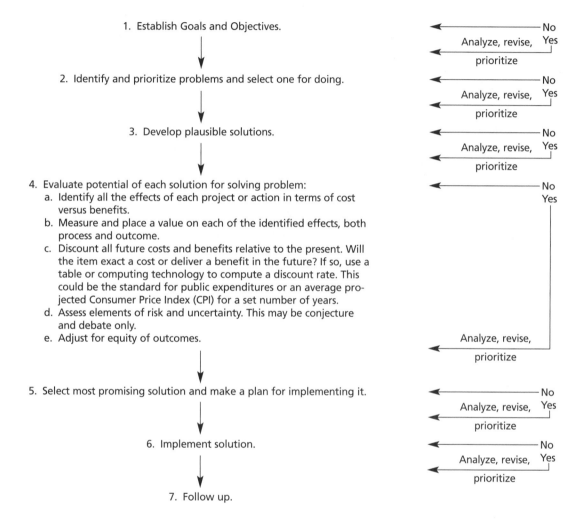

FIGURE 6-1 THE DECISION-MAKING PROCESS, INCLUDING COST–BENEFIT ANALYSIS

1. Establish Goals and Objectives.

    No
    Analyze, revise, Yes
    prioritize

2. Identify and prioritize problems and select one for doing.

    No
    Analyze, revise, Yes
    prioritize

3. Develop plausible solutions.

    No
    Analyze, revise, Yes
    prioritize

4. Evaluate potential of each solution for solving problem:
   a. Identify all the effects of each project or action in terms of cost versus benefits.
   b. Measure and place a value on each of the identified effects, both process and outcome.
   c. Discount all future costs and benefits relative to the present. Will the item exact a cost or deliver a benefit in the future? If so, use a table or computing technology to compute a discount rate. This could be the standard for public expenditures or an average projected Consumer Price Index (CPI) for a set number of years.
   d. Assess elements of risk and uncertainty. This may be conjecture and debate only.
   e. Adjust for equity of outcomes.

    No
    Yes

    Analyze, revise, prioritize

5. Select most promising solution and make a plan for implementing it.

    No
    Analyze, revise, Yes
    prioritize

6. Implement solution.

    No
    Analyze, revise, Yes
    prioritize

7. Follow up.

Establishing goals and objectives requires that decisions are made as to how they will be achieved. A first decision may be setting the priority in which the goals are carried out. Decisions do not relate only to problems. They relate to development of plans and programs to accomplish nursing goals and objectives. When the best alternative does not work, another decision on whether to start over from step 1 is required, especially if other alternatives have less chance of success. The cost versus the benefit of the solution is introduced at step 4.

Source: Author.

Strategic Model.

Strategic decision making usually relates to long-term planning. As an example, hospitals merge and nursing departments are affected. Among the decisions that are made are whether to hire one top manager or department head versus two or more, whether to decentralize and eliminate middle managers, and what operational strategies prevent duplication and maximize scarce resources, providing for their efficient use. Nagelkerk and Henry used a model by Mintzberg, Raisinghani, and Theoret, known as the MRT model, to design and test the nature of strategic decision making that entails substantial risk. They worked with chief nurse executives employed in six acute care hospitals with 400 or more beds each.[21] In applying this model, participants used mixed scanning of general and specific information from associates to identify complex problems. To develop potential solutions, they gathered facts from hospital documents. They made their selection of the best single solution by "(1) screening solutions using predetermined criteria, (2) identifying the costs and benefits as nearly as possible, and (3) selecting the single best solution."[22]

It was concluded that top managers make these final choices using intuition, formal analysis, and knowledge of organizational politics. In making good choices, top managers do extensive planning, communicating, and politicking.

In this research project, successful strategies for decision making were reported as follows:[23]

1. Building extensive networks of individuals and groups who would provide resources at local, state, and national levels
2. Searching the nursing, hospital, and business literature
3. Being knowledgeable and involved in the politics of one's organization and professional organizations
4. Communicating regularly and repeatedly about decision-making activities to organization members, especially those in the hospital's dominant coalition—usually the chief executive officer, finance manager, and chief of the medical staff
5. Directing most of their time and energy toward the accomplishment of their plans

Because the model proved promising in strategic decision making, it needs further testing, particularly in the area of human resource development and investment in human capital. As described in this work, strategic decision making was the domain of top management. With healthcare organizations becoming flatter and leaner, input from self-managed work teams may be profitable.

Steps in the Process

From these and other models of decision making, seven general steps of the process have been identified. Goals and objectives may be set before beginning the general process to answer the question, "What do we want the outcome or results of this decision to be?" When new products or services are the outcome, the goals and objectives are established first and problems or decisions are then forecast (step 1 of Figure 6-1). (Managers who wish to reverse steps 1 and 2 may do so.)

The problem must be identified (step 2 of Figure 6-1). Although this step may seem simple, recognizing and defining the problem is complex because of the diversity of individual perceptions. Because all individuals affected by the problem should be involved in discussing it, authority for decision making should be delegated to individuals at the level of impact. When this is impossible, representatives of various affected groups may provide input. Each representative may have a different perspective as to what the outcome should be. Nurses should make certain that the identified problem is one that requires their attention and cannot be handled alone by those involved. Collecting factual information in addition to subjective perceptions is essential. Logical and systematic fact finding includes questioning all sources for divergent opinions and objective data. When the difference between desired and present situations or outcomes is significant, it may signal recognition of the problem.

The third step in decision making is gathering and analyzing information related to the solution (step 3 of Figure 6-1). This step involves defining, through a series of activities, the specifications to be met by the solution. A thorough information search may be needed to validate that the problem has been correctly identified. This search should include knowledge of organizational policy, prior personal experience or training, or the experience of others. Externally, the nurse begins to identify alternatives, comparing the potential solutions to the desired outcome and the desired outcome to available resources. In organizational settings, database information systems may provide this information quickly. Establishing goals with measurable objectives helps focus the search for alternatives. When comparing potential alternatives, one should certainly consider the cost, the time required and available, and the capabilities of those who will be involved in implementing a decision.

It is essential to involve in these discussions the individuals who will be affected by the choice. Irrelevant, insignificant, and extraneous factors must be eliminated from consideration. Gaining a commitment to implement a decision before the choice is made supports the process. It is possible to reach a point of overload when the searcher has received information too quickly or in too great a quantity to process. Research indicates that the quantity of information sought has a direct, positive correlation with the degree of anticipated risk in the decision to be made. The personal confidence of the decision maker also affects the amount of information required to support decision-making choices. Less searching is required by the nurse who recognizes patterns or similarities to previously encountered problems and confidently makes a choice of alternatives.

The fourth and fifth steps in decision making are evaluating all alternatives and selecting one for implementation (Figure 6-1, steps 4 and 5). In the evaluation of alternatives, possible positive and negative consequences and the estimated probability of each choice are identified. A common approach involves identifying the best and worst possible outcomes to an alternative and then the outcomes that fall between the two extremes. As each alternative is evaluated, additional options may become apparent. Disagreement may stimulate the imagination and produce better solutions.

The effects of making no decision must be weighed against the effects of each proposed solution. Each alternative must be systematically evaluated for its efficiency and effectiveness in accomplishing the desired outcome and for the likelihood of achieving it with available or obtainable resources. The advantages and disadvantages of each alternative are identified during these steps to determine risk factors in possible outcomes. One should identify the solution that best satisfies specifications before any compromises, concessions, or revisions are made by involved parties. The alternative that provides the greatest probability of an acceptable desired outcome using available resources is most likely to be selected.

A sixth step in the decision-making process is to act on or implement the selected alternative (step 6 of Figure 6-1). The knowledge and skills of the decision maker transform the alternative into action by completing any necessary plans involving sequencing steps and preparing individuals to implement the solution while effectively communicating the process with all involved.

Orton suggests asking seven questions to increase the success of one's decision:[24]

1. Does the quality of the decision really make a difference?
2. Do I have all the information I need to make the decision alone?
3. Do I know what I'm missing? Do I know where to find the information? Will I know what to do with the information I'm given?
4. Do I need anybody's commitment to make sure this succeeds?
5. Can I gain commitments without offering participation in the decision?
6. Do those involved in the decision share the organization's goals?
7. Is there likely to be conflict about the available alternatives?

A final step in the process of decision making is to monitor the implementation and evaluate the outcomes (step 7 of Figure 6-1). The nurse compares actual results with anticipated outcomes and makes modifications as needed to accomplish the desired outcome. Evaluation criteria obtained from measurable objectives provide feedback for testing the validity and effectiveness of the decision against the actual sequence of events in the process. Determination of flaws or gaps in the process may assist the decision maker to monitor the process more closely in the future and prevent the recurrence of problems. The effective decision maker consciously follows these seven steps in a logical sequence.

Cost–Benefit Analysis

Cost–benefit analysis has a major role to play as a decision-making tool. Is the expenditure justified in terms of the return or benefit on the investment? Figure 6-1 illustrates the addition of cost–benefit analysis to the decision-making process. Cost–benefit analysis should be as objective as possible. Many actions can be quantified and a value placed on them. Others are qualitative and should be evaluated on a rational basis.[25]

Prescriptive Decision Theory

Prescriptive decision theory uses decision-making rules that are more clearly related to the rational modes of thinking (left-brain thinking). Descriptive decision theory, on the other hand, looks for patterns, regularities, or principles related to the process by which people actually make decisions.

The defining attributes of a decision are the following:[26]

- Making a deliberate mental choice
- Taking action based on indication or evidence
- Choosing between two or more options
- Bringing doubt or debate to an end by committing to certain actions or inactions
- Expecting to accomplish certain goals

The antecedents of a decision are the following:

- Consideration of a matter that causes doubt, wavering, debate, or controversy
- Awareness of choices or options
- Gathering information about alternatives
- Examination and evaluation of the feasibility of the various alternatives
- Weighing the risks and possible consequences of each option

The consequences of a decision are the following:

- A stabilizing effect, with an end to the doubt, wavering, debate, or controversy
- An action with one of the following goals: to reaffirm the decision with full implementation, to reverse the decision, to stand by the decision but to curtail full implementation, and to consider subsequent decisions in response to ever-changing circumstances and desires

Issues in Decision Making

Information technology increasingly affects decision making; pitfalls in the process originate more frequently in individuals than in computers. Individuals are still resistant to change involving risk and new ideas. Such attitudes stifle not only individuals but also groups. When nurses find themselves resisting, they should analyze their behavior with the goal of becoming more imaginative and creative. It is important to move away from becoming authoritarian and controlling. If the nurse chooses to control decision making and omit from the process those affected by the decision, a weaker commitment to implementing the decision is a natural result. When feasible, the nurse may use a team approach to decision making, as in a matrix organization. Group decision making usually produces greater commitment to putting the selected alternative into action and working for success. Team decision making is especially effective in patient care.

Other pitfalls of decision making include inadequate fact finding, time constraints, and poor communication. Failing to systematically follow the steps of the decision making process will likely result in unanticipated results.

Improving Decision Making by Improving Communication

Basic precepts other than those already mentioned include educating people so they know how to make decisions, securing top management support for decision making at the lowest possible level, establishing decision-making checkpoints with appropriate time limits, keeping informed of progress by ensuring access to first-hand information, using statistical analysis when possible to pinpoint problems for solution,[27] and staying open to the use of new ideas and technologies to analyze problems and identify alternatives. Computers can be used to support decision making through data-based management systems. Strategies and tools are available to improve decision-making abilities.

A successful nurse is one who stays informed about decisions being made at different levels of the organization after appropriately delegating these responsibilities, who deals only with those decisions requiring his or her level of expertise, who supports decision implementation, and who credits the decision maker. McKenzie purports that managers who make all decisions themselves convey a lack of trust in the ability or loyalty of their associates. Selective delegation of decision making gains the support of staff members and enhances their confidence. This can facilitate a sense of belonging and loyalty. Delegation leads to leadership. Leaders share authority and power rather than impose it. This is not to say that leaders never make decisions without input from associates. This may be necessary on occasion and is acceptable to associates who know they participate in decisions that rely on their level of knowledge and experience.[28]

Consensus Building

A positive strategy of decision making by Japanese leaders is consensus building. When a major change is to occur, Japanese leaders may spend months and even years gaining consensus of internal customers and even of some external customers such as suppliers. When change is initiated, concerned parties have had input into the decision-making process and get behind it to make it successful. They are stakeholders with a perception of a shared future. Kanter would probably label this a synergy, because it encourages cooperation of all groups. Partnerships among groups require consultation and cooperation. Such partnerships are egalitarian, with members talking about work and its tasks. These members search for consensus on goals that lead to successful outcomes for the corporation, the employees, and the shareholders.[29]

Groupthink and consensus building are somewhat in conflict. To build consensus, one listens to all parties, uses their ideas, and brings them onto the team by involving them in critical thinking and realistically considering their ideas. Groupthink aims for fast solutions with minimal critical thinking and participant input.

Role of Intuition

Intuitive reasoning abilities have a place in the decision-making process. Intuition is a powerful tool for guiding decision making. So-called left-brain activities, such as analytical and logical thinking, mathematics, and sequential information processing, are essential in decision making and problem solving. But right-brain functions allow people to simultaneously process information, conceive and use contradictory ideas, fantasize, and perceive intuitively. Intuition is defined as the power to apprehend the possibilities inherent in a situation. It is a subspecies of logical thinking and integrates information from both sides of the brain—facts and feeling cues.[30] Nurses who can think intuitively have a sense of vision; they generate new ideas and ingenious solutions to old problems. Agor reported research involving 2,000 managers using a Myers-Briggs type indicator. The Myers-Briggs type indicator is widely used to measure intuition. Initial findings showed intuitive ability varying by managerial level, with higher ability in top-level managers than in middle- or lower-level managers.

Factors cited by middle- and lower-level managers that impeded the use of intuition included lack of confidence, time constraints, stress factors, and projection mechanisms such as dishonesty and attachment. Follow-up of the 200 top executives who scored in the top 10% of the first study revealed that all but 1 used intuitive ability as a tool in guiding decisions. These managers stated that their intuitive ability stemmed from years of knowledge and experience. From this research, Agor identified eight conditions in which intuitive ability seems to function best:[31]

1. A high level of uncertainty exists.
2. Little previous precedent exists.
3. Variables are less scientifically predictable.
4. Facts are limited.
5. Facts do not clearly point the way to go.
6. Analytical data are of little use.
7. Several plausible alternative solutions exist to choose from, with good arguments for each.
8. Time is limited, and there is pressure to come up with the right decision.

Nurses are able to identify with these decision-making situations. Evidence supports the use of intuition in decision making. Research findings suggest that decision making in clinical practice is both a rational and intuitive process.[32] Evidence suggests "that intuition occurs in response to knowledge, is a trigger for action and/or reflection and thus has a direct bearing on analytical processes in patient/client care."[33] Intuition is based on rational factors of knowledge and experience.[34] However, it is stressed that there are appropriate times for using intuition as an adjunct to the logical steps of decision making—not situations in which objective data are complete. Because basic nursing education stresses the need for assessing facts and avoiding personal opinions, it may be difficult for some nurses to activate intuition for decision making. Agor identified techniques and exercises used by executives to activate and expand their intuitive decision-making abilities, including relaxation and mental/analytical techniques. A full account of Agor's research is beyond the scope of this chapter; the reader is referred to Agor's extensive writings on the subject of intuitive decision making.[35]

Intuition is observed in individuals and in groups and is a creative and powerful attribute. Groups use intuition to reach consensus, particularly when information is incomplete. Consensus in a group leads to selection of a solution to a problem or to the making of a decision. Intuition can be developed through group brainstorming sessions, group visualization, reflective practices, visualization, and quiet thinking time.[36]

The human brain has a specialized region for making personal and social decisions, which is located in the frontal lobes at the top of the brain and is connected to deeper brain regions that store emotional memories. Injury or stroke damage to this area causes personality changes, and the injured person can no longer make moral decisions. This knowledge has implications for behavior related to intuitive versus rational decision making.[37]

Decision making involves critical thinking. As the nurse becomes more expert, the process becomes more intuitive, and the expert nurse automatically processes the decision-making action as a consequence of a high level of knowledge and experience. The decision-making process is fostered by training, feedback, and the expansion of nursing knowledge. Case studies, value clarification exercises, and debates are good vehicles for teaching critical thinking.[38]

Nurses make critical decisions about resources affecting patient care. Resources include staff, equipment, supplies, bed space, time, and patient assignments to staff. Expert nurses make different decisions than do novice nurses. Nurses make decisions requiring intelligence and judgment, personal and professional values, ethics, law, political reality, organizational culture, norms of classes, and economics.[39] Intuitive nurses have clinical skills, incorporate a spiritual component in their practice, are interested in the abstract nature of things, are risk takers, are extroverted, and express confidence in their intuitions.[40]

Organizational Versus Personal Decisions

Organizational decisions relate to organizational purpose; constant refinement of organizational purpose is required because the organizational environment changes. This process provides opportunities for participative management styles, thereby giving associates the prerogative and responsibility of professional decision making.[41]

When are organizational decisions necessary? It would be easy to say we deal with professionals who are capable of making decisions related to their practice. An effective manager would not make decisions for competent professionals. However, limited decision-making skills of associates, uncertain instructions, novel conditions, conflicts, or failure of authority to make effective decisions or to make decisions at all may cause decisions to be appealed to a higher authority. Effective organizational decisions require collaboration and consultation with those having specialized knowledge.

From an organizational standpoint, decisions may be analyzed on the basis of futurity, impact, or qualitative (or value) factors and on whether the decision is recurrent, rare, or unique. Futurity is defined as the length of time over which the decision will affect the organization in the future and the time required to reverse its impact. Impact refers to the number of individuals or departments affected and is a determinant of the level at which the decision is made. When qualitative or value factors of philosophy or ethics are involved, decisions must be made at a higher level. The last characteristic refers to the uniqueness of the decision; recurrent decisions are made following a rule or principle already established.[42]

Historically, decision making in nursing has been authoritarian and centralized, with minimal input from nursing staff, particularly when it involves institutional policy. Nurses have also been limited in their professional autonomy. Literature on the sociology of professions indicates that a professional person has an ultimate or independent decision-making authority granted by society on the basis of unique knowledge and skill. This viewpoint gives physicians control over nurses. The traditional definition of autonomy no longer applies: Patients now demand more input in decision making, and, increasingly, patient care technology requires nurses to make independent life-and-death decisions. McKay redefined professional autonomy as "both independent and interdependent practice-related decision making based on a complex body of knowledge and skill."[43] Primary nursing promotes nurse accountability, intraprofessional and interprofessional consultation, and an assertive synthesis of nursing and medical care plans. Interdependent decision making promotes professional autonomy. The American Nurses Credentialing Center, Magnet Recognition Program, Force 9, emphasizes autonomy, specifically, the expectation of the Magnet Organization:[44]

> Autonomous nursing care is the ability of a nurse to assess and provide nursing actions as appropriate for patient care based on competence, professional expertise, and knowledge. The nurse is expected to practice autonomously, consistent with professional standards. Independent judgment is expected to be exercised within the context of interdisciplinary and multidisciplinary approaches to patient/resident/client care.[45]

Professional nurses are functioning with increasing professional autonomy, and nurse managers are moving into more executive positions in healthcare administration. Nurse managers recognize the advantages of nurses being involved in strategic institutional decisions such as those concerning major programs, policies, promotions, personnel, and budgets. Additionally, enhancing professional autonomy and the involvement of nurses in decision making have resulted in higher job satisfaction, better morale, lower turnover, improved communication, improved professional relationships with peers and colleagues from other disciplines, and higher productivity.[46]

Evidence-Based Practice 6-1

Blegen and others at the University of Iowa studied nurses' preferences for decision-making autonomy in Iowa hospitals. They found that nurses wanted a more independent level of authority and accountability in 12 of 21 patient care decisions, including those that concern patient teaching, pain management, preventing complications, clarifying and advancing orders, scheduling and discussing the plan of care with the patient, consulting with other providers, and arranging daily assignments and schedules. They also found that nurses wanted to make group decisions about such matters as setting policies, procedures, unit goals, job descriptions and standards, quality improvement, and job performance. Nurse managers wanted to increase decision making by staff nurses. It would appear that nurse managers should provide the impetus for more involvement in decision making by staff nurses by asking them what they want and actively involving them. The latter would include training and education. Staff nurses may want decision making autonomy in areas in which they are expert and competent.[47]

Many nurses equated decision-making autonomy with nurse professionalism. Most nurses are not autonomous because they are not self-employed. Research studies do not always support the premise that decision-making autonomy increases job satisfaction or performance or decreases nurse turnover.[48]

The nurse manager can maximize the opportunity for staff nurses to be involved in interdependent decision making by involving them at all levels of patient-care decision making, especially on interdisciplinary institution-wide committees. Strategies that have proven successful in involving nurses in accomplishing this include decentralization to the unit level, committee systems, and governance systems.[49]

Nurses who pursue holistic nursing practice encourage clients to make decisions about health and healthcare issues. Decisions about healthcare policy are not all controlled by healthcare professionals. They are made by the business sector and according to sociopolitical and economic variables. Nurses need to become policy analysts, because analysts use communication networks or structures as strategy to action. Communication with decision makers is crucial to effecting decision making. Nurses use networking and professional relationships to influence decision makers. They arrive at positions on healthcare policy through interest groups. Membership in professional associations, committees, and interest groups, plus communication with or as analysts, leads to participation in policy decision making and changes in the primary healthcare system.[50]

Shared governance is an organizational administrative model that has been used as a vehicle for increasing staff-nurse participation in decision making and problem solving. It often involves multidisciplinary groups. Shared governance has as its object the provision of a trusting and nonjudgmental environment in which nurses, along with others, use the decision-making and problem-solving processes to make productive changes in organizations. Improved communication is a product of the shared governance process.[51] Professional models of care are the expectation of magnet organization. Components of this expectation include care delivery models that define and promote the professional role of the registered nurse, including accountability for practice and care continuity. Professional practice models incorporate evidence-based practice and contemporary management concepts and theory. Adequate consideration relating to care delivery models are expected as well as staffing systems that incorporate patient needs, staff member skill sets, and staff mix.[53]

> *Research indicates that promotion of decision making by nurse managers is a factor in retention of critical care nurses.[51] Research also indicates that increased academic education is associated with better decision making in practice.[52]*

PROBLEM-SOLVING PROCESS

Decision making and problem solving are related. The first step in decision making is to identify the problem. But problem solving can involve making several decisions. The best way to define the relationship between the two is to define the steps of problem solving.

Steps in the Process

The steps of the problem-solving process are the same as the steps of the nursing or scientific process and the decision-making process: assess and analyze, plan, implement, and evaluate. Assessment includes systematic collection, organization, and analysis of data related to a specific problem or need. It involves logical fact finding, questioning all sources, and differentiating between objective facts and subjective feelings, opinions, and assumptions. Knowledge and experience guide the data collection and analysis of data. Before the process goes any further, assessment should also determine whether a commitment exists to implement a decision or an action.[54] Making certain that there is no readily apparent solution also saves the time of all people who may become involved in problem solving. Once the problem is identified, it must be determined whether it requires other than routine handling—that is, whether it is a rare or unique situation rather than a recurrent one.

This leads to the second step of problem solving: planning. Planning involves several phases. In nursing terms we determine priorities, set goals and measurable objectives, and plan interventions. Management literature essentially describes the same process: break the problem down into components and establish priorities; develop alternative courses of action; determine probable outcomes for each alternative; decide which course is best in relation to resources, goals, risks, and the like; and decide on and make a plan of action with a time table for implementation.[55]

When determining priorities, nurses should relate the problem to the corporate mission. Decisions involve choosing among alternative courses of action. They must have an acceptable effect on those directly involved, other areas affected, and the entire organization. Plans should include when and how to alter a course of action when undesired results occur.

The third step is implementation of the plan. The nurse should keep informed of the status of the process because it is unlikely that he or she will be directly involved. This is the one step in the process most likely to be delegated to associates. Implementation requires knowledge and skills appropriate to the specific alternatives selected.

Evaluation, the final step in problem solving, includes determining how closely goals and objectives were met, the success or failure of actions taken in resolving the problem, and whether the plan should be terminated because the problem has been resolved or whether it should be continued with or without modification.

Effective problem solving requires that the practitioner frequently work at a high cognitive level: the level of abstract thinking. The essential difference between problem solving and decision making is that in the former, the thinking process works to solve a problem, whereas in the latter, it serves to reach a goal or condition. Students learn to do problem solving by actually solving client's problems. In doing so, student and client collaborate. Computer simulations are available for problem solving. Students progress through several levels of cognitive problem solving and practice: novice, advanced beginner, competent, and proficient. Interactive videos are available for practice in solving clinical problems.[56] Many strategies are available through the Internet.

Shared Problem Solving

Although each step of the problem-solving process can be approached by an individual, input from all affected individuals or areas promotes more complete data collection, creative planning, successful implementation, and evaluation indicating problem resolution. Managerial problem-solving groups or teams are often formed in organizations, with the expectation that the team's effectiveness will prove to be greater than that of its individual members. Brightman and Verhoeven state that "[a] team of problem solvers has greater potential resources than an individual, can have a higher motivation to complete the job, can force members to examine their own beliefs more carefully, and can develop creative solutions."[57]

Grounded in decision-making and problem-solving skills, the nurse administrator uses expert communication skills to advance the organization's mission and goals.

Clark provides a problem-solving format which is a useful tool for professional nurses to drill down problem issues and to improve critical-thinking skills.[58]

COMMUNICATION TO ENHANCE DECISION MAKING AND PROBLEM SOLVING

To answer the question of who is involved in communication one could simply say, "everyone." Several aspects must be considered. The first of these is that the person who wants to be heard is involved in communication. For example, Exotic Winery wants to sell wine and wants people to know that it has wine and specialty products to sell. Its manager therefore advertises in an effort to communicate this desire to sell an appetizing product. The manager advertises through media such as newspapers, billboards, radio, television, and the Internet. A variety of tempting pictures is portrayed in these advertisements. If the manager is successful and people buy lots of wine and specialty cheeses as a result of the advertisements, then the message has been received and the manager has communicated to them.

A second aspect of communication occurs when a person seeks out desired information. Suppose someone plans a dinner party and want to serve specialty wines and cheeses. That person knows where the nearest store is, having heard or seen it advertised. He or she may have driven past the shop and observed signs that identify the product. That person may have been reminded of the product in the Sunday paper that morning. Even if the person cannot remember the address, he or she can always refer to the Yellow Pages for an address and phone number, call directory assistance, or search the World Wide Web. When a person wants information, there are many sources from which to obtain it. All these sources are mediums for communication.

Elements of Communication

At least two people are involved in communication: a sender, or provider, and a receiver. A sender usually has something he or she wants to communicate, even if the information is distasteful. A receiver usually has need of some information, whether good or bad. Regardless of the medium, information is transmitted from sender to receiver, and a communication occurs.

Whether or not money is exchanged, communication always involves a "buyer" or a "seller." The buying or selling is based on a need. Sometimes the receiver's need to hear is not as acute as the sender wants it to be. An example of this is the communication between a manager and an associate. A manager communicates the critical nature of patient safety goals to the staff, with policies established to ensure that mechanisms are in place to guarantee safety checks and ongoing monitoring. This message continues to be reinforced in staff meetings, by quality improvement data that is circulated, and on bulletin boards throughout the facility. Failure to adhere to policy is noted to result in serious consequences, possibly termination. However, when a staff member violates a safety standard and the patient is put in harms way, there are no consequences. As a result, now the staff member does not even hear the manager, because he or she has no reason to listen. When the staff member (and possibly the entire unit) is made aware of the unsafe nature of the actions and receives consequences, there is a reason to listen. Communication now takes place, because the staff member(s) finds sufficient reason for listening.

Communication is a human process involving interpersonal relationships, and therein lays its difficulty. In the workplace, some managers view their knowledge of events as power; sharing knowledge through communication is sharing power, and the manager does not want to share. Other managers do not realize the importance of communication in an information age because they are not up-to-date on the advantages of decentralization and participatory management. These managers frequently fall into crisis management, treating the symptoms of poor communication and never identifying the root causes. A third group of managers recognizes that communication is like the central nervous system in that it directs and controls the management process.

More than 80% of a higher-level manager's time is spent on communication: 16% of that time is spent reading, 9% on writing, 30% on speaking, and 45% on listening. Is there any question that communication skills are absolutely essential to career advancement in nursing?[59] Effective communication has three basic principles:

1. Successful communication involves a sender, a receiver, and a medium.
2. Successful communication occurs when the message sent is received.
3. Successful nurse managers achieve successful communication.

Climate for Communication

Organizational climate and culture are discussed in Chapter 7, Organizational Structure and Analysis. The communication climate should be in harmony with the corporate culture and should be used to encourage positive values, such as quality, independence, objectivity, and client service, among nursing employees. Communication is used to support the mission (purpose or business) and vision of the nursing organization and to tell the consumers or clients that nursing is of high quality. The media used include performance, nursing records, and marketing. Communication is objective when it is accurately portrayed with descriptions of factual outcomes judged on the basis of objective outcome criteria.

Nursing literature abounds with evidence of nurses' desire for autonomy and knowledge that they may use to communicate their support of autonomy. Nurses also may provide a climate in which the nursing business remains as free as possible of political constraints. When political considerations are imperative, the imperative is communicated to employees, who make decisions based on the institution's values and beliefs.

Organizational culture is more difficult to change than organizational climate, but both can be modified with managerial effort and skill. The first step for nurse managers is to sample employees' attitudes or ideas of how they receive information and effect communication. Managers and employees know the formal structure, including roles and modes of operation used to inform and communicate. What is the informal structure? It involves people who are heroes or role models who can be involved in communication if they are positive and enthusiastic. Otherwise, they may have to be replaced, particularly if these role models are destructive.

Cultural Agendas

Cultural agendas publicize the mission or business of the organization. They tell what the organization stands for and on what the nursing division, department, or individual unit places value.

Cultural agendas are used to communicate promotions, new hires, marriages, deaths, and other news about personnel. Heroes are highlighted with features that illustrate support of desired values and beliefs: the nurse who presents a paper, authors a book, or achieves prominence in the profession or the community; the nurse who is a champion bowler, an elected officer in an organization, or an appointed official in the healthcare system; and the nurse who is a volunteer in community activities. The cultural agendas also are used to publicize nursing units and special achievements such as ongoing research in burn care or rehabilitation.

Cultural agendas are publicized using various media, including newsletters, memorandums, awards ceremonies, and external communications, such as publications, radio, television, and organizational meetings. Such communications are most effective when they depict the people who are directly involved in the publicized events.

Cultural agendas can be effectively used to change the organizational climate and culture.[60] The nurse leader must establish the climate for effective communication. Wlody recommends the following:[61]

- Step I: Review your own communication technique.
- Step II: Concentrate the staff's attention on communication as a needed skill that everyone can develop.
- Step III: Lead the staff into more positive interaction within the unit.
- Step IV: Make daily rounds with the whole team.
- Step V: Form a group to reduce stress.

To be an effective communicator, a manager should develop close professional relationships with customers on their own turf. Nurse managers can do this by identifying their customers and visiting them. Their customers include their employees, other professionals, patients, families, suppliers, and others. Being a role model shows that the manager cares. Success is ensured through partnerships between managers and front-line employees.[62]

Nature of an Effective Climate for Communication

Important communication occurs between supervisor and employees at the work level, where climate is set. A supportive climate encourages employees to ask questions and offer solutions to problems. Additionally, a supportive climate facilitates equality, spontaneity, empathy, and respect. Conversely, a defensive climate emphasizes control, traditional hierarchical structures, superiority, and one-way communication. Nurse leaders should strive for a supportive climate.

Although research in the area of organizational attributes has been limited and the results inconclusive, some evidence shows that organizational size (number of employees) influences communication among associates but not between supervisors and associates. The climate is more open at the top, where higher-level supervisors are more likely to involve associates in decision making.

A supportive climate produces clear communication to support productive nursing workers and effective teamwork. It provides for identification of communication problems by designing instruments to collect data during specified periods of time. Real communication patterns and problems are diagnosed from analysis of the data and can be related to the communication climate and solved by using problem-solving techniques.

A strong relationship exists between good communication skills and good leadership.

Communication problems have been described as a major source of job dissatisfaction. Organizational communication systems are powerful determinants of an organization's effectiveness. Communication rules are organization specific and are either explicit or implicit. Explicit rules are codified. They govern formal activities such as access to managers or supervisors. Violation of explicit rules may result in sanctions. Implicit rules mimic norms of behavioral expectations and are not codified but mutually shared. Conformation to rules reduces dissonance and maintains stability. A questionnaire may be used to assess communication in six areas:

1. Accessibility of information
2. Communication channels
3. Clarity of messages
4. Span of control
5. Flow control/communication load
6. Individual communicators.[63]

Open-Door Policy

Communication climate influences the success of an open-door policy. An open-door policy of a nurse manager implies that an employee can walk into the manager's office at any time. Because nurse managers follow schedules, however, it usually is more convenient for both parties when the employee makes an appointment.

The communication climate associated with some organizations has made employees wary of the open-door policy. Line managers sometimes feel threatened when they see their employees in the boss's office. They find out the reason for the visit by any means possible. Some managers punish the employee by telling them to use the chain of command, adjusting performance evaluations, ostracizing the employee, adjusting pay increases, or working to fire the employee. This climate quickly teaches the employee not to use the open-door policy.

A nurse manager who believes in the open-door policy clearly states the rules, including whether the employee needs someone else's permission to make an appointment with the manager. A democratic manager who believes in setting a climate for open communication encourages visits. Such a manager knows how to deal with confidential communication to protect employees and their supervisors.

During negotiation, a supportive environment includes a favorable location.

Communication as Perception

In nursing, as in other disciplines, communication is perception. A person perceives only that which he or she is capable of hearing. A communication must be uttered in the receiver's language, and the sender must have knowledge of the receiver's experience or capacity to perceive.

Conceptualization conditions perception; a person must be able to conceive to perceive. In writing a communication, the writer must work out his or her own concepts first and ask whether the recipient can receive them. The range of perception is physiological, because perception is a product of the senses. However, the limitations to perception are cultural and emotional. Fanatics, for instance, cannot receive a communication beyond their range of emotions.

Different people seldom see the same thing in a communication, because they have different perceptual dimensions. Drucker said that to communicate the sender must know what the recipient, the true communicator, is able to see and hear, and why. Perhaps if we focus on the recipient as the "true" communicator, we can improve communications. The unexpected is not usually received at all or is ignored or misunderstood. The human mind perceives what it expects to perceive; to communicate, the sender must also know what the recipient expects to see and hear. Otherwise, the recipient has to be shocked to receive the intended message.[64]

People selectively retain messages because of emotional associations and receive or reject messages based on good or bad experiences or associations. Communication makes demands on people. It is often propaganda and so creates cynics. It demands that the recipient become somebody, do something, or believe something. This is powerful when the demand fits aspirations, values, and goals. Communication is most powerful when it converts, because conversion demands surrender.

Communication as perception indicates the value of a stated mission, philosophy, and goals. If statistical quality control is practiced, it should be applied to organizational communication as part of the total system and to prevent misconceptions.

Communication is the process by which time management, skills, prioritization, planning, and personal involvement are transmitted by managers to establish a statistical quality control program that implements change effectively. As managers effectively implement statistical quality control, they inspire conviction, commitment, and conversion of their workers. The workers are first motivated with conviction of the desirability of change; they are inspired by the leader's attitudes. This leads to commitment to the change and internal conversion to a personal attitude that results in high productivity.

"There is a major difference in perceptions between patients and clinic managers of patients' accessibility to healthcare clinics.[66] *Patients with less education, a history of chronic heart disease, and a diagnosis of stable angina need special follow-up."*[67]

Statistical quality control succeeds in a climate that fosters open communication among all managers and workers, commitment to employee involvement, and recognition of individuals and the unit or organization. The climate should be nonthreatening and positive.[65]

Communication Direction

For effective communication, start with the perceptions of the recipients. Listeners do not receive the communication if they do not understand the message. Nurse managers need to know what listeners are able to perceive before formulating a message. Many nurse managers focus on what they want to say and then cannot understand why the recipient does not understand the message.

The information load should be kept to a minimum to help increase communication. Management by objectives focuses on perceptions of both recipients and senders. Recipients have access to the experience of the manager. The communicative process focuses on aspirations, values, and motivations: the needs of the subordinates. Performance evaluation or appraisal should focus on the recipient's concerns, perceptions, and expectations. Communication then becomes a tool of the recipient and a mode of organization for the employee to use.

"Communication requires mutual respect andconfidence."

Information

Although they are interdependent, communication and information are different. Communication is perception; information is logic. Information is formal and has no meaning. It is impersonal and not altered by emotions, values, expectations, and perceptions.

Computers allow us to handle information devoid of communication content (e.g., personnel information). Information is specific and economical, based on a need of a person and for a purpose. Information in large amounts beyond that which meets a person's needs is an overload.

Communication may not be dependent on information; it may be shared experience. Information should be passed to the person who needs to know it, and that person must be able to receive it and act on it. Perception and communication are primary to information, and as information increases the communicator or receiver must be able to perceive its meaning. In the interest of time management, nurse managers need skills that sort information according to its importance. These skills require clear communication and acute perception.

Feedback

Feedback completes or continues communication, making it two-way. Today's workers are better managed in a climate that promotes theory, participation, or involvement. Most workers are more affluent and better educated than workers of the past, have increased leisure time, and retire earlier—all indications of their changed values.

Feedback is one of the most important factors influencing behavior. People want to know what they have accomplished and where they stand. Feedback works best when specific goals are set to note the improvements sought, measurable targets, deadlines, and specific methods of attaining goals.

Effective communication includes giving and receiving suggestions, opinions, and information. If this two-way interaction does not occur, little or no communication takes place.

One-way communication prevents input or feedback and interaction. It causes nurses to depersonalize their relationships with patients and families and serves as a barrier between nurses and physicians. It causes distorted communications that result in distorted and inaccurate feedback; scapegoating of peers, patients, and families; emotional blowups, skepticism of all messages; frustration and stress; delay of therapeutic interventions; and negative socioeconomic consequences.[68]

Evidence on Feedback

Evidence supports that feedback increases productivity. One study showed an 83% increase in productivity as measured by staff treatment programs and client hours, using the technique of private group feedback. Using the technique of public group feedback, productivity increased 163% in 38 weeks.[69]

When suggestions were answered promptly in a mental health organization of 80 employees, the number of suggestions increased by 222.7% over a 32-week period. In other studies, feedback plus training have been found to be even more effective. A review of 27 empirical studies indicated that objective feedback worked in virtually every case.

Evidence-Based Practice 6-2

A study was done to test the effect of feedback on process versus outcomes of reality orientation in a psychiatric hospital serving elderly patients. Subjects were psychiatric nurses and were divided into three groups: two groups were given appropriate feedback, whereas the third group did not receive any feedback. The nurses in the process feedback group showed "substantial increases" in process behavior over the control group that did not receive feedback. The nurses in the feedback group had increased patient contacts, but it was not determined whether their patients had increased reality orientation.[70]

Innovation and experimentation may be reduced by feedback that causes people to concentrate on process, methods, and procedures. Nurse managers should focus on outcomes or accomplishments that show that clinical nurses have been creative. New ideas as well as application of results of nursing research should be encouraged, and clinical nurses should be supported to develop proposals and conduct new nursing research. Levenstein recommends the following:[71]

- Be clear in your own mind about the criteria you are using to assess staff performance.
- Clarify the ends, and the means are more likely to fall into place.
- Emphasize flexibility in getting results rather than ritualistic observance of rules and procedures.

Successful synergies require leadership, cooperative management plans, joint incentives, information sharing, computer networks, face-to-face relationships, shared experiences, mutual need, and a shared future.[72] Communication is involved in almost every one of these activities. Kanter goes on to say that the communication imperative is that "[m]ore challenging, more innovation, more partnership-oriented positions carry with them the requirement for more communication and interaction."[73]

Difficult Conversations

Much has been written on the topic of difficult, fierce, and crucial conversations.[74–76] Patterson, Grenny, McMillan, and Switzler define a crucial conversation as "a discussion between two or more people when (1) stakes are high, (2) opinions vary, and (3) emotions run high."[77] The authors purport that we can handle these crucial conversations in three ways by avoiding them, facing them and handling them poorly, or facing them and handling them well. Crucial conversations can take many forms, including evaluating a colleague's work, talking to an associate about a personal hygiene problem, giving feedback, and talking to a team member who is not keeping their commitments. In their work on *Crucial Conversations,* Patterson et al. outline and define practical strategies, providing ways of "mastering crucial conversations" as well as ways to influence outcomes to make powerful changes. The power of dialogue is underscored in their work.[78]

Scott defines a fierce conversation as "one in which we come out from behind ourselves into the conversation and make it real."[79] Scott offers seven principles of fierce conversations:

1. Master the courage to interrogate reality.
2. Come out from behind yourself into the conversation and make it real.
3. Be here, prepared to be nowhere else.
4. Tackle your toughest challenge today.
5. Obey your instincts.
6. Take responsibility for your emotional wake.
7. Let silence do the heavy lifting.

Each principle is described with strategies to develop skills in handling fierce conversations. For example, in principle 4, tackle your toughest challenge today, Scott identifies skills in naming the problem, identifying and confronting the real obstacles in your path, and staying current with individuals important to the work of organization. She recommends that one "travel light, agenda-free." In principle 7, let silence do the heavy lifting, Scott offers the need for breathing space, slowing down the conversation so that insight can occur in the space between words. This affords the opportunity to discover what the conversation really means and what it needs to be about. Scott offers tools for questioning on one-to-one conversations, a decision tree, a confrontation model, and an outline for preparing an issue for discussion.[80]

Communication and Conflict Management

Conflict is often a result of poor communication. Supervisors sometimes react to employee outbursts in any of the following ways:

- Overriding their better judgments
- Becoming defensive
- Reprimanding the individual
- Cutting off further expression of feelings
- Monopolizing the conversation

The result is increased frustration for both the employee and the manager.

Baker and Morgan suggest the following techniques for dealing with employee outbursts:[81]

1. Tune into the real message the employee is trying to communicate. Interpret it correctly, and direct a response at the feeling level of the employee.
2. Determine the nature of the feelings being expressed. Be sensitive to them because they are subjective and express the employee's values, needs, and emotions. Feelings are neither right nor wrong, but they represent absolute truth to the individual and usually are disguised as factual statements. Determine if they disguise anger, frustration, hurt, or disappointment.
3. Let the feelings subside by encouraging venting. Listen and give emotional support, and then summarize what you have heard and interpreted from the outburst.
4. Clarify issues with questions that can be answered yes or no.
5. When impasses occur, try linking the ideas or feelings the employee has expressed.
6. Allow the employee to save face.
7. Be sure perceptions are accurate by summarizing them and checking them with the employee.
8. Verbalize your feelings as a supervisor by using positive "I" statements.

Negotiation

When disagreements about the intent of a communication occur, negotiation is needed to prevent conflict, resignation, or avoidance between supervisor and employee. Negotiation requires knowledge of human behavior and is based on human needs. When there is lack of confidence between supervisor and employee or among employees, nurse managers can solve the communication problem through a climate of openness that restores confidence through agreement and promotes individual autonomy as well as esprit de corps.[82]

Communication and change require negotiation; two basic types are cooperative and competitive. Agreement is the objective in both types. For nurse managers, cooperative or win–win negotiation is best. Nurse managers and employees negotiate cooperatively for win–win outcomes for employees and the institution.

The principles of negotiation are as follows:

- Maintain self-identity and insight into your own motives, values, perceptions, and skills.
- Understand others' values without judging them to be better or worse but only different from your own.
- View issues as potentially solvable.
- Use personal flexibility in analyzing and reacting to issues and behaviors.
- Use skills to repair damaged relationships, including the ability to retreat and regroup in a manner that allows for perceptual openness.

In the win–win negotiation process, the nurse manager will state these principles so that both manager and employee are on equal footing.

The following are the steps of the negotiation process:[83]

1. Preparing for negotiation (e.g., introducing a topic at a meeting)
2. Communicating a general overview of what is to be accomplished during the process
3. Relating the history of why negotiation is required
4. Redefining the issue to be addressed
5. Selecting when issues will be worked on
6. Encouraging discussion during the conflict stage of the issue
7. Addressing the fallback or compromise for both parties on the issue
8. Agreeing in principle during the settlement stage
9. Recapping and summarizing the agreement
10. Monitoring subsequent compliance of the agreement (after settlement)

During the negotiation process, the nurse manager is always positive in explaining ideas, suggestions, and benefits. The nurse manager actively listens to employee responses, gaining perceptions, identifying concerns, and explaining obstacles to these ideas. The manager encourages explanations and suggests ways of overcoming obstacles. Questions are phrased to obtain doubtful discussion and answers.

Successful negotiators achieve win–win outcomes that indicate progress, maintain self-respect, leave positive feelings, are sensitive to each other's needs, achieve a majority of each other's objectives, and facilitate future negotiation.

Change theory is involved in negotiation.[84]

Listening

Communication takes place between employer and employee. To have satisfied, productive employees, an employer must hear what employees are saying as well as what they are not saying. To really hear someone requires concentration. Many managers do not listen effectively to what employees are saying to them and thus discourage the person who may want to point out a problem but knows that either he or she will not be heard or that the suggestion will have no effect.

One reason nursing personnel find it difficult to listen to a change-of-shift report is that a person can listen four times faster than the 125 to 150 words per minute that are being spoken. The listener who is tuned out may not hear a message about an appointment or a directive regarding a patient. As a result, it is usually more efficient for the person to read a change-of-shift report or listen to it on a tape recorder.

Most working persons are engaged in some form of verbal communication 70% of the waking day, or approximately 11 hours and 20 minutes out of 16 hours. Of that time, 45% is spent listening to what will be 50% forgotten within 24 hours. Another 25% is forgotten in the next 2 weeks.[85] If this is true of nursing personnel, they will forget 75% of what they hear today within the next 2 weeks. Some researchers claim that immediately after a 10-minute speech we remember only 50% of what we hear; 25% is considered a good retention level.[86]

By learning the art of listening and observing, managers better understand what employees mean by what they say. They receive cues from employees' words and actions. Managers learn that men and women communicate differently. Learning the art of listening creates a better organization with better relationships and better outcomes.[87]

Causes of Poor Listening

Remember that it is an ineffective strategy to call a subject uninteresting or boring. Listen for useful information from what is considered a dull subject. Sift and screen, separate wheat from chaff, and look for something useful. Be an interested person, and make the subject interesting. Good listeners attempt to hear what is said.

It is also an ineffective strategy to criticize the delivery. Concentrate on finding out what the speaker has to say that is interesting or useful. Keep from being over-stimulated by the subject. Otherwise, you mentally prepare an argument or rebuttal and miss what the speaker says. Hear the speaker out before making judgments. Listen for the main idea rather than the facts; identify principles, concepts, and generalizations. Facts merely support the generalizations. Accept the face value of the message rather than evaluate it.

Avoiding eye contact with the speaker is ineffective and decreases trust. Communication is both verbal and nonverbal. Body language such as gestures, postures, and tone of voice may give stronger messages than the spoken word.

Defensive listening occurs when the speaker's message threatens the listener with blame or punishment for something. It prevents accurate listening and perceptions. Defensive listening is stimulated when a person's speech implies that a listener's behavior is being evaluated. Defensive response is reduced when the speaker describes behavior objectively. Speech that indicates the sender is trying to control the receiver evokes defense. People do not want their values and viewpoints controlled and shut out such messages. They want to have freedom to choose. When the sender solicits the collaboration of the receiver in solving mutual problems, the receiver responds positively.

Receivers defend themselves against perceived strategies to change their behaviors or control them, which they regard as deceitful. They respond to spontaneity and honesty, which they perceive as free of deceit.

Speech perceived as being unconcerned about the group's welfare evokes defense, whereas speech perceived as being empathetic evokes acceptance. People want to hear speech that indicates they are valued. Gestures can also communicate neutrality or empathy.

Communication, verbal or nonverbal, that indicates superiority evokes defense, whereas speech indicating equality is accepted and supported. Certainty indicates dogmatism and evokes defense. A defensive reaction is reduced by professionalism; such speech indicates the sender wants help, information, data, or input from the listener.[88]

Other reasons supervisors give for not listening include the following:[89]

- Employees do not expect them to listen.
- Employees have nothing of value to say.

- Listening is not part of their jobs.
- Employees should listen to them.

Techniques to Improve Listening

Improving listening ability can be accomplished in many ways. One method is to summarize what is being said for better understanding and retention. The listener should give empathetic attention to the speaker and try to understand the substance of what is being said; seek to be objective and to apply creativity; go beyond the speaker's dialect, stance, gestures, and attire to understand the meaning of the speaker's words; and try to counter his or her own emotions or prejudice even though the speaker may have opposite convictions.

It is important to discriminate among those to whom one listens. Listen to people who keep you informed and lighten your work load or save time. Listen to those who argue constructively and use those judgments to sharpen your own judgment. Know the kind of people who want to listen to you and the situation in which they will try to make you hear. Learn to recognize when you are prone to listen and when you are not.

Some people give good information, and others should listen to them. These people are trusted troubleshooters, line managers in charge of the bread-and-butter functions of primary patient care, staff specialists who have been delegated special tasks, or reliable decision makers. Graciously avoid exaggerators, opportunists, office politicians, gossips, and chronic complainers.[92]

The speaker's appearance, facial expression, posture, accent, skin color, or mannerisms can turn off the listener. A person who wants to hear must thus put aside all preconceived ideas or prejudices and give the speaker full attention so that the speaker is motivated to do a better job of communicating. While the person is talking, the listener analyzes what is said for ideas and facts. The receiver must also listen for feelings, which are the background to the performance—tone of voice, gestures, and facial expressions.

Mnemonics

A mnemonic is a device used to help one remember. The following are two examples of mnemonics:

1. AIDA: Capture **a**ttention, sustain **i**nterest, incite **d**esire, and get **a**ction.
2. PREP: **P**oint, **r**eason, **e**xample, and **p**oint.[93]

Such formulas are useful for preparing impromptu comments. The AIDA formula causes the speaker to focus on the listener's needs, interests, and problems. The PREP formula is ideal for spur-of-the-moment speaking. The first point reminds the speaker to clearly express a point of view on the subject. In giving the reason, the speaker explains why this is his or her point of view. These reasons should be illustrated with specific examples to clarify and substantiate the point: statistics, personal experiences, authoritative quotes, examples, analogies, anecdotes, and concrete illustrations. In the final point, the speaker brings the speech to a close with a restatement of the initial point of view. These formulas are intended to gain the attention of the listener and to elicit a positive response.

The following are some practical suggestions for encouraging people to listen:

- Be prepared by answering the questions who and what.
- Identify and evaluate the purpose of your remarks.
- Organize and outline the report or speech to convey the facts.
- Make efficient notes, and use them.
- Remember that you are part of the presentation.

> *Active listening is a skill for recognizing and exploring patients' clues, thereby giving healthcare providers a deeper understanding of the true reasons for the visit, which should result in increased patient satisfaction and improved outcomes.*[90]

> *The speech-comprehension difficulties of aging persons primarily reflect declines in hearing rather than in cognitive ability.*[90]

- Make your voice work for you with proper breathing and pitch.
- Communicate with your eyes.

Because critical thinking skills require interpretation of events based on present experience and factual data collection, they are also communication skills. Conceptualizing, which is a part of both communication and critical-thinking processes, supports this conclusion. Also, the set of information, belief-generating, and processing skills and abilities and the habit (based on intellectual commitment) of using these skills and abilities to guide behavior support the integration of critical-thinking ability and communication skills. Managers use their critical-thinking ability to identify feelings and become aware of beliefs, values, and attitudes of employees to communicate and respond to their needs. Active listening through use of all the senses is required of managers who need to recognize and respond to verbal and nonverbal messages from employees.[94]

> **66** *Peters says that managers should become obsessed with listening.* **99**[95]

To become a good listener requires practice. Listening to the patient can prevent errors. For example, during a patient's temporary stay in a skilled nursing facility, a medication error was made because the nurse refused to listen to the patients, a husband and wife admitted to the same room. The nurse communicated with a physician who did not know either patient. Unneeded laboratory tests were done and reported late. A further irony was the wife was a registered nurse, the husband was a medical doctor, and both were mentally alert. Every nurse manager and practicing nurse should work at improving his or her listening skills.

Good listeners get out from behind the desk and circulate with their customers. Good listening turns people on. Good listeners provide quick feedback, act on what they hear, and listen intensely and without preconceived notions.

> **66** *Managers who are good listeners may want to reward acts of meritorious listening.* **99**

Listening provides information that facilitates work, notes changes in patients' conditions more quickly, and speeds up responses to changes. It brings closure to action and problems, and it involves everyone.[96]

People tend to change the focus from listening to talking and telling. They perceive education as a solution to communication problems, whereas listening and adapting are the real solutions.

Listen informally at meals and coffee breaks, and listen formally to feedback from informative newsletters. Listen at no-holds-barred meetings. Listen rather than preach. Train people to listen. Provide employees with opportunities and places to talk and solve problems.

Listening to employees empowers them. A good listener is an engaged listener and takes notes. It is okay to ask "dumb" questions when one needs information. Knowledge is power and should never be hoarded. Because information is frequently leaked before it happens, managers should provide it to the first-line people who need it. Providing information does many things:[97]

- Motivates employees by making them potent partners
- Facilitates continuous improvement
- Discourages unneeded controls and delays
- Speeds up problem solving and decision making
- Stirs competition by stimulating ideas
- Begets more information
- Abets the flattened organizational pyramid

In *Crucial Conversations*, the authors describe power listening tools: ask, mirror, paraphrase, and prime. These tools are called power listening because they can best be remembered by the acronym AMPP. Briefly, these tools are as follows:[98]

1. <u>A</u>sk to get things rolling: Common questions might be, "What's going on?" "I'd really like to hear your opinion on this." "Don't worry about hurting my feelings. I really want to hear what you have to say."

2. <u>M</u>irror to confirm feelings: Common questions might be, "You seem angry to me. You say you're okay, but by the tone of your voice, you seem upset."

3. <u>P</u>araphrase to acknowledge the story: This tool allows for a summary of what the receiver understands. "Be careful not to simply parrot back what was said. Instead, put the message in your own words—usually in an abbreviated form."[99]

4. <u>P</u>rime when you are getting nowhere: This strategy comes from "priming the pump." The authors purport that, "when it comes to power listening, sometimes you have to offer your best guess at what the other person is thinking or feeling. You have to pour some meaning into the pool before the other person will do the same."[100]

To get information flowing requires extensive training in basic management skills.[101] The results of effective listening are that two people hear each other, beneficial information is furnished on which to base right decisions, a better relationship between people is established, and it is easier to find solutions to problems.[104]

❝Techniques to improve communication and prevent malpractice claims include documenting telephone advice to patients, determining when and how to terminate patients, improving communication and listening styles, knowing how to effectively obtain the patient's consent, and implementing careful oversight mechanisms with the receipt of outside diagnostic test results. ❞[102]

❝Some providers are being taught active listening techniques because malpractice suits are considered an expression of anger about some aspect of patient–provider relationships and communications. ❞[103]

❝Communication across settings is needed to understand nurses' contribution to the care of elderly patients making the transition from hospital to home.[105] Knowledge of the communication dynamics of caring for patients may help providers to design strategies to attain the basic goals of continuity of care. ❞[106]

COMMUNICATION MEDIA

Meetings

Meetings of all kinds are a medium for communication, often for purposes of information dissemination as well as for true communication.

To make his company successful, Robert Davies, founder and president of SBT Corporation, changed his management style. To keep his employees motivated, he decided to include two employees in all management meetings to provide ideas from the production level of the organization. Davies encourages employees to risk telling what they really think through an e-mail suggestion system. This computer suggestion box is connected to all employees via more than 100 stations. It ensures anonymity, and in 6 months it has spawned more than 100 suggestions, which must be read and answered. For example, employees kept requesting relaxation of the dress code, which was done and is successful. Even Robert Davies dresses casually, and employees are more comfortable talking with him. Technology, combined with listening, results in consensus, support for decisions, and a company in which employees do their best.[107]

Managers

Managers at all levels are also a medium for communication. To be successful in a complicated work environment, the nurse manager should be out and about. Communication includes gathering information for decision making, spreading the management vision, and letting employees know that leaders care for them. Communication is visibility. By walking around among employees and other customers, the nurse manager can prevent information distortion. This requires visiting and chatting with these knowledgeable people. The vision stamp is applied on the front line. By walking around, managers facilitate and coach; they do not give orders and conduct inspections. That is the work of the hands-on team.

Peters recommends the following actions for increasing management visibility:[108]

1. Put a note card in your pocket that says, "Remember, I'm out here to listen."
2. Take notes, promise feedback, and deliver. Fix things.
3. Cycle your actions through the chain of command and give managers the credit for fixing things.
4. Protect informants.
5. Be patient.
6. Listen, but preach a little, too, by killing unneeded red tape.
7. Give some, but not much, advance notice and travel alone. Take your own notes.
8. Work some night shifts; take a basic training course.
9. Watch out for the subtle demands you put on others that cut down on their practice of visible management.
10. Use rituals to help force yourself and your colleagues to get out and about.

We live in an information society; communication is the necessary ingredient for accomplishing missions and objectives. An effective communicator is an effective leader. Some managers use models or drawings to get their meanings across. Use synesthesia, the technique of transforming one sense to another, to communicate. Synesthesia helps one think "outside the box" by involuntarily joining real information from one of our senses to a perception in another sense. It stretches the mind to perceive reality from a more vivid sphere and range. Learn to express ideas graphically to engender employees' understanding, trust, and support. Use symbols of success, not symbols of defeat.

> *Some corporate executives have dismantled their offices. They maintain work areas at unit levels, with a system to correspond on the phone or computer and handle mail. They are visible.*

> *A nurse manager who holds information as a source of power is not an effective manager or leader.*

Effective communication creates meaning. It should be an act of persuasion. The right metaphor connects with the listener. The effective manager as leader acts and personifies the message transmitted via the metaphor. This leader transmits the message over and over.[109]

Effective nurse leaders share all the information possible. Employees cannot have too much information about the company. The only information a manager does not share is that protected by law, ethics, and decency.

Recognition programs promote communication. Nurse managers recognize fairly mundane actions, send written notes for work well done, and offer special recognition, such as serving a box of doughnuts or a cake to celebrate an individual or a group achievement. Nurse managers should be sure that all acts of special effort are heartfelt, that is, they should not be phony. Nurse managers should do a few big rewards and many small ones, be systematic, and celebrate events they would like to have repeated.[110]

Questions

Asking questions is an important method of communicating. Questions are asked to obtain information; the goal is mutual understanding. The tone of voice must encourage confidence and trust from the person questioned. Facial expression is important as the physical conduct of the questioner. The nurse manager should always go beyond the answer to a primary question and not flatly agree or disagree with the question.

The following types of questions should be used:

1. Open questions that give the other person the opportunity to freely express thoughts and feelings, rather than closed questions that force the receiver to become the sender of information.

Questions that can be answered yes or no do not give information or explanation. In the courtroom, attorneys use these questions to trap people or to clarify a point.

2. Leading questions that give direction to the reply, rather than loaded ones that restrict by putting the respondent on the spot
3. Cool questions that appeal to reason, rather than heated ones reflecting the emotional state of asker and answerer
4. Planned questions that are reflective and asked in logical sequence, rather than impulsive ones that just happen to occur to the asker
5. Complimentary or "treat" questions that tell the respondent that he or she can make an important contribution to the asker's views, rather than trick ones that place the respondent on the spot
6. "Window" questions that elicit the respondent's true thoughts and feelings, rather than "mirror" ones that reflect the point of view of the questioner

Successful questioning consists of creating and maintaining a climate for communication, asking the right questions in the right way, and listening to the responses.

Questions can be used to improve listening, with their use serving to clarify unclear statements. The questioner should take care not to overawe or threaten the speaker. Questions should be worded and spoken in a nonthreatening way, for example, "I am sorry I did not hear your comment clearly. Would you mind repeating it, please?" or "I do not quite understand what you mean by 'capital resource.' Would you explain further, please?"

A listener should never be embarrassed to ask questions that improve his or her understanding of a person's communication. Serious questions that result in clarification of or additional information increase comprehension and clear up misperceptions, thus helping senders and receivers. If the medium is an oral presentation, questions can be written down for use at appropriate times, such as during question periods and breaks, after meetings, and even later at an interview. Thus the listener can construct thoughtful questions.

When questions are used to clarify a point made by the sender, they can be closed yes-or-no questions. An example is, "Do you support the position on nurse autonomy you have just described?"[111]

Oral Communication

Oral communication is the most common form of communication used by executives, who spend 50% to 80% of their time communicating. Because oral communication takes so much time, a nurse manager should use the most effective words. Verbal messages are said to be 7% verbal (word choice), 38% vocal (oral presentation), and 55% facial expression.[112]

An advantage of face-to-face communication is that a person can respond directly to another or others. The larger the group, the less effective is face-to-face communication. An effective message requires knowledge of words and their various meanings as well as of the contexts within which the words can be used. Thus, effective communication may depend on use of the dictionary for correct vocabulary.

When giving a speech, one needs to keep in mind that the members of the audience are usually informed and sophisticated and have access to information. The members of the audience want the speaker to talk things over with them, not to talk to them. The speaker must be sincere and respect the listeners.

To present an effective speech, the speaker needs to do the following:

- Develop an outline and hold to four or five main ideas.
- Put other ideas under the main topic as subordinate ones.
- Open with an introduction.

- Close with a brief summary.
- Type the speech for easy reading.
- Practice by reading the speech.
- Maintain eye contact during the speech.
- Keep voice and manner informal and conversational.

A speaker should know the audience and its members' knowledge of the subject, intellectual level, attitudes, and beliefs. Former Vice President Hubert Humphrey said, "The necessary components to build a speech are full understanding of the facts of the subject, thorough understanding of the particular audience, and a deep and thorough belief in what you are saying."[113]

Figure 6-2 lists other techniques to use in preparing and giving an effective oral presentation.

FIGURE 6-2 TECHNIQUES FOR EFFECTIVE PUBLIC SPEAKING

1. Prepare carefully. What is the goal of your presentation? Is it to inform? Persuade? Entertain? It can be a combination of these and, to be effective, should probably combine at least two, such as entertainment with information or persuasion.

2. Prepare the presentation carefully. Make an outline and develop the content to fit the outline. Start well in advance so that you can read and adjust the material for a smooth flow of ideas.

   a. What is the purpose of the presentation? Did you select the topic, or was it given to you? In either instance, clarify the purpose with the organizers of the event or whoever engaged you to do the presentation.
   b. Prepare an introduction that gains the attention of the audience. Spark their interest. Humor often helps, but be careful of using cynicism or making derogatory remarks. References to religion, sex, and other controversial subjects should be carefully selected, if used at all. They are better avoided if you wish to persuade or inform, unless they are a part of your topic. Remember, words convey feelings, attitudes, opinions, and facts. Use them to turn the audience on, not off.
   c. Make the main points in the body of the presentation. Support them with appropriate and specific examples.
   d. Prepare or select visual aids to support the key points of the presentation. They are an extension of your presentation designed to appeal to the senses and increase reception.
   e. Know who the audience is and tailor the message to it. Provide useful material.
   f. Plan for audience participation with questions or appropriate exercises to involve listeners.
   g. Tie the message together with interval summaries and an effective conclusion. How do you want to leave the audience?
   h. If you plan to speak extemporaneously, make notes on cards or put outlines on a visual aid such as a poster, a chalkboard, an overhead transparency, or a slide projection screen.

3. Prepare the environment beforehand. Surroundings are important and should be as attractive as possible. Bear this in mind when you have input into selection.

   a. If you want to speak from a podium, make sure it is in place. If you want to sit, have a table and chair in place.
   b. Check lighting and sound equipment.
   c. Check audiovisual equipment.
   d. Remove unneeded barriers such as screens, furniture, and other movable objects. If pillars are in the way, rearrange your position or the audience seating, if this is possible. Arrange your proximity to the group to facilitate a feeling of closeness.
   e. Prepare your person for the presentation. Wear clothes that present you best. Conventional clothes are best because the audience should focus on your words and not your appearance. Be well groomed.
   f. Good preparation will help you to be relaxed. Get a good night's sleep the night before the presentation. Plan your schedule so as not to be excited beforehand. Eat and drink moderately. Sit and do deep-breathing exercises immediately before.

4. Be on time and use time effectively.

5. Speak to be heard.

    a. Use your voice, varying pitch, volume, rate, and tone for planned effect.
    b. Practice pronouncing words with which you have trouble.
    c. Pause to enhance your delivery. Short silences emphasize points and allow the audience to think about them.
    d. Make your presentation sound natural even if you read it.

6. Use body language effectively.

    a. Slowly develop the audience's awareness of your nonverbal behavior. Be aware of it yourself.
    b. Maintain eye contact.
    c. Plan your movements: walking, standing. Your posture should convey energy, interest, approval, confidence, warmth, and openness.
    d. Keep the space between you and the audience open.
    e. Use positive gestures.
    f. Use head movements for effect.
    g. Use facial expression for effect.
    h. Know where your hands and feet are at all times.
    i. Be genuine! An audience can quickly identify a fake.

7. Adapt to audience feedback, being sensitive to listeners' interests and moods.

    a. Listen for unrest, shifting in seats, whispering, muttering.
    b. Watch for nonverbal responses. Pay attention to body language, facial expressions, gestures, and body movements. Leaning backward or away is perceived as a negative response.
    c. Be prepared to answer questions if there are breaks in the presentation. You may want to plan for them. Repeat them before answering, regardless of whether they are oral or written. You are giving additional information.
    d. Treat your audience with respect in every way, and they will view you as genuine.

Source: Author.

Interviews

An interview is essential to practicing management by objectives. When good counseling and guidance techniques are practiced, interviews also are used to apprise current employees of their performance as well as to interview prospective employees. In disciplining an employee, it is necessary to interview the individual. When an employee leaves, an exit interview is desirable to learn why the person is leaving and to gain ideas for strengthening the personnel management program. Interview questions should be worded to obtain the most beneficial information. The following are suggestions for conducting effective interviews:

1. Use plain and direct language rather than technical, professional, or slang terms.
2. Keep questions short.
3. Use familiar illustrations.
4. Do not assume that the person being interviewed knows what you mean or are saying. Check the extent of the interviewee's knowledge beforehand.
5. Avoid improper emphasis so as not to indicate the answer you hope to elicit.
6. Be sure the interviewee attaches the same meaning to words that you do.
7. Be precise in choosing words. Use accurate synonyms and words with one pronunciation.

Written Communication

Writing is a common medium of communication. It comes in massive quantities: memos to be read and passed on, even if they go into someone else's wastebasket; letters and e-mail that need to be answered; newspapers and magazines that collect in stacks; junk mail; posters and flyers; and notices and newsletters. How should one handle all this material? First, make a mental decision to deal with each piece of paper. Establish a system for assigning priorities to the mass of written communications; skim through everything, and then answer or delegate that which can be handled immediately. Put aside whatever can be taken care of at a future date, but do not put things where they will be forgotten. Papers can be placed in a folder according to priority.

When writing, remember that you are writing for a receiver: a reader, viewer, listener, observer, or member of an audience. The receiver is not interested in you as a writer but only in the message being conveyed. Direct your message to the reader, use good marketing techniques, and sell your product.[114]

Figure 6-3 lists nine rules to follow when writing. The writer should put the reader's interest first, begin with a provocative question or striking statement, and get right to the point: the purpose of the written communication and the request for action. A personal letter is always better than a form letter. One should use a friendly tone, with first names and personal pronouns, which express an interest in the reader.

The following are some simple suggestions for communicating effectively through writing:[115]

- Use the active voice to give strength to written communication. About 10% of total words should be verbs.
- Use strong nouns.
- Use the subject and main verb early in the sentence.
- Avoid overuse of adjectives and adverbs; be specific when using adjectives. State a specific amount such as 100 instead of much, any, or a lot.
- Be as brief as possible.
- Use short words.
- Use sentences that contain one idea and are no longer than 16 to 20 words. Vary sentence length.
- Write naturally, using friendly conversational language. Use contractions such as "didn't" and "aren't" with discretion.
- Reread and revise your written communication. Look at the nouns and verbs. Evaluate your sentences; they should be simple, not complex. Determine whether you have said what you mean. Eliminate unneeded words.
- You may want to add a personal handwritten note at the bottom.

Written Reports

Written reports should indicate how the nursing objectives are being met. If a 24-hour nursing report is made from the patient units to the director of nursing, the information provided should show progress in relation to the achievement of unit and department objectives. The information should be provided in a simple, functional or practical, and qualitative (rather than complex and quantitative) manner. In providing information, the reporter should consider its relative value and purpose, eliminate overlap and duplication, and put the report in perspective. The report should indicate the work load and state pertinent facts describing the patients' status, the reason for hospitalization, and the nursing diagnosis and prescription. The following are other factors to consider in writing useful reports:

1. Size and cost should not exceed the need or strength of the objective or operation.
2. A strong report will not be contaminated with individual bias. For that reason, a computer printout has value over a hand-prepared report.
3. A strong report will be useful to many people, providing them with vital information to run the operation.
4. A strong report will have authentic and reliable sources of information, that is, people with the knowledge and skills required to judge what information needs to be transmitted. Some informa-

FIGURE 6-3   NINE RULES TO FOLLOW WHEN WRITING

1. Empathize. Be sensitive to the needs and desires of those who will read what you are writing. Arouse and maintain the reader's interest by appealing to the mind and emotions. For example, compose a message that transmits respect for the nurse while offering a credible and unique inspiration to taking nursing histories or preparing nursing care plans. When giving orders, explain why you are asking for the task to be done. You-centered (rather than I-centered) communications are interesting to the reader or listener. Give people honest and deserved praise, the kind of flattery that makes them feel that they are worth flattering. If you are addressing a particular person, put that person's name in the salutation as well as in the body of the letter or memo. Make an effort to please the receiver by using tact, respect, good manners, and courtesy.

2. Attempt to avoid the COIK ("clear only if known" to the reader or listener already) fallacy. Think of the misunderstandings that could occur in a written message that uses abstract terms. Your aim should be to create mental pictures using language that is suitable to the experience and knowledge level of the receiver.

3. Do not repeat anecdotes frequently, or the reader will be insulted. Avoid over-communication, over-detailing, and redundancy. Necessary repetition can be achieved by using pleasant and meaningful examples, illustrations, paraphrasing, and summaries. Repetition is essential to the mastery of a skill.

4. Express yourself in clear, simple language. Lincoln's Gettysburg Address contains 265 words, three fourths of them with just one syllable. Abstract, technical-sounding jargon, clichés, and trite platitudes may cover up insecurity in a writer afraid of committing herself or himself in writing. Avoid archaic commercial expressions, specialized in-house jargon, and fading "journalese" by writing clearly and concisely.

5. Make yourself accessible to the reader by positively and courteously requesting a response. You can ask a direct question and expect a reply by a certain date. You can also encourage response by giving a special return address, a private box or phone number, writing instructions, a postcard, or a return envelope. Make it easy, desirable, and pleasant for the reader to reply.

6. Use the format of the newspaper story: accuracy, brevity, clarity, digestibility, and empathy. Arouse the reader with a headline opener. Follow it with a summary that tells significant highlights in the opening paragraph. Then tell the details. Here is an example of a memo form that has worked for others.

Date_____ Time_____
To:_____ Subject:_____
From:_____
Objective:
1._____
2._____
3._____

7. Break up a solid page of print with a variety of forms: underline, space, italicize, capitalize, enumerate, indent, box, summarize, and illustrate. Make your reading attractive and digestible.

8. Back up what you write by what you do; build a reputation for integrity.

9. Organize your material.
   a. Outline key points.
   b. Compile data into groups according to commonality.
   c. Arrange materials in a logical sequential order:
      (i) Chronological
      (ii) Cause–effect relationship
      (iii) Increasing complexity
   d. Tie the groups together using transitional devices:
      (i) Time-order words (first, later, finally)
      (ii) Guide words (as a result, therefore, on the other hand)
   e. Link the communication with the previous message by referring to the following:
      (i) Date
      (ii) Subject
      (iii) Sender of correspondence
   f. Furnish appropriate excerpts from past correspondence.

Source: Author.

tion can be given by clerks, some by technicians, and some, of necessity, by the nurse manager.

5. If the report is going to a group of people with limited time, such as a board of directors, the writer should add an executive summary at the beginning of the report and highlight items on which he or she wants the readers to act. This may speed up the response.

Sometimes managers have a tendency to eliminate reports. Although the busy nurse manager may hope that all reports would be eliminated, doing so without consensus sometimes drives reports underground. Because reports and forms tend to proliferate, each should have an elimination date, at which time it will be eliminated unless it is rejustified.

Time is an element common to all reports. The perpetual report shows up-to-date events for a full year. As the latest month or quarter is added, the oldest is dropped. This time base deals with the realities of the present and provides consistency, completeness, and effectiveness in reporting.

If top management cannot extract the information it wants from reports, then either the information is unnecessary or the procedures need to be improved. Persons who design reports and reporting procedures should do the following:

1. Gain access to all documents listing the short- and long-term objectives of the unit, department, division, and institution. Objectives should be in agreement and clearly stated in writing. Progress is reported.
2. Establish priorities for reports.
3. Categorize reports, indicating which objectives are supported by each.
4. Determine what top management needs and wants to know, and then screen reports.
5. Test reports for logical patterns that avoid complexity and unwieldy clumsiness.
6. Classify reports according to frequency.
7. Determine the levels through which reports will pass.
8. Determine the point of origin.
9. Coordinate reports with the organizational structure.
10. Check for accuracy and consistency.
11. Account for the total cost of reporting.
12. Obtain the concurrence of all levels of management.

Reports form the nucleus of all management communications, and successful communications depend on an intelligently conceived report structure. The reader should be able to read from top to bottom and laterally as well as from bottom to top.

Organizational Publications

Barnard states that the first function of an executive is to develop and maintain a system of communication.[116] The bigger the organization, the more difficult it is for the director of nursing to communicate with the employees who give direct care to patients. This problem is further complicated by the requirement that services be provided 24 hours a day, 7 days a week. One medium for communication between nurse executives and employees is an organizational publication such as a newsletter or in-house magazine. This procedure does not have to be confined to nursing but can be supported and used by nursing staff. Certainly, the nurse executive will have input into the development and evaluation of such an organizational publication.

According to Tingey, a successful organizational publication will fulfill six requirements:[117]

1. It will meet clearly stated objectives related to the process of communications. These objectives will state what the executives of the institution or organization, including those in nursing, want to accomplish through the publication.

2. The publication will need a competent editor who can provide professional editing and who will ensure that the objectives are met.

3. The editor will need access to the ideas of top management. The nurse executive must provide the editor with the information needed to inform nursing personnel of changes in policy and procedures.

4. The objectives of the publication will be developed into a master management plan. This plan will indicate articles and story themes to be used to accomplish each objective.

5. Information about future events will provide personnel with articles that give an anticipatory viewpoint. In nursing this could include the organization's role in supporting continuing education, expected problems involved in collective bargaining, changes in organizational structure, and changes that will affect practice, such as new equipment, new supply products, and new support activities.

6. The editor should know the audience, including its members' educational level, interests, problems, and attitudes. The publication should be interesting to family members and contacts. An unread publication is useless.

Specific objectives of the publication will be related to the internal technologic environment, the internal social environment, the external environment, company social responsibilities, and organizational dynamics.

Electronic Media

Electronic media are key to a successful management strategy. To increase productivity in the workplace, nurse managers need to be aware of development within the telecommunications industry. For example, fax machines provide quick and accurate transmission of orders from physicians to nurses. Nurse managers should consider the following questions:

- Will fax machines improve the output of clinical nurses if they can use faxes to get drugs from the pharmacy more quickly and accurately?
- Will fax machines improve response times and the accuracy of diagnostic testing by providing an electronic link to the medical laboratory, radiology, and other departments?
- Will fax machines increase therapeutic response times among clinical nurses, physicians, physical therapists, respiratory therapists, and others?

Numerous other electronic media are available, including computer bulletin boards for fast memos and software programs that can be used to control supply inventories and provide just-in-time supplies. Electronic networks provide sources of instant up-to-date information about diagnoses and treatments. Cellular phones, electronic memo pads, and all the latest in telecommunications technology should be evaluated by nurse managers for use within and among patient care units. Evaluation should be a part of the strategic planning process. Adoption of new tools should be evaluated on the basis of value added to individual and corporate performances and cost–benefit analysis.

Even though sophisticated communications technology is in place, managers and employees often fail to communicate. Good communication is the key to achieving personal and organizational effectiveness. To be effective, information must be transferred in a timely fashion. Managers are responsible for using available information technology and therefore need to have related competencies. To communicate effectively, managers and employees need training in the skills of information technology.[118] The management information system or nursing information system should be transformed into a customer information system. Lack of electronic memos or faxes or other communications may indicate to personnel and patients that a nurse manager is not listening.

Figure 6-4 summarizes the different forms of communication media.

FIGURE 6-4	COMMUNICATION MEDIA

Meetings

Managers

Questions

Oral communication

Written communication

Interviews

Organizational publications

Electronic media

Source: Author.

THE FUTURE

People as Capital

Specialization, division of labor, and economics of scale do not work in a service organization. People are the capital resource, and return on people is the measurable outcome, not capital in buildings and machines. The cost basis of service organizations will continue to be in people.

- Good employees want ownership. They want to own stock in the company. They also want psychic ownership in the company. They believe they are entrepreneurs. Within the corporation, "intrapreneurship" is already creating new products and new markets, revitalizing companies from the inside out.
- The service economy produces to meet unique human needs. Ideas come from employees, who have a rich mix of cultures. Customer demands and needs spur intuition and creativity, leading to new products and services. Medical problems, including nursing problems, are not neatly packaged. They are organic and interdependent, requiring workers who integrate the specialties to meet the needs of the people.
- Capital must be compounded through education and software. Training and education reduce general and administrative costs to maintain and increase competition. Information should be bought as a direct cost because a productive employee must be up-to-date and have information to be competent and productive.

Organizational Best Practices

Organizations that foster personal growth and communication best practices will attract the best and brightest people. Work enlargement yields greater productivity from such people. They want health and fitness and education programs from their employers. They want work integrated into their lives. They want to work in environments that are democratic and that allow them to network and to work in small teams. They want work to be fun. This is the cornerstone to creating and sustaining healthy work environments.[119]

The American Organization of Nurse Executives in their work on *Healthy Work Environments* noted the following six critical factors essential for achieving work environment excellence:[120]

1. Leadership development and effectiveness
2. Empowered collaborative decision making

3. Work design and service delivery innovation
4. Values-driven organizational culture
5. Recognition and rewards system
6. Professional growth and accountability

Each of these factors is described in this important work. For example, factor 2, empowered collaborative decision making, supports the essential nature of working with multidisciplinary teams and sharing decision making. "Job satisfaction, productivity, and retention are positively related to the professional recognition nurses enjoy in a work environment that supports nursing practice autonomy and meaningful nurse participation in operational decisions. The shared governance model represents one approach to nurse empowerment that many organizations are using to create the structural and cultural conditions necessary to enhance the professional status and influence of nursing."[121]

To grow and profit, organizations have to eliminate their hierarchical orientation and become team oriented. They must emulate the positive and productive qualities of small business. The infrastructure of the organization will give way to networking and people orientation.

Many businesses are striving for monopoly through mergers, acquisitions, and coalitions to control their environments. Though success evolves from market feedback, market forces demand change from people and are brutally destructive when people fail. The market will become the arbiter of power, obliterating layers of bureaucracy unless seized by political means.

A successful organization has effective communication at all levels, including the managerial level. Managers are skilled in managing human resources to effect communication. Communication makes employees valuable, contributing members of the corporate team (an important perception). Successful communication reduces conflict by reducing litigation and external intervention by labor unions and regulatory governmental agencies.

A good communication system does the following:

- Aids in cost savings, improves efficiency, and enhances productivity. People who know the system uncover and fix any problems.
- Keeps management better informed as it supports trust
- Keeps employees informed of the company's plans, policies, goals, philosophies, and requirements. Informed employees act positively.
- Improves morale. Information means a satisfied employee not swayed by outside influences.
- Makes employees believe they are part of a team. Again, spirit and trust support common goals.
- Maintains a work environment free of outside adversaries and unwanted third-party influences
- Provides some confidentiality for mutual trust and respect
- Responds promptly and completely
- Provides a means for employees to vent
- Provides sufficient information
- Recognizes employees as individuals

Employee attitude surveys may be a means of evaluating the effectiveness of company communication. These surveys cover employees' feelings about job duties, working conditions, supervisory and managerial skills, communications, pay, benefits, training, promotional opportunities, personnel policies and procedures, morale, and job security. Analyze results, and make and implement a plan to resolve problems. Resurvey after a sufficient period.[122]

Managers

Managers should be retrained to be coaches and facilitators. Some organizations are already doing this. W. L. Gore & Associates has 38 plants, 5,000 employees, and no plant managers. Plant size is limited to 150 employees. As employees develop a following, they become the chosen leaders. Employees have sponsors when they are employed. If a job is not learned within 90 days, the employee is no longer paid. Advocate sponsors are consulted by a compensation sponsor to determine salary based on accomplishment.

Thirty-five percent of American corporations pay managers more than they deliver as value added, that is, the increased production and profit they add as a result of their performance. The manager's new role is that of coach, teacher, and mentor.[123]

Technology

Technology will be linked to the service orientation of surviving, adaptive, customer-oriented organizations. It will shift the cost curve, with labor continuing to have high income because of increased productivity. Quality will be paramount, requiring that the organizational design and the technology be brought together as enablers for human resources. Computers can supplement, not replace, human capital.

Technology will become overhead. Information technology will be used to solve problems for which there is little intelligence and very little collective knowledge. When available, information should be bought and not generated directly to decrease overhead costs and hierarchy. Otherwise, managers must establish entire teams of experts to develop and implement a system that may already be available. It will be cheaper to pay the experts by the minute, because many will be available electronically. Thus contract or consultative labor will replace hired labor, especially in the technologic sphere.

Artificial intelligence will be a key enabler that will create generalists. It replaces experts and encapsulates and capitalizes knowledge. Knowledge will be added to machines to become an extension of the user. A symbiotic relationship will exist between the manager and the expert machine.

Survival in the information age will depend on a combination of technology and strategic insights. Service organizations will have to find people who need services and deliver these services to them. During the past 6,000 years, information has belonged to the power structure, which did not trade it, market it, or give it away. The service industries of the information age will market services that are heavily information based.

People and technologic systems can quickly become obsolete. Managers should go after strategic, not technical, gains. They should not computerize what does not work or maintain obsolete technology in hiring people. Employers must be developed and updated, adjusted to the system, or they will "career hop" within and outside of the organization. Turnover is expensive because it throws away assets. Human resource assets generate more value added when they are managed, enriched, and involved in the enterprise.[124]

Evidence-Based Practice 6-3

Kelly, Ryan, Bailey, and Thompson in their work on the 2001 Arkansas State Planning Grant included qualitative methods to guide the development of options to expand health insurance coverage in the state. To understand the processes surrounding decisions related to health insurance coverage, focus groups were conducted with employers and household decision makers. The authors used qualitative research methods, and focus groups targeting small to moderately sized employers and household decision makers were conducted to outline steps in the decision-making process related to health insurance coverage. Analysis of qualitative data collected from both employers and household decision makers led to the development of a single model that described the decision-making process regarding health insurance. These findings provided key opportunities for policy development and intervention. Short-term interventions focused on the precipitating event and strategies available to individuals. Long-term research and educational opportunities focused on influencing the assessment of issues and the valuation of health insurance. The implication for policy, delivery, and practice is awareness of the decision-making about health insurance, and knowledge of external factors likely to influence that process. This provides policy-makers with the ability to develop targeted and timely strategies to expand health insurance coverage.[125]

SUMMARY

Creative decision making and problem solving occur concurrently with all major functions of nursing. Four models of the cognitive thinking skills involved in decision making are presented: the normative model, the decision-tree model, the descriptive model, and the strategic model.

Decision making involves having an objective, gathering data pertaining to the objective, analyzing the data, identifying and evaluating alternative courses of action to achieve the objective, selecting an alternative (the decision), implementing it, and evaluating the results. Nurses make the best decisions through knowledge and use of the theory of decision making combined with intuitive ability developed over years of experience.

Although problem solving is not the exact equivalent of decision making, it uses a similar thinking process. Decision making is different from problem solving in that its objective does not have to pertain to a problem. It can be an objective that relates to change, progress, research, or implementation of any operational or management plan.

Communication occurs between government and the governed, between governments, between buyers and sellers, between manufacturers and consumers, between pupils and teachers, between parents and children, and between neighbors. Most importantly, communication occurs between people only if they want it to. The products of lack of communication are too costly to accept: misinformation, misunderstanding, waste, fear, suspicion, insecurity, and low morale.

People have difficulty accepting that communication is not the answer to all problems of human relations and personnel management. A gap exists between senders and receivers that must be recognized before it can be bridged—a gap in background, experience, and motivation.

Good communication is frequently an illusion. It is not achieved only with open doors, geniality, or jokes. Communication is aided by listening to what people are really saying and perceiving what they are projecting through their words, facial expressions, tone of voice, and actions. To induce people to accept direction, one must encourage them to participate. They will listen for genuineness in the word of the boss as demonstrated by actions. Crucial conversations and crucial confrontation offer valuable tools to influence positive organizational outcomes.

APPLICATION EXERCISES

Exercise 6-1
From your communications (calls, memos, etc.), follow up on complaints or problems. Help resolve them.

Exercise 6-2
Have a group of internal and external customers meet with you to discuss communication and information problems. Listen to them. Guide them to good solutions. Facilitate action.

Exercise 6-3
The following exercises may be done individually or as a group. You may want to work with a group of your peers.

Case Study: You are Ms. Carrie Platt. You have been director of nursing at Mason General Hospital for 1½ years. Mason General is a 500-bed general hospital in a metropolitan area, serving a population of 700,000. The city has four other hospitals and a University Medical Center. A local ADN nursing program is affiliated with your hospital. Today is Monday, March 20. During the past week, on Thursday, March 16 and Friday, March 17, you were away from the hospital to conduct a 2-day workshop. It is 8 A.M. and you have just arrived at the hospital. You must leave the hospital at 8:50 A.M. to be at the airport at 9:10 A.M. There has been an unexpected death in the family and you will be gone the entire week. You notice that the in-basket contains several items. You should make decisions about these things before leaving.

INSTRUCTIONS: Three decision-making exercises appear on the following pages. Each exercise is composed of a memorandum or other medium and a decision worksheet format. Use the worksheet format to list ideas for action and arrive at a decision. If the information given lacks essential details, make any assumptions necessary. Possible examples of decisions include the following:

1. Take immediate action and state what the action is.
2. Delegate the action to another person and state who the person is.
3. Postpone the action; state to what time.
4. Other course; please specify.

A. MEMORANDUM

TO: Ms. Platt   SUBJECT: Poor charting of I&O
FROM: Kay Campbell, Nurse Manager–5 N   DATE: March 17

The I&O record on Mrs. East in 517 is incomplete for evening and night shifts for her postoperative period. She went into shock in the recovery room and is in renal failure. Dr. Blake is extremely upset about the lack of thorough charting of I&O. One of the evening aides heard Mr. East call his lawyer about the possibility of a lawsuit. We thought you needed to be aware of this situation.

DECISION WORKSHEET

SUBJECT DECISION ALTERNATIVES	ANALYSIS	DECISION SELECTED	DECISION

B. MEMORANDUM

TO: Ms. Platt   SUBJECT: Uniform Regulations
FROM: Mrs. Back, In-service Instructor DATE: March 17

The meeting with the nursing assistants regarding uniform regulations has been scheduled for March 21 at 10:00 A.M. in In-service Room 406. We appreciate your offer to discuss this matter with the nursing assistants.

DECISION WORKSHEET

SUBJECT DECISION ALTERNATIVES	DECISION ANALYSIS	DECISION SELECTED	DECISION

C. MEMORANDUM

SUBJECT DECISION ALTERNATIVES	DECISION ANALYSIS	DECISION SELECTED	DECISION

Exercise 6-4

Check your inbox. If you are not receiving communications from your customers (clinical nursing personnel, patients, and others), start a personal listening ritual. Call three customers a day and ask how they are doing and what their problems are. Listen to their responses.

Exercise 6-5

Use a group of coworkers to evaluate your current recognition program. Discard those activities that are not working if they cannot be fixed. Infuse the others with excitement. Consider having an "attaboy" and "attagirl" award for which customers can pick up a short form and fill it out when they feel especially good about something an employee has done. Recognize the employee immediately at change-of-shift report, breakfast, lunch, dinner, or whenever. Send out 10 thank-you notes a month to employees and 10 more to customers.

Exercise 6-6

Make notes of calendar events and bring a fresh fruit and vegetable tray, whole-grained breads, and crackers and cheeses to them.

Exercise 6-7

Be the first to make a contribution to the United Way or other community agency. Lead the charge when supporting a voluntary effort for a community activity. Recognize those who put forth community effort.

Exercise 6-8

Walk around your area of responsibility. Note at least one hassle that can be fixed each day (or week or month). Fix it! Use your crucial conversation and confrontation skills.

Exercise 6-9

Identify and analyze your worst failure each month. How can it be fixed? Fix it!

Exercise 6-10

Visit customers who call you on the phone. These include employees, patients, suppliers, peers, and others.

Exercise 6-11

Make a list of all the information you want employees to have. Schedule meetings with all of them. Give them the information, and leave them with a printed version.

Exercise 6-12

Consider a major project that your preceptor is working on. Drill down on the steps in decision making with your preceptor, identifying how decisions are made, rationales are given, and budgets are determined to ensure that such will be carried out.

Notes

1. Page, A. (Ed). (2004). *Keeping patients safe, transforming the work environment of nurses* (p. 118). Washington, DC: Institute of Medicine of the National Academies.

2. Ingersol, G., Fisher, M., Ross, B., Soja, M., & Kidd, N. (2001). Employee response to major organizational redesign. *Applied Nursing Research, 14,* 18–28.

3. Rousseau, D., & Tijoriwala, S. (1999). What's a good reason to change? Motivational reasoning and social accounts in organizational change. *Journal of Applied Psychology, 84,* 514–528.

4. Heifetz, R., & Laurie, D. (2001). The work of leadership. *Harvard Business Review, 79,* 131–140.

5. Ibid., Page, 2004.

6. Ibid., Page, 2004.

7. Lancaster, W., & Lancaster, J. (1982). Rational decision making: Managing uncertainty. *Journal of Nursing Administration,* 23–28.

8. Peters, T. (1992, March 3). This is CNN: Chaos is the future of business. *San Antonio Light,* p. B9.

9. Wah, S. S. (2001, July 1). Chinese cultural values and their implications to Chinese management. *The Free Library* (2001). Retrieved February 28, 2008, from http://www.thefreelibrary.com/. Chinese Cultural Values and their Implication to Chinese Management.-a077417369

10. Ibid., 2001.

11. Nolan, P. (1998). Competencies drive decision making. *Nursing Management, 9*(46), 27–29.

12. Arora, N. K., & McHorney, C. A. (2000). Patient preferences for medical decision making: Who really wants to participate? *Medical Care,* 335–341; Babic, S. H., Kokol, P., Zorman, M., & Podgorelec, V. (1999). The influence of class discretization to attribute hierarchy of decision trees. *Student Health Technology Information, 68,* 676–681.

13. Shankar, R. D., & Musen, M. A. (1999). Justification of automated decision making: Medical explanations as medical arguments. Proceedings of the AMIA Symposium, Nov 10 to 11 at Buena Vista Palace, Orlando, Florida, pp. 395–399; Jamieson, P. W. (1990). A new paradigm for explaining and linking knowledge in diagnostic problem solving. *Journal of Clinical Eng, 19*(1), 371–380; Gerdtz, M. F., & Bucknall, T. K. (1999). Why we do the things we do: Applying clinical decision-making frameworks to triage practice. *Accident Emergency Nursing, 35*(4), 50–57; Dowie, J. (1999). What decision analysis can offer the clinical decision maker: Why outcome databases such as KIGS and KIMS are vital sources for decision analysis. *Hormone Research, 51*(Suppl. 1), 73–82; Taylor, C. A., Draney, M. T., Ku, J. P., Parker, D., Steele, B. N., Wang, K., Feinstein, J. A., & LaDisa, J. F. (1999). Predictive medicine: Computational techniques in therapeutic decision making. *Computer Aided Surgery, 4,* 231–247; Balneaves, L. G., & Long, B. (1999). An embedded decisional model of stress and coping: Implications for exploring treatment decision making by women with breast cancer. *Journal of Advanced Nursing, 30*(6), 1321–1331; Mazumdar, M., & Glassman, J. R. (2000). Categorizing a prognostic variable: Review of methods, code for easy implementation and applications to decision making about cancer treatments. *Statistical Medicine, 90*(4), 113–132.

14. Offredy, M. (1998). The application of decision making concepts by nurse practitioners in general practice. *Journal of Advanced Nursing, 31*(2), 988–1000; McGuinness, S. D., & Peters, S. (1999). The diagnosis of multiple sclerosis: Peplau's interpersonal relations model in practice. *Rehabilitation Nursing, 24,* 30–33.

15. Lancaster & Lancaster, 1982, p. 23.

16. Vroom, V. H. (1973). A new look at managerial decision making, organizational decision making. *Organizational Dynamics, 34,* 66–80.

17. Brown, R. V. (1970). Do managers find decision theory useful? *Harvard Business Review, 15,* 78–89; Magee, J. (1964). Decision trees for decision making. *Harvard Business Review, 42,* 126; Magee, J. (1964). How to use decision trees in capital investment. *Harvard Business Review, 42,* 79.

18. Simon, H. A. (1976). *Administrative behavior* (3rd ed.). New York: The Free Press.

19. Ibid.

20. Lancaster & Lancaster, 1982.

21. Nagelkerk, J. M., & Henry, B. J. (1990). Strategic decision making. *Journal of Nursing Administration, 20* (7/8), 18–23.

22. Ibid., p. 21.

23. Ibid.

24. Orton, A. (1984). Leadership: New thoughts on an old problem. *Training, 28,* 31–33.

25. Harrison, K. (1991). Cost benefit analysis: A decision-making tool for physiotherapy managers. *Physiotherapy, 37,* 445–448.

26. Matteson, P., & Hawkins, J. W. (1990). Concept analysis of decision making. *Nursing Forum, 25,* 4–10.

27. Graham, D, & Reese, D. (1984). There's power in numbers. *Nursing Management, 30,* 48–51.

28. McKenzie, M. E. (1985). Decisions: How you reach them makes a difference. *Nursing Management, 31,* 48–49.

29. Kanter, R. M. (1989). *When giants learn to dance* (pp. 114, 153–155). New York: Simon & Schuster.

30. Agor, W. H. (1986). The logic of intuition: How top executives make important decisions. *Organizational Dynamics, 14,* 5–18.

31. Ibid., p. 9.

32. Watkins, M. P. (1998). Decision-making phenomena described by expert nurses working in urban community health centers. *Journal of Professional Nursing, 14*(1), 22–23.

33. King, L., & Appleton, J. V. (1997). Intuition: A critical review of the research and rhetoric. *Journal of Advanced Nursing, 26,* 194–202.

34. Easen, P., & Wilcockson, J. (1996). Intuition and rational decision making in professional thinking: A false dichotomy? *Journal of Advanced Nursing,* 667–673.

35. Agor, 1986.

36. Rew, L. (1986). Intuition: Concept analysis of a group phenomenon. *Advances in Nursing Science,* 21–28.

37. Blakeslee, S. (1994, May 30). Seat of morality inside the brain. *San Antonio Express-News,* p. 24A.

38. Casebeer, L. (1991). Fostering decision making in nursing. *Journal of Nursing Staff Development, 66,* 271–274.

39. Botter, M. L., & Dickey, S. B. (1989). Allocation of resources: Nurses the key decision makers. *Holistic Nursing Practice,* 44–51.

40. Miller, V. G. (1995). Characteristics of intuitive nurses. *Western Journal of Nursing Research,* 305–316.

41. Barnard, C., & Beyers, M. (1982). The environment of decision. *Journal of Nursing Administration,* 25–29.

42. Swansburg, R. C. (1976). *Management of patient care services* (pp. 149–170). St. Louis, MO: C.V. Mosby.

43. McKay, P. S. (1983). Interdependent decision making: Redefining professional autonomy. *Nursing Administration Quarterly,* 21–30.

44. American Nurses Credentialing Center. (2005). *Magnet recognition program.* Silver Springs, MD: AACN.

45. Ibid., p. 54.

46. American Hospital Association (AHA). (1984). *Strategies: nurse involvement in decision making and policy development* (pp. 1–10). AHA.

47. Blegen, M. A., Goode, C., Johnson, M., Maas, M., Chen, L., & Moorhead, S. (1993). Preferences for decision-making autonomy. *Image,* 339–344.

48. Dwyer, D. J., Schwartz, R. H., & Fox, M. L. (1992). Decision making autonomy in nursing. *Journal of Nursing Administration,* 17–23.

49. AHA, 1984.

50. Murphy, N. J. (1992). Nursing leadership in health policy decision making. *Nursing Outlook,* 158–161.

51. Anderson, B. (1992). Voyage to shared governance. *Nursing Management,* 65–67; Ide, P., & Fleming, C. (1999). A successful model for the OR. *AORN Journal,* 805–808, 811–813; Bell, H. M. (2000). Shared governance and teamwork: Myth or reality. *AORN Journal,* 631–635; Boyle, D. K., Bott, M. J., Hansen, H. E., Woods, C. Q., & Taunton, R. L. (1999). Managers' leadership and critical care nurses' intent to stay. *American Journal of Critical Care,* 361–371.

52. Girot, E. A. (2000). Graduate nurses: Critical thinkers or better decision makers? *Journal of Advanced Nursing,* 288–297.

53. Ibid., American Nurses Credentialing Center, 2005.

54. Scharf, A. (1985). Secrets of problem solving. *Industrial Management,* 7–11.

55. Blai, B., Jr. (1986). Eight steps to successful problem solving. *Supervisory Management,* 7–9.

56. Klaasens, E. (1992). Strategies to enhance problem solving. *Nurse Educator,* 28–30.

57. Brightman, H. J., & Verhoeven, P. (1986). Why managerial problem solving groups fail. *Business,* 24–29; Shaddinger, D. E. (1992). Digging for solutions. *Nursing Management,* 96f, 96h.

58. Clark, C. C. (2009). *Creative nursing leadership and management* (p. 117). Sudbury, MA: Jones and Bartlett.

59. Morgan, P., & Baker, H. K. (1985). Building a professional image: Improving listening behavior. *Supervisory Management,* 34–36; Griver, J. A. (1979). Communication skills for getting ahead. *AORN Journal,* 242–249.

60. Corbett, W. J. (1986). The communication tools inherent in corporate culture. *Personnel Journal,* 71–72, 74.

61. Wlody, G. S. (1984). Communicating in the ICU: Do you read me loud and clear? *Nursing Management,* 24–27.

62. Bice, M. (1990). Behavior is the most effective communicator. *Hospitals,* 78.

63. Farley, M. J. (1989). Assessing communication in organizations. *Journal of Nursing Administration,* 28.

64. Drucker, P. F. (1973). *Management: Tasks, responsibilities, practices* (p. 483). New York: Harper & Row.

65. Crosby, P. (1987). *Running things: The art of making things happen.* New York: NAL-Dutton.

66. Sanchez, J., Byfield, G., Brown, T. T., LaFavor, K., Murphy, D., & Laud, P. (2000). Perceived accessibility versus actual physical accessibility of healthcare facilities. *Rehabilitation Nursing,* 6–9.

67. Missik, E. (1999). Personal perceptions and women's participation in cardiac rehabilitation. *Rehabilitation Nursing,* 158–165.

68. Wlody, 1984.

69. Levenstein, A. (1984). Feedback improves performance. *Nursing Management,* 64, 66.

70. Levenstein, A. (1984). Back to feedback. *Nursing Management,* 61.

71. Ibid.

72. Kanter, 1989, pp. 108–114.

73. Ibid., p. 275.

74. Patterson, K., Grenny, J., McMillan, R., & Switzler, A. (2002). *Crucial conversations: Tools for talking when stakes are high.* New York: McGraw-Hill.

75. Stone, D., Patton, B., & Heen, S. (1999). *Difficult conversations: How to discuss what matters most.* New York: Penguin Books.

76. Scott, S. (2002). *Fierce conversations.* New York: Penguin Books.

77. Ibid., Patterson et al., 2002.

78. Patterson, K., Grenny, J., McMillan, R., & Switzler, A. (2005). *Crucial confrontations: Tools for resolving broken promises, violated expectations and bad behavior.* New York: McGraw-Hill.

79. Ibid., Scott, 2002.

80. Ibid., Scott, 2002.

81. Baker, H. K., & Morgan, P. (1986). Building a professional image: Using "feeling-level" communication. *Supervisory Management,* 25.

82. O'Sullivan, P. S. (1985). Detecting communication problems. *Nursing Management,* 27–30.

83. Smeltzer, C. H. (1991). The art of negotiation: An everyday experience. *Journal of Nursing Administration,* 26–30.

84. Bazerman, M. H., Curhan, J. R., Moore, D. A., & Valley, K. L. (2000). Negotiation. *Annual Review of Psychology, 51,* 279–314.

85. Haakenson, R. (1964). How to be a better listener. *Notes & Quotes,* 3.

86. Morgan & Baker, 1985.

87. Sousa, L. (1993, May 1). We need to teach life 101. *San Antonio Express-News,* p. 6B; Foster, N. J. (2001). *Good communication starts with listening.* Retrieved July 25, 2005, from www.mediate.com/articles/ foster2.cfm

88. Gibb, J. R. (1982). Defensive communication. *Journal of Nursing Administration,* 14–17.

89. Shields, D. E. (1984). Listening: A small investment, a big payoff. *Supervisory Management,* 18–22.

90. Lang, F., Floyd, M. R., & Beine, K. L. (2000). Clues to patients' explanations and concerns about their illnesses: A call for active listening. *Archives of Family Medicine,* 222–227.

91. Schneider, B. A., Daneman, M., Murphy, D. R., & See, S. K. (2000). Listening to discourse in distracting settings: The effects of aging. *Psychology of Aging,* 110–125.

92. Stewart, N. (1963). Listen to the right people. *Nation's Business,* 60–63.

93. Guncheon, J. (1967). To make people listen. *Nation's Business,* 96–102.

94. Woods, J. H. (1993). Affective learning: The door to critical thinking. *Holistic Nursing Practitioner,* 64–70.

95. Peters, T. (1981). *Thriving on chaos.* New York: Harper & Row.

96. Ibid.

97. Ibid., pp. 524–532.

98. Ibid., Patterson et al. (2005).

99. Ibid., Patterson et al. (2005), p. 150.

100. Ibid., Patterson et al. (2005), p. 152.

101. Peters, 1981.

102. Irving, A. V. (1998). Twenty strategies to reduce the risk of a malpractice claim. *Journal of Medical Practice Management,* 130–133.

103. Virshup, B. B., Oppenberg, A. A., & Coleman, M. M. (1999). Strategic risk management: Reducing malpractice claims through more effective patient-doctor communication. *American Journal of Medical Quality,* 153–159.

104. Sigband, N. B. (1969). Listen to what you can't hear? *Nation's Business,* 70–72.

105. Bowles, K. H. (2000). Patient problems and nurse interventions during acute care and discharge planning. *Journal of Cardiovascular Nursing,* 41.

106. Anderson, M. A., & Helms, L. B. (2000). Talking about patients: Communication and continuity of care. *Journal of Cardiovascular Nursing,* 15–28.

107. Davies, R. (1992). Managing by listening. *Nation's Business,* 1–6.

108. Peters, 1981, pp. 608–613.

109. Bennis, W., & Nanus, B. (1985). *Leaders: The strategies for taking charge* (pp. 14, 33–43, 106–108). New York: Harper & Row.

110. Ibid., pp. 366–367.

111. Nathan, E. D. (1966). The art of asking questions. *Personnel,* 63–71; Pulick, M. A. (1983). How well do you hear? *Supervisory Management,* 27–31; Morgan & Baker, 1985.

112. St. John, W. D. (1985). You are what you communicate. *Personnel Journal,* 40–43; Caruth, D. (1986). Words: A supervisor's guide to communication. *Management Solutions,* 34–35.

113. Zelko, H. P. (1965). How to be a better speaker. *Notes & Quotes,* 3.

114. Wilkinson, R. (1986). Communication: Listening from the market. *Nursing Management,* 42J, 42L.

115. Dulik, R. (1984). Making personal letters personal. *Supervisory Management,* 37–40.

116. Barnard, C. I. (1938). *The functions of the executive* (p. 226). Cambridge, MA: Harvard University Press.

117. Tingey, S. (1967). Six requirements for a successful company publication. *Personnel Journal,* 638–642.

118. Nalley, E. A., & Braithwaite, J. E., Jr. (1992). Communication: Key to a vital future. *Phi Kappa Phi Newsletter,* 1–3.

119. American Organization of Nurse Executives (2003). *Healthy work environments: Striving for excellence* (Vol. II). Manassas, VA: McManus & Monslave Associates.

120. Ibid.

121. Ibid.

122. Gilberg, K. L. (1993). Open communication provides key to good employee relations. *Supervision,* 8–9.

123. Strassman, P. A., & Zuboff, S. (1985). Conversation with Paul A. Strassman. *Organizational Dynamics,* 19–34; Rutigliano, A. J. (1985). Naisbitt & Aburdene on "re-inventing" the workplace. *Management Review,* 33–35.

124. Ibid.

125. Perry, D., Ryan, K., Bailey, M., & Thompson, J. W. (2002). A health insurance decision making model. *Academy of Health Services Research Health Policy,* 17 (5), 19, 21.

References

Barrick, I. J. (2009). *Transforming health care management: Integrating technology strategies.* Sudbury, MA: Jones and Bartlett.

Brafman, O., & Beckstrom, R. A. (2006). *The starfish and the spider: The unstoppable power of leaderless organization.* New York: Penguin Books.

Collette, C. L. (2000). Understanding patients' needs is the foundation of perioperative nursing. *AORN Journal,* 71 (3), 629–630.

Dilenschnedier, R. L. (2007). *Power and influence.* New York: McGraw Hill.

Foster, N. J. (2000). *Barriers to everyday communication.* Retrieved July 25, 2005, from www.mediate.com/ articles/ foster2.cfm

Hansten, R. I., & Jackson, M. (2004). *Clinical delegation skills: A handbook for professional practice* (3rd ed.). Sudbury, MA: Jones and Bartlett.

Institute of Medicine. (2003). *Health professions education: A bridge to quality.* Washington, DC: The National Academies Press.

Iyengar, S., & Simon, A. F. (2000). New perspectives and evidence on political communication and campaign effects. *Annual Review of Psychology, 51,* 149–169.

Kleinman, C. S. (2004). Leadership and retention. *Journal of Nursing Administration, 34,* 111–113.

Levitt, S. D., & Dubner, S. J. (2006). *Freakonomics.* New York, NY: Harpercollins.

Macrae, C. N., & Bodenhausen, G. V. (2000). Social cognition: Thinking categorically about others. *Annual Review of Psychology, 51,* 93–120.

Martin, R. (2007). *The opposable mind.* Boston: Harvard Business School Press.

Patterson, F., Ferguson, E., Lane, P., Farrell, K., Martlew, J., & Wells, A. (2000). A competency model for general practice: Implications for selection, training, and development. *British Journal of General Practice, 50,* 188–193.

Watson, C. A. (2004). Evidence-based management practices. *Journal of Nursing Administration, 34,* 207–209.

PART II

LEADING THE BUSINESS OF HEALTHCARE: PROCESSES AND PRINCIPLES

7 ORGANIZATIONAL STRUCTURE AND ANALYSIS

Denise Danna, RN, DNS, NEA, BC, FACHE

LEARNING OBJECTIVES AND ACTIVITIES

- Describe the basic principles of organizing.
- Examine the key components in developing an organizational structure.
- Evaluate the various types and the characteristics of organizational structures with an emphasis on participatory management style.
- Analyze the various types and characteristics of successful teams.
- Evaluate indicators for evaluating committee effectiveness.
- Explore the concept of group dynamics with an emphasis on functional roles of group members, group techniques, and groupthink.
- Synthesize the characteristics of a culture, in particular a culture of safety.
- Compare the culture and climate of an organization.
- Examine several types of nursing care delivery systems models and professional practice models of care.
- Discuss the characteristics of a healthful work environment.
- Analyze organizational structures in a nursing division as well as departmentation.
- Describe the informal organization.
- Synthesize the indicators used in monitoring organizational effectiveness.

CONCEPTS

Organizational theory, chain of command, unity of command, span of control, specialization, bureaucracy, line and staff, coordination, delegation, system of polices, role theory, organizational structure, organizational charts, hierarchical structure, matrix structure, decentralization structure, participatory management, shared governance, job enrichment, personalization, primary nursing, entrepreneurship, gain sharing, pay equity, organizational development, autonomy, accountability, organizational culture, team building, self-managed teams, committees, ad-hoc committees, standing committee, group dynamics, focus group, groupthink, culture of safety, organizational climate, nursing care delivery system, functional nursing, team nursing, case method, professional nursing practice environment, professional models of care, departmentation, informal organization

QUOTE

Our life is frittered away by detail . . . Simplify, simplify.

—Henry David Thoreau

NURSE MANAGER BEHAVIORS

The nurse manager maintains the nursing organization to support an organizational structure through adherence to basic principles of organizing and by appointing nursing personnel to all organization committees; ensures shared accountability for professional practice; collaborates in the design and improvement of systems and the identification of resources that ensure interventions are safe, effective, efficient, age relevant, and culturally sensitive; collaborates in the design and improvement of systems and processes that ensure interventions are implemented by the appropriate personnel. The nurse manager advocates for a work environment that minimizes work-related illness and injury.

NURSE EXECUTIVE BEHAVIORS

The nurse executive works with nursing employees to develop a decentralized and participatory management organizational structure that supports a professional practice environment that endorses autonomy, accountability, shared governance, and decision making through committee structure and group dynamics. The nurse executive evaluates systems and processes of nursing services to ensure achievement of nurse-sensitive patient, client, or family-centered outcomes and a safe working environment.

Introduction

Organizations consume most of our daily lives, whether we are going to school, church, or work. It is important for nurse executives to identify and function effectively within different types of organizational structures, delivery systems, and professional practice environments and models. To get work done and improve patient outcomes in a culture of quality and safety, individuals need to work together with clear expectations and a common goal. Teams, groups, and committees are critical elements within the framework of professional nursing administrative practice that accomplish these goals.

Healthcare delivery has changed dramatically over the years, and it is imperative that nurse executives lead the way to identify, develop, and implement delivery models that are appropriate for both the nursing profession and to the patients served. Challenges in the nursing work environment have come from such issues as changes in patient demographics, technological advances, biomedical advances, and the distribution of delivery of care to different and various clinical sites.

The American Organization of Nurse Executives (AONE) identified the required skill set for nursing leaders in the *AONE Nurse Executive Competencies*.[1] These competencies are critical for the nurse executive to master to succeed in today's healthcare environment. The second domain, Knowledge of the Healthcare Environment, identifies the nurse administrator as the person who is accountable for the professional environment where nurses practice (Figure 7-1). Wolper[2] describes the changes in the

FIGURE 7-1	AONE COMPETENCIES FOR NURSE EXECUTIVES. II. KNOWLEDGE OF THE HEALTHCARE ENVIRONMENT

- Clinical Practice Knowledge
  - Delivery Models/Work Design
    - Maintain current knowledge of patient care delivery systems and innovations.
    - Articulate various delivery systems and patient care models and the advantages and disadvantages of each.
    - Serve as a change agent when patient care work/workflow is redesigned.
    - Determine when new delivery models are appropriate, and then envision and develop them.

- Healthcare Policy
  - Governance
    - Evidence-based Practice/Outcome Measurement
    - Patient Safety
    - Utilization/Case Management
    - Quality Improvement/Metrics
    - Risk Management

Source: Copyright © 2005 American Organization of Nurse Executives.

nurse executive's role and responsibilities by comparing the nursing department and patient care focus (Figure 7-2).

ORGANIZATIONAL THEORY

Organizations exist to bring people and material resources together to accomplish the work of the organization. "Organizing is the process of grouping the necessary responsibilities and activities into workable units, determining the lines of authority and communication, and developing patterns of coordination."[3] Once plans are made, the mission, purpose, or business for which the organization exists has been established; the philosophy and vision statements have been developed and adopted; the objectives have been formulated; and resources are organized to sustain the philosophy, achieve the vision, and accomplish the mission and objectives of the organization. Organizations develop as goals become too complex for the individual and must be divided into units that individuals can manage.[4]

Fayol[5] referred to the organizing element of management as the form of the body corporate and stated that the organization takes on form when the number of workers rises to the level requiring a supervisor. It is necessary to group people, distribute duties, and adapt the organic whole to requirements by putting essential employees where they are most useful. An intermediate executive is the generator of power and ideas.[5] The body corporate of the nursing organization includes executive management and its staff, departmental managers (middle managers), operational managers (first-line managers), and practicing professional and technical nursing personnel. Reformed organizations eliminate middle management, with operational managers becoming the department heads. Professional nursing personnel manage the performances of technical nursing personnel. In a theory of nursing management, nurse managers have as their object the development of a nursing organization that facilitates the work of clinical nurses.

Definitions of Organizing

Urwick referred to organizing as the process of designing the machine. The process should allow for personal adjustments, but these are minimal if a design is followed. It should show the part each person will play in the general social pattern as well as the responsibilities, relationships, and standards of

| FIGURE 7-2 | AONE NURSE EXECUTIVE COMPETENCIES |

The American Organization of Nurse Executives (AONE) believes that managers at all levels must be competent in:

Communication and relationship-building:
- Effective communication
- Relationship management
- Influence of behaviors
- Ability to work with diversity
- Shared decision-making
- Community involvement
- Medical staff relationships
- Academic relationships

Knowledge of the healthcare environment:
- Clinical practice knowledge
- Patient care delivery models and work design knowledge
- Health care economics knowledge
- Health care policy knowledge
- Understanding of governance
- Understanding of evidence-based practice
- Outcome measurement
- Knowledge of and dedication to patient safety
- Understanding of utilization/case management
- Knowledge of quality improvement and metrics
- Knowledge of risk management

Leadership skills:
- Foundational thinking skills
- Personal journey disciplines
- The ability to use systems thinking
- Succession planning
- Change management

Professionalism:
- Personal and professional accountability
- Career planning
- Ethics
- Evidence-based clinical and management practice
- Advocacy for the clinical enterprise and for nursing practice
- Active membership in professional organizations

Business skills:
- Understanding of healthcare financing
- Human resource management and development
- Strategic management
- Marketing
- Information management and technology

Source: Copyright © 2005 American Organization of Nurse Executives.

performance. Jobs should be put together along the lines of functional specializations to facilitate the training of replacements. The organizational structure must be based on sound principles, including that of continuity, to provide for the future.[6]

Organizing is the grouping of activities for the purpose of achieving objectives, the assignment of such groupings to a manager with authority for supervising each group, and the means of coordinating appropriate activities horizontally and vertically with other units that are responsible for accomplishing organizational objectives. Organizing involves the process of deciding which levels of organization are necessary to accomplish the objectives of a nursing /division, department or service, or unit. For the unit, it would involve the type of work to be accomplished in terms of direct patient care, the kinds of nursing personnel needed to accomplish this work, and the span of management or supervision needed. Understanding key organizational principles is an essential step in developing an organizational structure (Figure 7-3).

Bureaucracy

Bureaucracy, a term coined by Max Weber, evolved from the early principles of administration, including those of organizing. These structures do not work in pure form and have been greatly adapted in today's organization.

FIGURE 7-3   KEY ORGANIZATIONAL PRINCIPLES

- Chain of command: This principle supports a mechanistic structure with a centralized authority that aligns authority and responsibility. Communication flows through the chain of command or channel of communication and tends to be one-way—downward.

- Unity of command: The unity of command principle states that an employee has one supervisor and that there is one leader and one plan for a group of activities with the same objective. This principle is still followed in many nursing organizations but is increasingly being modified by emerging organizational theory.

- Span of control: The span of control principle states that a person should be a supervisor of a group that he or she can effectively manage in terms of numbers, functions, and geography. This original principle has become elastic—the more highly trained the employee, the less supervision is needed. Some management experts recommend up to 75 employees answering to one supervisor.[7]

- Specialization: The principle of specialization is that each person should perform a single leading function. Thus there is a division of labor: a differentiation among kinds of duties. Specialization is thought by many to be the best way to use individuals and groups.

- Bureaucracy: Bureaucracy is highly structured and usually includes no participation by the governed. The principles of chain of command, unity of command, span of control, and specialization all support bureaucratic structures.

- Line and staff: Line authority refers to direct supervision of employees, whereas the staff function is associated with an employee that has an advisory role.

- Coordination: Coordination is when all departments and employees work together for achieving the overall purpose, mission, and goals of the organization.

- Delegation: Allowing decisions to be made at the lowest possible level within the organization. This does not, however, relieve the managers from their responsibility.

- A system of policies: Organizations, especially hospitals, operate with a set of policies, procedures, and guidelines.

Source: Author.

Among the historic strong points of bureaucratic organizations is their ability to produce competent and responsible employees. These employees perform by uniform rules and conventions; are accountable to one manager who is an authority; maintain social distance with supervisors and clients, thereby reducing favoritism and promoting impersonality; and receive rewards based on technical qualifications, seniority, and achievement. The characteristics of bureaucracy include formality, low autonomy, a climate of rules and conventionality, division of labor, specialization, standardized procedures, written specifications, memos and minutes, centralization, controls, and emphasis on a high level of efficiency and production. These characteristics frequently lead to complaints about red tape, procedural delays, and general frustration.[8]

Using the bureaucratic model as a reference, Hall studied 10 organizations evaluating the following six dimensions: division of labor, hierarchy of authority, employee rules, work procedures, impersonality, and technical competence. He found varying degrees of each of these dimensions. An organization could be highly bureaucratized in one dimension but not in others. Highly bureaucratic structures have a high degree of bureaucracy in each of the six dimensions. Similar organizations may have similar degrees of bureaucracy.[9]

Hall also found that age and size of an organization do not relate to its degree of bureaucratization. The "technical competence" dimension did not appear to correlate with the other five dimensions. It is the rational aspect of bureaucracy. A high degree of impersonality develops in organizations that deal with large numbers of customers or clients.[10] Hall's study has significance for nursing administration; the scale can be used for testing in healthcare organizations and in nursing divisions. Hall also studied the relationship between professionalism and bureaucratization and found a relationship between structural aspects and attitudinal attributes of a profession (Figure 7-4).[11]

The conclusion would be that the less bureaucratic the organization, the more nurses in it perceive themselves as professionals. Nurse managers need to move from bureaucratic management to transformational leadership, thereby empowering professional nurses in a world in which technology,

---

| **FIGURE 7-4** | **RELATIONSHIP BETWEEN PROFESSIONALISM AND BUREAUCRATIZATION** |

- Attitudes are strongly associated with behavior, particularly as they are related to membership in professional organizations and obtaining specialty certifications.

- Nurses are high in professionalism in terms of belief in service to the public, belief in self-regulation, and sense of calling to the field but are low in feeling of autonomy and using the professional organization as a reference point.

- Nurses are high in bureaucratization, except for technical competence.

- Autonomous organizations have less hierarchy of authority.

- An organization's size does not affect hierarchy.

- Autonomous organizations have less division of labor.

- Autonomous organizations have fewer procedures.

- Autonomous and heteronymous organizations emphasize technical competence.

- Professionalism increases with decreased division of labor, decreased procedures, decreased impersonality, and increased autonomy. Hierarchy is accepted if it serves coordination and communication functions.

- Bureaucracy inhibits professionalism.

Source: Author.

communication, and political, economic, demographic, and social forces are constantly reshaping the healthcare system.[12]

Organizational Components

Role Theory

Role theory claims that when employees receive inconsistent expectations and little information, they experience role conflict, which leads to stress, dissatisfaction, and ineffective performance. Role theory supports the chain of command and unity of command principles. Multiple lines of authority disrupt, divide authority between profession and organization, and create stress. They force employees to make choices between formal authority and professional colleagues. The result is role conflict and dissatisfaction for employees and reduced efficiency and effectiveness for the organization. Role conflict reduces trust of and personal liking and esteem for the person in authority; it reduces communication and decreases employee effectiveness. If management creates an environment that provides the needed support and guidance for employees, role conflict and ambiguity can be minimized (Figure 7-5).

The implications for nurse managers are obvious. Role conflict and role ambiguity are separate dimensions; role conflict is more dysfunctional. In a changing work environment nurses are required to perform in new roles and under new circumstances. Managers provide the education and support needed by nurses who are coping with their role changes. Management support addresses the potential and real need deficits nurses confront. The goal is to prevent role insufficiency by thoroughly preparing nurses to function in new roles. Managers may opt to do this through role modeling. Clear understanding of role changes and planned programs to support them reduce role stress and prevent role strain.[13]

FIGURE 7-5   **ACTIVITIES THAT REDUCE ROLE CONFLICT AND AMBIGUITY**

- Certainty about duties, authority, allocation of time, and relationship with others
- Guides, directives, policies, and the ability to predict sanctions as outcomes of behavior
- Increased need fulfillment
- Structure and standards
- Facilitation of teamwork
- Toleration of freedom
- Upward influence
- Consistency
- Prompt decisions
- Good, prompt communication and information
- Use of the chain of command
- Personal development
- Formalization
- Planning
- Receptiveness to ideas by top management
- Coordination of work plans
- Adaptation to change
- Adequacy of authority

Source: Author.

Effective use of role theory has a positive impact when making changes in a nursing care delivery system. Role ambiguity, role stress, and role strain are minimized through educational programs aimed at socializing nurses into their new roles. Effective communication improves role changes.[14] Nurses acquire more personal power and incentives as they move up the managerial hierarchy. Nurse managers are motivated by the content of their work and the tasks and responsibilities assigned to their positions. Upper-level managers and supervisory-level nurses have firm beliefs in their competence and regard their roles as meeting professional goals.[15] With the restructuring of healthcare organizations, particularly hospitals, a whole new approach to organizing is required that will include applications of organizational theory as related to culture, climate, team building, and role theory, among others.

Developing an Organizational Structure

A structure for an organization must meet the needs of that organization as written in the statements of mission, philosophy, vision, values, and objectives. Most existing institutions already have an organizational structure, which is typically a pyramid or hierarchical form of organization.[16] However, before the structure is changed, the management team should engage in a systematic analysis and do some sound thinking about altering the organization's design and structure, starting with objectives and strategy.

A newer concept in the theory of organizations is that the organizational structure affects the strategic decision-making process. Historically, changes in organizational structure have followed changes in strategy such as unit volume, geographical dispersion, and vertical and horizontal integration. The organizational form determines the decision-making environment: It delimits responsibilities and communication channels, controls the decision-making environment, and facilitates information processing.[17] Strategic decision making requires wide expertise from numerous levels. In nursing, managers should seek broad input from clinical nurses. This can be done through task forces, committees, project teams, or ad-hoc groups.

In developing or changing an organizational structure, results from research should be considered. In the report *To Err is Human: Building a Safer Health System for the 21st Century*, the Institute of Medicine (IOM) found that approximately 98,000 patients who are hospitalized each year die as a result of medical errors.[18] In a response to this report, the U.S. Department of Health and Human Services' Agency for Healthcare Research and Quality requested that the IOM conduct a study to identify the opportunities to improve the work environment of healthcare staff, especially nurses, to improve patient safety.[19] Several of the recommendations that were given by the IOM included changes in the organizational structure and culture. By analyzing the current practices and structure in organizations, recommendations such as the following can be implemented to ultimately change the structure of an organization:[20]

- Ensure that direct-care nursing staff participates in the decisions relating to design of work processes and work flow.
- Organizations should support and develop interdisciplinary collaboration throughout the organization.
- Organizations should provide the resources necessary to create a work environment for nurses to reduce errors.
- Organizations should create a culture of safety.

Organization Charts

Most nursing organizations have made graphic representations of the organizing process in the form of organization charts. These charts usually show reporting relationships and communication channels. Line charts show supervisor and employee relationships from top to bottom of the nursing organization. Hierarchical relationships exist on which communication channels follow the line of authority to and through the chief nurse executive.

Organization charts distribute the nursing responsibilities, and lines connect the positions. These responsibilities may be divided according to one function or a combination of functions: contiguous geography, similar techniques, similar objectives, or similar clientele. The solid lines on an organizational chart represent line positions. Lines of authority can be either horizontal or vertical. An example is that all the nurses in the intensive care unit report up to one nurse manager who has the authority over all the nurses in the intensive care unit and where the nurses are accountable to the one manager. The horizontal lines represent the communication patterns between individuals with similar responsibilities in the organization. For example, a solid horizontal line would exist between the nurse manager of an oncology unit and the nurse manager on the intensive care unit. Both nurse managers have the same responsibility in their job duties, report to the same supervisor, and have to work together to achieve the overall objectives of nursing and the organization.[21] The dotted lines on an organizational chart represent staff positions. Staff positions provide support and assistance to others. For example, the cardiovascular clinical nurse specialist and the intravenous nurse hold staff positions.[22]

Organization charts are sometimes referred to as schemas. Decentralized schemas are flatter because there are fewer levels of control or management. Managers have more freedom to act, and the emphasis is on results.

There are advantages and limitations to having a current organization chart (Figure 7-6). Also, organizational charts can be used in an organization to plan, develop policies, implement organizational changes, and identify strengths and weaknesses of the current organizational structure.[23]

The success of nursing and of healthcare organizations depends on service to the customer. The focus then is on job function, and the organization chart should reflect this rather than show titles or names. The traditional organization chart tells the employee who the boss is, and it often becomes a plan for empire building and for abdication of responsibility. Figure 7-7 shows how to evaluate an organization chart of a nursing division, department, or unit using standards for evaluating the effectiveness of line and staff relationships in a hierarchical organization.

Context

Certain contextual variables relate to an organization's structure, such as organizational charter or social function, size, technology, environment, inter-dependence with other organizations, structuring of activities, concentration of authority, and line of control of work flow (Figure 7-8).[24]

FIGURE 7-6	ADVANTAGES AND LIMITATIONS OF ORGANIZATIONAL CHARTS

Advantages	Limitations
Depict clear relationships	Depict only formal authority structure
Facilitate coordination	Often outdated and obsolete
Facilitate communication	Confuse authority with status
Utilize to implement organizational changes	No informal relationships shown
Facilitate organizational planning	
Use as instructional tool in orientation	
Promote decision making	
Identify inconsistencies and complexities	

Source: Author.

FIGURE 7-7   **STANDARDS FOR EVALUATING THE EFFECTIVENESS OF LINE AND STAFF RELATIONSHIPS IN A HIERARCHICAL ORGANIZATION**

Standards

1. Line authority relationships are clearly delineated and defined by the organizational and/or functional charts and policies.

2. Staff authority relationships are clearly delineated and defined by the organizational and/or functional charts and policies.

3. Functional authority relationships are clearly delineated and defined by the organizational and/or functional charts and policies.

4. Staff personnel consult with, advise, and provide counsel to line personnel.

5. Service personnel functions are clearly understood by line and staff personnel.

6. Line personnel seek and effectively use staff services.

7. Appropriate staff services are being provided by line nursing personnel and other organizational departments or services.

8. Services are not being duplicated because of line and staff authority relationships.

Source: Author.

FIGURE 7-8   **CONTEXTUAL VARIABLES OF AN ORGANIZATIONAL STRUCTURE**

- Organizational charter/social function: Nursing organizations exist within institutions that are either government owned, private not-for-profit, or private for-profit. Government-owned organizations are impersonally founded and highly centralized, with concentrated authority. Impersonality of origin increases the level of control of work flow. Because many healthcare organizations are impersonal in origin, they are highly centralized with increased line control of work flow of professional nurses.

- Size: Larger organizations tend to have more specialization and more formalization than small ones. The larger the size, the more decentralized the organization and the more standardized the procedures for selection and advancement of personnel.

- Technology: Technology can be defined as the steps or ordering of physical techniques used for organizational work flow, even if the physical techniques involve only the formulation of the plan. The more rigid and highly integrated the technology, the greater the structuring of activities and procedures and the more impersonal the control.

Source: Author.

Contingency theory was used to study the technology, size, environment, and structure in 157 nursing subunits located in 24 hospitals in the Canadian province of Alberta. The theory postulated that the wide range of differences in organizational structure varies systematically with such factors as technology, size, and environment. It was found that increased subunit beds decreased the registered nurse ratio and increased the measure of bureaucratization of professionals. There was no relationship between decentralization of the subunit and size and little relationship between size and role specificity.[25] These findings support those of Pugh and others, who found no relationship between size and concentration of authority, between size and line control of work flow, or between size and autonomy.[26]

Forms of Organizational Structures

A structure enables an organization to get the work done. It helps ensure that the purpose, goals, and objectives of the organization are achieved. The framework supported by the Magnet Recognition Program is an organizational structure that is flat, tall, and decentralized, allowing decision making by the nurse closest to the delivery of care to occur.27 Before selecting an organizational structure for an organization, it is critical to know the characteristics of each of the structures (Figure 7-9).

Hierarchical (Tall, Centralized, Bureaucratic) Structure A hierarchical structure is commonly called a line structure (Figure 7-10). It is the oldest and simplest form of management and is associated with the principle of chain of command, bureaucracy and a multitiered hierarchy, vertical control and coordination, levels differentiated by function and authority, and downward communications. These structures have all the advantages and disadvantages of a bureaucracy. Most line structures have added a staff component. In nursing organizations, both line and staff personnel are usually professional nurses.

FIGURE 7-9 **CHARACTERISTICS OF ORGANIZATIONAL STRUCTURES**

Decentralization	Hierarchical (Centralized)	Matrix
Flat organizational structure	Oldest and simplest form of management	Maintenance of old-line authority structures
Authority shifted downward within the organization to its divisions, services, and units	Use of such concepts as chain of command, vertical control, and coordination	Specialist resources obtained from functional areas
Delegates decision-making responsibilities to the ones doing the work—participatory management	Levels in organization differentiated by function and authority	Promotion of formation of new organizational units
Involves more people in making decisions at the level at which an action occurs	Downward communication pattern	Decision making at the organizational level of group consensus, first-line management level
Delegate authority from top managers downward to the people who report to them	Multitiered hierarchy	Exercise of authority by matrix manager over the functional manager
Employee is accountable for results	Company larger in number of employees.	Cooperative planning, program development, allocation of resources to accomplish program objectives
Increased productivity, improved morale, decreased absenteeism	Uniformity of policies and procedures	Assignment of functional managers to teams that respond to the chief of the functional discipline and matrix manager
Employee and relationship centered	Power and authority prevails	Usually focuses on specific product line or services

Source: Author.

| FIGURE 7-10 | A TYPICAL HOSPITAL ORGANIZATION CHART |

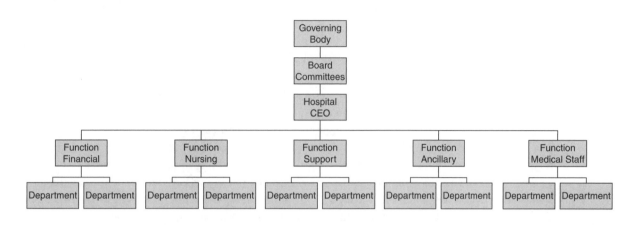

Source: Author.

Line functions are those that have direct responsibility for accomplishing the objectives of a nursing department (or service or unit). For the most part, they are filled with registered nurses, licensed practical nurses, and nursing technicians. Staff functions are those that assist the line in accomplishing the primary objectives of nursing. They include clerical, personnel, budgeting and finance, staff development, research, and specialized clinical consulting. The relationships between line and staff are a matter of authority. Line has authority for direct supervision of employees, whereas staff provides advice and counsel. There may be line authority within a staff section. Management is responsible for defining these positions clearly.

Functional authority takes place when an individual or department is delegated authority over functions in one or more additional departments. This has occurred in the development of infection control and quality assurance systems in which professional nurses have line authority to hospital management and staff authority to nursing management or line authority to nursing management and staff authority to other divisions. The functional staff does this through delegated authority to consult and prescribe procedures, and sometimes policies, for the function as it is to be carried out in the other departments. These delegated authority functions are clearly defined and carefully restricted. They are usually limited to procedures and time frames and do not include personnel or context. They should not weaken or destroy the authority and thus the effectiveness of line managers. For example, staff personnel might be assigned authority to recruit nurses, with line managers retaining final authority over hiring. The nurse administrator should ensure effective use of staff functions by line managers to make effective use of the advice of experts and reduce duplication of effort of line managers. Staff gives information that facilitates the solution of problems. Line managers in an effective and cooperative relationship seek such information.

Service departments are not necessarily staff in their authority relationships. Usually, they are a grouping of activities that facilitate the work of other departments through their operating functions. An example of this is the hospital's maintenance department, which provides the service of a functioning plant in which patient services are provided. It has the authority for performing its functions and may provide some staff advice and counsel. Within a hospital, as in any business, there may be many service departments, such as word processing centers and learning resource centers.

Activities are grouped together to provide for economical specialization. There may be service units for labor relations, contracts, legal matters, purchasing, and others. They may have functional authority, but care must be taken to keep them from causing divided loyalties, from delaying performance, and from displaying arrogance. They should provide for uniformity of procedures, policies, and standards for skilled service and a smooth operation.

Matrix Structure   A matrix management structure superimposes a horizontal program management over the traditional vertical hierarchy. Personnel from various functional departments are assigned to a specific program or project and become responsible to two bosses—a program manager and their functional department head. Thus an interdisciplinary team is created with core and extended team members. A longitudinal study of geriatrics matrix team program showed initial increased costs offset after a year by decreased acute care readmission rates, emergency room use, and nursing home placement. Mortality was significantly decreased and the functional ability of patients increased.[28]

The matrix organization design enables timely response to external competition and facilitates efficiency and effectiveness internally through cooperation among disciplines. Matrix nursing organizational structures have both advantages and disadvantages, as listed in Figure 7-11, Figure 7-12.[29,30]

Decentralization (Flat, Horizontal, Participatory) Structure   Flat organizational structures are characteristic of decentralized management. Decentralization refers to the degree to which authority is shifted downward within an organization to its divisions, services, and units. Decentralization is delegating decision-making responsibilities to the ones doing the work—participatory management. Implementation of a philosophy of decentralized decision making by top management sets the stage for involving more people—perhaps even the entire staff—in making decisions at the level at which an action occurs. Both decentralized management and participatory management delegate authority from top managers downward to the people who report to them. In doing so, objectives or duties are assigned, authority is granted, and an obligation or responsibility is created by acceptance. The employee is accountable for results.[31] In a decentralized participatory management structure, key attributes are integrated throughout the organization, management, and workforce. Such attributes consist of trust, commitment, goal setting, and autonomy.

FIGURE 7-11	**ADVANTAGES AND DISADVANTAGES OF MATRIX STRUCTURE**

Advantages	**Disadvantages**
Improved communication (vertical and horizontal)	Conflict due to multiple lines of authority, responsibility, and accountability
Improved coordination between healthcare teams	Loss of control over functional discipline
Increased organizational response to changes	Challenge to manage
Increased employee satisfaction	
Fewer organizational levels	
Enhanced decision making at bedside	
Improved collegial relationships	

Source: Author.

FIGURE 7-12

ESSENTIAL CONDITIONS FOR EFFECTIVE DECENTRALIZATION

- Freedom to function effectively
- Support from peers and leaders
- Concise and clear expectations of the work environment
- Appropriate resources

Source: Author.

In nursing, as in other organizations, delegation fosters participation, teamwork, and accountability. A first-line manager with delegated authority contacts another department to solve a problem in providing a service. The first-line manager does not need to go to his or her department head, who in turn would contact the department head of the other service, creating a communication bottleneck. The people closest to the problem solve it, resulting in efficient and cost-effective management. Research conducted on magnet hospitals found that most of the hospitals have a decentralized structure in which nurses had a feeling of control over their unit work environment.[32] Porter O'Grady identified several conditions as essential for effective decentralization (Figure 7-13).[33]

Role of the Nurse Executive

What is the role of the nurse executive under a decentralized system with participatory management? Its role is directed toward results. The nurse executive and nurse management team shares in planning and implementing the program. The nurse executive has a position of influence and attends the organization's highest decision-making body, the board of directors.

In one research study, 18 of 20 hospitals had some decentralization; 77% had some decentralization down to the unit level. The overriding purpose of decentralization was to increase worker satisfaction. Decentralization resulted in increased morale and job satisfaction and greater motivation among managers and workers. Personnel development, flexibility, and effective decision making all increased; conflict decreased, along with operational costs, negative attitudes, and underuse of managers. The workforce stabilized and became more effective and efficient. The study indicated that most managers do not understand the concept of delegation, are not effective communicators, do not concentrate on goals, and do not delegate according to the abilities and interests of their employees.[34] With the dynamics of decentralization, each unit works with its own budget; job descriptions are clear, concise, flexible, and current; in-service training is effective; performance standards are clear; employee recognition occurs; and accountability is enforced at all times. Figure 7-13 outlines standards for evaluating decentralization of authority in a nursing division, department, service, or unit and employee, together developing goals and objectives that are challenging, clear, consistent, and specific. Nurses and managers both will be motivated, healthy stress will be increased, and undesirable stress will be reduced.

Managers at all levels of nursing should subscribe to the philosophy of participatory management if it is to be successful. All managers and employees must unfreeze the present system of attitudes and values. This unfreezing process requires a comprehensive, well-planned, training program. Training promotes a sense of job security by preparing everyone for changed roles. Staff members at every level learn the reasons for participatory management, the advantages and disadvantages (Figure 7-14), and the roles they will play.

Good communication within the nursing organization is essential to an effective employee participation program. Good communication is effective communication; it is evident in employees who are

FIGURE 7-13	STANDARDS FOR EVALUATING DECENTRALIZATION OF AUTHORITY IN A NURSING DIVISION, DEPARTMENT, SERVICE, OR UNIT

Standards

1. Authority for decision making is delegated to the lowest operating level consistent with:
   a. Competence of subordinate managers
   b. Responsibility and accountability
   c. Economic management of enterprise
   d. Costs involved
   e. Need for uniformity and innovation of policy
   f. Management philosophy
   g. Subordinate managers' desires for independence
   h. Development of subordinate managers
   i. Need for evaluation and control
   j. Physical location of subordinate managers
   k. Organizational dynamics

2. Delegated authority is clear, specific, certain, and written. It is known by each subordinate manager.

3. Delegated authority supports the organizational, departmental, service, and unit goals, policies, standards, and plans.

4. Delegated authority is consistent with requirements of regulatory agencies, private and governmental.

Source: Author.

FIGURE 7-14	ADVANTAGES AND DISADVANTAGES OF PARTICIPATORY MANAGEMENT

Advantages	Disadvantages
High trust, mutual support	Increased time and money
Improved accountability and decision making	Decrease in management status
Enhanced communication	More competitiveness among departments
Increased morale and motivation	Duplication of functions
Improved effectiveness and productivity	Underutilization of management
Higher job satisfaction	Lack of teamwork
More teamwork	Revisions of policies and procedures
Decreased absenteeism	Lack of involvement by employees
Improved recognition of employee contributions	Self-evaluation threatening to employees
Better quality of work	Lack of understanding of change process

Source: Author.

informed about the business of nursing. Such employees know what management is saying and what management's intentions are. Management knows what employees are saying and how that agrees with the perceptions that management is working to develop. Broken communication contributes to stress and leads to direct economic losses through low productivity, grievances, absenteeism, turnover, and work slowdowns or strikes.

Flat organizational structures promote effective communication. Managers plan the vehicles, content, and intent of effective communication, and they monitor the process. Supervisors are important to effective communication and (as another aspect of their changed roles) work to ensure its openness. Management attitudes should promote truth, frankness, and openness. More than 1,000 businesses in the United States are involved in some form of participatory management. Many nursing organizations subscribe to the notion of participatory management to some degree. Centralized management and authority are becoming history in the development of the science of human behavior.[35] Because they have been subjected to centralized authoritarian management for so long, nursing personnel need to be schooled in the process of participatory management (Figure 7-15). This includes training to make input into collaborative decision making.[36]

Trust

Participatory management is based on a philosophy of trust. The employee is trusted to complete the task, with periodic progress reports and a final review with management. The time and rate of participation should be managed to control stress. Managers who empower and facilitate employee performance communicate trust. This process demonstrates the employee's capabilities and reveal shortcomings.

Motorola has had a participatory management program in effect since 1968, with almost all of its thousands of U.S. employees involved in it at some stage. These three basic ideas of their program embody trust:[37]

1. Every worker knows his or her job better than anybody else.
2. People can and will accept responsibility for managing their own work if that responsibility is given to them in the proper way.
3. Intelligence, perspective, and creativity exist among people at all levels of the organization.

Commitment

Personal involvement in managing a nursing service requires commitment from the chief nurse and other nurse managers. Managers should be highly visible to the staff, supporting and nurturing them. In turn, the staff should also be committed, a characteristic they develop from association with the

---

FIGURE 7-15 **CHARACTERISTICS OF PARTICIPATORY MANAGEMENT**

- Trust
- Commitment
- Goals and objectives
- Autonomy

Top Management

- Vertical versus horizontal integration
- Training
- Changed roles of supervisors
- Communication

Source: Author.

committed managers. They gain this commitment from seeing their bosses out at the production level where patients are being treated, from cooperating with their colleagues and managers in a spirit of teamwork, and from acquiring feelings of accomplishment.

Nursing commitment comes from knowing that the purpose of the organization is patient care and that the managers are working with the nurses to produce that care. Staff members share in making decisions and in coming to consensus with their bosses. This experience in participation "turns them on and tunes them in" so that they do not want to be lazy or mediocre. Commitment inspires staff to be industrious, outstanding, and productive. Under participatory management commitment is elicited, not imposed.

Professional nurses are motivated to develop their human skills, resulting in increased self-esteem. They have a sense of accomplishment and believe that management has supported their accomplishments. They believe they are expanding their worth through their work.

Goals and Objectives

Conflict resolution is a major requirement or goal of participatory management. Conflict is inevitable when human beings work together, but it is not productive to process or outcomes. In nursing, as in other occupations, conflict produces stress and results in turnover and absenteeism. Employees can be sensitized to deal with potential and real conflict and to take action to reduce its destructive consequences: fear, anger, distrust, jealousy, and resentment. Reducing the destructiveness of conflict can be accomplished by establishing a climate of openness with procedures for problem solving, persuasion, bargaining, and dealing with organizational politics. The goal is to reduce adversarial relations, which is accomplished through joint planning and problem solving and facilitating employee consultation.[38]

A key goal for a nursing organization is to keep itself healthy. Participatory management encourages a healthy work environment. Participation makes maximum use of employees' abilities without relinquishing the ultimate authority and responsibility of management. Professional nurses want to have input into decisions but do not want to do the job of managers. They want the support of managers, to talk with them, and to be informed. Without this support, nurses develop anger and hostility, which results in absenteeism and lower productivity.

Goal-setting activities can occur with reasonably frequent performance review and feedback. Nursing personnel bring their goals and objectives to conferences with managers. The process is reciprocal, with the manager and employee together developing goals and objectives that are challenging, clear, consistent, and specific. Nurses and managers both will be motivated, healthy stress will be increased, and undesirable stress will be reduced.

Career development programs for professional nurses help to reduce conflict and inspire loyalty to an organization. Provided with job information, nurses can set goals for themselves that relate to promotion, tenure, and job security. Differences in work attitudes and personal aspirations are recognized. There is less professional role conflict. New employees, who are young and fresh out of college, should be given information about the nature of the organization, current and future availability of jobs, career opportunities and career ladders, and management goals and responsibilities. Managers learn about the professional nurse employees' aspirations and expectations and should help them set a course and monitor it.[39]

Autonomy

Autonomy is the state of being independent and of having responsibility, authority, and accountability for one's work and personal time. Professional employees indicate they want autonomy for practicing their profession and in making decisions about their work. They do not want their decisions made for them by hospital administrators, physicians, or others. They want to be treated as equal partners and colleagues in the healthcare delivery system. This desire for autonomy has increased as nurses have developed increasingly sophisticated knowledge and skills and have used them with effective results.

Professional nurses want autonomous control over conditions under which they work, including pace and content. Such decisions are often in conflict with management's coordination role, a conflict that can be mitigated by involving professional nurses in delegating coordination of activities.[40]

Professional nurses are willing to assume and accept responsibility and to be held accountable for a charge. They want authority, the rightful and legitimate power to fulfill the charge. This authority comes from their expert knowledge and skill, their license, their position, and their peers.[41]

The autonomy of professional nurses is evident in an organization in which management trusts nurses by giving them freedom to make decisions and take actions within the scope of their knowledge. Nurses are thus free to exercise their authority. This freedom is legitimized in the bylaws of their departments and in job descriptions, performance appraisals, and management support of their decisions. Nurses' independent behavior includes acknowledging mistakes, taking action to correct them, and preventing them from happening again.

The professional nurse is accountable for the consequences of his or her actions. Relationships exist between responsibility, authority, autonomy, and accountability.

To have autonomy, nursing employees should be involved in setting their own goals and be allowed to determine how to accomplish their goals. This principle applies to all nursing employees. When professional nurses work with other nursing employees, they should facilitate participation and input from these groups. This approach promotes interest, trust, and commitment.[42]

A study of nurse autonomy found variations in perceptions of whether the nurses were expected to exhibit autonomy and of whether they were supported in exhibiting it. The typical nurse exhibiting the highest level of autonomy was a female with a master's degree practicing in a clinical administrative role in the emergency room who perceived an expectation to function autonomously to a high degree. The typical nurse exhibiting the lowest level of autonomy was a male staff nurse in the operating room or postanesthesia with less than a master's degree who perceived an expectation to practice autonomously to a low extent or was unsure of the expectation for autonomy. No change was found in the perceived levels of autonomy from studies done 15 years before. Highest scores were found among nurses practicing in the emergency room, psychiatry, and critical care, areas in which institutions and physicians grant the greatest autonomy. Nurses at the master's level had the highest scores in autonomy. Below that level, poor role definition, role confusion, and poor role modeling contribute to a socialization process that encourages all nurses to act the same. Conversely, nurses in administrative roles have clearer role expectations and correspondingly higher scores on autonomy. Apparently, they are not empowering their practice staff to have the same level of autonomy. The authors found from the results of their study that their findings may indicate that autonomy is not expected or supported by hospitals.[43]

To foster greater autonomy, nurses need to be included in decision making, policy setting, and financial decisions. They need to have role clarity and to be educated at a higher level for autonomous practice. Greater attention needs to be paid to role modeling to facilitate understanding of nursing independent, dependent, and interdependent aspects. When elements are identified within one area of practice that promote autonomy, they need to be incorporated into other areas as well.[43]

Evidence-Based Practice 7-1

A study of graduating students at one university indicated that the students ranked high on individual autonomy. It would appear that lack of professional status is not due to lack of autonomy in individual nurses. Therefore consideration must be given to the denial of autonomy by employing institutions as the root cause. Nurses probably arrive at their first job with more autonomous attitudes than do workers in other industries. Serious consideration should be given to the role that institutions play in blocking nurses' efforts at achieving professional autonomy. Nursing education should address this issue by looking critically at existing programs and working to educate nurses who will be able to claim their rightful professional status.[44]

Top Management

What is the role of top management under a decentralized system with participatory management? Its role is directed toward results. Because effective controls are needed to monitor performance of lower-level units, top managers use computers to assist in making decisions and developing controlling techniques for decentralization.

In one research study, 18 of 20 hospitals had some decentralization; 77% had some decentralization down to the unit level. The overriding purpose of decentralization was to increase worker satisfaction. Decentralization resulted in increased morale and job satisfaction and greater motivation among managers and workers. Personnel development, flexibility, and effective decision making all increased; conflict decreased, along with operational costs, negative attitudes, and underuse of managers. The workforce stabilized and became more effective and efficient.

Vertical Versus Horizontal Integration

Vertical integration combines decentralization with integration. When businesses and industries decentralize operations into product lines and subsidiaries, each unit maintains its partnership and identity within the corporate structure. Before the advent of the prospective payment system and competition among hospitals, the industry was largely characterized by horizontal integration of departments within divisions. Some examples are nursing; operations related to patient care services, such as pharmacy, physical therapy, and occupational therapy; operations related to plant management, including housekeeping; and finance.

As competition increased, hospitals began the quest to diversify into new markets. New corporate structures that included umbrella corporate management with subsidiary companies were formed. As hospitals struggle for survival, many choose vertical integration as a means of capturing lost revenues through control of input and output. Whether all efforts at vertical integration will be successful depends on the market share of products and services captured. Moderate effects on operating costs as a result of hospital mergers have been reported. Certain objectives for vertical integration can be found in Figure 7-16.[45]

From the viewpoint of function rather than structure, organizations have focused on the vertical dimension of decentralized decision making. This vertical dimension aims for representation by levels of employees, thereby restricting decentralization to a single function or issue considered to be of primary importance to the organization. Health care has sometimes focused on issues of marketing and quality control, in which decisions are made up or down the hierarchy.

Horizontal integration is also important to the success of participatory management. Integration of the decentralized decision-making process horizontally or laterally links traditionally separate functional hierarchies. The organizational structure and functions require adaptation to models that support participatory processes.[46] Organizational integration requires a merger of information technology that reports results for all organizational entities.[47] Healthcare systems are sometimes horizontally and vertically integrated for maximum service integration, service delivery, patient capture, and medical education.[48]

FIGURE 7-16	OBJECTIVES OF VERTICAL INTEGRATION AND HORIZONTAL INTEGRATION

Vertical Integration	Horizontal Integration
Conversion of internal cost centers into revenue producers	Improved communication across functions
Development of new and expanding markets for hospitals	Links separate functional hierarchies

Source: Author.

Training

Managers at all levels of nursing should subscribe to the philosophy of participatory management if it is to be successful. All managers and employees must unfreeze the present system of attitudes and values. This unfreezing process requires a comprehensive, well-planned, training program. Training promotes a sense of job security by preparing everyone for changed roles. Staff members at every level learn the reasons for participatory management, the advantages and disadvantages, and the roles they will play.

Managers might be threatened by the concept of participatory management if they perceive their authority is being diminished. Their training program requires that their competencies be assessed. This training will include developing managers' abilities to be frank with employees, to be willing to admit to past failures, and to encourage contributions from their workers and to be influenced by them. Managers need to learn to deal with justifying the existence of their jobs.[49]

Centralized management and authority are becoming history in the development of the science of human behavior.[50] Because they have been subjected to centralized authoritarian management for so long, nursing personnel need to be schooled in the process of participatory management. This includes training to make input into collaborative decision making.

In participatory management a complementary relationship exists between managers and practitioners, rather than a hierarchical one. Training is done to prepare staff and prevent insecurity. Availability of managers qualified to function in participatory management increases decentralization. Training of supervisors should focus on changes in their needs as well as their functions. Supervisors will learn to gain self-fulfillment from delegating and team building.[51]

Management training of supervisors includes group dynamics, problem solving, planning, and decision making. Such training can occur through conferences, workshops, and seminars. It should be rewarding and continuous to be successful. It will relieve the threats supervisors feel from challenges by employees, from exposure of their weaknesses, from perceived loss of prestige and power, and from "digging in" to keep control.[52]

Changed Roles of Supervisors

Decentralization with participative management means that roles must be redefined and coordinated to prevent conflict. Nurse managers and primary nurses have increased management responsibility. For some, this means decreased hands-on clinical responsibility. Supervisors of nurse managers have decreased responsibility for unit management and become mentors, role models, and facilitators. With a flattened organizational structure, some may lose jobs, whereas others have the overall scope of their responsibility increased.[53]

Evidence-Based Practice 7-2

In one experiment in decentralized patient education, all clinical nurses caring for patients became the teachers. The assistant head nurse became the facilitator, that is, the person responsible for planning and developing objectives for patient education programs and for promoting staff interest and participation in all phases. The education department became the resource available to coordinate teaching programs in support of the primary nurse. The advantages of decentralized versus centralized patient education include using all nursing and health personnel for education, providing education to a maximum number of patients and families, and having each nurse assume professional responsibility for patient education.[54]

As supervisors learn to delegate authority, they modify the climate that promotes deviant behavior by giving professional nurses what they want: the authority to manage themselves. Because authority gives the supervisors initiative in performing their jobs and freedom to question managers, managers should expect loyalty in return. The profession of nursing does not employ nurses; organizations do. Participatory management is a process in which there must be an ongoing dialogue with constraints: nurses will control their profession, and management uses its input to set objectives and priorities and to review output. Nurse employees cannot control the enterprise, and management cannot compromise the professional or ethical standards of professional nurses.[55]

In participatory management, the supervisor facilitates rather than directs the workforce. Traditional supervising functions are delegated downward. There must be clear delineation of a manager's basic responsibilities, distinct from behavioral or management style. Managers can gain satisfaction from their ability to make clinical nurses successful and satisfied. The interpersonal skills and conceptual abilities demanded of supervisors increase. Supervisors should be challenged and should have a future. Supervisors promote implementation of committee decisions, listen, and offer assistance.[56]

Because fewer supervisors are needed, career development programs for college-educated nurses must provide them promotional opportunities as clinical practitioners, managers, teachers, or researchers. Supervisors are important to the success of decentralized decision making and employee involvement in the management of nursing and the healthcare system. They should be taught to manage under employee involvement programs. They need to learn that they will have more time to plan and organize work and to be creative. Their jobs can be expanded upward, but they should keep in contact with employees and encourage participation by everyone.

Communication

Good communication is effective communication; it is evident in employees who are informed about the business of nursing. Such employees know what management is saying and what management's intentions are. Management knows what employees are saying and how that agrees with the perceptions that management is working to develop. Broken communication contributes to stress and leads to direct economic losses through low productivity, grievances, absenteeism, turnover, and work slowdowns or strikes.

Flat organizational structures promote effective communication. Managers plan the vehicles, content, and intent of effective communication, and they monitor the process. Supervisors are important to effective communication and (as another aspect of their changed roles) work to ensure its openness. Management attitudes should promote truth, frankness, and openness.

Participation enhances commitment and interdepartmental and intradepartmental communication. In medium-sized and large organizations, a communication center will operate 24 hours a day. Message delivery will be facilitated. Computers will be used to communicate instantly, nurse to nurse, nurse to manager, manager to nurse, and nurse to others. Messages will be hand-delivered when necessary.

Decentralization requires a movement away from mainframe information processing toward distributed systems of smaller computers. This change increases flexibility and control at lower organizational levels, giving users heightened feelings of ownership of the system. Packaged software then offers fast relief for specific application needs. End-user involvement with computer applications increases.[57]

With direct communication, the middle person is eliminated and time is saved. The problem of missing medical laboratory or radiology reports is taken up between the primary nurse or the nurse manager and the manager of the department immediately responsible.[58] Increased representation of clinical nurses on hospital and departmental committees improves communication. The goal is to facilitate the flow of information, not to embody it in the authority of a management position. Objectives, group brainstorming, and self-directed work teams are vehicles of effective communication used in participatory management.

Activities Involving Nurses in Participatory Management

Some of the programs and structures that can be used to involve nurses in participatory management are job enrichment, personalization, primary nursing, shared governance, entrepreneurship, gain sharing, and pay equity (Figure 7-17).

| **FIGURE 7-17** | **PARTICIPATORY MANAGEMENT ACTIVITIES** |

- Job enrichment: Job enrichment satisfies the motivation to fulfill higher-order needs, including variety within and among jobs and a strategy that challenges by emphasizing performance output over job processes. Job enrichment creates jobs with greater responsibility and more flexibility and promotes personal development.

- Personalization: A strategy that focuses on people and knowledge, not numbers and politics. Those who use personalization stress empathy and involve professionals in making critical decisions that affect them.

- Primary nursing: Primary nursing as a modality of nursing care delivery makes nursing worthwhile work, enhances nurses' self-esteem through performing a complete function, produces results of a personal endeavor, and realizes collegial and collaborative relationships.[59] In a hospital setting where primary nursing is practiced, decentralization of patient care delivery systems provides the most efficient nursing care. Primary nurses are accountable. The ideal environment for self-governance is primary nursing with a stable, mature, self-directed, skilled, and committed staff trained in leadership skills.[60] Other nursing modalities that are compatible with participatory management are modular nursing, team nursing, case management, and collaborative practice models.

- Shared governance: Shared governance is defined as the allocation of control, power, or authority among mutually interested parties. The principles of shared governance are more consistent with the principles of professionalism than are the principles of participatory management.

- Entrepreneurship: As decentralization and vertical integration strategies are implemented in healthcare organizations, a great opportunity exists for professional nurses to be involved in entrepreneurship. Nurses can form small companies with the support of government agencies and private businesses. Such companies require venture capital that can, with sufficient preparation, be obtained from the government and the private healthcare industry. Entrepreneurship in nursing will be good for professional nurses and the healthcare industry because it will create independent thinkers who are motivated to be productive, creative, and more competitive in the marketplace. They will become like other business people who have a strong desire to control their own careers.

- Gain sharing: Gain sharing is a group incentive program in which employees share in the financial benefits of improved performance. It has many of the same advantages and disadvantages as other methods of participatory management. Top management is sensitive to the employees' goals, and employees identify with the organization through greater involvement. The results of gain sharing are measurable: sav-

(continues)

ings, improved labor-management relations, fewer grievances, less absenteeism, and reduced turnover. Gain sharing adds money to intrinsic rewards. Stock ownership and profit sharing are economic rewards similar to gain sharing. Gain sharing, stock ownership, and profit sharing may not be legally possible in not-for-profit organizations. However, increased financial benefits can be made available through legal means such as merit pay, certification pay, and clinical promotions.

- Pay equity: Pay equity between management and employees is an issue of participatory management. Professional nurses, like other professional workers, frequently respond negatively to the strategy of linking financial benefits to promotion into management. They want financial reward for accomplishing personal and organizational objectives that increase productivity and reduce turnover and absenteeism. These rewards can be in the form of nonmanagerial advancement of salary, status, recognition, autonomy, and responsibility. This can be accomplished through dual ladders, that is, clinical promotions that match management promotions. Such promotions preserve nurses' professional career opportunities with financial rewards based on graduated pay scales that can be objectively measured through levels of achievement culminating in mastery.

Source: Author.

Shared Governance

Data supporting reduction in turnover and increases in levels of nursing satisfaction are evidence of successful outcomes of shared governance processes. There are main principles of shared governance that should be reviewed before deciding to implement this structure (Figure 7-18).[61]

Three models of shared governance are the congressional model, the unit-based model, and the councilor model. All three models delineate four broad areas of accountability: practice, quality, education, and management. Accountabilities of practice include practice standards, job descriptions, care delivery systems, and nursing representation in hospital-wide committees. Additional quality issues include practice standards, job descriptions, the care delivery system, and nursing representation in hospital-wide committees. Accountabilities for quality include delineation of data sources, evaluation criteria, evaluation processes, and mechanisms for quality improvement, credentialing, peer review, and research. Education accountabilities include needs assessment, incorporation of new standards of research, and evaluation of educational endeavors. Accountabilities of management include provision

FIGURE 7-18 PRINCIPLES OF SHARED GOVERNANCE

- Shared governance is not a form of participatory management. Participatory management means allowing others to participate in decisions over which a line manager has control.

- Shared governance is not management driven. All activities that are neither direct caregiving nor related to that process are in support of it.

- Shared management has no locus of control. Accountabilities of a role are attributed to the role from within the role; they can never be assigned, nor can they be given away.

- Models should be based on a clinical rather than an administrative organization.

- Governance should be representative in nature, not democratic.

- Representatives should be elected, not selected.

- Bylaws should provide a system of checks and balances, and they should be passed by a majority vote of the entire nursing staff.

Source: Author.

of resources, including human and financial resources; implementation of council or committee decisions; interdepartmental problem solving; and facilitation of staff problem solving, decision making, and leadership.[62]

Under collaborative governance, managers become integrators, facilitators, and coordinators. Clinical managers are educated in decision making, team building, group dynamics, goals and objectives development, interviewing skills, budgeting, disciplining, and rewarding. Unit personnel develop policy. Structure is kept informal except for areas governed by law, regulations, and efficiency, in which representative central committees operate. Unit personnel decide whether their unit will be "open," in which case personnel float in and out, or "closed." For the system to work, all unit employees must buy into it. It takes years to build successful collaborative governance. A successful system is in a constant state of flux and chaos. This system is based on shared beliefs, including such assumptions as knowledge is power; risk taking, with or without success, is growth; individuals are unique in their contributions; and maximum productivity results when organizational and personal values are congruent.[63]

To prepare for self-management, there must be a committed administration, a prepared staff, time, a willingness to make mistakes and move on, and managers who are able to relinquish decision-making power over daily operations. Those responsible for fostering self-management must prepare for a fundamental change in the perception of "self as manager" and "subordinate" roles and responsibilities. In self-management, it is more important than ever for management to set and communicate clear expectations. Without a safe environment, self-management will fail because people will avoid changing or taking risks. Ongoing training and information sessions, with feedback and practice, are fundamental to the success of the new model. Gaining trust of staff and first-line supervisors and managers is made possible through modeling self-management principles and practices in the administrative structure of the organization.[64]

Although it appears that shared governance is expanding, a persistent question relates to whether its benefits are being objectively evaluated. Research studies show that nurses gain job satisfaction and growth satisfaction from working in a nurse-managed special care unit with a shared governance management model.[65] Surveys of nurses involved in horizontal integration through hospital acquisition indicate that nurses value shared governance and professional nursing autonomy.[66] Descriptive reports of shared governance organizations report the following:

- Shared governance decentralizes decision making, disperses power, increases participatory management, and enlarges the span of control. It can be unit based, department based, or organization based.[67]
- Shared government involves staff in management, education, quality, and practice issues that support changes in skill-mix and patient-focused care systems.[68]
- Shared governance as an organizational structure supports vertical integration, product line development, and an organizational culture with strong relationships.[69]

One way to develop support for a self-governance structure is to create nursing bylaws or a set of principles or statements that govern the internal affairs of the nursing division.[70] The nursing bylaws are based from the mission, philosophy, goals, and objectives from both the organization and specific to nursing services and should contain essential elements (Figure 7-19).

Organizational Development

Organizational development deals with changing the work environment to make it more conducive to worker satisfaction and productivity. An underlying premise is that "people planning" is as important as technical and financial planning. Organizational development allows managers to attend to the psychological as well as the physical aspects of organizations. Change is the terrain to which organizational

FIGURE 7-19	ESSENTIAL ELEMENTS IN A SET OF NURSING BYLAWS

- Mission, vision, philosophy of the professional nursing organization
- Core values of the professional nursing organization
- Definition of nursing
- Governance functions of the professional nursing organization
- Role of the professional nurse
- Professional nurse staff membership
- Advancement opportunities for professional nurse
- Credentials review process
- Description of the governance structure
- Discipline, appeals, and parallel levels processes
- Bylaw review and revision process

Source: Author.

development applies. Some of the common types of organizational development interventions that can be used are teams, process improvement, work redesign, training, performance management systems, and structural change.[71]

Organizational development can sustain the favorable or desirable aspects of bureaucracy. Change can be used to modify the undesirable aspects of bureaucracy. There is room for directive and nondirective leadership within organizations. Nurse managers have to be strong and tough in supporting the values of clinical nurses. They have to be proactive in planning, designing, and implementing new organizational structures and work environments. The object is to develop people, not to exploit them. Organizational development emphasizes personal growth and interpersonal competence.[72]

Autonomy and Accountability

Among the psychological and personality attributes of organizational development are autonomy and accountability, both crucial elements of nursing professionalism. A professional nurse is obliged to answer for decisions and actions. This is achieved using a management by results approach. This approach defines performance standards incorporating acceptable behavior and results. It includes tracking for progress, performance feedback, making adjustments, and personnel accountability.[73]

Characteristics of professional autonomy include self-definition, self-regulation, and self-governance. Professional nurses respond to demographic changes in society by defining and reshaping the content of nursing practice. They address societal needs, including the needs for increased care for the elderly and the control of resources. Autonomy is strengthened by unbundling the hospital bill and by direct reimbursement for nursing services by third-party payers.

Self-governance for nursing includes a nursing administrator hired or elected with input from nurses, self-employment of nurses, approval of nursing staff privileges by peer review with privileges revoked by the nursing staff organization, and case management.[74]

Argyris describes people as complex organizations who work for an organization for their own needs or gains. These needs exist in varying degrees or at varying depths that must be understood by organizations. People seek out jobs to meet their needs. They develop and live on a continuum from infancy to adulthood that is reflected throughout life and work and leisure.[75]

Ridderheim describes a particular hospital administrator's action to change a management style that was paternalistic, used downward communication, encouraged dependency, and inhibited management development. In an opinion survey, the hospital's employees scored high on patient care and personal pride in work but low in decision-making ability. The following are among the changes made by the administrator after organizational assessment and consultation:[76]

- Decisions were turned back to operating managers, giving them freedom to act within broad policy guidelines.
- Operating management was restructured in an executive operating committee that included the administrator and assistants for medical staff affairs, operations, facilities, patient care, personnel, and finance. Each assistant had policymaking status.
- A core group was established at lower levels of management to focus on the technical interests and objectives of the hospital.
- Task forces were established for special projects.
- A team was set up to monitor terminations, retirements, recruitments, advancements, and demotions.
- Performance standards were developed for each manager.
- Team-building seminars were held.
- After 9 months, progress was critiqued at a retreat, first by the executive operating committee and then by subordinate managers.
- Achievement in relation to goals, individual growth, and teamwork was stressed over seniority.
- Subsequent surveys showed improvement in job satisfaction, supervisory concern for employees, supervisory emphasis on goal achievement, and work group emphasis on teamwork, decision-making practices, and motivational conditions.

Team Building

Team building is an essential process in today's healthcare environment. As healthcare organizations are faced with intense pressure to control cost and increase productivity and efficiency with continued regulatory and legislative constraints, effective team building can produce the ultimate outcome of improved health care. For example, one study concluded that the amount of involvement and interaction between the nurses in an intensive care unit and the physicians directly influenced the differences in patient mortality.[77] In the *Scope and Standards for Nurse Administrators*, interdisciplinary collaboration (team building) is threaded throughout the standards of practice: assessment, diagnosis and identification of outcomes, planning, and implementation.[78] In the *Standards of Professional Performance, Standard 12. Collaboration*, the nurse administrator is identified as the one who should collaborate with nursing staff, interdisciplinary teams, all departments, and the community.[79] Collaboration should be focused on developing, implementing, and evaluating programs and services; enhancing care delivery; and increasing employee satisfaction.[80] As the nursing workforce continues to intensify and the shortages increase, nursing is called on to develop interdisciplinary collaborative solutions.[81] One way to achieve this expectation is through team building and the effective use of interdisciplinary teams, work groups, and committees.

Team building is a method of participative management that encourages commitment, creativity, support, and growth of the individual, the unit, and the organization. The objective of team building is to establish an environment of cohesiveness among healthcare workers, whether among different shifts on one unit or among other units and departments throughout the facility. This cohesiveness enables organizations to develop patient care teams, committees, or work groups that use problem-solving techniques and demonstrate a commitment to the organization and each other to reach the goals and objectives of the organization.

One continually hears such remarks as "This organization does not care about the employees!" or "This organization really cares about its employees!" Nurse managers want to hear the positive statement. A person who works courageously and confidently, with the discipline and willingness to endure hardship, manifests high morale. Morale is a motivation factor related to productivity and product or service quality indicators. A person with low morale is not satisfied with his or her work. Low morale is evident in the person who is timid, cowardly, devious, fearful, disorderly, unruly, rebellious, turbulent, or indifferent as a result of job dissatisfaction and organizational milieu. Dissatisfied workers do not contribute positively to esprit de corps. Companies want high morale and cohesiveness among employees, and they use different strategies, such as team building, to address the issue.

The principle of synergy underlies team building. Synergy puts the thinking power of a selected group together for the most effective outcome. To sustain synergy, there are six basic rules to follow, as listed in Figure 7-20.[82]

The value of team building is to improve such processes as goal setting, relationships among people performing the work, group collaboration, and the allocation of the work that needs to be done.[83] Nurse managers should create a humanistic environment for nursing employees, one that fosters trust and cooperation—the synergy. Such an environment treats employees, rather than technology and buildings, as the most important asset. Nurses who have high self-esteem or self-worth are energetic and confident, take pride in their work, and have genuine respect and concern for their patients, visitors, peers, and others. Their behavior reflects this self-worth expressed in high morale, job satisfaction, and a commitment to each other and to the organization.

Today's nurse managers will be effective if they are informed about nursing staff's personal values and concerns. Work conflicts, type of shifts, child care services, and family responsibilities are examples of what is important to staff nurses. By knowing such information, the nurse manager can be knowledgeable about the issues and provide whatever guidance and assistance is needed to promote a positive work climate for staff.

Before team performance can be improved, the nurse manager must assess how the current team is functioning.[84] To facilitate team building and successful teams, the nurse manager should use steps similar to the problem-solving process, listed in Figure 7-21.[85]

A nurse manager may begin team building by asking for volunteers from every shift to work together on an issue. One example is to work on improving the response time of answering patients' call lights. The team is asked to present its recommendations to the staff on that unit.[86] Once the team

---

FIGURE 7-20	**SIX BASIC RULES TO SYNERGY AND TEAM BUILDING**

1. Define a clear purpose. Each team member must clearly be knowledgeable about the reason they are together. The team members must be able to articulate the goals, objectives, and purpose of the team.

2. Actively listen. Each team member must be focused on each individual and listen to what is being said. Active listening is not judgmental and means being completely absorbed and attentive to the speaker.

3. Maintain honesty. Each team member must be objective in providing feedback to the speaker. No one should make the speaker feel belittled or that his or her views are not correct or important.

4. Demonstrate compassion. Each team member should listen in a caring manner to the other's viewpoint.

5. Commit to resolution of conflicts. Each team member must agree to disagree even though his or her view or opinion is not the same. Team members must work toward a common understanding and acceptance of the issue at hand.

6. Be flexible. Each team member must be open and flexible to another individual's perspective. Everyone works together to accomplish the goal or objective.

Source: Author.

FIGURE 7-21   STEPS TO FACILITATE TEAM BUILDING

1. Assess the functioning of the team through such methods as direct observation, employee interviews or meetings, and questionnaires.

2. Identify the problem(s) resulting in team dysfunction, such as negativism, poor goal setting, poor interpersonal relationships among the members, and lack of commitment and disengagement.

3. Analyze the team's strengths and weaknesses.

4. Develop an action plan to develop strategies for the team.

5. Implement the strategies that should be communicated to the entire staff.

6. Evaluate the results of the team-building effort on a continuous basis.

Source: Author.

functions well, team building then can focus on work production. Some meeting time should always be dedicated to morale, motivation, and team skills and discussion of team direction.[87]

Recognition of the individual worth of each nurse is an important morale builder. It gives the individual self-esteem. Managers can stimulate self-esteem with praise that promotes a sense of competence, success, and worth. Nurse managers have to believe they are worthy before they can nurture that belief in subordinates. Each nurtures each other. Managers who have self-esteem are not afraid to explore their personal feelings with their peers or subordinates.

Most professional nurses spend many hours in the workplace, and they depend on their jobs as a major source of self-esteem. For this reason, nurse managers should aspire to build a work environment that enhances the self-esteem of all nurses. Such an environment promotes outstanding performance. This is even more important in times of stress and with particular challenges: downsizing, declining patient days, and workforce shortages. Recognition can be made through many avenues, and even a simple "thank you" can increase the self-esteem of an individual. Nave and Thomas suggest 50 specific techniques to boost employee morale, including such strategies as snacks during breaks, potluck suppers, annual parties, birthday cards, and other strategies that acknowledge the individual and teams.[88]

Team development is a complex and tough job. The team leader identifies training needs of the team and the individual members. The team leader also runs interference for the team, acts as liaison in negotiation for scarce resources, arranges publicity for accomplishments, and keeps abreast of information on outside events affecting the team. When conflicts arise from perceptions that some team members are doing more than their share of work or that the wrong members are getting promoted, the team leader manages them. The dream team collaborates with enthusiasm to get a job done well.

Teams

The team organization has been tried in nursing since the 1950s. It has been used mainly at the operating or primary care level rather than at top or middle management levels. A team is a number of people—usually fairly small and with different backgrounds, skills, and knowledge, and drawn from various areas of the organization (their home) who work together on a specific and defined task. There is usually a team leader or team captain.[89]

In healthcare institutions, patients see the physician as team leader. However, the team leader uses the resources of the entire organization; in many cases it is the nurse who identifies, recommends, and coordinates these resources.

A team must have a continuing mission, which nursing has. The team should be highly flexible without a rigid chain of command. Like all organizational structures in business, industry, or health-care institutions, the team organization needs clear and sharply defined objectives. Leadership decides on decision and command authority, and the team is responsible for accomplishing the tasks or mission. Team members know each other's functions, but leadership must first establish clarity of objectives in everybody's role. Everyone on the team should know the whole work and be adaptable and receptive to innovation. The team leader gives continuing attention to clear communications and clear decision making. A team should be kept small for top management work and for innovative work. Otherwise, the team design complements the functional design. A combination may consist of employees who work in teams but produce work organized on the functional principle. This approach seems to work best in nursing and is probably better than either organizational structure in its pure form. Team organization is a difficult structure requiring great self-discipline.

Self-Managed (Self-Directed) Work Teams   One specific type of team that has been used effectively is the self-managed (self-directed) work team. A self-directed work team is a functional group of typically 8 to 15 employees. The team shares responsibility for a particular unit of production, including units of service or information. Members are cross-trained in all the technical skills necessary to complete the tasks assigned. Members have the authority to plan, implement, and control all work processes. Members are responsible for scheduling, quality, and costs, and responsibilities have been clearly defined in advance. There are nine characteristics of a self-directed work team:

1. Bottom-up communication
2. Consensus
3. Big picture
4. Ongoing diverse training
5. Mobility
6. Empowerment
7. Challenge/innovation
8. External competition
9. Work and celebration

Employers indicate that self-directed work teams improve quality, increase productivity, decrease operating costs, and foster greater commitment from workers. Employees state that they feel "in on things," involved in decisions, challenged, and empowered, and they also have increased job satisfaction.

Self-directed work teams have leaders. During early phases, upper management appoints the leader. As the team grows and changes, it selects its leader. Eventually, the role rotates. The team leader is an internal facilitator. Middle managers are trained to become external facilitators.[90]

Self-managed work teams are empowered to make all decisions about the work they do. For example, Federal Express and IDS claim productivity is up 40% with self-managed work teams. A survey of Fortune 1,000 companies indicates that 68% use self-managed work teams, although only 10% of workers are in them (Figure 7-22).[91]

The change to self-managed work teams requires training of management personnel who are uncomfortable with the process and find their status and power threatened. Managers have to unlearn traditional autocratic approaches with punitive emphasis and tight controls on the workforce. Managers are trained to overcome feelings of threat and resentment to change, to perceive workers as mature and responsible, to believe that workers can train each other, to believe that peer pressure can overcome absenteeism and that a self-managed team gives them time to develop key people, and to believe they can be a resource to team members and a support group among themselves. They are facilitators who work with the group. Leaders are key to the success of self-directed work teams, and

FIGURE 7-22 ELEMENTS OF SUCCESSFUL SELF-MANAGED TEAMS

- Empower the teams with decision making.

- Provide teams with e-mail communication systems so teams can talk with each other.

- Create teams only for work that can be done by teams.

- Make teamwork the centerpiece of a pay-for-performance system.

- Inspire teams to increase morale, productivity, and innovation.

- Use the right team for the right job. Form a problem-solving team to solve a problem, and then disband it. Use work teams to do the day-to-day work. Work teams should be self-managed, have power to change the order of things, and have budgets.

- Create a hierarchy of teams that make decisions on the spot. To build the 777, Boeing used three layers of teams: a top management team to see that the plane was built correctly and on time, leader teams from engineering and operations to oversee the work teams, and cross-functional work teams. A fourth layer of airplane integration teams with access to everyone in the organization was added later. Problems were identified and solved early.

- Maintain trust and morale. When restructuring, bring employees into the process. Plan for job loss by re-training, reassigning, retiring, and attrition.

- Tackle people problems head on by spending time to get people to work together.

Source: Author.

their use of power is crucial in breaking down the organizational barriers preventing effective teams. Managers can make the transition to new roles with modified behavior and attitudes, but this is not a simple task for them.[92]

One of the activities that self-managed work teams can do effectively is problem solving, a powerful service strategy that gets everyone working toward top performance. Employees believe their ideas and efforts are valued. Once the self-managed work teams are formed, problem solving may be introduced in five steps, shown in Figure 7-23.[93]

FIGURE 7-23 FIVE STEPS FOR PROBLEM SOLVING

1. Brainstorm to identify problems. Team members are asked to describe problems they have observed or experienced.

2. Once all problems are listed, team members are asked to vote on paper for the three problems they believe are most significant. The votes are tallied and the most important problem is presented.

3. Brainstorm for possible solutions to the problem. The most promising solution is selected. Team members are assigned to investigate the solution and gather further information to report on later. The meeting is then closed.

4. At the next meeting, the team reports their findings, which are discussed, including positive and negative aspects.

5. The team chooses the solution through discussion and general agreement. Team members share the responsibility for putting the solution to work.

Source: Author.

Self-directed work teams and work groups are successfully used to reduce cost per unit of service, improve service and customer satisfaction, determine optimal staffing levels, and reduce the number of layers of organization. These teams perform tasks that require technical and management skills, thereby increasing productivity.[94]

Committees

A committee is a group that evolves out of a formal organization structure. Committees are formed to make collective use of knowledge, skills, and ideas. They blend the good characteristics of several individuals' reason to make careful appointments or selections. Committees can serve useful functions in the organizational process of nursing and administration. In addition to being organizational entities, committees are a part of managerial planning, and, in turn, they make plans. They are directed by leaders who are appointed by management or elected by constituents determined by management. Because professional nurses want autonomy but are mostly employed by organizations, formal groups, including committees, are a medium for promoting autonomy by giving these nurses a voice in managing the organization. Research conducted on magnet hospitals in the early 1980s revealed that nursing staff was significantly involved in committees throughout the hospital. Committees included medical staff, hospital, and nursing committees in which nurses were viewed as active participants and contributors to the committees.[95] Figure 7-24 outlines standards for evaluating nursing committees.

Types of Committees   Two of the most common types of committees in which nurses participate are ad-hoc/task force and standing committees. Committees are used by organizations to provide a mechanism to bridge communication gaps between departments or units. Standing committees are advisory in authority, although some may have collective authority to make and implement decisions. An example of a standing committee is the nurse practice committee or the infection control committee. Ad-hoc committees, or task forces, are groups of several individuals who work together on a specific project that is time limited—for example, a group of nurses selected by their peers to develop a preceptor program for graduate nurses. Ad-hoc committees are very important in healthcare organizations because they bring together in a short time frame individuals who have the expertise to work on the projects.

FIGURE 7-24   STANDARDS FOR EVALUATING NURSING COMMITTEES

1. The committee has been established by appropriate authority: bylaws, executive appointment, or other.

2. Each committee has a stated purpose, objectives, and operational procedures.

3. There is a mechanism for consultation between chairs and persons to whom they report.

4. Each committee meeting has a published agenda.

5. Committee members are surveyed beforehand to obtain agenda items, including problems, plans, and sharing of news.

6. Each committee has an effective chair.

7. Recorded minutes of each committee's meetings are used to evaluate the committee's effectiveness in meeting stated objectives.

8. Committee membership is manageable and representative of the expertise needed and the people affected.

9. Nurses are adequately represented on all appropriate institutional committees.

Source: Author.

Making Committees Effective

Purposes of Committees   Organizations promote communication through meetings. In 1 year the cost of meetings in U.S. companies is several billion dollars, and executives spend as much as 60% of their time in meetings. For this reason, nurse managers should evaluate the purposes and functions of committees, particularly of standing committees. Evaluation should be both normative and summative and should determine whether committees are accomplishing their purpose or are wasting the time and talents of many people who are required to attend the meetings. Are unnecessary meetings being held?

Meetings fulfill deep personal and individual needs. Their effective use by groups improves productivity. Types of committees are determined by organizational objectives and functions. Committees can be effectively used to implement major policy changes, to accomplish a job, and to plan strategically. Problems requiring research and planning are better assigned to individuals. Day-to-day decisions should be handled by line managers.[96]

A major purpose of using groups or committees is to involve personnel in participatory management that gives representation of employees at all levels a share in the decision-making process. According to Dixon,[97] this goal can be accomplished by having the following:

- Enough groups to ensure representation at all levels.
- Standing committees, ad-hoc committees, town hall meetings, and small meetings so that all levels are represented.
- Representation by visible managers to ensure support.
- Control of employees.
- Planned absence of managers at selective meetings to encourage discussion.
- Stimuli to employee participation with tangible results.
- Members solicited as volunteers, appointed by managers, or selected by employees.
- Technical assistance to identify problems, promote communication, and solve problems.
- A focus on the power of the group to act on its own recommendations, have its own budget, or access company resources.

Organization of Committees   Committees and work groups are effective when they are formally organized, have a purpose, designate a leader, keep written minutes of their work, and achieve results (Figure 7-25).

FIGURE 7-25   **SUCCESS FACTORS FOR EFFECTIVE COMMITTEES**

- Every committee should have a purpose and short-term objectives.

- Committee members should be chosen according to their expertise and their capacity to represent the larger group.

- The committee members must contribute in terms of commitment, time, and energy.

- Committees should be of manageable size for discussion and disagreement. Six to eight members are usually recommended.

- Committee chairs should be accountable to a specific administrator who provides guidance to the chair through consultation.

- Committees should have prepared agendas and effective chairs. Figure 7-24 contains standards for evaluating nursing committees.

Source: Author.

Nursing should be represented on most healthcare institution committees and always on those whose activities affect nursing. It should have representation that is effective in determining the outcomes of a health team approach to patient care services. In effect, nurses should determine how they would practice nursing. The organizational standards presented in Appendix 7-1 meet the goals of shared governance.

Improving Committee Effectiveness   There is no one way to measure group effectiveness, but multiple indicators can provide a framework to measure effectiveness of groups and committees:[98]

- Productivity of the work group or committee
- Satisfaction of group members
- Quality of work produced
- Opportunity for the work group or committee to work together toward one common goal

Nurse managers can improve the effectiveness of standing and ad-hoc committees by establishing minimal ground rules, shown in Figure 7-26.[99]

FIGURE 7-26   **GROUND RULES FOR IMPROVING COMMITTEE EFFECTIVENESS**

- Establish clear stated objectives (see Appendix 7-1)
- Establish a committee structure to support the clearly stated objectives (see Appendix 7-1)
- Plan all meetings and events to meet the goals and objectives
- Keep committee to a manageable size
- Define membership:
  - Councils: 40–50 persons
  - Committees: 10–12 persons
  - Assemblies: 100+ persons
- Draw up point-to-point agenda and send to attendees
- Tailor the meeting room to the group and prepare it beforehand
- Draw up a point-by-point agenda and send it to the attendees. Include the purpose of the meeting. Key points in developing agenda include
  - Put dull items early and "star" items last
  - Decide whether to place divisive items early or late
  - Plan a time for starting important items
  - Limit committee meetings to 2 hours or fewer.
- Schedule meetings to begin 1 hour before lunch or 1 hour before the end of the workday.
- Avoid putting extraneous business on the agenda.
- Read the agenda and write in comments before the meeting.
- Prepare for the meeting by learning the subject matter and by preparing audiovisual materials to support it.
- Time the agenda items. New or controversial subjects usually take more time. Attention spans diminish after the first hour. Use time efficiently, including mealtimes.
- Referee and set the pace of the meeting. Summarize and clarify as needed.

(continues)

- Promote lively participation by involving attendees in the program with a warm-up "getting acquainted" phase, a conflict phase, and a total collaboration phase. Bring out the personal goals of the individuals.

- Listen to what others have to say so there will be a sharing of knowledge, experience, judgments, and folklore.

- Bring the meeting to a definite conclusion by obtaining decisions and commitments.

- Follow-up as necessary to eliminate loose ends. Evaluate whether the meeting's purpose was achieved.

- Circulate useful information with the minutes. Keep the minutes brief, listing time, date, place, chair, attendance, agenda items and action, time ended, and the time, date, and place of the next meeting. Figure 7-27 provides a checklist for evaluating meeting effectiveness.

Source: Author.

FIGURE 7-27	CHECKLIST FOR EVALUATING MEETING EFFECTIVENESS

Standards	Yes	No
1. The meeting started on time.	_____	_____
2. A quorum existed.	_____	_____
3. The meeting agenda is on a schedule.	_____	_____
4. The agenda for the meeting reflects the purpose of the committee.	_____	_____
5. The chair acts as an equal member of the group, taking no special considerations.	_____	_____
6. The chair follows the agenda.	_____	_____
a. Dull items are scheduled early, star items last.	_____	_____
b. Divisive items are strategically placed.	_____	_____
c. Important items have a starting time.	_____	_____
d. The agenda avoids "any other business."	_____	_____
e. Meetings are scheduled for one hour before lunch or one hour before end of work day.	_____	_____
f. The chair is well prepared for the meeting.	_____	_____
g. The chair referees, paces, summarizes, and clarifies discussion.	_____	_____
h. The meeting concludes with definite decisions and a commitment to them.	_____	_____
i. The chair follows up on necessary items.	_____	_____
j. Useful information is circulated with the minutes.	_____	_____
7. The chair allows adequate time for discussion.	_____	_____
8. The chair facilitates participation by all members.	_____	_____
9. Items requiring further study are referred to smaller groups as projects. Timetables for results are established.	_____	_____
10. Managers attend meetings when needed to ensure support.	_____	_____
11. Managers plan absences from selected meetings to encourage discussion.	_____	_____
12. Technical assistance is provided to facilitate meeting success.	_____	_____

Source: Author.

Group Dynamics

Because the work of organizations is accomplished by groups, teams, or committees, many researchers have studied the dynamics of group function. Nurse managers need to be well grounded and knowledgeable about group dynamics, because group work is such a time commitment. Although not all groups are committees, the management of a group of employees whose goal is to accomplish the objectives of the enterprise is similar to the leadership and management of a committee whose goal is to accomplish selective objectives. In the 1920s researchers at Harvard Business School found that worker morale and productivity were positively influenced by small, informal work groups.[100]

In the world of the nurse manager, work is performed by individuals and by groups. Primary nursing is a frequently used modality of practicing nursing because it gives professional nurses more autonomy than do other modalities. It adds accountability, because nurses are continuously responsible for patients from admission through discharge. Case management adds group dynamics to the autonomy, because the case manager is responsible for functioning in a collaborative practice with other professional nurses and with physicians. Case management also uses managed care as a medium to keep the patient on the critical path from admission through discharge. Case management can extend through the illness episode to include home care, even at the critical care level.

Stevens advocates the use of groups for management and states that they can greatly increase productivity when used effectively. Nurse managers need to function in groups to promote problem solving and acceptance of responsibility. The group can function within an administrative council and demonstrate its ability to manage itself by preparing agendas, reviewing status of agenda topics, obtaining and using learning aids, and handling meetings. In short, it is possible to structure the business of groups and to direct and control the behavior of group members.[101]

Each member of a group plays a role in achieving the work of the group. Because each member has a unique personality and individual abilities, the group leader needs to know how groups function to facilitate effectiveness. Original studies of group dynamics were done through observations of informal groups. The Hawthorne studies of 1924–1932 were conducted in four phases designed to discover what would make workers increase their output. The results of the studies indicate that employees respond to identification with their groups and to the interpersonal relationships with members of their small groups by increasing their output.

Through interpersonal relationships, group members perform task roles, group-building and maintenance roles, and individual roles. In the performance of these roles, the group members share the power of the organization and its management. Benne and Sheats identify functional roles of group members, shown in Figure 7-28.[102–104]

FIGURE 7-28   **BENNE AND SHEATS' FUNCTIONAL ROLES OF GROUP MEMBERS**

Group task roles: Each member of a group performs a role related to the task of the group or committee to arrive cooperatively with the other group members at a definition of and solution to a common problem:

- Initiator-contributor: A group member who proposes or suggests new group goals or redefines the problem
- Information seeker: A group member who seeks a factual basis for the group's work
- Opinion seeker: A group member who seeks opinions that reflect or clarify the values of other members' suggestions
- Information giver: A group member who gives an opinion indicating what the group's view of pertinent values should be
- Elaborator: A group member who suggests by example or extended meanings the reason for suggestions and how they could work

(continues)

- Opinion giver: A group member who states personal beliefs pertinent to the group discussion
- Coordinator: A group member who clarifies and coordinates ideas, suggestions, and activities of the group members or subgroups
- Orienter: A group member who summarizes decisions or actions and identifies and questions differences from established goals
- Evaluator critic: A group member who compares and questions group accomplishments and compares them to a standard
- Energizer: A group member who stimulates and prods the group to act and to raise the level of its actions
- Procedural technician: A group member who facilitates the group's action by arranging the environment
- Recorder: A group member who records the group's activities and accomplishments

Group-building and maintenance roles: Individual members of the group work to build and maintain group functioning:

- Encourager: A group member who accepts and praises the contributions, viewpoints, ideas, and suggestions of all group members with warmth and solidarity
- Harmonizer: A group member who mediates, harmonizes, and resolves conflicts
- Compromiser: A group member who yields his or her position within a conflict
- Gatekeeper and expediter: A group member who promotes open communication and facilitates participation to involve all group members
- Standard setter or ego ideal: A group member who expresses or applies standards to evaluate group processes
- Group observer and commentator: A group member who records the group process and uses it to provide feedback to the group
- Follower: A group member who accepts the group members' ideas and listens to their discussion and decisions

Individual roles: Group members also play roles to serve their individual needs:

- Aggressor: A group member who expresses disapproval or vetoes the values or feelings of other members through attacks, jokes, or envy
- Blocker: A group member who persists in expressing negative points of view and resurrects dead issues
- Recognition seeker: A group member who works to focus positive attention on himself or herself
- Self-confessor: A group member who uses the group setting as a forum for personal expression
- Playboy: A group member who remains uninvolved and demonstrates cynicism, nonchalance, or horseplay
- Dominator: A group member who attempts to dominate and manipulate the group
- Help seeker: A group member who manipulates members to sympathize with expressions of personal insecurity, confusion, or self-deprecation
- Special interest leader: A group member who cloaks personal prejudices or biases by ostensibly speaking for others

Source: Author.

Nurse managers with a working knowledge of group dynamics can use their knowledge to assemble groups. Such knowledge is important in the selection of chairs of committees, task forces, and other groups of clinical nurses. It is equally important in selecting nurses for organization committees if nursing is to gain power and recognition for its contributions to the mission and objectives of the corporate entity.

Group training gives members awareness of the roles they play and the opportunity to manage themselves so that they become more productive. Group training has evolved into a science that contributes to a theory of nursing practice and nursing management. Self-analysis or self-evaluation and development of sensitivity to others to make oneself productive within group settings are a part of these theories. Nurse managers benefit from training in group dynamics and may include it in a continuing staff development program for professional nurses. This can be done through actual role playing of group missions.

Group Leaders

Group leaders may be formal, informal, or specialized. Formal leaders are appointed by management or elected by management directive; they carry line authority and the power to discipline and control group members. Informal leaders emerge from the group process. Their influence inspires cooperation and mediation, and group members reach consensus about their contributions to the effective functioning of the group in their quest of goals. Specialized leaders are often temporary leaders who have a special skill or ability that is needed by the group at a particular point in time.

Participative management requires commitment of individuals to work toward shared goals as well as profitability. A dynamic leader inspires people to put spirit into working for a shared goal. The leader can use symbols, posters, slogans, T-shirts, and memorable events. The leader must believe in people and support a theory of leadership that espouses self-direction, self-control, commitment, responsibility, imagination, ingenuity, creativity, and effort. How the leader behaves toward peer group members demonstrates these beliefs.[105] Leaders can make committees and meetings effective by having an extensive knowledge of group dynamics. They keep the group on course by convincing each member of the genuine need for input and by personal sensitivity to group processes. They draw in the shy and the quiet. They politely cut off the garrulous and protect the weak. While controlling the squashing reflex in themselves, they encourage a clash of ideas by mitigating domination by cliques. They refrain from being judgmental. Group leadership requires a thinking, skilled performance based on knowledge and ability acquired through management education and training.[106]

Phases of Groups

Groups have a natural history of development. Some groups move through all five stages, whereas other groups, due to factors such as leadership or membership experience, may never experience each phase. The following are five generally accepted phases of a group.

1. *Forming or orientation phase.* This is the phase during which group members discover themselves. They want uniqueness; they want to belong while maintaining personal identity. They test each other for appropriate and acceptable behavior. This is the time to exchange information, discover ground rules, size each other up, and determine fit. When forming these groups, the nurse manager includes experts, affected constituencies, people who implement the solution, persons with different problem-solving styles, and equal numbers of sensing/thinking and intuitive/feeling individuals. The group leader develops the explicit norm of constructive conflict: disagreement, multiple definitions, minority opinions, devil's advocate, professional management, and a "group wins" psychology. Implicit norms are avoided because they bring bias to the group process by imposing individual values and beliefs. The leader helps members fit into the group, providing structure, guidelines, and norms, and making members comfortable.
2. *Conflict or storming phase.* During this phase, group members jockey for position, control, and influence. Leadership struggle and increased competition take place. The leader helps members through this phase, assisting with roles and assignments.
3. *Cohesion or norming phase.* Roles and norms are established, with a move toward consensus and objectives. Members reach a common understanding of the true nature of the opportunity to reach the group's goals. They diagnose the root cause of the problem, the deviation from expected performance. They are open to alternative definitions with multiple views. Morale and trust improve, and the negative is suppressed. The leader guides and directs as needed.

4. *Working or performing phase.* Members work with deeper involvement, greater disclosure, and unity. They complete the work. The leader may intervene as needed.

5. *Termination phase.* Once goals are fulfilled, the group terminates. The leader guides the members to summarize discussions, express feelings, and make closing statements. The group is reluctant to break up. A celebration can help.[107]

Group Cohesiveness

Group cohesiveness includes the forces (bundle of properties) acting on the members of a group to preserve group integrity. These forces deal with and overcome disruption and conflict. Among the forces are such beliefs as the power of influence of the group, the personality of individual members of the group, and the mission or goals of the group. Cohesiveness is demonstrated by mutual understanding and support, improvements in self-esteem, and successful completion of the mission and goals of the group. Cohesive groups have a positive valence, with the combination of members' inputs leading to a strengthening of group processes and outcomes.[108]

Knowledge of group dynamics is needed by nurse managers to improve leadership competencies and to facilitate group discussion and communication. Groups are a common feature of a majority of experiences of all nurses in such roles as outcome management, team coordination, and teaching of students, patients, and families.[109]

Selected Group Techniques

A number of group techniques have been developed to make groups effective and productive. Among these are the Delphi technique, brainstorming, the nominal group technique, and focus groups (Figure 7-29).

FIGURE 7-29 | **GROUP TECHNIQUES**

- Delphi: Originally developed by the Rand Corporation as a technological forecasting technique, the Delphi technique pools the opinion of experts. This technique can be used in nursing management to pool the opinions of a group of leaders in the field. Each round of questioning has three phases. For example, the group is polled for input, which is analyzed, clarified, and codified by the investigator and given as feedback to the experts; the experts are then polled for further commentary on the composite of the first round. This process can continue for three to five rounds.[110] Members of the group using the Delphi technique may never have the opportunity to meet personally, because most of the activities are done through correspondence or electronically.

- Brainstorming: As a group technique, brainstorming seeks to develop creativity by free initiation of ideas. The object is to elicit as many ideas as possible. The following are the steps in the brainstorming technique:

  ○ The leader instructs the group, giving the member the topic or problem and telling him or her to respond positively with any ideas or suggestions relative to it. No critical responses are allowed.

  ○ The leader lists on a poster or chalkboard all ideas and suggestions as they are given and encourages their generation.

  ○ Ideas and suggestions are evaluated only after each group member has contributed all possible ideas and suggestions.

- Nominal group technique: The problem or task is defined. Members independently write down ideas about it, trying to make the ideas more problem-centered and of higher quality. Each member presents ideas to the group without discussion. The ideas are summarized and listed. Next, the members discuss each recorded idea to clarify, evaluate, and assign a priority to each decision. The results are averaged and the final group decision is taken from the pool. The process takes about 1.5 to 2 hours and results in a sense of accomplishment and closure.[111] Nominal group technique is a reliable evaluation tool and an efficient group teaching technique.[112]

(continues)

- Focus groups: Focus group methods stem from consumer market research. They do not provide quantitative research but a phenomenologic approach to qualitative research. Focus groups offer descriptions of the vicarious experiences of the participants. Groups of 8 to 12 participants meet as a group with a moderator who facilitates focused discussion on a topic. Focus groups have been used to develop nurse retention programs. Some of the objectives of focus groups are as follows:[113]

  - To provide an intellectual forum for innovative solutions to chronic problems

  - To encourage a specific communication process whereby a different breadth and depth of interaction, spontaneity, and cross-fertilization can occur, allowing participants to pick up ideas from one another. Ultimately, group ownership of ideas occurs.

  - To allow for necessary venting of workplace irritants

  - To provide an excellent opportunity for management to hear and translate constructive criticism in a neutral, nonemotional environment

  - To provide an environmental process whereby groups can visualize, define, and appreciate the size and complexity of the problem as well as that of the solution[114]

Source: Author.

Groupthink

One of the potential disadvantages of team building and working in committees or other work groups is the possibility of groupthink among members of the team or committee. Groupthink is inappropriate conformity to group norms. It occurs when group members avoid risk and fear to disagree or to carefully assess the points under discussion. The symptoms of groupthink are listed in Figure 7-30.[115]

Groupthink will not occur when members are aware of the potential for it. Groups are considered effective when their resources are well used; their time is well used; their decisions are appropriate, reasonable, and error-free; their decisions are implemented and supported by group members; problem-solving ability is enhanced; and group cohesion is built by promoting group norms and structuring cooperative relationships. The group's leader should teach group members cures for groupthink that include the following:[116]

- Acting as devil's advocate
- Considering unlimited alternatives

FIGURE 7-30 **SYMPTOMS OF GROUPTHINK**

- Illusions of invulnerability, leading to overconfidence and reckless risk taking
- Negative feedback ignored and rationalized to prevent reconsideration
- A belief of inherent morality
- Stereotyping of the views of people who disagree as wrong or weak and badly informed
- Pressure on members to suppress doubts
- Self-censorship by silence about misgivings
- Unanimous decisions
- Protection of members from negative reaction

Source: Author.

- Thinking critically
- Providing increased time for discussion
- Changing directions
- Surveying people affected by the problem under discussion
- Seeking other opinions
- Constructing challenging group measures
- Including input from people in the group who do not agree with you

Some of the programs and structures that can be used to involve nurses in participatory management are job enrichment, personalization, primary nursing, shared governance, entrepreneurship, gain sharing, and pay equity.

Culture

Organizational culture is the sum total of an organization's beliefs, norms, values, mission, philosophies, traditions, and sacred cows. It is a social system that is a subsystem of the total organization. Organizational cultures have artifacts, perspectives, values, assumptions, symbols, language, and behaviors that have been effective. Organizational cultures include communication networks, both formal and informal. They include a status/role structure that relates to characteristics of employees and customers or clients. Such structures also relate to management styles, whether authoritative or participatory. Management style impacts individual behavior. In a healthcare setting, these structures promote either individuality or teamwork. They relate to classes of people and can be identified through demographic surveys of both employees and patients. In addition, there is a technical or operational arm for getting the work done and an administrative arm for wages and salaries; hiring, firing, and promoting; report making and quality control; fringe benefits; and budgeting. Figure 7-31 illustrates aspects of organizational culture.

The artifacts of an organizational culture may be physical, behavioral (rituals), or verbal (language, stories, myths). Verbal artifacts result from shared values and beliefs. They include traditions, heroes, and the party line, and they result in ceremonies that embody rituals. These include ceremonies to reward years of service, the annual picnic, the Christmas party, and the wearing of badges and insignia.[117] Culture is created by such rites and rituals as follows:[118]

- Casual day (e.g., workers wear jeans and sport shirts on Friday to create an atmosphere of creativity and friendship)
- Birthing rooms and sibling birth participation programs to promote family health
- Focus on quality, service, and reliability
- A strong communication network
- Face-to-face contacts

FIGURE 7-31   ORGANIZATIONAL CULTURE

ARTIFACT	Dress, office space, office décor, logos, pictures
VALUES, ASSUMPTIONS	Language, stories, verbal communication, nonverbal communication, rites
BEHAVIORS	Ceremonies, hiring and terminating practices

Source: Author.

A nurse manager needs to be aware of the culture of his or her unit, department, and organization. A successful manager identifies and accepts the prevailing culture before making changes. It is more difficult to change a culture at the level of basic beliefs, values, and perspectives. It is easier to change technical and administrative systems. Managers and personnel who survive in a culture learn how to support the values and norms of that culture. Their conformity impedes change and innovation. The social, technical, and managerial systems are changed through organizational development. To change the culture may require changing the leader.[119]

When nurse executives from magnet hospitals were asked to identify nursing's top three current challenges, one of their responses included culture—"identifying, reassessing, changing the culture of nursing in my organization."[120] Nurse executives reported that culture issues were related to the changing role of the registered nurse and effects of mergers and consolidations. Other notable issues identified by the nurse executives were their concern about educating new staff to the organization's culture and values and how financial awareness and responsibility is so ingrained into healthcare organizations.[121]

Culture of Safety

In today's healthcare environment quality and safety are paramount. Building a culture of safety is a strategic goal for all healthcare organizations, especially since the seminal report *To Err is Human: Building a Safer Health Care System in the 21st Century*.[122] This report focused in on the fact that healthcare environments, especially hospitals, require a substantial improvement in quality and safety whereby nurses play a critical role in achieving this goal. Nurses are the closest to the patient and can easily identify the problems and issues encountered in the work environment. The report provides the haunting statement that medical errors are responsible for 44,000 to 98,000 patient deaths per year,[123] costing an estimated $17 billion to $29 billion per year.[124] Four specific recommendations were made from the report, listed in Figure 7-32.

Crossing the Quality Chasm was the next critical report from the IOM that focused on changes in the healthcare system to improve safety and with the outcome of protecting patients from harm. The report addressed the outdated systems used in healthcare organizations and called for healthcare providers to come together to redesign healthcare processes. The report outlined 10 principles to guide healthcare redesign, listed in Figure 7-33.[125]

The third report from the IOM, *Keeping Patients Safe: Transforming the Work Environment of Nurses*,[126] identified factors in the work environment for nurses that impacted safety and made specific recommendations for improving the work environment to improve safety. Figure 7-34 lists the areas identified for improving safety in the work environment.

FIGURE 7-32 | **TO ERR IS HUMAN: IOM GOALS**

- Establish a national focus to create leadership, research, tools, and protocols to enhance the knowledge base about safety.

- Identify and learn from errors through immediate and strong mandatory reporting efforts as well as encouragement of voluntary efforts to ensure the system continues to be made safer for patients.

- Raise standards and expectations for improvements in safety through the actions of oversight organizations, group purchasers, and professional groups.

- Create safety systems inside healthcare organizations through the implementation of safe practices at the delivery level.

Source: Reprinted with permission from To Err Is Human: Building a Safer Health System. Copyright 1999 by the National Academy of Sciences. Courtesy of the National Academy Press, Washington, D.C.

FIGURE 7-33 | **10 PRINCIPLES TO GUIDE THE REDESIGN OF THE HEALTH-CARE SYSTEM**

1. Care should be based on continuous healing relationships.

2. Care should be customized based on patient needs and values.

3. Patients should have control with shared decision making.

4. There should be shared knowledge and a free flow of information.

5. Evidence-based decision making should be evident.

6. Safety should be designed in as a system priority.

7. There should be transparency to promote informed decision making.

8. The system should anticipate patient needs, not just respond.

9. There should be a continued decrease in waste within the system.

10. There needs to be cooperation among clinicians.

Source: IOM, Crossing the Quality Chasm.

FIGURE 7-34 | **AREAS IDENTIFIED FOR IMPROVING SAFETY IN THE WORK ENVIRONMENT**

- Nurse staffing ratios and practices

- National data reporting of staffing

- Increased resources for knowledge and skill development from orientation through length of tenure

- Support for interdisciplinary activities that promote collaboration

- Limits on hours worked

- Design of work environments and care processes with a recommendation to first focus on medication administration and hand washing

- Creating an overall culture of safety within healthcare organizations

---

Source: IOM, Keeping Patients Safe.

Critical components and processes that relate to a culture of safety within an organization include such aspects as identifying sentinel events, implementing the national patient safety goals, improving communication, developing teamwork, enhancing clinical systems, patient inclusion, providing ongoing staff education, and discovering staff perceptions related to safety.

How do you build a culture of safety and what role does nursing, in particular the nurse executive, have in this process? The culture of an organization determines whether patient care delivered in the setting is safe or not. If the organization cultivates an environment open to identifying and reporting errors, the organization will be headed in the right direction on building the infrastructure necessary for a safe environment. It is imperative for organizations to move from a culture of blame to a culture of safety and quality. In *The Nurse's Role in Promoting a Culture of Patient Safety*, Friesen and coworkers compare the characteristics between a culture of safety and a culture of blame.[127] In a culture that promotes safety, the organization has a leadership team that is supportive, expects open communication, requires a root cause analysis when errors occur, and encourages reporting of events in a nonpunitive environment. In a culture that promotes blame, the organization has a leadership team that is not visible, exhibits closed communication, and demonstrates a punitive approach to errors.

Page identifies three stages for implementing a culture of safety:[128]

- Stage 1: Emphasis on compliance with regulatory standards and meeting technical requirements
- Stage 2: Valuing a culture of safety and achieving the performance expectation of safety
- Stage 3: The culture of safety becomes inherent throughout the organization where there is a culture supporting continuous improvement.

Nurse Executive's Role in Patient Safety   Nurse executives are challenged to create a practice environment that fosters multidisciplinary collaboration, professional development, and a culture of safety. For nurse executives to accomplish such a task, they must achieve and develop competencies that specifically address culture of safety skills, knowledge and commitments. The AONE developed a toolkit outlining the nurse executive's role in patient safety, *Role of the Nurse Executive in Patient Safety: Guiding Principles Toolkit*. AONE identifies guiding principles to assist the nurse executive in developing an organizational culture of safety:[129]

- Lead cultural change
- Provide shared leadership
- Build external partnerships
- Develop leadership competencies

To address the competencies needed by nurse executives to build a culture of safety in their organizational, AONE developed the AONE Nurse Leader–Patient Safety Competency Model. This model is designed to support an environment that promotes safe, high-quality patient care through leadership (Figures 7-35, 7-36, and 7-37).[130–132]

| **FIGURE 7-35** | **PATIENT SAFETY LEADERSHIP COMPETENCIES** |

- Active and disciplined listening
  - Use of active and effective listening behaviors, such as questioning and summarizing. Encourage participation, discussion, and engagement.
- Engagement and inclusiveness
- Vigilance for error identification
  - Continuously scan organization for patient safety risk trends and identify areas of opportunity and create plans to intervene and improve. Develop a system to track events and patient safety concerns so that data can be assessed and trended.
- Integrator of people and task
  - Encourage participation, discussion and engagement from a variety of team members. Connect people together that are working on similar objectives.
- Interdisciplinary coleadership and collaboration
  - Collaborate with leadership at the top of the organization and members of the interdisciplinary team to create a partnership to support patient safety as a priority within the organization
- Action orientation
  - Define a plan for patient safety with a timeline. Assign responsible parties, objectives, and a timeline to complete specific action plan toward improving patient safety.
- Art of championing

(continues)

- o Communicate vision of safety to all staff throughout the organization. Serve as a positive and encouraging role model for a safe patient care environment.
- Collaborative practice agreements
  - o Define a vision, mission, goals, and objectives for patient safety within the organization. Work collaboratively with leaders in the organization to meet defined goals and objectives including adequate and appropriate resources, human as well as material/supply.
- Team leading and participation
  - o Form partnerships with individuals with expertise and competence in the realm of patient safety. Foster a single team of engaged staff with mutually agreed upon goals and expectations.
- Importance of top down leadership culture of safety
- Senior leaders must embrace patient safety as a priority, determine a plan, align resources, motivate, and encourage others throughout the organization.

Source: Copyright © 2005 American Organization of Nurse Executives.

FIGURE 7-36	CORE PATIENT SAFETY TECHNOLOGY COMPETENCIES SYSTEMS

- Systems: process management and process improvement
  - o Determine critical indicators and system to measure performance and opportunities for improvement. This requires a defined process.
- Human factors
  - o Focus on systems, but understand characteristics of human behaviors to understand errors.
- Root cause analysis
  - o Review variations in process with involved staff to determine cause of error. Continue to ask why to find potential cause of error.
- Safety rounding
  - o Conduct patient safety rounds by senior leadership to identify safety risk trends; ensure follow-up.
- Teaming
  - o Work collaboratively with key leaders and staff members allows for communication and information sharing and requires accountability. Need to develop outcome-based solutions.
- Risk management
  - o Intention is to create and maintain a safe and effective environment for patients, visitors, and staff to prevent or reduce loss.
- Error mitigation
  - o Explore patient care scenarios, identify potential sources of error, and recommend specific solutions, knowledge and practice in Failure Mode Effect Analysis (FMEA)
- Error recovery at the sharp edge
  - o Establish processes to make it easier to recover or back out if a wrong action is taken by practitioners at the patient that is closest to the process breakdown.
- Victims of error
  - o Apology to patient/family, support staff at sharp edge
  - o Need to have timely, full disclosure with a sincere apology. It is the provider's moral obligation to do this. Acknowledge stress of error to patient, family, staff—everyone will need support and intervention.
- System thinking and quality improvement methods
  - o Method to improve processes, safety and care delivery through assessing systems, and how individuals function within the system (not focused solely on the individual)

Source: Copyright © 2005 American Organization of Nurse Executives.

FIGURE 7-37	CULTURE OF SAFETY COMPETENCIES

- Patient and family centered care
  - Care that is focused on the patient's and family's needs and expectations.
- Fair and just principles
  - Timely, fair, appropriate actions that are carried out equitably when blameworthy behaviors have occurred (see http://www.justculture.org)
- Practice environment of autonomy and shared decision making
  - Respect for individual's ability and right to determine what happens. A team-oriented structure that gives everyone the authority to make decisions for themselves.
- Accountability vs. blame
  - Assign accountability. Determine goals. Avoid blame. Thank those that share concerns and perceived patient safety risk.
- Safety over convenience orientation
  - Resources—acquire resources needed for patient safety (personnel, systems, finances)
  - Supports—patient safety requires significant commitment, resource, and support
  - Communication—patient safety requires excellent, intense communication among care providers (SBAB) and leaders
- Shouldering the burden of improvement vs. external blame
  - Start somewhere and always seek process improvement. Avoid finding excuses/hindrances. Determine and manage a timeline. Set goals and priorities.

Source: Author.

Healthcare organizations want a culture that provides the customer with a positive experience through an organizational commitment and attention to quality and safety that permeates to each employee. Organizations achieve a culture of safety when they are challenged to be the best they can be and promote a sense of pride in the organization. Leaders work collaboratively with all members of the healthcare team to lead a commitment to patient safety.

Climate

Organizational climate is the emotional state, perceptions, and feelings shared by members of the system. It can be formal, relaxed, defensive, cautious, accepting, trusting, and so on. It is the employees' subjective impression or perception of their organization. The employees of major concern to nurse managers are the practicing nurses. Practicing nurses create or at the very least contribute to the creation of the climate perceived by patients.

Managers create the climate in which practicing nurses work. If managers trust them, practicing nurses provide good information to keep their managers informed. This climate promotes the concept that most hands-on employees can perform routine management, accounting, engineering, and quality tasks. Well-trained, well-equipped, and self-managed work teams, the members of which are also good salespersons, can perform 90% of expert staff work. The object of expert staff is to spread knowledge quickly.[133]

Organizational climate relates to the personality of an organization and can be changed. Following are six sociological dimensions of organizational climate:

1. Clarity in specifying certification of the organization's goals and policies. This is facilitated by smooth flow of information and management support of employees.
2. Commitment to goal achievement through employee involvement
3. Standards of performance that challenge, promote pride, and improve individual performance
4. Responsibility for one's own work fostered and supported by managers
5. Recognition for doing good work
6. Teamwork and a sense of belonging, mutual trust, and respect[134]

Practicing nurses want a climate that gives them job satisfaction through good working conditions, high salaries, and opportunities for professional growth through counseling and career development experiences and opportunities. Nurses achieve job satisfaction when they are challenged and their achievements are recognized and appreciated by managers and patients. They achieve satisfaction from a climate of collegiality with managers and other healthcare providers and in which they have input into decision making. Just as importantly, nurses want a climate of administrative support that includes adequate staffing and shift options. Personnel shortage, frustration, failure, and conflict in nursing have required sweeping changes in intrinsic and extrinsic rewards, including career development programs that increase the ability of professional nurses to develop their self-esteem through self-actualization. This is particularly relevant in today's environment of constrained resources and nursing shortages.

Management climate surveys measure clarity and understanding of an organization's goals, effectiveness of decision-making processes, integration, cooperation, vitality, leader effectiveness, openness and trust, job satisfaction, opportunities for growth and development, level of performance, orientation and accountability, effectiveness of teamwork and problem solving, and overall confidence in management. Surveys may be used to make a diagnosis and to achieve the following:[135]

- Establish new strategic directions
- Clarify an organization's mission, objectives, and goals
- Identify managers' and supervisors' training and development needs
- Reallocate resources
- Prepare a foundation for cultural change
- Revise hiring priorities using a patterned interview as well as peer interviewing to select the best fit for the unit and organization

Many studies have been done to determine work climate within business, industry, and healthcare organizations. Climate and philosophy result from the corporate culture, and changing the culture leads to climate change. One head nurse designed and implemented a project to motivate the nursing staff of a medical unit to better service and greater self-satisfaction. She designed an "employee of the month" motivational strategy that included measurable performance criteria. Though the staff was initially disinterested, they eventually increased their interest and participation. Productivity increased, as did emergence of talents. The strategy culminated in a recognition ceremony. The employee of the month received a free lunch or dinner, and his or her picture was put on the bulletin board. By the end of 6 months, 25 of 144 employees had earned the title of employee of the month, their voluntary participation indicating that it met some of their needs.[136] Figure 7-38 lists several activities that promote a positive organizational climate.

Organization of Work

Work is organized according to the stages in the process. In some areas the work moves to the skills and tools; examples are coronary care nursing and operating room nursing. Sometimes a team moves different skills and different tools to the work, for example, when an operating room team moves to a delivery room to perform a caesarean section. We certainly find combinations in nursing.

FIGURE 7-38	ACTIVITIES TO PROMOTE A POSITIVE ORGANIZATIONAL CLIMATE

- Develop the organization's mission, philosophy, vision, goals, and objectives statements with input from practicing nurses, including their personal goals.

- Establish trust and openness through communication that includes prompt and frequent feedback and stimulates motivation.

- Provide opportunities for growth and development, including career development and continuing education programs.

- Promote teamwork.

- Ask practicing nurses to state their satisfactions and dissatisfactions during meetings and conferences and through surveys.

- Market the nursing organization to the practicing nurses, other employees, and the public.

- Follow through on all activities involving practicing nurses.

- Analyze the compensation system for the entire nursing organization and structure it to reward competence, productivity, and longevity.

- Promote self-esteem, autonomy, and self—fulfillment for practicing nurses, including feelings that their work experiences are of high quality.

- Emphasize programs to recognize practicing nurses' contributions to the organization.

- Assess unneeded threats and punishments and eliminate them.

- Provide job security with an environment that enables free expression of ideas and exchange of opinions without threat of recrimination, which may manifest as downscaled performance reports, negative counseling, confrontation, conflict, or job loss.

- Be inclusive in all relationships with practicing nurses. Trends affecting the delivery systems of care are as follows: changes in patients and providers, medical advances, technology, care delivery, professional relationships, and recognition and rewards, patient demographics and characteristics, financial constraints, and clinical trends. Demand for competency and quality continues to be a driving force, as the healthcare environment becomes more complex and experiences rapid change.

- Help practicing nurses to overcome their shortcomings and to develop their strengths.

- Encourage and support loyalty, friendliness, and civic consciousness.

- Develop strategic plans that include decentralization of decision making and participation by practicing nurses.

- Be a role model of performance desired of practicing nurses.

Source: Author.

Much of the work in nursing is accomplished by a functionally structured organization. Clarity is an advantage of the functional structure, because the individuals know where they stand, and they understand their tasks. Functional structures are usually stable. A disadvantage is that sometimes the task neither relates to the whole structure nor contributes to the common purpose. Functional structures are rigid, and frequently they neither prepare nurses for the future nor train or test them. Functional organizations become costly when friction builds up and requires coordinators, committees, meetings, troubleshooters, and special dispatchers. Functional organizations make low psychological demands on people; people in such organizations tend to focus on their efforts only. Small functional organizations are economical and foster good communications. These organizations are good when one kind of work is done. Usually, they require that decisions be made at the top. Nurses within them have narrow visions, skills, and loyalties. Employees of such organizations focus on function rather than on results and performance. The functional process does not usually apply to top management positions or to performance of innovative work by employees.

Managed care and case management appear to be leading innovations in healthcare delivery. Benefits are controlled costs, improved outcome monitoring, reduced bureaucracy, less travel time for patients, and fewer people to sort out or confront. Patient care needs and outcomes should be assessed and evaluated by nurses. Nurses who refer needs to others should determine priority of patient care tasks. This is the essence of work redesign that retains nursing autonomy and influence.[137]

Some healthcare institutions integrate standards of practice into their nursing care delivery systems. Structure and process standards are stated as outcome standards and are used to measure the overall effectiveness of the nursing division. The integration is accomplished throughout the core committees of the nursing division, including quality assessment, policy and procedure, job description, and other committees. This is done through nursing care plans and the computer system. The nursing care plans may be generic or individual and include nursing diagnosis/problems, intervention/discharge plans, and goals.[138]

RESTRUCTURING NURSING ORGANIZATIONS

The survival of many hospitals is threatened as they compete for growth and a competitive edge in the marketplace. Consumers and payers are searching for organizations that are efficient in producing positive, cost-effective health care. For this reason, Flarey indicates that the governing boards may need to be reconstituted. Members of governing bodies should focus on patient care. Many hospitals include the chief nurse executives in governing board meetings as active participants.[139] Figure 7-39 provides questions through which to evaluate organizational function.

FIGURE 7-39	EVALUATING ORGANIZATIONAL FUNCTION

Answer the following questions as a final evaluation of your organizing function within a department or unit. For those checked No, plan changes so that they will result in effective organizing. Then implement the management plan.

	Yes	No
1. Is there evidence that organizing is an intentional and ongoing function of the division, department, service, or unit?	_____	_____
2. Is there evidence that organizing changes as plans, goals, or objectives change?	_____	_____
3. Is there evidence that managers are developed or replaced to fit organizational changes emerging from changed plans and objectives?	_____	_____
4. Are organizational managerial relationships clearly structured to give security to individual managers?	_____	_____
5. Has authority been delegated to appropriate levels of managers?	_____	_____
6. Is there evidence that delegation of authority has been balanced to retain control of appropriate administrative functions by the chief nurse executive?	_____	_____
7. Is information dissemination clearly separated from decision making?	_____	_____
8. Is the authority delegated commensurate with the responsibility?	_____	_____
9. Is there evidence of acceptance of responsibility and authority by subordinate managers?	_____	_____

(continues)

10. Is there evidence that subordinate managers have the power to accomplish the results expected of them? _____ _____

11. Is there evidence that authority and responsibility have been confined within divisional, departmental, service, or unit boundaries? _____ _____

12. Is there evidence of balance in support and use of staff functions? _____ _____

13. Is there evidence of balance in support and use of functional authority? _____ _____

14. Is there evidence of maintenance of the principle of unity of command? _____ _____

15. Is there evidence of efficient and effective use of service departments? _____ _____

16. Is there evidence of too many levels of managers (overorganization)? _____ _____

17. Is there evidence of unneeded line assistants to managers (overorganization)? _____ _____

18. Is there evidence that the nursing division, department, service, or unit is organized to facilitate accomplishment of its specified objectives by its personnel? _____ _____

19. Is there evidence that the nursing division, department, service, or unit structure has been modified to fit human factors after being organized to accomplish its specified objectives? _____ _____

20. Is there evidence that the nursing division, department, service, or unit is organized to accomplish planning for recruiting and training to meet present and future personnel needs? _____ _____

21. Is there evidence that the organizational process is flexible enough to adapt to changes in its external and internal environment? _____ _____

22. Are changes in organization justified, based on deficiencies, experience, objectives, purpose, and plans? _____ _____

23. Is there evidence that the organizing process is balanced between inertia and continual change? _____ _____

24. Is there evidence that all nursing personnel know the organizational structure and understand their assignments and those of their co-workers? _____ _____

25. Is there evidence that the nursing organizational charts are widely used? _____ _____

26. Is there evidence that nursing organizational charts provide comprehensive information to all workers? _____ _____

27. Is there evidence that there are job descriptions and job standards for every job and that they are widely used by nursing managers? _____ _____

28. Is there evidence that nursing employees are all oriented to the nature of the nursing organizing process? _____ _____

29. Is there evidence that the organizing process within the nursing division, department, service, or unit prevents waste or unplanned costs? _____ _____

30. Is there evidence that the nursing organization has an effective span of control by managers? _____ _____

31. Are the lines of authority within the nursing organization clear? _____ _____

32. Is there evidence that the management information system is effective? _____ _____

33. Is there evidence that each employee has only one supervisor? _____ _____

34. Is there evidence that the CNE has absolute responsibility for subordinate nursing managers? _____ _____

35. Is there evidence that all nursing managers are able to effect their leadership abilities? _____ _____

Source: Author.

Kanter defines synergies as "interactions of businesses that would provide benefits above and beyond what the units could do separately."[140] Synergies are a positive consequence of restructuring in which organizations are downsized (employees cut), demassed (middle management cut), and decentralized. The aim of restructuring is to achieve synergies from the value of adding up the parts to create a whole.[141] One of the elements of restructuring is to build a synergistic model of a governing body. A synergistic model for the governing body as suggested by Flarey considers governing body functions such as defining mission, quality of care, strategic planning, financial viability, community relations, policy development, and decision making.

Old organizational forms do not work in today's healthcare environment. Sovie recommends development of special project teams to design the required structure and system change using five steps of restructuring shown in Figure 7-40. The goals are improvement of patient care, organizational success, and staff satisfaction.[142]

Restructuring of organizations includes downsizing and elimination of middle managers. The hands-on workers are thus empowered to provide clients (customers, patients) what they need and want. Before they can be empowered, hands-on nursing workers need to have management training for their new roles. The span of control is greater when hands-on workers are educated, trained, motivated, stable, and empowered. Such workers neither want nor need micromanagement. The manager with a widened or expanded span of control now becomes mentor, guide, facilitator, and coach.

Small departments can be consolidated under one department head through empowerment. Examples are physical therapy, occupational therapy, endoscopy, neurodiagnostics, sleep disorders, social services, and respiratory therapy. Issues of loss of power and authority arise and must be resolved so that job shrinking and empowerment can occur. Managers who spend time protecting their turf decrease productivity of their workers. Nurse managers of their units can do all hiring, resolve patient complaints, have budget authority associated with staffing and patient losses, and provide orientation to new managers. Clearly, the span of control for top managers can increase as first-line managers are empowered.

Downsizing is a common organizing activity in the corporate world, including healthcare organizations and institutions. The goals of downsizing are to decrease costs and increase profits. Although decentralization and participatory management are identified with downsizing, the goals are not always the same. Decentralization and participatory management have increasing job satisfaction and increased productivity as primary goals.

FIGURE 7-40 | **FIVE STEPS OF RESTRUCTURING NURSING ORGANIZATIONS**

- Create an organizational culture marked by commitment to high-quality care and superior, responsive service to all users including patients, families, physicians, nurses, and other staff.

- Redesign the organizational structure to flatten it and eliminate or reduce barriers among departments, disciplines, and services.

- Empower the staff, invest in employee education and training, and create mechanisms to ensure information flow.

- Develop special project teams to design the required system changes; nurture and promote innovation and pilots of new approaches.

- Celebrate accomplishments and innovators, and champion care for the caregivers; support, recognize, and reward.

Source: Author.

Companies are now reporting that the anticipated results of downsizing have not occurred. There have been huge emotional and financial costs to employees and significant costs to American corporations. Between 1983 and 1993, Fortune 500 companies eliminated 4.7 million people from their payrolls. Job cuts do not necessarily lead to improved productivity. Gains in production are frequently traced to firms with growing employment. Mass layoffs do not inspire worker loyalty; workers should be well prepared for restructuring.[143]

Business must adapt organizational structures because of marketplace demands related to greater rates of change, higher competitive intensity, and information technology. Healthcare organizations should do the same. What services should a business offer, and what should it divest? Hospitals are high cost producers. The excessive vertical integration since diagnosis-related groups may be to blame. The emerging organizational structure is messy: Some resources need to be centralized to improve productivity by responding to customers' needs. A good organization has key aspects of both consistency and inconsistency.[144]

When reengineering organizations, leaders should use key strategies such as emotional management, professional empowerment, and empowerment by values. Staff members are given room to grow and to learn from their mistakes.[145]

Excessive organizational structures are inhibitors to quick responses to change. Get staff out into the field. This includes accounting, purchasing, personnel, and others. There should be only three to five layers of management in the total organization. Every chief executive officer should look at the corporate structure from the perspective of increasing the span of control through reduction of layers of management. Matrix organization brought about de facto centralization as groups were connected to groups by dotted lines on organization charts. The most effective management structure is supervisor, department head, and boss. In healthcare organizations, this would be nurse manager, nurse executive, and hospital administrator.

Winning companies have three to nine fewer levels of management. Winning companies have workers doing their own maintenance, self-inspection, direct costing, and just-in-time inventory management. Winning companies have few people at headquarters level. They decentralize database management, eliminate approval signatures, retrain middle managers, and increase spending authority at unit level.[146]

Mergers and acquisitions result in unified management teams with single executive managers. As examples, one chief executive officer replaces two to several, one assistant administrator for nursing replaces two to several, and one department head replaces two to several. Desirable characteristics include a highly visible chief nurse executive, a professional practice model of patient care, nursing diagnosis as the basis for nursing care delivery, and collaborative practice among professions.

An organizational analysis should be done to gain the theory and skills needed to intervene in complex organizational systems. Areas analyzed include formal organizational structure, power bases, leadership, communication system, and organizational climate (see Figure 7-37). Used to prepare clinical nurse specialists, an organizational analysis can be used by nurse managers and practicing clinical nurse specialists.[147]

Models of Nursing Care Delivery Systems

Nurse executives are responsible for both promoting a professional nursing practice environment and identifying and implementing an effective care delivery model that achieves positive outcomes for the organization and patient. A nursing care delivery model is one component of the professional practice model.[148] Traditional models of care delivery have been useful to nursing over the years; however, with such challenges and trends affecting the delivery systems of care, including changes in inpatients and providers, medical advances, technology, care delivery, professional relationships, patient demographics and characteristics, financial constraints, and clinical trends, these traditional models may not be as effective as they once were. In addition, the demand for competency and quality continues to be a driving force, as the healthcare environment becomes more complex and rapidly changes.[149]

Wolf and Greenhouse suggest that nursing care delivery systems should be sustainable over time, fit within the strategic framework of the organization and are evidence based.[150] These authors indicate the nursing care delivery models should be structure, process, and outcome driven. Wolper identified key aspects of nursing practice 20 years ago that have remained central in today's healthcare environment (Figure 7-41).[151]

Several authors have identified specific elements of innovation in newer care delivery models that include the following characteristics: an elevated registered nurse role, increased focus on the patient, improving patient transitions and handoffs, leveraging technology, driven by results, early and regular involvement of caregivers in the design and implementation of the models, and involvement in patient in decision making.[152]

Several nursing care delivery models that are emerging in today's environment are discussed below:

1. *Parish nursing:* One of the oldest types of nursing whereby patients are provided with healthcare services in their church or church-related settings. This nursing care delivery model delivers care in a holistic approach with spirituality at the core, which makes this model unique.[153] The role of the parish nurse includes health educator, community liaison, personal health counselor, and volunteer counselor.[154]

2. *Community-based nursing centers:* Originated to (1) serve the poor and uninsured in areas that were difficult to reach and (b) initiate faculty practice in nursing graduate programs.[155] Community-based nursing centers can be found in underserved areas and also in school-based clinics and faith-based clinics. Community-based nursing centers usually have nurse practitioners providing patient care with emphasis on health promotion, wellness, and provision of services for designated populations.[156]

3. *Patient- and family-centered care:* Nine elements are espoused:

   - Recognize family and professional collaboration
   - Honor diversity of families
   - Recognize family strengths
   - Share complete and unbiased information
   - Promote family-to-family support and networking
   - Incorporate developmental needs
   - Implement comprehensive policies and programs
   - Design accessible health care systems

FIGURE 7-41   KEY ASPECTS OF NURSING PRACTICE MODELS

- Create the environment for practice.

- Establish and ensure the standards of nursing care delivery.

- Coordinate patient care with inputs from all types of health professionals.

- Select and develop the nursing workforce.

- Evaluate and plan the work of nursing to meet patient requirements for care.

- Provide adequate staffing.

- Evaluate and develop relationships within and external to the hospital services.

Source: Author.

Patient- and family-centered care emphasized collaboration with families and patients at all ages and in all settings. Both the families and patients take an active role in their health care and develop a partnership with healthcare providers to overall improve their health care outcomes.

4. *Collaborative patient management model:* High Point Regional Health System in High Point, North Carolina designed a multidisciplinary, population-based, case management model as their delivery model of patient care.[157] The purpose of this model was to link quality, cost, and care delivery processes. High Point Regional Health System built a nursing care delivery model that was designed for specific population-based groups targeting high-volume, high-risk, and high-cost patients. This model included patient care coordinators who had oversight of the interdisciplinary teams. A nurse-initiated patient education focus was central to this model.

5. *Partnership clinical model:* This nursing care delivery system uses unlicensed assistive personnel in direct patient care in partnership with a registered nurse. The partnered model includes the following:[158]

   - Cross-trained unlicensed assistive personnel to work one-to-one with a registered nurse in direct patient care
   - Registered nurse accountable for all patients and included in all decision making
   - Unlicensed assistive personnel trained to draw labs, administer electrocardiogram and assist with respiratory and physical therapy

6. *Hospital at home:* This model was developed at Johns Hopkins Bayview Medical Center in Baltimore, Maryland and is an acute home-based program. Elderly patients who are seen in the emergency room or referred by their personal physician may be eligible to participate. A multidisciplinary team that includes a physician, registered nurse, and nursing assistant provide hospital-level care to the patient in the home.[159] This model was tested as a demonstration project with the Veterans Administration medical system with the assistance of computerized medical system (CMS). Results to date have shown a 75% reduction in complications for patients receiving services in this care delivery system.[160]

Professional Nursing Practice Environment

There are many challenges the national health care system is facing that render the nursing workplace a less-than-optimal environment to recruit and retain registered nurses. Problems such as nursing shortages resulting in increased work loads, intergenerational staff, unpredictable payment systems, technological advances, new delivery systems, along with the multiple and complicated quality and safety initiatives all play a part in shaping organizations with a sense of complexity, chaos, and instability. The nursing practice environment consists of specific organizational characteristics that either facilitate or constrain professional nursing practice.[161] Several professional nursing organizations address the characteristics or elements of a positive work environment where nurses practice, such as AONE's *Principles and Elements of a Healthful Practice/Work Environment,*[162] Texas Nurses Association's *Nurse-Friendly Hospital Criteria,*[163] the American Nurses Credentialing Center's Magnet Recognition Program,[164] or American Association of Critical Care Nurses' white paper, *Hallmarks of the Professional Nursing Practice Environment*[165] (Figure 7-42).

FIGURE 7-42 **CHARACTERISTICS OF A HEALTHFUL WORK ENVIRONMENT**

- Support professional development through educational and clinical advancement programs.
- Develop a culture emphasizing accountability, collaboration, quality, and safety.

- Recognize nurses' contributions to practice.
- Enhance nursing leadership through training and development.
- Ensure that an adequate number of qualified nurses are available to provide quality care.
- Encourage decision-making at all levels in the organization.

Source: Copyright © 2005 American Organization of Nurse Executives.

Evidence-Based Practice 7-3

A research project conducted by McManis & Monsalve Associates in collaboration with the AONE examined the characteristics of healthy work environments of 21 hospitals. The study revealed six critical factors that are essential for creating an excellent work environment:[166]

1. Leadership development and effectiveness
2. Empowered collaborative decision making
3. Work design and service delivery innovation
4. Values-driven organizational culture
5. Recognition and reward systems
6. Professional growth and accountability

These success factors are familiar to those organizations that have achieved Magnet Recognition Program and those who are working toward that achievement. The report provides the reader with in-depth discussions and presentations of the creative and effective strategies that these 21 hospitals implemented to achieve a work environment of excellence.[167]

Professional Models of Care

The professional practice model is the structure that allows nursing to accomplish defined goals within the context of a client-centered healthcare plan, and evaluating responses to nursing care and treatment.[168] Hoffart and Woods identify five subsystems in a professional practice model:[169]

1. Professional values
2. Professional relationships
3. A care delivery model
4. Management or governance
5. Professional recognition and rewards

According to the Magnet Recognition Program, professional models of care support the following:[170]

- Promotes the professional role of the registered nurse to include accountability for one's own practice
- Incorporates evidence-based practice
- Includes contemporary management concepts and theory
- Staffing systems
- Address patient needs, patient population demographics, nursing of nursing staff members, and ratio of nurses serving in various roles and levels
- Continuity of care
- Care delivery model

Several professional models of care are discussed below.

1. *Transforming care at the bedside:* This model was created by the joint efforts of the Institute for Healthcare Improvement and the Robert Wood Johnson Foundation to develop and validate interventions for transforming care in acute care hospital medical-surgical units. The model is built on a four-point framework (IHI) that guides managers and staff in implementing specific interventions to transform care at the bedside (Figure 7-43).[171]

2. *Nursing practice model:* Valley Baptist Medical Center in Harlingen, Texas built a nursing practice model that included unit action committees on each nursing unit, a comprehensive integrated tool called the restorative care path, variance analysis, permanent care teams with clinical managers, assistant clinical managers, licensed vocational nurses, nursing assistants, and collaborative nurse physician practice with a physician–nurse liaison committee. Because credentialing and recredentialing of physicians is considered the ultimate form of peer review, it should be considered for peer review of nurses.[172]

3. *Group practice:* Nursing group practice at Catherine McAuley Health System "is a formal membership of professional nurses who contract to provide nursing care for a specific patient population." Nurses may contract privately or as employees of an organization. They provide 24-hour coverage 365 days a year. The group's staffing for cardiothoracic surgery includes 16 nurses, two certified surgical technologists, and one clinical nurse manager who reports to the clinical director of operating room services. The group eliminated the first-line manager, making the clinical nurse manager a resource facilitator, liaison, and mentor. A supportive climate emphasizes trust, accountability, and responsibility. The criteria for group practice membership include clinical competence and leadership ability. Evaluating peers use a clinical ladder with described behaviors. The practice model is shared governance: practice, education, and performance improvement assurance councils.

The following are suggested activities to implement a group practice:

- Define roles and organization structure.
- Determine program costs.
- Decide on membership criteria and staffing mix.
- Set salary guidelines (e.g., hourly or salaried status).
- Work with the hospital administration in writing policies and planning for implementation.
- Plan to evaluate the success of the program using specific, predetermined instruments.

| FIGURE 7-43 | TRANSFORMING CARE AT THE BEDSIDE |

- Safe and reliable care: Care for moderately sick patients who are hospitalized is safe, reliable, effective, and equitable.

- Vitality and teamwork: Within a joyful and supportive environment that nurtures professional formation and career development, effective care teams continually strive for excellence.

- Patient-centered care: Truly patient-centered care on medical-surgical units honors the whole person and family, respects individual values and choices, and ensures continuity of care. Patients will say, "They give me exactly the help I want (and need), exactly when I want (and need) it."

- Value-added care processes: All care processes are free of waste and promote continuous flow.

Source: Author.

Staff satisfaction, cost, and quality assurance all improved. Turnover rate decreased. Problems such as surgical complications and poor communications were prevented. Products and techniques were changed to reduce costs. Turnaround times were faster. Financial recognition was made quarterly. Incorrect sponge and instrument counts were reduced 25%.[173]

4. *Helper model:* The helper model of healthcare delivery is widespread. It matches registered nurses with nurse aides. To work efficiently, the helper model requires the following:[174]

- Experienced registered nurses at the competent or proficient levels of practice
- Permanent registered nurse–nurse aide pairs
- Enhanced primary nursing
- Support for agency and float nurses
- Policy for attendance that targets incentive and reward programs
- Thoroughly prepared registered nurses/nurse aides
- Support systems
- Follow-up in-services

5. *Differentiated practice:* Role theory underlies the concept of differentiated practice, which defines the levels of competence within which two categories of registered nurses practice: nurses with bachelor's degrees and those with associate degrees. The BSN (bachelor of science in nursing) level is the professional practice level; the ADN (associate degree in nursing) is the associate or technical practice level. These practice levels can function within a variety of different delivery systems, including team and primary systems. The premise for differentiated practice is that professional practice exercises the nurse's autonomous decisions, including personal acceptance of risks and responsibilities in making professional judgments. Extended education at a BSN level or higher is required preparation for this role at the professional practice level.[175] The differentiated group professional practice model has three major components, of which differentiated care delivery is one:[176]

- Group governance
- Differentiated care delivery
- Shared values

A differentiated practice system or delivery model has the following components:

- Differentiated registered nurse practice
- Use of nurse extenders
- Primary case management

Differentiated care delivery is designed so that nurses with varying educational preparation and work experience can most efficiently use their knowledge and skills while delegating non-nursing tasks to assistive personnel. Nurse extenders are delegated tasks rather than patient assignments.[177]

The differentiated practice role has three basic components:

- Provision of direct care
- Communication with and on behalf of patients
- Management of patient care

A differentiated practice maximizes available registered nurse resources for efficiency and effectiveness. "Differentiated practice is a strategy that calls for licensed and practicing nurses to be used in accord with their respective experience, ability, and formal and continuing education. Further, differentiated practice is defined as both a human resource deployment model and an alternative to primary nursing and case management." It is role differentiation. More education and experience are needed for cognitive skills.[178]

In an ethnographic study of differentiated practice in an operating room, it was found that introduction of a new role requires insight into setting and an emphasis on staging and orientation of employees to the new role.[179] Otherwise, introduction of a new role can create turmoil and job insecurity. To use the differentiated practice mode, the nurse's knowledge and skills are assessed (Figure 7-44).

Styles and others advocate differentiated credentialing. What are the goals of differentiated credentialing and what would it accomplish? In the practice environment, cost-effectiveness often calls for varied nursing personnel. It is essential that the professional level be designated. To gain public respect and rights of self-determination, nursing must adhere to the professional norm. Role-delineated relationships with other health professionals and incentives for improvement depend on identification of professional status. In brief, higher standards of care; clear public recognition and specificity in authority, accountability, roles, and responsibilities; and rewards for the professional nurse are the goals of the entry effort.

The proposed solution might work like this: BSN education, registered nurse licensure, followed with national generalist certification with the title CPN (certified professional nurse), and then a differentiated practice with recognition/reimbursement.[180]

6. *Relationship-based care model:* Creative Health Care Management consultants developed a nursing practice model called relationship-based care.[181] The model is based on theories of caring and relationships, relationships between the healthcare employee and the patient and family, the healthcare employee's relationship with self, and his or her relationship with peers.[182] The model is structured on the following dimensions:[183]

- Teamwork
- Professional nursing
- Leadership
- Care delivery

FIGURE 7-44   **DIFFERENTIATED PRACTICE ASSESSMENT**

RN Professional	**RN Associate or Technician**
BSN prepared	Non-BSN RN
Makes complex decisions and interactions	Assists the professional nurse
Cost management of supplies, clinical alternatives, flexible scheduling of personnel, and case loads	Performs high-skill tasks such as chemotherapy
Structures the unstructured	Special tests and procedures
Cognitive role and highly skilled tasks	May lead self-managed work team coached by professional nurse
Care manager	Direct care provider
Independent judgments, initiative, problem solving	Uses common, well defined diagnoses
Coaches self-managed work team	Works in structured settings and situations
Manages all resources, fiscal and material	
Consults with other disciplines	
Discharges patients	

Source: Author.

- Resources
- Outcomes

Analyzing Organizational Structures in a Division of Nursing

Analyzing the organizational structure of a division of nursing entails six main steps, which should be used when major organizational problems occur, such as friction among department heads over authority, staffing problems, and the like. These steps also apply to organizing a new corporation, division, or unit and to reorganizing.

Step 1

Compile a list of the key activities determined by the mission and objectives of patient care. The written philosophy and vision statements will help by indicating important values to be considered. Once this list is completed, it must be analyzed. Group similar activities together. What are the central load-carrying elements? Most will be related to primary care, and philosophy usually dictates that excellence of patient care is a requirement for the accomplishment of objectives.

Whenever the strategy changes, the organizational structure should be reviewed and analyzed. This includes changes in mission, philosophy, vision, objectives, and the operational plan for accomplishing the objectives. The analysis of key activities can be done according to the kinds of contributions made, including the following:

- Results-producing activities related to direct patient care, such as training, recruiting, and employment
- Support activities, which may include those related to vision or future, values and standards, audit, advice, and teaching
- Hygiene and housekeeping activities
- Top management activities to include "conscience" activities such as vision, values, standards, and audit as well as managing people, marketing, and innovation

Service staff such as those performing advisory and training support should be limited. They should be required to abandon an old activity before starting a new one. Prevent them from building empires as a career. Informational activities are the responsibility of top management though they stem from support such as controller and treasurer. There must be a system for disseminating information. Hygiene and housekeeping need the attention of nurses if they are to be done well and cheaply. This does not mean that nurses will do these tasks but rather that nurses will recognize their importance and support and facilitate their being done by the appropriate departments. Contract services are the answer in some instances. Consider whether the groups of key activities should be rank ordered in the sequence in which they will occur.

Step 2

Based on the work functions to be performed, decide on the units of the organization. Decision analysis is important here, because it must be decided which kinds of decisions will be required and who will make them. Decisions involving functions of future commitments may have to be a top management function, depending on the degree of futurity of a decision and the speed with which it can be reversed. It will be necessary to analyze the impact of decisions on other functions; the number of functions involved will be an important factor. Qualitative factors such as decisions involving ethical values, principles of conduct, and social and political beliefs will have to be analyzed. The frequency of the decision will influence its placement: Is it recurrent or is it rare? In principle, all decisions should be placed at the lowest level and as close to the operational scene as possible.

Step 3

Decide which units or components will be joined and which separated. Join activities that make the same kind of contribution. This requires relations analysis and will be related to the sequence of key activities or functions.

Step 4

Decide on the size and shape of the units or components.

Step 5

Decide on appropriate placement and relationships of different units or components. This will result from the relations analysis (see step 3). There should be the smallest possible number of relationships, with each made to count.

Step 6

Draw or diagram the design and put it into operation. This results in an organizational chart or schema.

Minimum Requirements of an Organizational Structure

Minimum requirements of an organizational structure should be taken into consideration to achieve organizational success (Figure 7-45).

To apply design principles that are appropriate, the nurse manager uses a mixture of all that are productive, including the following:

- Organizational needs derive from the statements of mission and objectives and from observation of work performed.

FIGURE 7-45 | **MINIMUM REQUIREMENTS OF AN ORGANIZATIONAL STRUCTURE**

- Clarity: Nurses need to know where they belong, where they stand in relation to the quality and quantity of their performances, and where to go for assistance.
- Economy: Nurses need as much self-control of their work as they can possibly be given. They need to be self-motivating. There should be the smallest possible number of overhead personnel necessary to keep the division and units operating and well maintained.
- Direction of vision: Nurse managers must direct their vision and that of their employees toward performance, toward the future, and toward strength. Nurses must understand their own tasks and the common tasks of the organization. They should see that their tasks fit the common tasks so that the structure helps communication.
- Decision making: Nurses should be organized to make decisions on the right issues and at the right levels. They should be organized to convert their decisions into work and accomplishments. The chair of the department of nursing and the staff make all nursing decisions and see that nursing work is done.
- Stability and accountability: Nurses should be organized to feel community belonging. They can adapt to show objectives requiring changes in their functions and productivity.
- Perception and self-renewal: Nursing services should be organized to produce future leaders. The organizational structure should produce continuous learning for the job each nurse holds and for promotion.

Source: Author.

- Organizational design and structure develop to fit organizational needs, so that people perform and contribute to achieving the work of the division of nursing.
- A formal organization should be flexible and based on policy that promotes individual contributions to the achievement of organizational objectives.
- A formal organization is efficient when it promotes achievement of objectives with a minimum of unplanned costs or outcomes. Most results should be planned, should give satisfaction to supervisors and employees, and should not occasion waste and carelessness. When grouping activities for organizing purposes, the supervisor or administrator should examine the benefits and disadvantages of alternate groupings.
- A formal organization should build the least possible number of management levels and forge the shortest possible chain of command. This eliminates stresses and levels of friction, slack, and inertia.

Figure 7-46 outlines standards for evaluating departmentation of authority in a nursing division, department, service, or unit.

FIGURE 7-46   **STANDARDS FOR EVALUATION OF DEPARTMENTATION**

1. Nursing activities have been grouped to attain goals and sustain the enterprise.

2. Nursing activities have been grouped for intradepartmental and interdepartmental coordination.

3. Personnel roles have been designed to fit the capabilities and motivation of persons available to fill them.

4. Personnel roles have been designed to help employees contribute to departmental or unit objectives.

5. Personnel roles provide optimum and economic job enlargement.

6. Nursing activities have been grouped for full use of resources, people, and material.

7. Nursing activities have been grouped for optimum cost benefits.

8. Nursing activities have been grouped to match special skills to special needs.

9. Nursing activities have been grouped to achieve an optimum management span.

10. Nursing activities and personnel have been grouped for optimum correlation for decision making and problem solving.

11. Nursing activities have been grouped to achieve minimal levels of management by providing for delegation of responsibility and authority to the lowest competent operational level.

12. Nursing activities and personnel have been grouped to eliminate duplication of staff services and centralized services of specialists.

13. Nursing activities and personnel have been grouped to facilitate production of products and services that will promote health of individuals and groups.

14. Nursing activities and personnel have been grouped to promote soundness of industrial relations programs and fiscal policies and procedures.

15. Nursing activities have been grouped to fulfill time demands of shifts.

16. Nursing activities have been grouped to achieve priorities and allow for change and flexibility in achievement of objectives.

17. Nursing activities have been grouped to facilitate training of employees.

18. Nursing activities have been grouped to facilitate communication.

Source: Author.

Departmentation

These steps should be used when major organizational problems occur, such as friction among department heads over authority and staffing problems. They also apply to organizing a new corporation, division, or unit and to reorganizing an established entity. Steps 3, 4, and 5 involve departmentation, the grouping of personnel according to some characteristic.

Departmentation is an organizing process. For departmentation purposes, functional specialties are formed from clusters of units with similar goals. In most of our healthcare institutions, the functions of nursing are grouped into a division or department. Within that division or department are further groupings of nursing personnel by specialization, such as medical, surgical, pediatric, and obstetric. Sometimes the grouping is further broken down into areas of subspecialization. This process is termed *functional departmentation*. Clients may also be grouped according to degree of illness, such as minimal, intermediate, or intensive care.

There are advantages and disadvantages of functional departmentation. Among the advantages are focus on the basic activities of the enterprise through a logical and time-proven method of organizing, efficient use of specialized personnel, simplified training, and tight control by top administration. A big disadvantage for nursing is that people tend to develop tunnel vision about their specialty and the service or unit within which they work.

Time departmentation is common within healthcare organizations. Personnel are grouped by shift. This has important implications for administration as the activities of shifts have to be grouped according to qualifications and numbers of personnel on any shift.

Territorial departmentation involves grouping of activities according to geography or physical plant. This is more common in merged organizations with geographically separated units. Some activities, such as staff development, may be assigned by territory and specialization and grouped by function.

Territorial departmentation should encourage participation in decision making in provision of health services to a wider population base and be of a nature that prevents illnesses and injuries. There may be justification for the exploration and formation of consortiums using the principle of territorial departmentation. For example, several small hospitals in an area could contract for consultant services in research, clinical nurse specialist services, or nursing education services.

In addition to functional, time, and territorial departmentation, there is the fourth option, product departmentation. This approach has implications for health care, although its ultimate achievement may not always be immediately practical. Increasingly, the products of nursing care are focused on the health needs of populations and those who need not only the illness care but also the care that keeps aging populations healthy; that maintains health and prevents injury and disease in the large group who take voluntary risks such as smoking, reckless driving, poor eating, poor exercising, or using artificial mood changers; that promotes a clean environment; that modifies the health risks associated with human reproduction; and that decreases the need for illness care. In the vertically integrated organization, product line departmentation is common.

Departmentation could be done on the basis of consumer needs or demands. There is a distinct possibility that healthcare institutions will offer people a choice of services in the future, thereby giving them the opportunity to select those services that are covered by third-party payers and those that are paid for out-of-pocket. Also, the times the services are given and who are giving them may well be part of the choice.

There may be no pure form of departmentation that will work in the healthcare institution. It may be more important to look at all the variables to group people to facilitate successful production of healthcare services. In the matrix organization, product and functional forms of departmentation are combined. Projects have managers who move products through production stages in coordination with managers of each production stage. We will see more use of matrix organizations in nursing as health care takes on new dimensions.

At the present, nursing services are usually organized using a mix of departmentations. As long as the system is based on logic, it will provide a viable and efficient organization. Figure 7-46 can be used to evaluate departmentation of nursing service activities and personnel.

Informal Organization

Every formal organization has an informal one. The informal organization meets the needs of individuals with similar backgrounds, values, hobbies, interests, and physical proximity. It meets their needs for sharing experiences and feelings. Some administrators try to hinder the effects of informal organizations because they facilitate the passing of information. The information may be rumor, but the best way to combat rumor is by free flow of truthful information. Only information that might violate individual privacy or the survival and health of the enterprise should be kept from subordinates. The informal organization can help to serve the goals of the formal organization if it is not made the servant of administration. It should not be controlled. A major shortcoming in its use is that not all employees are part of the informal organization.

Nurse managers should encourage and nurture informal organizations that do the following:

- Provide a sense of belonging, security, and recognition
- Provide methods for friendly and open discussion of concern
- Maintain feelings of personal integrity, self-respect, and independent choice
- Provide an informal and accurate communication link
- Provide opportunities for social interaction
- Provide a source of practical information for managerial decision making
- Are sources of future leaders

Problems can include creation of conflicting loyalties, restricted productivity, and resistance to change and management's plans.[184]

Organizational Effectiveness

The product or output of an organization is termed *organizational effectiveness*. There should be a relationship between organizational effectiveness and organizational performance. Nurse managers define the goals and provide the resources for both organizational effectiveness and organizational performance. There are multiple indicators to monitor in determining organizational effectiveness (Figure 7-47).

FIGURE 7-47	INDICATORS USED IN MONITORING ORGANIZATIONAL EFFECTIVENESS

- Patient satisfaction with care
- Family satisfaction with care
- Staff satisfaction with work
- Staff satisfaction with rewards, intrinsic and extrinsic
- Staff satisfaction with professional development: career, personal, and educational
- Staff satisfaction with organization
- Management satisfaction with staff
- Community relationships
- Organizational health

Source: Author.

Nurse administrators control these dimensions of organizational effectiveness. Proactivity is more successful in developing them than is reactivity.[185] The organizational effectiveness of hospitals could be improved if administrators would enter into general or limited partnerships with nurses. Hospitals have moved to vertical integration to capture the lost revenues of retrospective reimbursement. General hospitals have entered into services such as home care, long-term care, psychiatric care, rehabilitation, hospice care, rental and sale of durable medical supplies, and many other profit–making services. Although they call for general or limited partnerships with physicians, they ignore nurses as a potential source of partnerships for profit. Instead, the not-for-profit status of hospital inpatient beds is reputed to be maintained by policies that tie nursing to charity and idealism rather than to viability and profitability. Such statements as the following validate this tie: "Keeping nursing care in the not-for-profit hospital corporation preserves the oldest tradition of hospitals and their role in serving the needy."[186]

Nurses can overcome this attitude by themselves becoming proactive. As an example, nurses could plan a limited partnership that would provide contract nurses through a staffing agency owned by them. They could offer a hospital a contract to provide needed personnel on a first priority basis, with surplus personnel provided for other institutions. The contract could provide for up-to-date continuing education of the agency nurses through cooperative arrangements with the contracting hospital. Profits would be shared, and nurses would perceive that the hospital supported nursing entrepreneurship, thus contributing to their morale and professional esteem. Other ventures could be added to improve organizational performance as well as organizational effectiveness and to give nurses a sense of ownership.

Vertical integration, mergers, linkages, and multihospital systems have created more and new corporate nurse roles. The corporate nurse is physically and organizationally removed from daily nursing service operations. As such, the corporate nurse reviews data from a number of hospitals and organizations, comparing outcomes. Having access to much data and many specialties and serving on corporate committees, the corporate nurse creates a personal power base. She or he can develop systems for member organizations in such areas as management education, nursing division policy, search and selection of nurse executives, research, quality assurance, risk management, and others.[187]

Symptoms of Malorganization

Recurring problems signal malorganization. They indicate that the focus is on the wrong elements of the business when it should emphasize key activities, major business decisions, performance, and results rather than secondary problems. Another symptom of malorganization is too many meetings attended by too many people. Such meetings are poor tools for accomplishing work. An alternative is to give individual assignments, to meet only to report, and to avoid duplication. Committees are instruments of participation and communication and must be made productive. Too many management levels are another symptom of malorganization. Build the least possible number of management levels and forge the shortest possible chain of command. This eliminates stresses and levels of friction, slack, and inertia.

If people always have to worry about other people's feelings, there will be overstaffing. If the organization is put together to get the job done, layers of coordinators will not be needed. Fit the chart to the organization and its needs rather than drawing a chart and building the organization to support it.

SUMMARY

There are neither best designs for a nursing organization nor universal design principles. Nurse managers need to work for an ideal organizational structure, and they need to be pragmatic. They should build, test, concede, compromise, and accept. They should design the simplest organization for getting the job done. They should focus on key activities to produce key results. The organization is productive when the people are performing care that meets clients' needs and for which employees have a sense of accomplishment.

An organization can be shaped through the following:

- Enacting job enlargement that is qualitative and meaningful, interesting, and intellectually rewarding
- Making the structure more manageable. Increasing clinical nurses' autonomy reduces the organization's size.
- Increasing the span of control of the manager
- Shortening the hierarchy
- Involving the employees in participation
- Decentralization
- Increasing the employee's stake in his or her own performance
- Increasing creativity while maintaining fiscal responsibility
- Replacing direction and control with advice
- Meeting employees' needs

One main way to get employees involved in the shape of the organization is through committee work. Committees provide employees with a representative voice in the management of organizations. A standing committee has continuity as an organizational entity, whereas an ad-hoc committee is formed for a purpose and disbanded when that purpose is fulfilled. Committees can facilitate communication, promote loyalty, pool special human resources, reduce resistance to change, and give people opportunities to work together. They should have purposes, objectives, and operational procedures. Committees can waste time if they make a premature decision or do not accomplish their objectives. They can be made effective by application of the management functions of planning, organizing, directing (leading), and controlling (evaluating).

Chairs of committees need knowledge and skills of group dynamics, which can be provided through staff development programs for all nurses desiring it. Groups work in five phases:

1. Forming or orientation phase
2. Conflict or storming phase
3. Cohesion or norming phase
4. Working or performing phase
5. Termination phase

Group techniques include the Delphi technique, brainstorming, the nominal group techniques, and focus groups, among others. Group leaders either are appointed (formal leaders) or emerge from the group (informal leaders).

Self-directed work teams increase participatory management by broadening jobs and increasing employee cohesiveness. Self-directed work teams enable the employees to have more decision-making abilities, thereby improving employee satisfaction, productivity, and commitment to the organization.

Decentralization disburses authority and power downward to the operational units of an organization. Increased productivity, improved morale, increased favorable attitudes, and decreased absenteeism are the products of decentralized decision making. Decentralization supports participatory management, the characteristics of which are trust, commitment, involvement of employees in setting goals and objectives, autonomy, inclusion of employees in decision making, change and growth, originality, and creativity.

Decentralized and participatory organizations are usually flat or horizontal, employee- and relationship-centered. They are vertically integrated to enhance revenue production by developing new markets for healthcare organizations.

Training is essential to the success of participatory management because managers are often threatened by loss of authority. They have to be prepared for their new roles. Practicing nurses need to be able to perform as collaborators in the management of nursing organization and the healthcare institution. With their new roles comes increased accountability for practicing nurses. Managers become facilitators.

Although participatory management has numerous benefits or advantages, it also has some disadvantages. Among those disadvantages are occasional failures, occasional difficulty fixing responsibilities, and difficulty in changing employee perceptions of previously authoritarian management.

The nursing management function of organizing is an evolving one. It evolves as nurse managers learn and apply the knowledge gained from research and experience in business and industry. They further develop the organizing function through nursing research and experience in nursing management.

APPLICATION EXERCISES

Exercise 7-1
Use Figure 7-39 to evaluate the nursing organization chart of the organization in which you work as a student or employee.

Exercise 7-2
Use Figure 7-7 to evaluate the nursing division, department, service, or unit in which you work as a student or an employee.

Exercise 7-3
List characteristics of decentralization and participatory management evident in your organization.

List characteristics of centralized management evident in your organization.

List changes you would like to see implemented to increase decentralization of decision making in your organization.

Exercise 7-4
Describe the form of organizational structure of the nursing division and unit in which you work as a student or employee. Discuss the changes that could be made to make it more functional.

Exercise 7-5
Select two teams, one composed of experienced employees and the other composed of newer employees. Consider an emergency situation in which the fire alarm has gone off in a patient care area. Compare the two teams with regard to their working relationships, communication skills, and ability to prioritize and make decisions. Create a plan to develop the skills of the less effective team.

Exercise 7-6
Use Figure 7-27 and Figure 7-24 to evaluate a nursing meeting in the organization in which you work as a student or as an employee.

When the minutes of the same meeting have been distributed, use Figure 7-27 to evaluate them. Is there a difference between the actual meeting and the minutes? What is it? How can the process be improved?

Make a management plan to improve the committee's meetings and/or the minutes. Be tactful and use a positive approach in your planning.

Exercise 7-7
Examine the collective minutes of an ad-hoc committee. Identify the phases of the committee and link each phase with recorded behaviors. Summarize your findings.

Exercise 7-8
Attend meetings of several committees for the purpose of identifying behavior of members in the group task roles. Identify the role each member is playing. Write a brief summary of your observations. Do the same for members in group-building and maintenance roles and members in individual roles.

Exercise 7-9

Utilize Figure 7-32 and compare two nursing units, preferably on different shifts and determine the different rites and rituals that differ.

Exercise 7-10

Go to the Web sites of the IOM, Agency for Healthcare Research and Quality Response, Leapfrog, TJC, and QSEN and update the status of each. What is new? What is the evidence, if any, to demonstrate that any of the initiatives are working?

Exercise 7-11

Reflect on a recent error that resulted in serious harm in your organization. How was the situation managed? Did the questions asked focus on identifying someone to blame, like these: What is wrong here? Who was responsible for this? Or were they questions that would allow the organization and the provider to learn more about the situation and be better positioned to avoid recurrences of the error? Better questions for investigating an error include these: Why is this error occurring again and again? Am I missing a lesson here? How can I turn this situation into an opportunity for growth and learning for myself and the team?

Exercise 7-12

Differentiate between culture and climate of an organization. Support your answer.

Exercise 7-13

Describe the nursing care delivery model used at the hospital where you are a student or employee. Identify the role of the registered nurse in this model.

Exercise 7-14

Provide an example to illustrate the type of professional practice model used at the organization where you are a student or employee.

Notes

1. American Organization of Nurse Executives (AONE). *AONE nurse executive competencies.* Retrieved February 29, 2008, from www.aone.org/aone/resource/home.html
2. Wolper, L. (2004). Health care administration. Planning, implementing, and managing organized delivery systems (4th ed., p. 357). Sudbury, MA: Jones and Bartlett.
3. Liebler, J. G., & McConnell, C. R. (2004). *Management principles for health professionals* (p. 166). Sudbury, MA: Jones and Bartlett.
4. Argyris, C. (1973). Personality and organization theory revisited. *Administrative Science Quarterly, 18,* 141–167.
5. Fayol, H. (1949). *General and industrial management* (pp. 53–61) (C. Storrs, Trans.). London: Sir Isaac Pittman & Sons.
6. Urwick, L. (1944). *The elements of administration* (pp. 37–39). New York: Harper & Row.
7. Peters, T. (1987). *Thriving on chaos.* New York: Harper & Row.
8. Gibson, J. L., Ivancevich, J. M., & Donnelly, J. H., Jr. (1994). *Organizations: Behavior, structures, processes* (8th ed., pp. 539–541). Burr Ridge, IL: Richard D. Irwin.
9. Hall, R. H. (1963). The concept of bureaucracy: An empirical assessment. *The American Journal of Sociology, 10,* 32–40.
10. Ibid.
11. Hall, R. H. (1968). Professionalization and bureaucratization. *American Sociological Review,* 92–104.
12. Sofarelli, D., & Brown, D. (1998). The need for nursing leadership in uncertain times. *Journal of Nursing Management,* 201–207.
13. Warda, M. (1992). The family and chronic sorrow: Role theory approach. *Journal of Pediatric Nursing,* 205–210.

14. MacLeod, J. A., & Sella, S. (2002). One year later: Using role theory to evaluate a new delivery system. *Nursing Forum*, 20–28.

15. Miller, J. O., & Carey, S. J. (1993). Work role inventory: A guide to job satisfaction. *Nursing Management*, 54–62.

16. Wolper, 2004, p. 653.

17. Pugh, D. S., Hickson, D. J., Hinings, C. R., & Turner, C. (1969). The context of organization structures. *Administrative Science Quarterly*, 91–114; Leatt, P., & Schneck, R. (1982). Technology, size, environment, and structure in nursing subunits. *Organizational Studies, 3*, 221–242.

18. Institute of Medicine (IOM). (2000). *To err is human: Building a safer health system for the 21st century*. Washington, DC: National Academy Press.

19. Institute of Medicine (IOM). (2004). *Transforming the work environment of nurses* (p. 2). Quality Chasm Series. Washington, DC: National Academy Press.

20. Ibid., pp. 8, 9, 12, 13.

21. Marquis, B., & Huston, C. (1996). *Roles and functions in organizing. Leadership roles and management functions in nursing: Theory and application* (pp. 144–149). Philadelphia: Lippincott-Raven.

22. Ibid.

23. Rowland, H. S., & Rowland, B. L. (1997). Nursing Administrative Handbook (4th ed.). Sudbury, MA: Jones and Bartlett, Inc., p. 87.

24. Pugh et al., 1969.

25. Ibid.

26. Ibid.

27. American Nurses Credentialing Center. (2005). Magnet Recognition Program®. Application Manual, Silver Spring, MD: American Nurses Credentialing Center Publishers, pp. 38–39.

28. Newman, J. G., & Boisoneau, R. (1987). Team care and matrix organization in geriatrics. *Hospital Topics*, 10–15.

29. McClure, M. L. (1984). Managing the professional nurse: Part I. The organizational theories. *Journal of Nursing Administration*, 15–21; Timm, M. M., & Wavetik, M. G. (1983). Matrix organization: Design and development for a hospital organization. *Hospital & Health Services Administration*, 46–58; American Organization of Nurse Executives (AONE). (1984). *Organizational models for nursing practice*. Chicago: American Hospital Association.

30. Ibid.

31. Mosley, Pietri, & Megginson, 1996, pp. 274–277, 346, 582.

32. McClure, M., Poulin, M., Sovie, M., & Wandelt, M. (2002). Magnet hospitals: Attraction and retention of professional nurses (the original study). In M. McClure & A. Hinshaw (Eds.), *Magnet hospitals revisited: Attraction and retention of professional nurses*. Washington, DC: American Nurses Publishing.

33. Koloroutis, M. (2004). *Relationship-based care: A model for transforming practice* (p. 75). Minneapolis, MN: Creative Health Care Management.

34. Shoemaker, H., & El-Ahraf, A. (1983). Decentralization of nursing service management and its impact on job satisfaction. *Nursing Administration Quarterly*, 69–76.

35. Walton, 1985.

36. Gordon, G. K. (1982). Developing a motivating environment. *Journal of Nursing Administration*, 11–16.

37. Weisz, W. J. (1985). Employee involvement: How it works at Motorola. *Personnel*, 29–33; Poteet, G. W. (1984). Delegation strategies: A must for the nurse executive. *Journal of Nursing Administration*, 18–27.

38. Fine, R. B., & Walton, R. E. (1985). From control to commitment in the workplace. *Harvard Business Review*, 77–84.

39. Raelin, J. A., Sholl, C., & Leonard, D. (2002). Professional work environment. *Nursing Administration Quarterly*, 82–88.

40. Ibid.

41. Batey, M. V., & Lewis, F. M. (1982). Clarifying autonomy and accountability in nursing services: Part I. *Journal of Nursing Administration*, 13–17.

42. Bragg, J. E., & Andrews, I. R. (1984). Participative decision making: An experimental study in a hospital. In B. Fuszard (ed.), *Self-actualization for nurses* (pp. 102–110). Rockville, MD: Aspen.

43. Collins, S. S., & Henderson, M. C. (1991). Autonomy: Part of the nursing role? *Nursing Forum, 26,* 23–29.

44. Bough, S. (1992). Nursing students rank high in autonomy at the exit level. *Journal of Nursing Education,* 58–64.

45. Snail, T. S. (1998). Organizational diversification in the American hospital. *Annual Review of Public Health, 19,* 417–453.

46. Clegg, C. W., & Wall, T. D. (1984). The lateral dimension to employee participation. *Journal of Management Studies,* 429–442.

47. Friedman, B. A. (1997). Orchestrating a unified approach to information management. *Radiology Management,* 30–36.

48. James, D. M. (1998). An integrated model for inner-city health-care delivery: The Deaconess center. *Journal of the National Medical Association,* 35–39.

49. Weisz, 1985.

50. Walton, 1985.

51. Simons, B. J. (2002). Participatory management strategies. *Journal of Nursing Administration, 2,* 72–78.

52. Schuster, M. H., & Miller, C. S. (1985). Employee involvement: Making supervisors believers. *Personnel,* 24–28.

53. Simons, 2002.

54. Malkin, S., & Lauteri, P. (1980). A community hospital's approach: Decentralized patient education. *Nursing Administration Quarterly,* 101–106.

55. Raelin et al., 2002.

56. Walton, 1985.

57. Robinson, M. A. (1991). Decentralize and outsource: Dial's approach to MIS improvement. *Management Accounting,* 27–31.

58. Cox, C. L. (1980). Decentralization uniting authority and responsibility. *Supervisor Nurse, 28,* 32.

59. Bragg & Andrews, 1984.

60. Probst, M. R., & Noga, J. M. (1980). A decentralized nursing care delivery system. *Supervisor Nurse,* 57–60; Elpern, White, & Donahue, 1984.

61. Porter-O'Grady, T. (1992). *Implementing shared governance.* St. Louis, MO: Mosby.

62. Ibid.

63. Jacoby, J., & Terpstra, M. (1990). Collaborative governance: Model of professional autonomy. *Nursing Management,* 42–44.

64. Maldonado, T. (1992). *Lecture, senior management class.* San Antonio, TX: Incarnate Word College.

65. Pugh et al., 1969.

66. George, V. M., Burke, L. J., & Rodgers, B. L. (1997). Research-based planning for change: Assessing nurses' attitudes toward governance and professional practice autonomy after hospital acquisition. *Journal of Nursing Administration,* 53–61.

67. Prince, S. B. (1997). Shared governance. Sharing power and opportunity. *Journal of Nursing Administration,* 28–35.

68. Joiner, G., & Wessman, J. (1997). Expanding shared governance beyond practice issues. *Recruitment, Retention, Restructuring Research,* 4–7.

69. Aikman, P., Andress, I., Goodfellow, C., LaBelle, N., & Porter-O'Grady, T. (1998). System integration: A necessity. *Journal of Nursing Administration,* 28–34.

70. Rowland, H., & Rowland, B. (1992). *Nursing administration handbook* (3rd ed.: Sudbury, MA: Jones and Bartlett, p. 99).

71. Brorkowski, N. (2005). *Organizational behavior in health care.* Sudbury, MA: Jones and Bartlett.

72. Dunphy, D. (1983). Personal and organizational change—-Status and future direction. *Work and People,* 3–6.

73. Johnson, J., & Luciano, K. (1983). Managing by behavior and results—Linking supervisory accountability to effective organizational control. *Journal of Nursing Administration,* 19–26.

74. Dayani, E. C. (1983). Professional and economic self-governance in nursing. *Nursing Economic$,* 20–23.

75. Argyris, 1973.

76. Ridderheim, D. S. (1986). The anatomy of change. *Hospital & Health Services Administration,* 7–21.

77. Knaus, W., Draper, E. A., Wagner, D. P., & Zimmerman, J. E. (1986). An evaluation of outcome from intensive care in major medical centers. *Annuals of Internal Medicine, 104*(3), 410–418.

78. ANA, 2004, pp. 15, 16, 17, 19, 20.

79. Ibid., p. 28.

80. Ibid.

81. Ibid., p. 3.

82. Kowalski, K. (1995). Teambuilding. In P. Yoder-Wise (Ed.), *Leading and managing in nursing* (pp. 286–288). St. Louis, MO: Mosby-Year Book.

83. Ibid., in Dyer, W. (1987). *Team building issues and alternatives.* Boston: Addison-Wesley.

84. Schaffner, T., & Bermingham, M. (1993). Creating and maintaining a high-performance team. In *Nursing leadership: Preparing for the 21st century* (p. 80). Washington, DC: American Organization of Nurse Executives.

85. Ibid.

86. Ibid.

87. Russell-Babin, K. (1992). Team building for the staff development department. *Journal of Nursing Staff Development,* 231–234; San Juan, S. P. (1998). Team building: A leadership strategy. *Journal of the Philippine Dental Association,* 49–55.

88. Nave, J. L., & Thomas, B. (1983). How companies boost morale. *Supervisory Management,* 29–33.

89. Drucker, P. F. (1973). *Management: Tasks, responsibilities, practice.* New York: Harper & Row, 564.

90. Dumaine, B. (1994, September 5). The trouble with teams. *Fortune,* 86–88, 90, 92.

91. Caudron, S. (1993). Teamwork takes work. *Personnel Journal,* 76–84.

92. Manz, C. C., Keating, D. E., & Donellon, A. (1990). Preparing for an organizational change to employee self-management: The managerial transition. *Organizational Dynamics,* 15–26.

93. Seelhoff, K. L. (1992). Six steps to team problem solving. *Hotels,* 26.

94. Brandon, G. M. (1996). Flattening the organization: Implementing self-directed work groups. *Radiology Management,* 35–42; Yeatts, D. E., & Schultz, E. (1998). Self-managed work teams: What works? *Clinical Laboratory Management Review,* 16–26.

95. McClure et al., 2002, p. 12.

96. Stevens, B. J. (1975). Use of groups for management. *Journal of Nursing Administration,* 14–22.

97. Dixon, N. (1984). Participative management: It's not as simple as it seems. *Supervisory Management,* 2–8.

98. Fried, B., & Rundall, T. (1994). Managing groups and teams. In S. Shortell & A. Kaluzny (Eds.), *Health care management: Organization design and behavior* (3rd ed., pp. 144–147). New York: Delmar.

99. Jay, A. (1982). How to run a meeting. *Journal of Nursing Administration,* 22–28.

100. Mayo, E. (1946). *The human problems of industrial civilization.* Boston: Harvard Business School.

101. Stevens, 1975, pp. 14–22.

102. Benne, K. D., & Sheats, P. (1948). Functional roles of group members. *Journal of Social Studies,* 41–49.

103. Ibid.

104. Ibid.

105. Dixon, 1984, pp. 2–8.

106. Caramanica, L. (1984). What? Another committee? *Nursing Management,* 12–14; Jay, 1982, pp. 22–28.

107. Northouse, L. L., & Northouse, P. G. (1985). *Health communication: A handbook for health professionals.* Englewood Cliffs, NJ: Prentice Hall; Brightman, H. J., & Verhowen, P. (1986). Running successful problem solving group. *Business,* 15–23.

108. Beeber, L. S., & Schmitt, M. H. (1986). Cohesiveness in groups: A concept in search of a definition. *Advances in Nursing Science,* 1–11.

109. Tipping, J., Freeman, R. F., & Rachlis, A. R. (1995). Using faculty and student perceptions of group dynamics to develop recommendations for PBL training. *Academic Medicine,* 1050–1052; Cook, S. H., & Matheson, H. (1997). Teaching group dynamics: A critical evaluation of an experiential programme. *Nursing Education Today,* 31–38; Krejci, J. W., & Malin, S. (1997). Impact of leadership development on competencies. *Nursing Economic$,* 235–241; Abusabha, R., Peacock, J., & Achterberg, C. (1999). How to make nutrition education more meaningful through facilitated group discussion. *Journal of the American Dietetic Association,* 72–76.

110. Hodgetts, R. M. (1990). *Management theory, process and practice* (5th ed., p. 286). Orlando, FL: Harcourt Brace.

111. Northouse & Northouse, 1985, pp. 240–241.

112. Lloyd-Jones, G., Fowell, S., & Bligh, J. G. (1999). The use of the nominal group technique as an evaluative tool in medical undergraduate education. *Medical Education,* 8–13; Swansburg, R. C. (1995). Nominal group technique. In B. Fuszard (Ed.), *Innovative strategies in nursing* (2nd ed., pp. 93–100). Gaithersburg, MD: Aspen.

113. Ekblad, S., Marttila, A., & Emilsson, M. (2002). Cultural challenges in end-of-life care: Reflections from focus groups' interviews with hospital staff in Stockholm. *Journal of Advanced Nursing,* 623–630; Corring, D. J., & Cook, J. V. (1999). Client-centered care means that I am a valued human being. *Canadian Journal of Occupational Therapy,* 71–82; Hind, M., Jacjson, D., Andrewes, C., Fulbrook, P., Galvin, K., & Frost, S. (1999). Exploring the expanded role of nurses in critical care. *Intensive Critical Care Nursing,* 147–153; Dewar, B. J., & Walker, E. (1999). Experiential learning: Issues in supervision. *Journal of Advanced Nursing,* 1459–1467; Dreachslin, J. L. (1998). Conducting effective focus groups in the context of diversity: Theoretical underpinnings and practical implications. *Qualitative Health Research,* 813–820; Jinks, A. M., & Daniels, R. (1999). Workplace health concerns: A focus group study. *Journal of Management in Medicine, 13,* 95–104; Hildebrandt, E. (1999). Focus groups and vulnerable populations. Insight into client strengths and needs in complex community health care environments. *Nursing Health Care Perspectives,* 256–259; Reiskin, H., Gendrop, S., Bowen, A., Wright, P., & Walsh, E. (1999). Collaboration between community nurses and nursing faculty using substance abuse prevention focus groups. *Nursing Connections,* 31–36; Hirst, S. P. (2000). Resident abuse: An insider's perspective. *Geriatric Nursing,* 38–42; Lowry, R. J., & Craven, M. A. (1999). Smokers' and drinkers' awareness of oral cancer: A qualitative study using focus groups. *British Dental Journal,* 668–670.

114. DesRosier, M. B., & Zellers, K. C. (1989). Focus groups: A program planning technique. *Journal of Nursing Administration,* 20–25.

115. Rosenblum, E. H. (1982). Groupthink: The peril of group cohesiveness. *Journal of Nursing Administration,* 27–31; Rowland, H. S., & Rowland, B. L. (2002). *Handbook for nurse administrators.* Philadelphia, PA: Lippincott; Leo, M. (1984). Avoiding the pitfalls of management think. *Business Horizons,* 44–47.

116. Ibid.

117. del Bueno, D. J., & Vincent, P. M. (1986). Organizational culture: How important is it? *Journal of Nursing Administration,* 15–20.

118. Moore, W. W. (1991). Corporate culture: Modern day rites and rituals. *Healthcare Trends and Transitions,* 8–13, 32–33.

119. Dyer, W. G., & Dyer, W. G., Jr. (1986). Organizational development system change or culture change? *Personnel,* 14–22.

120. Kramer, M., & Schmalenberg, C. (2002). Staff nurses identify essentials of magnetism. In M. McClure & A. Hinshaw (Eds.), *Magnet hospitals revisited: Attraction and retention of professional nurses* (p. 52). Washington, DC: American Nurses Publishing.

121. Ibid.

122. IOM, 2000.

123. Ibid.

124. Ibid.

125. Institute of Medicine (IOM). (2001). *Crossing the quality chasm: A new health system for the 21st century.* Washington, DC: National Academy Press.

126. Institute of Medicine (IOM). (2004). *Keeping patients safe: Transforming the work environment of nurses.* Washington, DC: National Academy Press.

127. Friesen, M., Farquhar, M., & Hughes, R. (2005). *The nurse's role in promoting a culture of patient safety* (pp. 13–19). Silver Spring, MD: Center for American Nurses.

128. Page, T. (2003). Applying airline safety practices to medication administration. *Medical-Surgical Nursing, 12,* 77–93.

129. American Organization of Nurse Executives. *Role of the nurse executive in patient safety. Guiding principles toolkit.* Retrieved on June 26, 2008 from www.aone.org/aone/resource/home.html

130. Ibid.

131. Ibid.

132. Ibid.

133. Peters, T. (1991, September 24). Experts' strengths can be a weakness. *San Antonio Light*, p. B3.

134. Munn, H. E., Jr. (1984). Organizational climate in the health care setting. *Health Care Supervisor*, 19–29.

135. Desatnick, 1986.

136. Holt Ashley, M. (1985). Motivation: Getting the medical units going again. *Nursing Management*, 28–30.

137. del Bueno, D. L. (1993). Paradigm shifts—What's good and not so good for health care. *Nursing & Health Care*, 100–101.

138. McAllister, M. (1990). A nursing integration framework based on standards of practice. *Nursing Management*, 28–31.

139. Flarey, D. L. (1991). The nurse executive and the governing body. *Journal of Nursing Administration*, 11–17.

140. Kanter, 1989, p. 36.

141. Ibid., pp. 57–67.

142. Sovie, M. D. (1990). Redesigning our future: Whose responsibility is it? *Nursing Economics$*, 21–26.

143. Genasci, L. (1994, July 24). Downsizing not always effective, experts say. *San Antonio Express-News*, p. H3.

144. Kaestle, P. (1990). A new rationale for organizational structure. *Planning Review*, 20–22, 27.

145. Staring, S., & Taylor, C. (1997). A guide to managing workforce transitions. *Nursing Management*, 31–32.

146. Peters, T. (1987). *Thriving on chaos* (pp. 424–438). New York: Harper & Row.

147. Reddecliff, M., Smith, E. L., & Ryan-Merritt, M. (1989). Organizational analysis: Tool for the clinical nurse specialist. *Clinical Nurse Specialist*, 133–136.

148. Wolper, 2004, p. 359.

149. Ibid., p. 361.

150. Wolf, G., & Greenhouse, P. (2007). Blueprint for design. Creating models that direct change. *Journal of Nursing Administration, 37*, 381–387.

151. Wolper, 2004, p. 350.

152. Kimball, B., & Joynt, J. (2007). The quest for new innovative care delivery models. *Journal of Nursing Administration, 37*, 392–398.

153. Wolper, 2004, p. 363.

154. Ibid.

155. Wolper, 2004, p. 364.

156. Ibid.

157. Kimball & Joynt, 2007.

158. Lookingland, S., Tiedeman, M., & Crosson, A. (2005). Nontraditional models of care delivery. *Journal of Nursing Administration, 35*, 74–80.

159. Kimball & Joynt, 2007.

160. Ibid.

161. Wolf & Greenhouse, 2007, p. 382.

162. American Organization of Nurse Executives. (2004). *Principles and elements of a healthful practice/work environment.* Retrieved July 17, 2008 from www.aone.org/aone/resource/home.html

163. Texas Nurses Association. *Nurse-friendly hospital criteria™.* Retrieved July 17, 2008 from www.texasnurses.org

164. American Nurses Credentialing Center, 2005, pp. 45–46.

165. American Colleges of Nurses. (2002). *Hallmarks of the professional nursing practice environment.* Retrieved July 17, 2008 from www.aacn.nche.edu/publications/positions/hallmarkswp.pdf

166. McManis & Monsalve Associates. (2003) *Healthy work environments. Striving for excellence.* Retrieved July 17, 2008 from www.mcmanis-monsalve.com/assets/publications/healthy_work_environments_full.pdf

167. Ibid.

168. *Model nursing practice act.* Retrieved July 17, 2008 from www.ncsbn.org/312.htm

169. Hoffart, N., & Woods, C. (1996). Elements of a nursing professional practice model. *Journal Professional Nursing, 12*, 354–364.

170. American Nurses Credentialing Center, 2005, pp. 45–46.

171. Robert Wood Johnson Foundation, Retrieved on June 26, 2008, www.rwjf.org

172. Adams, R. A., & Rentfro, A. R. (1988). Strengthening hospital nursing: An approach to restructuring care delivery. *Journal of Nursing Administration,* 12–19.

173. Schmekel, C. E. (1991). Nursing/group practice. *AORN Journal,* 1223–1226, 1228.

174. Metcalf, K. M. (1992). The helper model: Nine ways to make it work. *Nursing Management,* 40–43.

175. Manthey, M. (1991). Delivery systems and practice models: A dynamic balance. *Nursing Management,* 28–30.

176. Milton, D., Verren, J., Murdaugh, C., & Gerber, R. (1992). Differentiated group professional practice in nursing: A demonstration model. *Nursing Clinics of North America,* 23–29.

177. Ibid.

178. Ehrat, K. S. (1991). The value of differentiated practice. *JONA,* 9–10.

179. Graph, C., Roberts, K., & Thorton, K. (1999). An ethnographic study of differentiated practice in an operating room. *Journal of Professional Nursing,* 364–371; Smith-Blair, N., Smith, B. L., Bradley, K. J., & Gaskamp, C. (1999). Making sense of a new nursing role: A phenomenological study of an organizational change. *Journal of Professional Nursing,* 340–348.

180. Styles, M., Allen, S., Armstrong, S., Matsurra, M., Stannard, D., & Ordway, J. S. (1991). Entry: A new approach. *Nursing Outlook,* 200–203.

181. Koloroutis, 2004, p. 11.

182. Ibid., p. 4.

183. Ibid.

184. Han, P. E. (1983). The informal organization you've got to live with. *Supervisory Management,* 25–28.

185. Cameron, K. (1986). A study of organizational effectiveness and its predictors. *Management Science,* 87–112.

186. Ibid.

187. Beyers, M. (1984). Getting on top of organizational change: Part 3. The corporate nurse executive. *Journal of Nursing Administration,* 32–37.

APPENDIX 7-1

Nursing Council Bylaws

ARTICLE I

NAME

1.1 The name of this Committee shall be the Nursing Council.

ARTICLE II

The purpose of this Council shall be:

2.1 To ensure excellence in nursing care which will return patients to their best possible state of health or will enable them to die with dignity.

2.2 To provide a climate which will promote and support the practice of professional nursing.

2.3 To provide a forum for the discussion of management and patient care concerns.

The function of the Council shall be:

2.4 To ensure excellence in nursing care.

    a. Through the development and support of ad-hoc committees.

    b. Through the support of XYZ Standards of Care.

2.5 To develop nursing service employees to their fullest potential.

    a. Through the development and support of ad-hoc committees.

    b. Through the support of XYZ Standards of Care.

ARTICLE III

MEMBER

The members of this Council shall be:

   3.1   All members of Nurse Manager Council Group, Clinical Council, Executive Council, committee chairs, and representatives from the XYZ College of Nursing.

ARTICLE IV

OFFICERS

The officers shall consist of:

   4.1   Chair, Vice-Chair, and Parliamentarian

      a.   All officers shall be elected by secret ballot.

      b.   A majority of votes cast will be required to be elected.

      c.   In the event a majority of votes is not achieved by the first ballot, a run-off between two candidates having the most votes shall be required.

      d.   Ballots shall be counted by the Administrative Secretary and RTN I.

      e.   Officers shall serve for one year and are eligible for reelection for one consecutive term.

   4.2   Officers, together with the Assistant Administrator of Nursing, shall constitute a governing board.

   4.3   In the event of a vacancy:

      a.   The Vice-Chair replaces the Chair.

      b.   The Parliamentarian shall replace Vice-Chair.

      c.   The new Parliamentarian will be appointed by the governing body.

   4.4   Duties of the officers:

      a.   The Chair shall work closely with the other officers of the Council. The Chair and other officers shall meet one week prior to each regular meeting for the purpose of developing and distributing the agenda and establishing time limits for discussion. The Chair is responsible to the Council for the smooth and effective functioning of its committees. The Chair is a voting member of the Executive Council and is responsible to the Council for communicating recommendations to the Executive Council. The Chair shall function according to the guidelines established in Robert's Rules of Order.

      b.   The Vice-Chair shall assume the duties of the Chair in his or her absence and shall serve as Chair of the nominating committee.

      c.   The Parliamentarian shall oversee that the Business of Nursing Council is conducted according to Robert's Rules of Order.

   4.5   Qualifications for office—Must be members of Nursing Council.

ARTICLE V

MEETINGS

   5.1   Regular meetings shall be held quarterly.

   5.2   The annual meeting shall be held in November, at which time annual reports of officers and Chair shall be read and officers elected.

   5.3   Special meetings shall be called by the Chair. The purpose of the meeting shall be stated in the call and at least two days notice will be given.

ARTICLE VI

QUORUM

A quorum of the Council shall be one-third of the membership. The presence of a quorum shall be documented in the minutes.

ARTICLE VII

COMMITTEES

7.1 Policy and Procedures Committee

    a. Purpose

        1. To establish guidelines, policies, and instructions for performance of procedures in accordance with the current standards of nursing practice for personnel of the Department of Nursing. The guidelines are specific and prescribe the precise action to be taken under a set of circumstances.

        2. To annually appraise policies and procedures followed by nurses, and to develop new policies to meet present and future needs.

        3. To assure compliance between nursing policy and hospital policy.

    b. Membership

        1. Members shall be appointed from each of the divisions within the Department of Nursing and from the XYZ College of Nursing. One member shall be appointed from each of the following: Executive Council, Staff Development, and Nursing Resources. Two members shall be appointed from the USA College of Nursing. Three members (one Nurse Manager or Clinical Specialist, one staff registered nurse, and one LPN) shall be appointed from each of the following divisions: Medical Surgical, Maternal Child, Critical Care, and Special Services.

        2. Each member shall have an alternate appointed to attend in the member's absence.

        3. Members are to be appointed to serve a two-year term, beginning January 1 of each year.

        4. Each representative may be reappointed for one consecutive term. Only one-half of the membership shall turn over annually.

    c. Meetings

        1. The policy and procedures committee shall meet at least six times annually.

        2. The time, date, and place of meetings shall be determined by the Chair.

        3. Minutes of the meeting shall be recorded and kept on file in Nursing Service.

        4. The Chair of this committee shall be elected by its membership.

    d. Duties

        1. To accept written recommendations from an individual or committee regarding the need for a policy or procedure.

        2. Identify independently the need for a policy or procedure.

        3. To research the literature and other resources to determine common, accepted nursing practice.

        4. To develop policy and procedures statements.

        5. To annually review and revise as necessary all current policies and procedures.

        6. To report to Nursing Council at each regular meeting.

        7. To prepare a written annual report outlining the accomplishments of the committee. The report shall be prepared by the Chair of the committee and submitted to the Chair of the Nursing Council.

7.2 Nominating Committee will meet during the last quarter prior to the annual meeting as called by the Chair. The slate of nominees shall be presented to Council for consideration one month prior to the annual meeting.

7.3 Bylaws

    a. Purpose—To review the bylaws of the Nursing Council and make recommendations to the Council for bylaws revision.

    b. Membership

        1. A Chair shall be elected from Nursing Council following the annual meeting.

2. Members shall be volunteers from Nursing Council.

    c. Meetings

        1. The Chair shall determine the frequency, time, date, and place of meetings.

        2. Minutes of the meeting shall be recorded and kept on file in Nursing Service.

7.4 Ad-Hoc Committees

    a. Purpose—To provide a vehicle by which specific tasks or programs can be assumed by a committee.

    b. Membership

        1. Membership shall follow the same format as for standing committees, unless the council decides that a smaller, more specific group will be more appropriate.

        2. Members can be appointed by Nursing Council or the committee may elect its Chair during its first meeting.

    c. Meetings

        1. During the first meeting, the committee shall:

          a. Define its purpose.

          b. Outline the necessary steps to achieve the purpose.

          c. Establish a tentative timetable.

        2. Minutes of the meetings shall be recorded and kept on file in Nursing Service.

          d. Duties

            1. The committee Chair shall report to Nursing Council during regular meetings.

            2. When the committee has completed its task, a final recommendation is made to Nursing Council for approval. Upon acceptance of this final recommendation, the Ad-Hoc Committee is dissolved.

7.5 RTN-I

    a. Purpose—To provide a forum for the discussion of topics relating to the practice of professional nursing at USAMC.

    b. Membership

        1. RTN from each unit or area and float pool for term of one year.

        2. Any RTN may attend as an observer.

        3. Adviser chosen by the committee and approved by administration. The adviser is a non-voting member.

        4. Officers are chosen by the committee.

    c. Duties

        1. To identify problems related to professional nursing and recommend solutions to Nursing Council.

        2. To disseminate information to coworkers.

        3. To review at monthly meetings all approved new and/or revised policies and procedures.

        4. To accept and assume responsibility for projects delegated by Nursing Council.

        5. To report to Nursing Council at each regular meeting. The report shall include:

          a. Problems identified concerning professional nursing.

  b. Recommendations for the solution of the identified problems.

  c. Progress on delegated projects.

  d. Summary of monthly committee activities.

6. To prepare an annual written report outlining the accomplishments of the committee. This report shall be prepared by the committee Chair and submitted to the Chair of Nursing Council.

7.6 Nurse Practice Committee

  a. Purpose

  1. To assist in identifying potential or actual problems related to quality of care, recommend corrective action, develop and plan for corrective action, and review effectiveness of corrective actions until an acceptable level of compliance is obtained. An additional charge of the committee is to develop and/or revise Nursing Standards of Care and Practice.

  b. Membership

  1. The Clinical Administrator for Nursing Practice shall assume position of Chair.

  2. The Nurse Practice Committee is comprised of a Registered Nurse from each nursing unit within the hospital.

  c. Duties

  1. To review and evaluate Quality Assurance monitoring.

  2. To evaluate the effectiveness of previous actions taken to improve care based on follow-up and tracking.

  3. To plan appropriate actions that will improve the delivery of nursing care and affect patient outcomes.

  4. To communicate and implement the planned action and follow-up at the unit level.

  5. To identify trends for potential monitoring and evaluation.

  6. To report Quality Assurance analysis to Nursing Council at each regular meeting.

  d. Meetings

  1. The committee will meet at least monthly or as called by the Chair.

  2. Each committee member will receive written notice prior to meetings for attendance.

  3. An annual written report summarizing the accomplishments of the committee shall be prepared by the Chair and shall be presented to Nursing and Executive Council.

ARTICLE VIII

PARLIAMENTARY AUTHORITY

The business of this group shall be conducted according to Robert's Rules of Order.

ARTICLE IX

AMENDMENTS

The bylaws may be amended at any regular meeting by a majority vote. Any member of Council may present an amendment for vote.

  The proposed amendment must be presented to the Committee in writing one month prior to voting.

8 HUMAN RESOURCE DEVELOPMENT:
Recruitment, Retention, and Managing Conflict

Elizabeth Thomas, MSN, RN
Kathy S. Thompson, MSN, RN
Robert W. Koch, DNS, RN

LEARNING OBJECTIVES AND ACTIVITIES

- Develop a list of strategies to use in recruiting students into nursing education programs.
- Develop an effective nurse recruitment advertisement.
- Conduct an effective simulated interview of a nurse applicant.
- Describe the assessment center process.
- Define the terms *human resource development, autonomy, empowerment,* and *andragogy.*
- Discuss the relevance of autonomy and empowerment in human resource development in nursing.
- Apply the concept of andragogy to human resource development in nursing.
- Discuss the promotion and termination policies of an employing organization.
- Analyze causes of conflict and its relationship to human resource issues.
- Make plans to manage conflict.
- Use techniques or skills for managing conflict.
- Discuss cultural diversity and its relationship to human resource issues.

CONCEPTS

Human resource management, recruiting, selecting, credentialing, assigning, assessment center, retaining, turnover, career planning, human resource development, autonomy, empowerment, andragogy, promoting and terminating, conflict, conflict management, cultural diversity, cultural sensitivity, cultural awareness, cultural competence

QUOTE

Try to learn something about everything and everything about something.

—Thomas Huxley

Plans, organizes, directs, and controls all aspects of the development of a human resource management program that meets all legal requirements governing personnel employment; manages people to reflect human resource management policies and procedures according to industry standards.

Establishes direction, aligns persons, stimulates motivation, and inspires people to make useful change in performing their nursing roles. Uses input from employees to identify those factors that recruit and retain the best personnel available. Promotes human resource management activities to reflect the cutting edge of advancements in the field. Uses research results to develop a model of human resource development that leads people and enhances their productivity by putting to use their specific knowledge and strengths.

Introduction

Human resource management is the activities an organization conducts to use its human resources effectively. The effective use of human resources enhances organization performance and fosters the attainment of strategic goals. Human resource management includes the activities of human resources planning, recruitment, selection, orientation, training, performance appraisal, compensation, and safety. Human resource management is the strategic and coherent approach to the management of an organization's most valued assets—the people working there, who individually and collectively contribute to the achievement of the objectives of the enterprise.[1] This chapter provides an overview of processes used in the management and the development of human resources.

RECRUITMENT

Recruiting Students into Nursing

Maintaining a steady pipeline of individuals into the profession of nursing should be a consideration of all nurse executives. As the existing nursing workforce ages, the number of individuals recruited into nursing as a profession is of utmost importance. The United States is in the midst of a nursing shortage that is expected to intensify as baby boomers age and their need for health care grows. Compounding the problem is the fact that nursing colleges and universities across the country are struggling to expand enrollment levels to meet the rising demand for nursing care.

Some projections estimate that the U.S. shortage of registered nurses (RNs) will increase to 340,000 by the year 2020.[2]

Evidence-Based Practice 8-1

Based on findings from the Nursing Management Aging Workforce Survey, 55% of surveyed nurses reported their intention to retire between 2011 and 2020. The majority of those surveyed were nurse managers.[3] Furthermore, in April 2006 officials with the Health Resources and Services Administration released projections that the nation's nursing shortage would grow to more than 1 million nurses by the year 2020.[4]

With these projections, it becomes every nurse executive's responsibility to initiate recruitment at the prelicensure level. The business of recruiting students into nursing requires long-term strategies for all educators and healthcare providers. Recruitment is more effective if potential consumers of nursing services are involved. Professional nurses can work through community organizations to involve the community in changing the image of nursing and in the recruitment effort. The image of nursing should reflect the qualifications and credentials of caregivers that provide safe, effective care to individuals and communities. However, nursing leaders must also consider that preconceived stereotypes of nursing exist and may negatively affect recruitment efforts.

Evidence-Based Practice 8-2

In a survey of 641 college-bound high-school seniors, investigators attempted to determine why nursing is not selected more frequently as a career option. Although the overall opinion about nursing was favorable, most of the students (86%) believed that nurses mainly followed doctors' orders. Only a few students believed that nurses do important work (5.4%); that nursing is challenging (9.4%), a real profession (9.3%), an important profession (5.4%); or that it provides a good opportunity to help people (3%).[5]

If the workforce issues related to the nursing shortage are to be managed, nursing leadership must consider what impressions are being portrayed of professional nurses. Healthcare agencies have tremendous opportunities in shaping the image of professional nursing. Some healthcare facilities have formed specific committees that focus on the recruitment of students into nursing education programs. From this work, a multitude of initiatives have been successful in recruiting individuals into the nursing profession. Figure 8-1 lists some activities that may be helpful recruiting into nursing education programs.

Recruiting Nurses into Employment

Pivotal in the role of nurse executives, the recruitment of qualified nursing professionals is paramount to ensuring safe and effective care delivery. The goal in recruiting is to attract the best and the brightest. However, many employers of nursing have settled for the "warm body" to fill the empty position. This unfortunately often leaves the selection of new nurses to chance and may result in both unhappy employee and miserable employer.

Employers of nurses must be willing to do what it takes to attract the best and brightest talent. Today's workforce is not as complex as some may believe. In fact, most nurses are merely looking for the basics: challenging assignments, opportunities to grow as professionals, authentic work–life balance, and economic rewards. The efforts to recruit nurses should be focused and intentional. Otherwise, recruitment efforts are left up to chance with disappointing results.

| FIGURE 8-1 | STRATEGIES FOR RECRUITING NURSING STUDENTS |

1. Form a committee to create a plan.
   a. Include clinical nurses
   b. Set goals
   c. Create a management plan for each goal

2. Obtain recruitment materials from organizations.
   a. National League for Nursing (NLN)
   b. American Nurses Association (ANA)
   c. American Organization of Nurse Executives (AONE)
   d. National Student Nurses Association (NSNA)
   e. American Association of Colleges of Nursing (AACN)
   f. State
   g. Local

3. Prepare additional recruitment materials.
   a. News stories for newspapers, TV, and radio
   b. Posters for schools
   c. Speakers' bureau
   d. Model speeches
   e. Tours

4. Coordinate with other nurse education programs and prospective employers of nurses.
   a. Associate degree programs
   b. Diploma programs
   c. BSN programs
   d. Hospitals
   e. Public health
   f. Staffing agencies
   g. Ambulatory care facilities
   h. Nursing homes
   i. LPN programs
   j. Other

5. Prepare and offer consultation programs for junior and senior high schools.
   a. Administrators
   b. Teachers
   c. Guidance counselors
   d. Students, including potential dropouts
   e. Financial advisers
   f. Language and cultural resource advisers

6. Coordinate activities of recruiters in schools of nursing.
   a. Sources of information by telephone and mail
   b. Target adults seeking second careers, men, minorities, and immigrants

7. Involve community agencies in recruitment efforts.
   a. Professional organizations
   b. Social organizations
   c. Service organizations
   d. Others

8. Evaluate results accomplished.
   a. Number and locations of programs presented
   b. Number of students counseled
   c. Number of follow-ups
   d. Number of applicants to local or other programs
   e. Homerooms visited
   f. Career days held by high schools, schools of nursing, and employers
   g. Inquiries to source persons by telephone or letter

9. Do work-study programs.
   a. High schools with employers
   b. High schools with schools of nursing
   c. Schools of nursing with employers
   d. Cooperative education

Source: Author.

Successful recruitment efforts begin with a strategic plan. Without a plan, what do employers tell prospective employees about the facilities' future? Bright people expect documented strategies and a game plan. One of the best ways to welcome developing nursing professionals into the workplace is to offer them a spot on a team. Generations X and Y, those born between 1965 and 1976 and 1977 and 1994, respectively, value the chance to be part of a group with a larger goal.[6] However, if the prospective workplace has no goals, the potential employee may find a more attractive and exciting place to work.

Another part of the strategic recruitment plan is to examine the needs of the workplace. In other words, the employer needs to know what talent and skills the job will require. Additionally, there should be written job descriptions for every position that reflect reality. There should be no hidden duties or assignments. Nurses in today's job market also consider availability of support staff when considering an employer. Healthcare facilities that protect the professional staff through the use of ancillary personnel to accomplish non-nursing functions are attractive to the potential nurse employee.[7]

Training and learning is no longer a benefit—it is an expectation. Today's nursing workforce expect more than just technical competence; they have been educated to insist on continuing education that will aid in their professional development. Nursing leadership must commit to' the investment. Additionally, the facility must provide up-to-date technology. The best employees expect the best tools.

Today's healthcare employers must be willing to offer the nurse the opportunity for work–life balance. One of the reasons many children of nurses shun the profession is the absence of work–life balance they witnessed while growing up. Today's nurses are no longer willing to work the long arduous work schedules that once dictated the lives of their professional predecessors. The successful employer who recognizes that nurses need time to rejuvenate will not only recruit but will maintain a healthy nursing workforce.

Finally, there must be room for advancement or bright nurses will not stay. The facility that is serious about recruiting will develop mechanisms that provide clear passageways for advancement. One example is the use of career ladders and clinical advancement programs. There are no magic formulas for recruiting nurses; a sound recruitment plan will clearly differentiate one healthcare facility from another and make it a strong contender in the fight for today's most talented nurses.

Nurse Recruiter

Critically important to the nursing organization is the nurse recruiter. The nurse recruiter is the person who is responsible for identifying and screening/evaluating qualified candidates for an open position within the organization. The recruiter generally works closely with the nurse executive to determine which candidates are best suited for open positions. Nurse recruiters are expected to have knowledge of health care and its practices, policies, environment, and culture. Additionally, the nurse recruiter must be familiar with federal, state, and local hiring laws.

A good nurse recruiter is an experienced interviewer and uses an array of interviewing techniques. Recruiters need outstanding sales and communication skills because many times they serve as the facilities' representative. Frequently, the nurse recruiter must "sell" the healthcare facility's career opportunities to applicants. The nurse recruiter must possess a strong ability to build internal and external relationships with multiple customers.

One function of the nurse recruiter is the development of an organizational recruitment plan. In many organizations, the nurse recruiter works closely with the leadership to create a formal nurse recruitment plan. The plan for workforce recruitment is influenced by factors such as structural reorganization, turnover and retention, and vacant positions. There are six steps of a formal recruitment plan:[8]

1. Gathering a database through situational scanning, forecasting, and variance audits comparing demand with supply data
2. Setting objectives
3. Designing strategies to accomplish the objectives
4. Establishing the annual nurse recruitment budget
5. Implementing the strategies through operational plans
6. Evaluating and using feedback to take corrective action

Marketing

An organization that is perceived to be the "employer of choice" retains their employees and is more capable of replacing their losses than are less sought-after employees. A variety of recruitment methods may be used for communicating nursing vacancies and when choosing a specific way to reach potential employees. Some popular options are internal job postings; newspaper, radio, and television advertisements; trade magazine advertisements; Internet job sites; college campus interviews; and current employee referrals. The choice of which option to use depends on the number of positions to be filled and the cost of each recruitment method.

In considering marketing and recruiting materials, it is important to remember that image matters. Recruitment brochures, pamphlets, and written material should be enticing and provide the applicant with a desire to work for the organization. Web sites, specifically, should be professionally designed and easy to navigate. Efforts should be directed toward providing the potential applicant with information that directly influences their intention to pursue employment.[9]

Some recruiting experts recommend a marketing approach to recruitment of nurses. Such an approach focuses on the nurse as the consumer of employment. Figure 8-2 presents a scheme for a marketing survey for recruiting and retaining nurses that includes some of these ideas. The marketing plan determines what needs to be done to sell employment to prospective professional nurses. Data are analyzed, objectives set and evaluated, and a plan made and promoted.[10]

Interview

Thompson defines an interview as "an equal level, face-to-face discussion between a job seeker and a person with full authority to fill the position under discussion."[11] Nurses, as the job seekers, want a face-to-face discussion with the person who has hiring authority. They may be considering several jobs, having narrowed the field down to those that specifically fit their career goals.

FIGURE 8-2 | CRITERIA FOR DEVELOPING AN EFFECTIVE NURSE RECRUITMENT ADVERTISEMENT

1. Target the population.

2. Catch the reader's attention.

3. Consider a picture that depicts a professional nurse in action, the kind of action nurses say they want.

4. List several factors that attract nurses:
   a. Opportunity for self-fulfillment
   b. Knowledge of helping others
   c. Intellectual stimulation
   d. Educational opportunity
   e. Fellowship with colleagues
   f. Adequate income
   g. Opportunity for innovation
   h. Opportunity to choose hours
   i. Opportunity for advancement
   j. Chance to be a leader
   k. Adequate support systems
   l. Child-care facilities
   m. Good fringe benefits
   n. Entrepreneurial opportunities

5. Involve clinical nurses in developing the advertisement.

6. Test the advertisement on the clinical nurse staff.

7. Run the ad in the Sunday newspapers, selecting those that are read by the target population.

8. Run the ad in nursing journals that are read by the target population.

9. Establish a Web site.

10. Provide for telephone and mail replies from applicants.
    a. Free telephone numbers
    b. Specific address
    c. Fax number and e-mail address

11. Provide for effective telephone and mail replies to be returned from the organization.
    a. The phone should be answered with positive responses that elicit interviews. Clinical nurses making immediate follow-up calls to prospective applicants can be effective.
    b. Effective packages of recruitment materials mailed to prospective applicants. (Depict and detail factors listed under number 4.)

12. Arrange for interview, including a visit to the organization.
    a. Contact person and sponsor
    b. Travel reimbursement
    c. Paid room and meals
    d. Interviews with person doing hiring; personnel specialists, including recruiter; and clinical nurses

13. Make a follow-up offer in writing.

14. Form a cadre of retired nurses (over 65 years of age)
    a. Establish with an appealing name
    b. Use a specific identification (a uniform or patch)
    c. Identify specialties needed
    d. Identify shifts needed
    e. Reward with good pay and continuing education

Source: Author.

The nurse recruiter or a human resources specialist will compile a personnel file that contains a completed application form, a resume or curriculum vitae, references, and any documents that are required by policy or law, such as a current, valid license to practice nursing and school transcripts. The interviewer should prepare for the interview by reading the information in the applicant's file. The interviewer should make notes of questions to ask the applicant about the information contained in the file. Adequate time should be set aside for the interview, which should take place in a private office where there will be no interruptions. An interview guide is helpful in conducting an interview satisfactorily to both the nurse manager and the applicant (Figure 8-3).

All candidates for nurse jobs should be treated as professionals. It is illegal to ask them certain questions, such as those listed in Figure 8-4. Information about age and date of birth may be necessary, for insurance or other benefits, can be obtained after the candidate is hired. Also, consider that many candidates have questions. When complete information cannot be given, the interviewer should make a note, get the information, and communicate it to the candidate as quickly as possible. Figure 8-5 lists questions that candidates may ask and that the interviewer should be prepared to answer. Eye contact, rapport, and follow-up after the interview are important strategies to incorporate into the interview process. Figure 8-6 outlines the nurse executive's responsibilities as well as those of the candidate.

Assessment Center Process

Hiring is an investment in the right and best-qualified person. Interviewing techniques are often cursory and do not result in hiring the right person. Assessment center techniques should be considered for the hiring of nursing professionals. Del Bueno, Weeks, and Brown-Stewart define the assessment center as "a comprehensive, standardized process by which multiple sampling techniques are used to determine an individual's actual or potential ability to perform skills and activities vital to success on the job."[12]

FIGURE 8-3	**INTERVIEW GUIDE**

Candidate:

Date and time of interview:

1. Arrange seating.

2. Make introductions and establish rapport.

3. Ask prepared questions.
   a. Tell me about yourself.
   b. What is your present job?
   c. What are your three most outstanding accomplishments?
   d. What is the extent of your formal education?
   e. What three things are most important to you in your job?
   f. What is your strongest qualification for this job?
   g. What other jobs have you held in this or a similar field?
   h. What were your responsibilities?
   i. Do you mind irregular working hours? Explain.

   j. Would you be willing to relocate? To travel?
   k. What minimum salary are you willing to accept?
   l. Are you more comfortable working alone or with other people?

4. Answer candidate's questions.

5. Note the following: Candidate was
   a. On time
   b. Well dressed
   c. Well mannered
   d. Positive about self

6. Maintain eye contact.

7. Note candidate's personal values.

8. Close the interview.
   a. Make an offer
   b. Obtain acceptance
   c. Set timetable for making offer or receiving response to offer

---

Source: Author.

FIGURE 8-4	ILLEGAL QUESTIONS

Employment interviewers are forbidden by law to ask the following questions:

1. Age

2. Date of birth

3. The length of time residing at present address

4. Previous address

5. Religion; church attended; spiritual adviser's name

6. Father's surname

7. Maiden name (of women)

8. Marital status

9. Residence mates

10. Number and ages of children; who will care for them while applicant works

11. Transportation to work, unless a car is a job requirement

12. Residence of spouse or parent

13. Whether residence is owned or rented

14. Name of bank; information on outstanding loans

15. Whether wages were ever garnished

16. Whether bankruptcy was ever declared

17. Whether ever arrested

18. Hobbies, off-duty interests, clubs

Source: Author.

FIGURE 8-5	CANDIDATE'S QUESTIONS AND INTERVIEWING TIPS

1. How much job security does this job have?

2. What previous experience does this type of job require?

3. What is the future of this type of job?

4. What is the growth potential for this particular job?

5. Where will the most significant growth for this type of job in the healthcare industry occur?

6. What is the starting salary for this job?

7. How do pay raises occur?

8. How does one find out when other job openings occur?

9. What are the fringe benefits of this job?

10. What are the requirements for working shifts and weekends?

11. What is the floating policy?

12. What are the opportunities for continuing education?

13. What are the opportunities for promotion?

14. What child care facilities are available?

15. What are the staffing and scheduling policies?

Tips

1. Keep the atmosphere positive, pleasant, and businesslike.

2. Focus on the essential goals.

3. Provide answers in a brief, factual, and friendly manner; use a soft and clear tone of voice; maintain a relaxed posture; and keep hands still.

4. Do not attempt to bluff answers to questions.

5. Review information sent to you before the interview.

6. Be prepared for questions related to personal philosophy and style, community relations, professional goals, clinical and administrative style, decision-making ability, flexibility in working with diverse groups, fiscal issues, personnel management, and group relationships.

7. Avoid controversial issues of religion, abortion, and politics; do not discuss confidential matters.

Source: Author.

| FIGURE 8-6 | WHAT HAPPENS DURING AN INTERVIEW? |

The hiring executive

1. Gives information about job and institution.

2. Assesses the competencies the candidate possesses in relation to the job opening.

3. Evaluates the candidate's personal characteristics in relation to the staff members with whom candidate will work (fit to staff).

4. Assesses candidate's potential to move organization toward its goals.

5. Assesses candidate's enthusiasm and state of health.

6. Forms impressions about candidate based on behavior, appearance, ability to communicate, confidence, intelligence, personality.

7. Assesses candidate's ability to do the job.

8. Determines facts about candidate.

The candidate

1. Gives information about self.

2. Assesses the opportunity for developing and using competencies on the job.

3. Assesses ability to relate to the employees with whom candidate will work.

4. Assesses potential for achieving personal career goals.

5. Assesses the institution's climate and the morale of the employees.

6. Assesses opportunities for promotion and success.

7. Assesses own ability to do the job.

8. Determines facts about the organization and working conditions.

Source: Author.

The assessment center process pools information from various sources. It may also be used to plan orientation programs, for promotions, and for placement in clinical and career ladders. The following are some other characteristics of the assessment center process:

1. Assessment center process exercises are developed to measure job dimensions.
2. Assessors are selected and specifically trained to rate the candidates.
3. Each candidate is assessed by at least two persons.
4. Reliability and validity of assessment centers are high.
5. The process is job specific.
6. The process is equitable to minorities and women.
7. The process has self-development value for participants.
8. The process is expensive and may favor conformists.
9. The process diminishes the risk of hiring or promoting inappropriate candidates.
10. The process is stressful, time-consuming, and tiring for assessors; it favors outsiders.

In a similar process, a master interview tool may be developed that categorizes content such as documented clinical and administrative expertise, research, education, and other significant factors. In this method, points are assigned according to the weight of each rating category for various positions. A pool of interview questions is developed to determine the applicant's ability to communicate, organize thoughts, solve problems, and relate to others; to assess the applicant's knowledge, philosophy, experience, and personality traits; and to reveal the applicant's frame of reference, level of expectation, attitudes, feelings, and management style. Interview panels consist of three members, the chair being appointed by the chief nurse executive. The tool is claimed to have fairly high interrater reliability, to decrease interview time, and to assist in selecting the most qualified applicant.[13]

Search Committee

A search committee is a group of individuals who serve as representatives of the employing agency and who participate in application screening, interviewing, and selecting the top job candidate(s). Many jobs that entail great responsibility in the organization result in the appointment of a search committee. The objective is to obtain input into the hiring process from the people who will be affected by the appointment. Such committees are widely used in higher education. The following is an outline of search committee procedures:[14]

1. A search committee is appointed by the chief executive officer with input from the population to be affected.
2. A chair is appointed by administration or elected by the search committee to serve as the liaison between the two.
3. The search committee's responsibilities are clearly laid out by policy or by the committee itself. Most committees recruit, screen, interview, and recommend applicants. Administrators generally make final decisions about appointments.
4. The search committee usually agrees at the outset to maintain all information about applicants confidential. It will not discuss any individual candidate outside the committee, except in general terms of progress reports to staff or faculty.
5. The search committee selects and implements a strategy for recruiting candidates.
6. Applications are screened after references and credentials have been obtained.
7. Applicants are scheduled for interviews and visits to the institution. Figure 8-7 contains a list of possible search committee interview questions.
8. Once all applicants have been interviewed, the committee analyzes the information and ranks the candidates.
9. A list of recommended applicants is sent to the chief executive officer.
10. The chief executive officer invites an applicant for a return visit and decides whether to make a job offer.

FIGURE 8-7   **PREPARATORY QUESTIONS FOR SEARCH COMMITTEE**

1. What style of management do you follow?
2. What are your personal weaknesses and strengths?
3. What are your perceptions of the role the person in this job will perform?
4. How can this organization benefit your career?
5. What are your ideas of what the relationship should be between nurses and physicians?
6. What job in nursing would you like most to have?
7. What do you view as the role of nursing in this organization?
8. What do you view as the role of nursing in the community?
9. What do you think of collective bargaining?
10. How would you go about determining that your department operates efficiently and effectively?
11. Why should I (we) hire you?
12. How would you go about meeting the goals of the organization?
13. How would your family adapt to this area?
14. What are your career goals?

Source: Author.

SELECTING AND ASSIGNING

Selecting

The consequences of poor hiring will be exaggerated in the coming years as the nursing shortage continues to grow. Furthermore, it will be more difficult and more expensive to replace nurses. As a result, healthcare organizations that make more hiring "mistakes" will have a multitude of critical negative consequences to address. There are specific steps the healthcare organization can take to help nurse executives and managers improve their ability to make better hiring decisions. These include training the nurse leader in appropriate hiring skills.

The importance of management training cannot be stressed enough. To increase the likelihood of making better hiring decisions, organizations must provide training for all managers. Although the human resource department in larger organizations generally partners with managers and takes the lead in screening many job candidates, the line managers still play a big role in the hiring process and almost always make the final decision.

Although the mechanics of the hiring process are important, soft skills development is equally important. These might include general interpersonal skills, communication, etiquette, and even the legal dos and don'ts of interviewing.

The organization must place an emphasis on good hiring. This can be achieved, in part, by including hiring effectiveness on the nurse leader's performance appraisal. With so many responsibilities pulling nurse executives in different directions, those job duties that are included on the performance appraisal are likely to be higher priorities. It communicates to nurse managers that it is an important organizational objective and deserves their attention.

A critical mistake occurs when the nurse leader "passes," or fails to hire a talented individual just because a few technical skills are missing. The manager must exercise judgment to ensure the "missing" skills are not essential for the effective performance of the current job and can, indeed, be acquired in a reasonable period of time. There is a fine line between hiring a marginal employee and hiring a talented employee with the untapped potential to be a star performer. One can drag the organization down and the other can contribute immensely to the company's successful performance.

The ability to hire top talent should be an integral responsibility of every manager. After all, it directly impacts the manager's own success (and, ultimately, the organization's as well). It has been said that one is only as good as the people one surrounds oneself with.

Assigning

During the initial assignment period the new nurse is oriented to the job description. Candidates should have a choice of the possible units to which they will be assigned. However, there are times when a requested job assignment is not available or a position is not open. For example, where can a candidate who wants to work in the operating room be assigned when no vacancies exist in this area? In this situation, the candidate can be offered a choice of vacant positions in a clinical area that may be similar, such as a postoperative surgical unit. Also, the employer may consider contracting with the employee with a promise to transfer to a vacated position when one becomes available. However, it is unethical and poor practice for the employer to make a promise that he or she cannot fulfill. Such practices result in mistrust and ultimately a poor reputation among the staff.

It is imperative that new employees not be surprised by their assignments on the first day of working a new job. When assignment policies are fair, reasonable, and acceptable, candidates start work with a positive attitude. Thorough orientation is essential to ensure competency, job satisfaction, and high productivity in the particular assignments the nurse is accepting.

RETENTION

The retention of competent professional nurses in jobs is a major problem of the U.S. healthcare industry, particularly for hospitals and long-term care facilities. Most Americans change jobs about 15 times by the age of 35, and nurses are no exception. Nurses change and achieve major career goals four or five times in their lifetime, including changing their specialty or the role they play in the profession.[15] However, it is clearly recognized that a wise strategy for nurse executives is to focus on making internal improvements rather than worrying needlessly about external labor market conditions that are outside of management control.

It is far better to retain nurses than to recruit them; the advantages include cost benefits, high morale, and high-quality care. One study indicated that nurses stayed in their jobs when they received peer support, participated in a professional practice model, received tuition reimbursement, and had input into decision making; when communication was open; and when medical staff was supportive.[16] Nurse executives are advised to incorporate the American Nurses Association RN Bill of Rights as part of the organization's nurse retention policies (Figure 8-8).

| FIGURE 8-8 | AMERICAN NURSES ASSOCIATION'S BILL OF RIGHTS FOR REGISTERED NURSES |

All registered nurses have

1. The right to practice in a manner that fulfills their obligations to society and to those who receive nursing care.

2. The right to practice in environments that allow them to act in accordance with professional standards and legally authorized scopes of practice.

3. The right to a work environment that supports and facilitates ethical practice, in accordance with the *Code of Ethics for Nurses* and its interpretive statements.

4. The right to freely and openly advocate for themselves and their patients, without fear of retribution.

5. The right to fair compensation for their work, consistent with their knowledge, experience, and professional responsibilities.

6. The right to a work environment that is safe for themselves and their patients.

7. The right to negotiate the conditions of their employment, either as individuals or collectively, in all practice settings.

Source: Copyright © American Nurses Association. Reprinted with permission.

Turnover

According to a study by Aiken and colleagues, more than 40% of nurses working in hospitals reported being dissatisfied with their jobs. The study indicates that one of every three hospital nurses under the age of 30 is planning to leave his or her current job in the next year.[17] In 2007 a report released by the Price Waterhouse Coopers' Health Research Institute found that though the average nurse turnover rate in hospitals was 8.4%, the average voluntary turnover for first-year nurses was 27.1%.[18]

Evidence-Based Practice 8-3

In a comprehensive report initiated by the Agency for Healthcare Research and Quality in 2007, the authors found that the shortage of registered nurses, in combination with an increased work load, poses a potential threat to the quality of care. Additional analysis has found that every 1% increase in nurse turnover costs a hospital about $300,000 a year. Furthermore, hospitals that perform poorly in nurse retention spend, on average, $3.6 million more than those with high retention rates. Considering these studies, it is apparent that nurse turnover is a monumental problem that not only affects quality patient care but also the costs of care.19

Job Expectations and Satisfaction

There is little doubt that the high turnover rate in nursing is a result of job dissatisfaction. Multiple studies have examined the determinants of turnover within nursing with inconclusive findings. However, it appears that organizational climate/culture is an important determinant of "intent to leave" among nurses.[20] Higher wages do not reduce intent to leave, and increased pay alone without attention to organizational climate is unlikely to reduce nurse turnover.

There is a direct correlation in retaining nurses and the leadership skills of the nurse manager. Skills that enhance nurse retention include transformation leadership style, extroverted personality traits, fostering of nurse empowerment, autonomy, and group cohesion.

For nurses, the lack of recognition or lack of advancement opportunities is also a likely reason to leave a job. It is too easy for nursing leaders to blame a lack of monetary compensation for nurse turnover, when in reality it is poor management and poor human relations. Nurses must feel valued and believe they make a difference in the organization. Nursing leaders must recognize and incorporate strategies to foster a culture where the nurse is valued for their contribution. Implementing interventions aimed at creating positive work environments is one of the most effective strategies to reduce nurse turnover.

Retention Strategies

Nurses leave an organization because they believe their nursing work is not adequately valued and they are not able to provide the level of care they know patients deserve. Many healthcare organizations have initiated interventions to decrease nurse turnover and create positive work environments that will satisfy nurses. Below are a few examples of nurse retention strategies.

Nurse Retention Coordinator

Indiana University Hospital developed a model with a designated full-time nurse retention coordinator. The duties of the coordinator include conducting exit/transfer interviews with nurses, holding one-to-one retention discussions, and leading unit interviews. The coordinator tackles such problems as schedule negotiation, employee reassignment, conflict resolution, and referring nurses for help with stress and burnout. The nurse retention coordinator also conducts educational sessions on team building and recognition of cultural and generational differences.[21]

Management Education

Worried by the severe shortage of nurses, one healthcare facility in Tennessee developed an action plan to educate nurse leaders in strategies to retain the nursing workforce. This facility based their intervention on the belief that nurse retention is directly related to the abilities of the nurse leaders in the organization. This hospital system tackled their retention problems by strengthening the nurse leadership through classroom and online instruction, external consultation with management experts, and an assessment of each manager's abilities for coaching and developing employees.[22]

Retaining the Older Worker

With a critical nursing shortage on the horizon, it is very important to keep older, experienced nurses in the workforce longer. To do this, several strategies may be used to keep the older nurse employed. One facility recognized that older nurses must be satisfied with their jobs and feel "job embeddedness," which includes feeling linked to the people and the institution. Some ways that increase embeddedness in older workers include offering flexible scheduling, mentoring opportunities, and allowing the older employee to represent the institution within the community.[23]

For some older nurses, the need to care for ailing parents or a spouse may cause them to exit the workforce. Some healthcare facilities consider offering "elder day care" to keep the senior nurse on the job. Other desired job attributes of older nurses include coworker support, teamwork, retirement benefits, adequate equipment, healthcare benefits, open door policy, respect from physicians, job security, shift of choice, paid time off, respect from administration, and educational opportunities. If healthcare organizations are to keep the most experienced nurses, nurse leaders must consider these attributes as necessities rather than fringe benefits. The loss of the most experienced nurses will no doubt affect quality care and have major effects on the organization.

Career Planning

Employees tend to stay longer in an organization where they are experiencing personal and professional growth. Employers who share their vision for the organization, including the growth plan, foster a climate of organizational connectedness and reduce intent to leave. When an employee feels challenged and cared for, he or she will more likely stay longer on the job. Nurse leaders must learn ways to assist professional nurses to achieve career satisfaction if they are to retain the workforce. To be successful in their careers, professional nurses need a sense of personal fulfillment and job significance.

Career Ladders and Career Development Programs

The career ladder is used to denote vertical job promotion. In business and human resources management, the ladder typically describes the progression from entry-level positions to higher levels of pay, skill, responsibility, or authority. Moving up the career ladder should be a function of three factors: time, performance, and skill set attainment. Advancing in the career development program should not be so easy that it becomes automatic simply by employment longevity. Most experts agree that employees should demonstrate a commitment to the organization before being considered for advancement within the career ladder. An employee should "put in" a designated amount of time before being eligible to climb the next level of a career ladder.[24]

A good employee development program must be based on performance over an extended period of time. Documentation typically includes the annual performance appraisal and more informal items, such as written commendations for outstanding service.

Continuing education is a critical component in an effective employee development program and career ladder. To climb the career ladder, the employee should participate in a specified amount of continuing education. This education can be in the form of advanced college credits or merely continuing education units acquired through workshops or seminars related to the nurse's area of expertise, thus enhancing the existing skill set.

Properly administered, a career ladder should result in a win–win situation for both employers and employees. By using career ladders the nurse may receive recognition, corresponding salary increases, or increased prestige. With career ladders, the organization benefits from a more stable, better educated workforce.

However, there is one caveat the nurse executive should consider with the implementation of career ladders. Not every nurse will participate in career ladder advancement. Some employees are comfortable, and function well, at a lower level of responsibility and still meet the requirements of the job. Advancement on the career ladder should never be mandatory.

A clinical career ladder should do the following:

1. Improve the quality of patient care.
2. Motivate staff in the following areas:
   a. Job proficiency and expertise, that is, motivate nurses to reach their highest level of professional competence.
   b. Pursuit of education, which is an important factor in mobility
   c. Development of career goals
3. Provide methods of objective and measurable performance evaluation, and reward clinical competence for the purpose of advancement.
4. Promote retention within the clinical area and reduce the turnover rate.[25]

Performance criteria in any clinical ladder system should be clearly differentiated and specific at each level. The evaluation process must be measurable, and salary differentials must be significant enough to provide motivation. Any system should involve evaluation of educational and leadership criteria as well as skill performance. Figure 8-9 is an example of a basic clinical ladder model.

FIGURE 8-9 — BASIC CLINICAL LADDER MODEL

A. Clinical/Staff Nurse I (beginner/novice)
   1. Experience and Education
      Current state licensure with less than one year of experience.
   2. Description
      a. Needs close supervision.
      b. Performs basic nursing skills/routine patient care.
      c. Begins to develop patient assessment skills/communication skills.

B. Clinical/Staff Nurse II (advanced beginner)
   1. Experience and Education
      a. Current state licensure with more than 1 year of experience.
      b. BSN with more than 6 months of experience.
      c. MSN without experience.
   2. Description
      a. Demonstrates adequate/acceptable performance.
      b. Can differentiate importance of situations and set priorities.
      c. Requires less supervision.
      d. Demonstrates interest in continuing education.

C. Clinical/Staff Nurse III (competent)
   1. Experience and Education
      a. Current licensure with 2 or more years of experience.
      b. BSN with more than 1 year of experience.
      c. MSN with more than 6 months of experience.
   2. Description
      a. Demonstrates unsupervised competency using the nursing process.
      b. Is able to plan and organize in terms of short-range and long-range goals.
      c. Demonstrates direction in actions.
      d. Accepts leadership responsibility readily.
      e. Demonstrates well-developed communication skills.
      f. Shares ideas and knowledge with peers.

D. Clinical/Staff Nurse IV (proficient)
   1. Experience and Education
      a. Current licensure with 3 years of clinical experience and pursuit of BSN.

    b. BSN with more than 2 years of experience.
    c. MSN with more than 1 year of experience.

  2. Description
    a. Demonstrates specialized knowledge and skills.
    b. Continues professional education.
    c. Assumes leadership/supervisory responsibility.
    d. Recognizes and adjusts to situations that vary from the norm.
    e. Delegates responsibility appropriately; uses wide range of alternatives in solving problems.

E. Clinical/Staff Nurse V (expert)
  1. Experience and Education
    a. MSN with more than 2 years of appropriate clinical experience.
    b. BSN required with more than 3 years of experience; pursuing MSN.

  2. Description
    a. Demonstrates expertise in clinical practice.
    b. Assumes/delegates personnel and management responsibility.

Source: Author.

Job Variety and Job Sharing

Rotating employees through different jobs has many advantages, such as keeping employees stimulated and productive and eliminating boredom and burnout. It also lets the employee gain other useful skills, which can increase organizational productivity. Job rotation can be used for entry level employees as well as employees with more work experience. It could even be used for employees nearing retirement by allowing them to teach newer employees valuable knowledge useful within the company.

Job rotation can be tailored to fit the organization by rotating employees through special projects, partial week rotations, internships, or temporary assignments. The outcome of a properly run job rotation program includes retaining, motivating, and educating employees.

However, the nurse executive should not confuse job rotation programs with shift reassignment (pulling) to another unit. The chronic reassignment of nursing personnel to cover vacancies is always viewed as a negative to nurses and has been the cause of a great deal of disgruntlement. One sure way to negate any positive recruitment and retention efforts is to allow perpetual shift reassignment within the healthcare agency.

Another option for nursing is job sharing, that is, two persons filling one full-time equivalent job at a ratio of work agreed on by them. This option is convenient for nurses who want and can afford to work part-time and need the personal time off. Less acceptable to nurses has been mandatory sharing of work in organizations in which technology and restructuring have reduced the amount of available labor for pay.[26]

HUMAN RESOURCE DEVELOPMENT

Human resource development (HRD) is the process by which corporate management stimulates the motivation of employees to perform productively. HRD provides the stimuli that motivate nursing personnel to provide nursing care services to clients at quality and quantity standards that keep the healthcare organization reputable and financially solvent, the nurses satisfied with their professional accomplishments and quality of work life, and the clients treated successfully.[27]

In HRD, people grow and prosper from learning to use the skills of problem solving, logic, inquiry, critical thinking, and decision making. HRD is a lifelong process. It is also a process of helping and sharing that leads to competence and satisfaction with both the process and outcomes. The HRD process facilitates self-direction, self-discipline, focus on immediate problems, and satisfaction related to employee participation in problem solving and decision making.[28]

Nurse executives and managers in today's workforce must be knowledgeable in developing the most precious resource—the nursing staff. HRD encompasses many concepts, including problem solving, decision making, leadership, motivation, and communication. In nursing, HRD should be a proactive program and part of strategic planning.

Healthcare organization administrators have discovered that efficiency and effectiveness are byproducts of formalized human development programs. Programs that facilitate human relationships, reliability, initiative, autonomy, and talents promote trust, reduce stress, and facilitate communication.

Empowerment and Autonomy

Empowerment of professional nurses can go a long way in developing employee autonomy and accountability. To increase the level of nurse accountability and autonomy, the leadership needs to increase the level of employee empowerment in the organization. Nurse executives must understand that the level of nurse autonomy and accountability seldom increase without leadership making efforts to increase the level of empowerment first.

To increase empowerment and thus nurse accountability, a program that starts with the executive leadership and then moves to management training and supervisor training is needed. Only when the leaders, managers, and supervisors have a common understanding for employee empowerment is it likely that that the level of employee autonomy will increase. Then, the next logical step is to educate employees who may need training in problem-solving skills.[29]

People want to be successful, perform well, learn new skills, and be involved in decisions about their work. Managers who support the professional autonomy of nurses support empowerment of this group. Through empowerment, professional nurses gain a sense of control and are capable of using their own strength and power to solve workplace problems. Empowerment is therapeutic and spiritual; it is healthy for both employees and the organization.[30]

Self-Awareness and Lifelong Learning

HRD is aimed at developing the employee to his or her optimal level of performance. One goal of HRD is the development of a self-reliant learner who remains a knowledgeable and skilled worker in the future. Humans are learning machines. We are most alive and functioning closest to our potential when we are learning, adapting, adjusting, and finding new ways, approaches, and techniques to improve our lives (or the lives of others) in some way.

The nurse executive should encourage self-awareness and lifelong learning among all levels of the staff. It is through HRD activities that employees think about what they are experiencing in one part of their work life and how it relates to and connects with challenges, problems, opportunities, and situations that occur in other parts. Effective HRD helps employees to realize that they must be willing to adapt and change if they want to grow. Successful HRD programs are attained through mentoring of the leaders, support from staff development professionals, and the use of adult education theory to accomplish these goals.

Andragogy and HRD

Developed as a leading educational theory, Malcolm Knowles popularized andragogy as one central consideration in educating the adult learner. Andragogy is the process of engaging adult learners in the structure of the learning experience. Knowles' theory can be stated as four simple postulates:[31]

1. Adults need to be involved in the planning and evaluation of their instruction (self-concept and motivation to learn).
2. Experience (including mistakes) provides the basis for learning activities (experience).

3. Adults are most interested in learning subjects that have immediate relevance to their job or personal life (readiness to learn).
4. Adult learning is problem centered rather than content oriented (orientation to learning).

In HRD learners are adults, and educational programs are based on theories of adult education. Nursing leaders who strive to promote HRD within an organization should consider principles of adult learning. A healthy environment must be established that allows adults to participate in making decisions that affect their work lives. HRD embraces the adult learner and assumes that education enriches one's life and promotes better employees.

Job Promotion and Advancement

A promotion is the advancement of rank or position in an organizational hierarchy system. Promotion may be an employee's reward for good performance. A promotion is when an employee is moved into a job with greater scope and responsibility than his or her current job. Promotions in and of themselves do not mean a monetary increase in salary. But in general, organizations adjust salaries with promotions when the monetary value of the new job is higher than the value of the job the incumbent currently holds. Before a company promotes an employee to a particular position, it ensures that the person is trained to handle the added responsibilities. This is marked by job enrichment and various training activities.

One way for nurse managers to ensure that all professional nurses have promotion opportunities is to develop a promotion system that indicates all promotion categories within the organization. Nurse managers should develop specific promotion policies with input from all categories of professional nurses and the human resource department. These policies should include the following:[32]

1. All vacant positions should be posted even if change in pay and rank does not occur.
2. Promotion rosters should be prepared that rank all candidates by education, experience, and performance with the best-qualified candidate at the top of the list.
3. Applicant interviews should be based on a set of established criteria.
4. The best-qualified candidates should be selected for promotion.
5. Unsuccessful candidates should be notified of the selection decision and individually counseled.
6. The promotion should be announced to appropriate employees within the organization.

Darling and McGrath write that some nurses may experience psychological trauma when moving upward from clinical to managerial positions. The newly promoted individual often is unaware of the transition process involved in a promotion, including the fact that social and professional ties are affected with other clinical nurses. Newly promoted individuals frequently take on more responsibilities and burdens and soon feel isolated and alone. To prevent or minimize anxiety associated with promotion, a transition program should include clear role descriptions and expectations, clear job descriptions, and classes in role transition strategies.[33]

Job Termination

Managers report that terminating employees is the job they most hate to do. Sometimes, however, terminating a staff person's employment is the best step to take for the organization. Sometimes terminating a person's employment is the kindest action the nursing leader can take for the person. In some circumstances, firing an employee is an immediate necessity for the safety and well-being of patients or other staff.

When terminating a worker, employers must take care to follow specific legal guidelines. By adhering to the necessary procedures, an employer can ensure that he or she avoids any legal entanglements and that the difficult situation is handled as smoothly as possible. Employees cannot be terminated at will. They are protected by public policy set forth in the National Labor Relations Act, the Civil Rights Act of 1964, the Age Discrimination in Employment Act, the Vocational Rehabilitation Act, and the Occupational Safety and Health Act. The legalities concerning job termination can be complicated and require the sage advice of a human resource specialist or legal counsel.[34]

In most cases, employees should be terminated only after all efforts to retain them have been exhausted. Disciplinary action should be progressive, moving from verbal conference, to written warning, to suspension, to discharge. Progressive disciplinary steps should be clearly defined by written policies and procedures.

Firing an employee is an unpleasant job. There are three major reasons for job termination: termination for cause, termination for poor performance, and job layoff.

Termination for Cause

One major reason for firing an employee is termination for cause. Included in this category are such actions as stealing from the organization or threatening another employee. In healthcare organizations, the endangerment of patients is another factor that warrants immediate termination. This type of termination occurs quickly because it is important to remove the problem employee from the workplace. Termination for cause is the easiest for the employer than other types of termination because the employee to be fired has committed a blatant offense.

Poor Performance

Most frequently, employees are fired because of poor work performance. This occurs when an employee performs poorly on the job consistently for some period of time. Employees fired for this reason are not entirely surprised. This is because a great deal of documentation, communication, and reevaluation is involved in making the decision to terminate employment because of poor performance.

The first time employees may be informed of a problem with their performance is at the employee evaluation. When an employee is given a poor evaluation, the supervisor should offer counseling so that the problem may be corrected. Often times, this nudge in the right direction is sufficient to correct the employee's errors. If an employee's performance does not improve with counseling, more steps must be taken to ensure that employee the opportunity to improve. The worker should receive a written document, explaining all deficiencies. It is important to thoroughly document both the offenses committed by the employee and steps taken to improve performance.

After counseling the employee and documenting the work-related problems, the employer should reevaluate the employee to ascertain the level of improvement. If all these steps are taken and there is little or no improvement in the employee's job performance, termination may be considered. In many cases, however, the struggling employee may realize that this job is not suitable to him or her. At that time, the employee may wish to resign of his or her own accord.

Layoffs

The final reason an employee may be terminated is the layoff. Employees are laid off when budget cuts or a lack of work compel the organization to sever the working relationship with one or more employees. This type of involuntary termination is unique, because the employee is not terminated because of his or her own actions. When considering layoffs it must first be determined that a reduction in staff is the only viable answer for the problem at hand.

Regardless of the reason, before terminating the employment of an individual, the manager must prepare carefully. First, the manager should consult with his or her supervisors. If the termination of the individual is not acceptable to the higher-ranking officials in the organization, the manager may not be able to fire that employee. The manager's supervisors should be kept abreast of all actions leading up to the decision to terminate employment.

In the termination process the manager should

- Review all written documents included in the individual's personnel file.
- Plan out and practice what will be said in the exit interview.
- Be able to answer any question the employee might have about the termination.
- Prepare a list of all company belongings that should be returned upon termination, such as keys or equipment.
- Consult legal counsel with questions about termination.
- Bring in a witness for the exit interview.

Document everything related to the employee's dismissal. If the employee takes legal action for unlawful termination, the manager will need a written record of the reason for termination and the exit conference with the employee. In the case of employees terminated for poor job performance, this means having on file all job evaluations, notices of deficiency, and a rough written transcript of what is said in the exit interview.[35]

CULTURAL COMPETENCE

The latest U.S. Census reports that one in every three Americans belongs to a racial/ethic minority group.[36] Developing respect for cultural diversity is essential for success in the workplace and is the foundation for building intercultural competence. "Culturally competent individuals value diversity and respect individual differences regardless of one's race, religious beliefs, or ethnocultural background."[37]

Culture can be described as the sum total of socially transmitted behavioral patterns, including the arts, beliefs, values, customs, and life-ways and other products of human work and thought of a population of people that focus on their world view and decision making.[38] Just as the expectation is that healthcare professionals is sensitive to the cultural influences of those for whom they care, the nurse administrator must also be culturally sensitive in recruitment, hiring, and retention strategies.

It is important to increase one's cultural awareness and sensitivity, because culture is largely unconscious and can be powerfully influential in communication, decision making, and handling conflict. The following outlines characteristics of cultural competence as described by Pernell and Paulanka.[39] Though these indicators are applied to clients, they may also be applied to healthcare providers.

- Developing an awareness of one's own existence, sensations, thoughts, and environment without letting them have an undue influence on those from other backgrounds
- Demonstrating knowledge and understanding of the client's culture, health-related needs, and culturally specific meanings of health and illness
- Accepting and respecting cultural differences
- Not assuming that the healthcare provider's beliefs and values are the same as the client's
- Resisting judgmental attitudes such as "different is not as good"
- Being open to cultural encounters
- Being comfortable with cultural encounters
- Adapting care (communication, decision making, conflict resolution) to be congruent with the client's culture
- Cultural competence is a conscious process and not necessarily linear.

Becoming culturally competent is a dynamic process between leadership, employees, and customers that requires cultural knowledge and skill development at all service levels, including strategic planning, policymaking, administration, and practice. Cultural competence and strong diversity management will help healthcare organizations effectively draw on talent and intellectual capital and motivate more employees.

CONFLICT MANAGEMENT IN A DIVERSE WORKFORCE

Dealing with conflict can be particularly challenging in the management of a culturally diverse workforce. Conflict management serves to improve communication, work relationships, and productivity outcomes. Creating a healthy work environment is critical to a culture of quality and safe healthcare delivery systems.

The American Organization of Nurse Executives strongly supports the identification and adoption of evidence-based management practices, which include attention to work redesign. An education and research priority of American Organization of Nurse Executives is creating positive and healthy work environments in nursing and health care. This is a challenge at best, requiring understanding of the organization's culture in handling conflict, costs of conflict, the impact of organizational complexity, barriers to managing conflict, and strategies for effective conflict resolution.[40]

Rapid changes in health care, including dismantling of the traditional structure in healthcare organization, have resulted in an atmosphere of the unknown. Additionally, uncertainties caused by changes in roles and role relationships and uncharted and evolving relationships with new categories of healthcare workers have added to the perplexing work environment. These factors often lead to conflict in the workplace.

Symptoms such as high levels of negativity and passivity; poor leadership; ineffective problem-solving skills; strangled communication flow; volatile emotions, with anger surfacing; difficulty accepting changes; and recruitment and retention difficulties further create conflicting individual and organizational goals.[41]

Conflict relates to feelings, including feelings of neglect, of being viewed as taken for granted, being treated like a servant, not being appreciated, being ignored, being overloaded, and other instances of perceived unfairness. Conflict relates to ignoring an individual's self-esteem and worth. The individual's feelings may build from anger to rage. During these times, overt negative behaviors such as brooding, withdrawing, arguing, instigating unrest among staff, or fighting can be observed. The individual can let feelings and behavior interfere with job performance, resulting in carelessness, mistakes in areas of responsibility, and reduced productivity for the unit of service.

Characteristics of Conflict

The characteristics of a conflict situation are as follows:[42]

- At least two parties (individuals or groups) are involved in some kind of interaction.
- Mutually exclusive goals or mutually exclusive values exist, either in fact or as perceived by the parties involved.
- Interaction is characterized by behavior destined to defeat, reduce, or oppress the opponent or to gain a mutually designated victory.
- The parties face each other with mutually opposing actions and counteractions.
- Each party attempts to create an imbalance or relatively favored position of power vis-à-vis the other.

Conflict in healthcare organizations can be viewed from a structural or political perspective. From the structural perspective, conflict interferes with the accomplishment of organizational purposes. Bolman and Deal note that hierarchical conflict raises the possibility that the lower the level of employee, the more likely that management directives may be subverted. Conflict among major partisan groups can undermine an organization's effectiveness and the ability of its leadership to function.[43]

Assessing Conflict

Hawkins and Kratsch describe different aspects of assessing a conflict situation, noting symptoms, underlying issues, and incorrect assumptions that can influence how the problem is defined. How this is handled may facilitate or hinder resolution of the true issue.[44]

Symptoms of conflict may include negative body language such as eye-rolling, turning away, repetition of story or request, disruptive behaviors (throwing objects, slamming doors), avoidance behaviors, turnover, compensation claims, and disability. Underlying needs and interest driving conflict may include needs not being met: resource needs (time, staff, space, information), psychological needs (recognition, respect, control, power, safety), emotional needs (fear, shame, sadness, loss, disappointment, support), and values in conflict (autonomy, dignity, honor, fairness or justice). Labels or inaccurate assumptions can also block resolution and are important to understand in assessing conflict. For example, labels such as "difficult family," "passive-aggressive coworker," "not a team player," "intellectual snob," "bully," "incompetent," and "uncooperative" may get in the way of true understanding of the issue and resolution.[45]

Antecedent Sources of Conflict

Conflict may develop from a number of antecedent sources:[46]

- Incompatible goals
- Distribution of scarce resources, when individuals have high expectations of rewards
- Regulations, when an individual's need for autonomy conflicts with another's need for regulating mechanisms
- Personality traits, attitudes, and behaviors
- Interest in outcomes
- Values
- Roles, when two individuals have equal responsibilities but actual boundaries are unclear, or when they are required to fill simultaneously two or more roles that present inconsistent or contradictory expectations
- Tasks, when outputs of one individual or group become inputs for another individual or group, or outputs are shared by several individuals or groups

Stress and Conflict

Conflict leads to stress, fear, anxiety, and disruption in professional relationships. These conditions can, in turn, increase the potential for conflict. Stressors include having too little responsibility, lack of participation in decision making, lack of managerial support, having to keep up with increasing standards of performance, and coping with rapid technological change.

Confrontations, disagreements, and anger are evidence of stress and conflict. Stress and conflict are caused by poorly expressed relationships among people, including unfilled expectations. Stress in patients leads to iatrogenic ailments, complications, and delayed recovery. It may be created by depression and anxiety. Stressed staff members cannot cope with stressed patients. Stressed staff display inefficiency, job dissatisfaction, and insensitive care.

Families, like patients, can add to stress when they are not managed appropriately. Increased stress for patients and staff members decreases effective use of staff time. These problems increase patient care costs because they increase the length of the illness and decrease nursing efficiency and effectiveness. In the future these patients may go somewhere else for care, whether on their own initiative or the recommendations of physicians, relatives, friends, or acquaintances.[47]

Conflict: Beliefs, Values, and Goals

Incompatible perceptions or activities create conflict. This is particularly evident when nurses hold beliefs, values, and personal goals different from those of nurse managers, physicians, patients, visitors, families, administrators, and so on. Nurses' values may boil over into conflicts related to ethical issues involving do not resuscitate orders, callous statements that belittle human worth, abortion, abuse, acquired immunodeficiency syndrome, and other problems. Personal goals may conflict with organizational goals, particularly with regard to staffing, scheduling, and the climate within which nurses work. Nurses who must violate their personal standards will lash out at the system.

Violating personal standards is demeaning to nurses and causes loss of self-esteem and emotional stress. Nurses must know they are valued and that their beliefs, values, and personal goals are respected. Like other people, nurses act to protect their personal or public image when confronted. They respond in terms of others' expectations of them because they want approval. They will defend their rights and their professional judgments. The ego is easily bruised and becomes a big problem in conflict. Defense becomes more heated when one or both parties to a conflict are uninformed or manipulated. When nurses are not recognized or respected, they feel helpless. They feel hopeless when they are unable to control the situation.[48]

Conflict Management Through Effective Communication

Effective communication is an art that is essential to maintaining a therapeutic environment. It is necessary in accomplishing work and resolving emotional and social issues such as conflict. Supervisors resolve conflict with effective communication. To promote effective communication that resolves conflict, the nurse leader should incorporate the following:[49]

- Teach nursing staff members their role in effective communication.
- Provide factual information to everyone: be inclusive, not exclusive.
- Consider all the aspects of situations: emotions, environmental considerations, and verbal and nonverbal messages.

Active Listening

Active or assertive listening is essential to managing conflict. To be sure that their perceptions are correct, nurse managers can paraphrase what the angry or defiant employee is saying. Paraphrasing clarifies the message for both. Paraphrasing can help cool off the situation because it gives the employee time and the opportunity to hear the supervisor's perceptions of the emotions expressed. Active assertive listening is sometimes called stress listening. Powell suggests these techniques:[50]

1. Do not share anger; it adds to the problem. Remain calm and matter-of-fact.
2. Respond constructively in both verbal and nonverbal language. Be cheerful but sober. Prevent interruptions. Bring problems into the open. Always be courteous and respectful and maintain eye contact.
3. Ask questions and listen to the answers. Determine the reasons for the anger.
4. Separate fact from opinion, including your own.
5. Do not respond hastily. Plan a response.
6. Consider the employee's perspective first.
7. Help the employee find the solution. Ask questions and listen to responses. Do not be paternalistic.

Resolving Conflict Through Negotiation

Negotiation is probably the most rapidly growing technique for handling conflict. According to Hampton, Summer, and Webber, negotiation includes bargaining power, distributive bargaining, integrative bargaining, and mediation. They are defined as follows:[51]

- *Bargaining power:* Refers to another person's inducement to agree to your terms
- *Distributive bargaining:* What either side gains at the expense of the other. Most labor management bargaining falls into this category.
- *Integrative bargaining:* Negotiators reach a solution that enhances both parties and produces high joint benefits. Each party looks out for its own interests, with the focus shifting to problem solving from reducing demands to expanding the pool of resources.

- *Mediation:* Mediators attempt to eliminate surrender as a demand. They encourage each party to acknowledge that it has injured the other but is also dependent on the other.

Mediation is a part of negotiation, but it also is a more intense strategy in its own right. The mediator is often brought into the process when the parties are locked in a positional posture. According to Marcus, the mediator must determine whether it is possible to get the parties to talk and to construct an adaptive process that moves them from confrontation, to cooperation, to resolution.[52]

Marcus says mediation includes "pre-meditation appropriateness, pre-meeting investigation and party buy-in, party meeting, issue clarification, option building, option assessment, movement toward mutually acceptable solutions, and resolution and implementation."[53] In each phase, the mediator simultaneously engages in investigation, empathy, neutrality, managing the interaction, inventiveness, and persuasion. Because mediation is voluntary, either party can suspend or postpone the mediation.

Results of Conflict Resolution

If attention is given to the role of the nurse manager in creating a climate for productive work by nurses, many of the causes of conflict are eliminated. Knowledge and skills related to managing conflict when it occurs are essential to the role of nurse manager.

Conflict can be a constructive and positive source of energy and creativity when properly managed. Otherwise, conflict can cause an environment to become dysfunctional and destructive, draining energy and reducing both personal and organizational effectiveness. It can destroy initiative or creativity. Conflict can cause hostile and disruptive behavior, loss of team spirit, and loss of desire to work toward common goals. It can result in deadlock and stalemate. Managed conflicts do not escalate.[54]

SUMMARY

Nurse leaders are challenged to create work environments that address the needs and respond to the opportunities of a diverse workforce. Effective leaders must move beyond their own cultural frame of reference to promote strong intercultural communication and create cultural synergy in the workplace. They must recognize and take full advantage of the productivity potential inherent in a diverse population. Experts caution organization leaders that developing an effective diversity management strategy is a long, challenging process that cannot be solved simply by attending a few half-day workshops. Managing a culturally diverse workforce does not happen haphazardly. Instead, it requires a deliberated and proactive approach.

APPLICATION EXERCISES

The following exercises can be done in groups of students or employees. Form groups of five to eight persons. Select a leader to keep the group moving and a recorder to write the plan or report. Refer to the chapter text for techniques and skills for assessing and managing conflict.

Exercise 8-1

A newly appointed CNO of a small rural hospital is experiencing staffing problems with the registered nurses. She discovers that within the community there are several retired nurses who might consider returning to work on a part-time basis. List strategies that this nurse executive might consider in the recruitment efforts of older nurses.

Exercise 8-2

Consider your present workplace (or a healthcare agency that you are familiar with) and create a list of strategies that would promote work retention of registered nurses. What resources are needed to implement these strategies?

Exercise 8-3

Case Study. During the P.M. change-of-shift report an RN calls in ill and the staffing office says she cannot be replaced. This leaves only one RN, Mrs. K, for 26 patients. Mrs. K says, "If you do not get another RN for this unit, I am going to quit this job. I will not do it this shift, but I will not put up with this constant shortage of help. I don't care if it is an RN, but I should have people with some skills to get the patients cared for. The reason everyone quits around here is because they are overworked, underpaid, and the hospital management does not give a damn. The place needs to be investigated."

Outline a plan to deal with this conflict. You may use the following format:

1. What is (are) the cause(s) of the conflict?
2. List aims, strategies, and specific skills for resolving the conflict.

Exercise 8-4

Case Study. A surgeon and a scrub nurse get into an argument during an operation. The surgeon tells the scrub nurse that she is stupid and that he does not want her to scrub for him again. The scrub nurse says she is totally competent but that he expects her to read his mind. She says, "If you don't quit badgering me, I'm going to sue you and this hospital!" The argument escalates into a shouting match.

Outline a plan to deal with this conflict. You may use the following format:

1. What is (are) the cause(s) of the conflict?
2. Assess the dimensions of the conflict.
3. List aims, strategies, and specific skills for resolving the conflict.

Exercise 8-5

Describe a recent instance of a conflict in which you were involved. Was it resolved satisfactorily? Can the group help in finding a better solution? Discuss.

Notes

1. Casicio, W. F., & Aquinis, H. (2005). *Applied psychology in human resource management* (6th ed.). Upper Saddle River, NJ: Prentice Hall.
2. Ibid.
3. Cohen, J. D. (2006). The aging nursing workforce. How to retain experienced nurses. *Journal of Healthcare Management, 51,* 233–245.
4. Health Resources and Service Administration. (2007). *Toward a method for identifying facilities and communities with shortages of nurses, summary report.* U.S. Department of Health and Human Services.
5. Degazon, C. E., & Shaw, H. K. (2007). Urban high school students' perceptions of nursing as a career choice. *Journal of National Black Nurses' Association, 18,* 8–13.
6. Hu, J., Herrick, C., & Hodgin, K. A. (2004). Managing the multigenerational nursing team. *Health Care Manager, 23,* 334.
7. Stuenkel, D. L., Nguyen, S., & Cohen, J. (2007). Nurses perceptions of their work environment. *Journal of Nursing Care Quality, 22,* 337–342.
8. Pattan, J. E. (1992). Developing a nurse recruitment plan. *Journal of Nursing Administration,* (2), 33–39.
9. Costello, D., & Vercler, M. A. (2006). Are your recruitment strategies up to date? *Nursing Homes* 6(1), 26–34.
10. Flynn, W. J., Mathis, R. L., & Jackson, P. J. (2004). *Healthcare human resource management.* Mason, OH: Thompson.
11. Thompson, M. R. (1975). *Why should I hire you?* (p. 94). New York: Jove Publications.
12. del Bueno, D. J., Weeks, L., & Brown-Stewart, P. (1987). Clinical assessment centers: A cost-effective alternative for competency development. *Nursing Economics,* 21–26.

13. Battle, E. H., Bragg, S., Delaney, J., Gilbert, S., & Roesler, D. (1985). Developing a rating interview guide. *Journal of Nursing Administration,* 39–45.

14. Alpern, S., & Shmuel, G. (2002). Searching for an agent who may or may not want to be found. *Operations Research, 50,* 311–327.

15. Spitzer-Lehmann, R. (1990). Recruitment and retention of our greatest asset. *Nursing Administration Quarterly,* 66–69.

16. Erenstein, C. F., & McCaffrey, R. (2007). How healthcare work environments influence nurse retention. *Holistic Nursing Practice, 21,* 303–307.

17. Aiken, L. H., Clarke, S. P., Sloane, D. M., & Sochalsk, J. A. (2004). An international perspective on hospital nurses' work environments: The case for reform. *Policy, Politics, & Nursing Practice, 4,* 255–263.

18. Author. (2007). What works: healing the healthcare staffing shortage. Price Waterhouse Coopers.

19. Author. (2007). Research news. Agency for Healthcare Research and Quality.

20. Rondeau, K. V., Williams, E. S., & Wagar, T. (2008). Turnover and vacancy rates for registered nurses: Do labor market factors matter? *Healthcare Management Review, 33,* 69–78.

21. Clevenger, K. (2007). The role of a nurse retention coordinator: One perspective. *Nursing Management, 38,* 8–10.

22. Herrin, D., & Spears, P. (2007). Nurse leadership development to improve nurse retention and patient outcomes: A framework. *Nursing Administration Quarterly, 31,* 231–243.

23. Cohen, J. (2006). The aging nursing workforce: How to retain experienced nurses. *Journal of Healthcare Management, 51,* 233–245.

24. Gaffney, S. (2005). Career development as a retention and succession planning tool. *Journal for Quality and Participation, 28,* 7–10.

25. Noe, R. A. (2005). *Employee training and development.* New York: McGraw-Hill.

26. Erenstein & McCaffrey, 2007.

27. Flynn et al., 2004.

28. Ibid.

29. Ibid.

30. Upenieks, V. (2005). Recruitment and retention strategies: A magnet hospital prevention model. *Medical-Surgical Nursing, 4,* 21–27.

31. Knowles, M. S. (1998). *The adult learner: The definitive class in adult education and human resource development.* Linacre House, Jordan Hill, Oxford, UK: Gulf Professional Publishing.

32. Boeehr, T. A., Vandana, N., Gudanowski, D., & Such, M. (2004). Perception of reason for promotion of self and others. *Human Relations, 57,* 413–438.

33. Darling, L. A. W., & McGrath, L. G. (1983). The causes and costs of promotion trauma. *Journal of Nursing Administration,* 29–33.

34. Casicio & Aquinis, 2005.

35. Dalton, C. (2002). Employment-at-will vs. wrongful discharge (employee termination, court cases). *Business Horizons, 45,* 3.

36. U.S. Census Bureau. (1999). Statistical abstract of the United States, p. 132.

37. Pernell, L. D., & Paulanka, B. J. (2005*). Guide to culturally competent health care* (p. xvi). Philadelphia: F. A. Davis.

38. Ibid.

39. Ibid.

40. Ibid.

41. Ibid.

42. Filley, A. C. (1980). Types and sources of conflict. In M. S. Berger, D. Elhart, S. C. Firsich, S. B. Jordan, & S. Stone (Eds.), *Management for nurses: A multidisciplinary approach* (pp. 154–165). St. Louis, MO: C. V. Mosby.

43. Bolman, L. G., & Deal, T. E. (1991). *Reframing organizations: Artistry, choice, and leadership* (p. 199). San Francisco: Jossey-Bass.

44. Hawkins, A. L., & Kratsch, L. S. (2004). Troubled units: Creating changes. *AACN Clinical Issues.* Apr–Jun; *15*(2):215–21.

45. Ibid.

46. Hermann, M. K., Alexander, J., & Kiely, J. T. (1992). Leadership and project management. In Decker & Sullivan, 571.

47. Murphy, E. C. (1984). Managing defiance. *Nursing Management,* 67–69.

48. Silber, M. B. (1984). Managing confrontations: Once more into the breach. *Nursing Management, 54,* 56–58.

49. Murphy, 1984.

50. Powell, J. T. (1986). Stress listening: Coping with angry confrontations. *Personnel Journal,* 27–29.

51. Hampton, D. R., Summer, C. E., & Webber, R. A. (1987). *Organizational behavior and the practice of management* (pp. 635–639). Glenview, IL: Scott, Foresman.

52. Marcus., p. 32

53. Ibid.

54. Hashem, A., & Alex, P. (2001). Conflict resolution using cognitive analysis approach. *Project Management Journal, 32,* 4.

References

Aiken, L., Haven, D., & Sloane, D. (2000). The magnet nursing services recognition program: A comparison of two groups of magnet hospitals. *American Journal of Nursing, 100,* 26–36.

American Hospital Association (AHA). (2002). *Hospital statistics 2002.* Chicago, IL: Author.

American Hospital Association Commission on Workforce for Hospitals and Health Systems. (2002). *In our hands: How hospital leaders can build a thriving workforce.* Chicago, IL: Author.

American Health Care Association (AHCA). (2002). *Results of the 2001 AHCA nursing position vacancy and turnover survey.* Washington, DC: Author.

Bradley, C. (2000, April 17). Building a workforce. *HealthWeek, 4,* 4.

Bradley, C. (2000, June 12). Taking our data to the street. *HealthWeek, 6,* 4.

Bolster, C., & Hawthorne, G. (2004). *Big raises all around. Hospitals and health networks* [electronic version]. Retrieved September 12, 2004, from http://www.hospitalconnect.com/hhnmag/jsp/articledisplay.jsp?dcrpath5 AHA/NewsStory-Article/data/httn0902Coverstory-salary&domain5HHNmag

Buerhaus, P. I., Staiger, D. O., & Auerbach, D. I. (2000). Implications of an aging registered nurse workforce. *Journal of the American Medical Association, 283,* 2948–2954.

Carpenter, J. E., Conway-Morana, P., Petersen, R., Dooley, B., Walters, B., & Wilder, M. (2004). Engaging staff in nursing recruitment and retention initiatives, a multihospital perspective. *Journal of Nursing Administration, 34,* 4–5.

Cook, C. (2004). The many faces of diversity: Overview and summary. *Online Journal of Issues in Nursing, 8* (1). Retrieved July 17, 2008 from http://nursingworld.org/MainMenuCategories/ANAmarketplace/ANAPeriodicals/OJIN/TableofContents/volume82003

Curtin, L. (2004). Adjusting to an aging workforce. Paper presented at the Conference on Solving the Nursing Shortage: Strategies for the Workplace and the Profession, June 1–4, 2004, Washington, DC: JCAHO.

Deutschendorf, A. (2003). From past paradigms to future frontiers: Unique care delivery models to facilitate nursing works and quality outcomes. *Journal of Nursing Administration, 33,* 52–59.

Drucker, P. F. (1999). *Management challenges for the 21st century.* New York: HarperCollins.

Fabre, J. (2004, February). Improve patient safety and staff retention by mentoring your staff. *Nursing News, 28,* 9.

Hensinger, B., Minerath, S., Parry, J., & Robertson, K. I. (2004). Asset protection: Maintaining and retaining your workforce. *Journal of Nursing Administration, 34,* 268–272.

Institute of Medicine (IOM). (2003). *Unequal treatment: Confronting racial and ethnic disparities in health care.* Washington, DC: National Academies Press.

Kirsch, M. (2000). The myth of informed consent. *American Journal of Gastroenterology,* 588–589.

Kleinman, C. S. (2004). Leadership and retention, research needed. *Journal of Nursing Administration, 34,* 111–113.

Mitchell, S. (2000, May 1). Raising the bar: Green light for accreditation agencies signals better nursing education. *HealthWeek,* 12.

Moore, A. (2004). Drive for diversity. *Nursing Standard, 18,* 18–19.

O'Brien-Pallas, L. Duffield, L. C., & Alksnis, C. (2004). Who will be there to nurse? Retention of nurses nearing retirement. *Journal of Nursing Administration, 34,* 298–302.

Page, A. (2004). *Keeping patients safe, transforming the work environment for nurses.* Washington, DC: National Academies Press.

Parson, M. L., & Stonestreet, J. (2004). Staff retention: Laying the groundwork by listening. *Nursing Leadership Forum, 8,* 107–113.

Platzer, H., Blake, D., & Ashford, D. (2000). An evaluation of process and outcomes from learning through reflective practice groups on a post-registration nursing course. *Journal of Advanced Nursing,* 689–695.

Snelgrove, S., & Hughes, D. (2000). Interprofessional relations between doctors and nurses: Perspectives from South Wales. *Journal of Advanced Nursing,* 661–667.

9 STRATEGIC PLANNING AND MANAGEMENT

Sandra Smith Pennington, PhD, RN
Elizabeth Simms, RN, MSN

LEARNING OBJECTIVES AND ACTIVITIES

- Define the mission or purpose statement as it pertains to nursing services.
- Use a set of standards to evaluate a purpose or mission statement for a nursing agency.
- Write a purpose or mission statement for a nursing agency. Identify the vision and values to be imparted to customers.
- Define philosophy as it pertains to nursing services.
- Use a set of standards to evaluate the philosophy statement of a nursing agency.
- Write a philosophy statement for a nursing agency.
- Define objectives as they pertain to nursing services.
- Apply a set of standards to evaluate the objectives statements of a nursing agency.
- Write objectives for a nursing agency.
- Define planning.
- Differentiate among examples of the purposes of planning.
- Differentiate among examples of the characteristics of planning.
- Differentiate among examples of the elements of planning.
- Describe strategy as it relates to the planning function of nursing services.
- Describe the strategic planning process.
- Describe operational planning.
- Define the operational plan (management plan) as it pertains to nursing services.
- Use a set of standards to evaluate an operational plan of a nursing agency.
- Differentiate among examples of strategic and tactical planning.
- Write a business plan.
- Describe a balanced scorecard.

CONCEPTS

Mission, purpose, vision, values, philosophy, objectives, planning, strategic planning, functional planning, venture planning, operational planning, divisional planning, unit planning, business plan

QUOTE

If anything is certain, it is that change is certain. The world we are planning for today will not exist in this form tomorrow.

—Philip Crosby

NURSE MANAGER BEHAVIORS

Directs senior managers in developing statements of mission (purpose), vision, values, philosophy, and objectives. Authors strategic and operational planning with key management personnel and uses on a daily basis.

NURSE EXECUTIVE BEHAVIORS

Involves representatives of all units of the organization in developing and implementing statements of mission (purpose), vision, values, philosophy, objectives, and operational plans. Includes a system for evaluation, feedback, and update of these statements. Develops a strategic plan with inputs from representative personnel of the entire organization. Coaches management staff in developing and implementing operational plans that support the strategic plan. With management staff, performs periodic audits and identifies the potential for the need for change.

Introduction

Strategic planning is a means by which an organization defines its future. The planning process involves strategies that provide direction for an organization's future as well as an operational plan for the business. Planning affords the opportunity to determine how capital and human resources are allocated. The mission, values, philosophy, and objectives are powerful tools in the planning process.

Mission (or purpose), vision, values, and philosophy (or beliefs) are the basic tools of management. Knowledge of their use is part of the theory of nursing management. These tools are part of the purposeful planning function of nursing management, and skill in using them successfully is part of the strategy of nursing management planning.

Written statements of purpose, vision, values, philosophy, objectives, and written strategic and operational plans are the blueprints for effective management of any enterprise, including a healthcare institution. These components of planning exist at each management level. Statements at the corporate level serve the top managers of the organization. Statements at the division level serve the managers and personnel of major divisions, such as nursing, operations, or finance. These statements evolve from and support those of the institution. Services, departments, and units each have written statements of purpose, vision, values, philosophy, objectives, and written operational plans that are developed from and support the documents at division and corporate levels (Figure 9-1).[1]

| FIGURE 9-1 | EVOLUTION OF MISSION, VISION, VALUES, PHILOSOPHY, AND OBJECTIVES STATEMENTS AND OPERATIONAL PLANS |

Mission (purpose) statements   Corporate
                                             ↓
Vision and value statements   Division
                                             ↓
Philosophy (beliefs) statements   Department
                                             ↓
Objectives statements   Unit
Operational (management) plans

Source: Author.

MISSION OR PURPOSE, VISION, AND VALUES

Mission or Purpose

The mission of an organization describes the purpose for which that organization exists. Mission statements provide information, direction, and inspiration that clearly and explicitly outline the way ahead for the organization. Mission statements provide vision.[2]

The purpose of any organization is to provide individuals with the means to lead productive and meaningful lives. Therefore the purpose of the organization and each unit should be defined, a teamwork approach should prevail, constituents should be properly trained, and all individuals should be treated with respect.[3]

Every organization exists for specific purposes or missions and to fulfill specific social functions. For healthcare organizations, this means providing healthcare services to maintain health, cure illness, and allay pain and suffering.

Articulation of a mission statement is the first step in the strategic planning process. Industry leaders have learned that customers are the most critical stakeholders and frequently note this fact in their mission statements.[4] Mission statements in successful business and industrial organizations incorporate socially meaningful and measurable criteria to provide a clearly defined reason for being. These simple yet crucial statements move the organization forward and are formulated for performance, products, and services. They contain statements of ethics, principles, and standards that are understood by workers. Workers who clearly perceive that they are pursuing meaningful and worthwhile goals through their individual efforts are more committed and dedicated than those who do not.[5]

The mission of an organization moves, guides, and delivers the organization to its perceived goal. The intent of the mission statement should be the initial consideration for an employee who is evaluating a strategic decision. It is widely held that the purpose or mission statement should be created from a vision statement that describes the things for which the company stands. The vision statement is created with the customer's needs in mind; to determine these needs, one must ask and listen to the customer. External customers are those who purchase the products or services of the organization. In nursing, external customers are prospective patients and families, accreditation and licensing officials, faculty and students, and even taxpayers and shareholders. Internal customers include employees, both departmental and intradepartmental. Appropriate current events should be noted through reading and meetings, highlighting those events that will enhance the mission of the organization and for which the clinical nurses will claim or share ownership.[6] The mission or purpose statement incorporates the culture of the organization, including strong leadership, rules and regulations, achievement of goals, and the notion that people are more important than work.[7]

Vision

The vision of an organization should be an image of the future the organization seeks to create; it is not an abstract tool but a practical tool offering goals to be accomplished in terms that can ultimately be assessed. It is a mental prediction of the fulfillment of the organization's success. Employees who participate in developing the vision statement believe in their own abilities and are more committed to the organization than employees who do not participate. The vision statement is shared company-wide so that

> **"Nurse leader-managers must find both the vision and the courage to move nursing forward as a knowledge-intensive profession."**

employees may live the vision. It is updated to keep pace with technology and trends.[8] A vision statement is sometimes considered more strategic than a mission statement.

Vision, values, mission, or purpose statements are initially meaningful only to their creators.[9] Translated for the community, these statements place value on the way nurses care for people. Nursing education teaches the meaning of values such as tolerance and compromise. Diverse populations should be considered in developing vision and values statements for nursing organizations.

Values

Values are concepts of perceived worth or importance that drive the institution and inform its mission, vision, and goals; examples of values are commitment, creativity, honesty, quality, respect, and caring. Values are the moral rationale for business. Value statements make employees feel proud and managers feel committed. They give meaning to the right way to do things; they give employees enthusiasm and energy. Values bond people and set behavioral standards.[10] At least half of U.S. corporations have a values statement. Agreement on values provides a mechanism for built-in quality; adherence to values makes organizations successful.[11]

Nursing Mission or Purpose

Defining a mission or purpose allows nursing organizations to be evaluated for performance. The mission articulates nursing's essential nature, its values, and what it should and will be; it describes the constituencies to be satisfied. The mission is the framework for the professional nurse manager's commitment to standards. How nursing is defined and conceptualized is important to its professional practice.

One of the major functions of a nursing entity is to provide evidence-based nursing care to clients, which can include promotion of self-care concepts. Thus the statement should include definitions of nursing and self-care as set by professional nurses.

Virginia Henderson defined nursing as follows[12]:

> The unique function of the nurse is to assist the individual, sick or well, in the performance of those activities contributing to health or its recovery (or to peaceful death) that he would perform unaided if he had the necessary strength, will, or knowledge. And to do this in such a way as to help him gain independence as rapidly as possible.

Yura and Walsh describe the nursing process as follows[13]:

> . . . an orderly, systematic manner of determining the client's health status, specifying problems defined as alterations in human need fulfillment, making plans to solve them, initiating and implementing the plan, and evaluating the extent to which the plan was effective in promoting the optimum wellness and resolving the problems identified.

King defined nursing as[14]

> . . . a process of action, reaction, interaction, and transaction whereby nurses assist individuals of any age group to meet their basic human needs in coping with their health status at some particular

point in their life cycle. Nurses perform their functions within social institutions and they interact with individuals and groups. Therefore, three distinct levels of operation exist: (1) the individual; (2) the group; and (3) society.

Orem defined nursing as follows[15]:

> Nursing is an art through which the nurse, the practitioner of nursing, gives specialized assistance to persons with disabilities of such character that more than ordinary assistance is needed to meet daily needs for self-care and to intelligently participate in the medical care they are receiving from the physician. The art of nursing is practiced by "doing for" the person with the disability, by "helping him to do for himself," and/or by "helping him to learn how to do for himself." Nursing is also practiced by helping a capable person from the patient's family or a friend of the patient to learn how "to do for" the patient. Nursing is thus a practical and didactic art.

Kinlein suggested that "nursing is assisting the person in his self-care practices in regard to his state of health."[16]

Emerging from these and other theories of nursing are common terms central to the definition of nursing: nurse, patient or client, individual, group, society, nursing process, self-care, and health.

A further mission of nursing is to provide a public good. This purpose should be indicated in the mission statement of the nursing entity. Because it gives the reason for their employment, the mission statement is written so that all people working within the organizational entity can understand and abide by it. An ultimate strategy is to have nursing personnel participate in developing mission statements and in keeping them updated so that they are empowered to fully support them.

The mission should be known and understood by other healthcare practitioners, by clients and their families, and by the community. A statement of purpose must be dynamic, giving action and strength to evolving statements of philosophy, objectives, and management plans. Statements of purpose can be made dynamic by indicating the relationship between the nursing unit and patients, personnel, community, health, illness, and self-care. Figures 9-2, 9-3, and 9-4 are examples of mission statements of an organization, the division, and the unit, respectively. Figure 9-5 lists the standards for evaluation of the mission statements of an organization.

FIGURE 9-2 | **MISSION STATEMENT OF AN ORGANIZATION**

SUBJECT: MISSION STATEMENT

It is the mission of the Metropolitan Medical Center to:

1. Provide a center of excellence in the provision of medical care to our patient population, regardless of age, race, religion, political beliefs, or sexual preference.

2. Provide a clinical setting in which physicians, nurses, and those of allied health services may experience enrichment of educational opportunities.

3. Create an atmosphere of innovation in practice and technology to benefit our clientele, internal and external.

4. Foster attitudes of creativity and compassion in care delivery in every person associated with the organization.

5. Develop and fund research opportunities to provide professional growth, and to seek improvements in evidence-based/best practice patient care.

Source: Author.

FIGURE 9-3	MISSION STATEMENT OF A DIVISION

SUBJECT: PURPOSE STATEMENT OF THE DIVISION OF NURSING

The mission and purpose of the Division of Nursing supports the Mission statement of the Metropolitan Medical Center. It is the purpose of the Division of Nursing to:

1. Uphold the written standards of quality nursing care for our patient population.

2. Encourage an atmosphere that will foster continuing professional development of the nursing staff through educational opportunities and mentoring.

3. Promote nursing research activities, utilizing staff in cooperation with postgraduate nursing and faculty nursing.

4. Provide a framework for the evaluation of the quality of nursing care delivered.

Source: Author.

Proprietary changes have brought innovation and competition to the healthcare industry. They have also brought business techniques that have moved the hospital industry from being facilities dominated to being market driven. The corporate structures of for-profit hospitals consider product line and function and focus on mission. This focus has been adopted by not-for-profit hospitals that now look at mission statements in relation to new markets, market share, and diversification. The organization of these new not-for-profit corporate structures can be compared with a chain, with regionalization and integration as links. The leadership of these organizations is dynamic and future oriented rather than focused on maintenance.[17]

"Good mission statements express the organization's vision and values, evoking passion in the employees. Good mission statements delineate the organization's uniqueness. Effective nurse leaders make sure that employees see, feel, and think the mission by following it themselves. They expect and accept resistance.[18]"

FIGURE 9-4	PURPOSE STATEMENT OF A UNIT

SUBJECT: PURPOSE: ACUTE CARE UNIT

The purpose of the Acute Care Unit is consistent with and supports the purpose of the Division of Nursing. The purpose of the Acute Care Unit is to:

1. Provide excellence in nursing care through physical, emotional, and spiritual care for clients and their families; they will be afforded privacy, dignity, and respect.

2. Enable nursing staff to act as patient advocates, coordinating care across the disciplines to provide an optimal level of care.

3. Provide every client an individualized plan of care, taking into account cultural customs particular to each.

4. Monitor quality of care/performance of staff on a continuous basis, with monthly audits, peer review, and annual evaluations.

Source: Author.

FIGURE 9-5	STANDARDS FOR THE EVALUATION OF MISSION STATEMENTS OF THE NURSING DIVISION AND ITS DEPARTMENTS, SERVICES, AND UNITS

1. The mission statement tells the reason for the existence of the nursing division, department, service, or unit in relation to the practice of nursing and of self-care as defined by the nursing staff and in relation to the service being provided to the community of clients. Once definitions of nursing and self-care have been developed by the nursing staff and ratified by the nursing administration, they may be quoted in the mission statement.

2. The nursing division mission statement supports the mission of the organization. Unit mission statements are customized by line personnel.

3. The statement indicates that the nursing organization exists to provide a public good.

4. The mission statement is developed by the people who will live by it.

5. It includes a set of core values held by the people who will live by it.

6. It is short, clear, and unambiguous; it has a clear meaning.

7. The mission statement describes the organization's uniqueness.

Source: Author.

PHILOSOPHY

A written statement of philosophy sets out values, concepts, and beliefs that pertain to nursing administration and nursing practice within the organization. It verbalizes the visions of both nurse managers and nurse practitioners regarding what they believe nursing management and practice to be. It states their beliefs as to how the mission or purpose will be achieved, giving direction toward this end. Statements of philosophy are abstract and contain value statements about human beings as clients or patients and as workers, about work that will be performed by nursing workers for clients or patients, about self-care, about nursing as a profession, about education as it pertains to competence of nursing workers, and about the setting or community in which nursing services are provided. Statements of philosophy are valuable and usable if they reflect the current practice of an institution with an eye to the future.

"The character and tone of service are set by planning that evolves purpose and philosophy statements, one from the other, for the organization and each of its units."

Hodgetts states that "all managers bring a set of values to the workplace." Managers have economic, theoretical, political, religious, aesthetic, and social values. Values are inherent in a management philosophy.[19] Nurse managers must be involved in outlining, implementing, and evaluating the unit philosophy which must reflect the values of the times in their statements of philosophy; their philosophy is crucial to the success of the organization, because a philosophy of caring from management pervades the patient care environment.[20]

Among the contents of a philosophy statement are the core values related to a nursing modality; the need for advanced preparation, continuing education, lifelong learning, students, research and best practice, and nursing management; and nursing's role in the organization. Philosophy statements pertain to patients' involvement in their care and to their extended families. Philosophy statements also pertain to nurses' rights, including commitment to staff promotion, and nurses' responsibility to the profession.[21]

From a business aspect, the philosophy statement is an outgrowth of the institutional culture. Most Fortune 500 companies have a philosophy statement; it is displayed on posters or plastic cards, in brochures, articles, annual reports, speeches, and books. People who believe in a company philosophy perform ethically, help employees make correct decisions, speak with one voice, have a sense of corporate purpose, and work more productively.[22]

Concerns prevalent in a business philosophy are customers and employees, quality, excellence, growth, profits, shareholders, and the society that the business serves. The philosophy statement supports the mission statement as the glue that binds the separate parts together as a cohesive, productive whole. It motivates employees to accomplish complex tasks in an intimate, relatively simple work environment.[23]

A philosophy must be communicated zealously and totally supported by top management. As with the mission statement, the philosophy statement is most effective when developed by those who will live by it. Unlike mission and objectives statements, the philosophy statement remains constant.

Figures 9-6, 9-7, and 9-8 are examples of the philosophy statement of an organization, division, and unit, respectively. Figure 9-9 lists the standards for evaluation of philosophy statements of an organization.

OBJECTIVES

Objectives are specific statements of goals to be accomplished. They are action commitments through which the key elements of the mission are achieved and the philosophy or beliefs sustained. Objectives are used to establish priorities. They are stated in terms of processes or results to be achieved and focus

---

FIGURE 9-6	**PHILOSOPHY STATEMENT OF AN ORGANIZATION**

SUBJECT: PHILOSOPHY OF THE METROPOLITAN MEDICAL CENTER

We believe that:

- The Metropolitan Medical Center is a center of excellence in care delivery, in educational opportunity, and in the development of research.

- We believe that we are the leaders in health care in our community; that health care entails prevention and wellness in addition to treatment of illness and injury.

- We strive to provide the most effective and innovative medical services to all clients.

- We must provide continual assessment of the quality of care provided by continuous evaluation of services; we will strive to improve performance based on Quality Assurance oversight.

- We will provide each patient with dignity, provide privacy and confidentiality, and permit the right to make choices in health care based on factual information provided by the medical/nursing staff.

- Metropolitan Medical Center employees are our major asset; they have the responsibility to perform their duties within the mission, vision and philosophy, and policies and procedures to strive toward the highest standard of care.

- Continued professional development of every employee, regardless of role served, is necessary to provide optimal patient care; it is a shared responsibility of the organization and each individual employee.

- Research is both necessary and beneficial to the continued growth of the healthcare professions; we will foster and fund research in conjunction with graduate nursing and medical personnel.

- We are committed to providing a safe environment to our clientele and to our employees through an active Risk Management department.

- It is the responsibility of the Metropolitan Medical Center to maintain fiscal integrity.

Source: Author.

FIGURE 9-7	PHILOSOPHY STATEMENT OF A DIVISION

SUBJECT: PHILOSOPHY OF THE DIVISION OF NURSING

We believe that:

- The philosophy of the Division of Nursing is and must be consistent with the philosophy of the Metropolitan Medical Center.
- Our function within the organization is to ensure the highest quality medical care is provided equally to each patient admitted for treatment.
- Health care begins with prevention and wellness, and must emphasize self-care. Nursing care delivery will be based on the work of nursing theorists and evidence-based practices.
- Our patients must be treated with dignity and care delivered on an individualized basis.
- A multidisciplinary approach to care is necessary to the physical, emotional, and spiritual well-being of our patients and their families.
- It is our responsibility to maintain qualified staff, in adequate numbers, to ensure the care needs of our clients and their families; "qualified" staff must be provided with the means of continuing professional development through mentoring and an active Education Department. The staff bears equal responsibility with the organization for continuing education.
- We must provide the framework, in conjunction with the Quality Assurance Department, for the continual evaluation of standards of care delivered.
- Research within our division is beneficial to patient care and staff development.

Source: Author.

FIGURE 9-8	PHILOSOPHY STATEMENT OF A UNIT

SUBJECT: PHILOSOPHY STATEMENT OF THE ACUTE CARE UNIT

- We believe that all patients deserve to be treated equally, with dignity and compassion, and provided with individualized plans of care.
- We believe that the goal of health care is the progression of the patient toward an optimal level of health, supported by education in self-care for the patients and their families.
- We believe that a multidisciplinary approach to care provides for complete services to our patients; it is the responsibility of the nursing staff to coordinate efforts among the disciplines.
- We believe that our staff is our greatest asset; preceptorships, mentoring, and organizational-based educational offerings give support toward continuing professional development.
- We believe that family is an extension of the patient and must be involved in the patient's progress. Information and education must be provided to allow optimal healthcare choices.

Source: Author.

on the provision of healthcare services to clients. Like the statements of mission and philosophy, they must be meaningful, relevant, and functional. They must be alive. Moore states, "If objectives are presented in terms of what can be observed, they can serve as useful tools for evaluation of nursing care and personnel performance, and as a basis for planning educational programs, staffing, requisition of supplies and equipment, and other functions associated with the nursing department."[24]

| **FIGURE 9-9** | **STANDARDS FOR EVALUATION OF PHILOSOPHY STATEMENTS OF THE NURSING DIVISION, DEPARTMENT, SERVICE, OR UNIT** |

1. A written statement of philosophy should exist for the nursing division and each of its units.

2. A written statement of philosophy should be developed in collaboration with nursing employees, the consumers, and other healthcare workers.

3. Nursing personnel should share in an annual (or more frequent) review and revision of the written statement of philosophy.

4. The written statement of philosophy should reflect these beliefs or values:

    (a) The meaning of the clinical practice of nursing.

    (b) Recognition of the rights of individuals and of the responsibility of nursing personnel to serve as advocates for those rights.

    (c) Selective other statements about humanity, society, health, nursing, nursing process, self-care relevant to external forces (community, laws, etc.) and internal forces (personnel, clients, material resources, etc.), research, education, and family as are deemed appropriate to accomplishing the mission of the division and each of its units.

5. The nursing philosophy should support the philosophy of the organization as expressed at all levels above the nursing division.

6. The statement of philosophy should give direction to the achievement of the mission.

Source: Author.

Objectives are concrete statements that become the standards against which performance can be measured. According to Moore, nursing organizations should have objectives for evaluation of patient care, evaluation of personnel performance, planning of educational programs, staffing, and requisition of supplies and equipment. Objectives are the basic tactics of any business, including the business of nursing management. Objectives must be selective rather than global, multiple rather than single to balance a wide range of needs and goals related to nursing services for clients or patients. They must demand productive use of people, money, and material resources and be updated through innovation. Objectives direct the discharge of a social responsibility to the community. Objectives must be used, and one way to use them is to develop them into specific management and operational plans.

Drucker writes that mission and purpose, as well as the basic definition of a business, must be translated into objectives if they are to become more than insight, good intentions, and brilliant epigrams never to be achieved.[25]

The nursing staff, and specifically the nurse manager, must decide where efforts will be concentrated to achieve results. Some areas of concentration have already been mentioned; others may be similar to those related to business and industry. These include marketing and the development of healthcare services in areas of need. Great potential exists in the area of prevention of disease and injury. Another area for objectives is innovation, which includes the introduction of new methods and particularly the application of new knowledge along with new technology.

Other areas for objectives are organization of and use of all resources: human, financial, and physical. Objectives address the need to develop managers as well as the needs of major groups within the division (such as nonmanagerial workers), labor relations, the development of positive employee attitudes, and maintenance and upgrading of employee skills. Objectives provide for attractive job and career opportunities and for activities to control worker assignment and productivity. They are the means by which productivity in nursing may be measured (Figure 9-10).

FIGURE 9-10 — EXAMPLES OF CATEGORICAL AREAS FOR WRITING OBJECTIVES

- *Evaluation of patient care.* To develop methods of measuring the quality of patient care.

- *Evaluation of personnel performance.* The patient benefits from close nursing supervision of all nonprofessional personnel who give patient care and from continuous appraisal of the nursing care given and the performance of all nursing personnel based on professional standards.

- *Planning educational programs.* The patient benefits from a continuous, flexible program of in-service education for all divisions of nursing personnel adapted to orientation, skill training, continuous education, and leadership development.

- *Staffing.* To establish a systematic staffing pattern for patient care so that all members of each department can function in accordance with their skill levels for the maintenance of continuity of nursing care and management of nursing service.

- *Requisition of supplies and equipment.* To supply nursing personnel with adequate resources to facilitate patient care; to anticipate future nursing needs and plan for the acquisition of needed resources.

- *Marketing.* To collaborate and consult with intradepartmental health team members for maximal effectiveness in promoting health care and disease prevention. New programs will be developed to meet identified needs.

- *Innovation.* To influence progressive nursing practices and research training programs in supporting changing trends that improve the quality of patient care.

- *Organization and use of all resources (human, financial, and physical).* To apply standards for decentralization of decision making and to increase efficiency and effectiveness of staffing and budgeting.

- *Social responsibility.* To support, publicize, and sustain service to the community in health endeavors.

- *Research and development.* To sustain the nursing profession and the organization.

Source: Author.

Management balances objectives. There are short-term objectives, with their accomplishment in easy view or reach; long-term objectives; and some objectives in the "hope to accomplish" category. The budget is the mechanical expression of setting and balancing objectives. The nurse manager plans two budgets, one for operations and one for future capital expenditures. Some priorities are set with the budget, as illustrated in Figure 9-11.

Objectives are a fundamental strategy of nursing, because they specify the end product of all nursing activities. They must be capable of being converted into specific targets and specific assignments,

FIGURE 9-11 — EXAMPLES OF BALANCED OBJECTIVES

- *Long-term objective.* Write a plan to develop patient teaching guides for all areas.

- *Short-term objective.* Establish procedures for safe nursing care by having fire department personnel hold classes on fire evacuation procedures for all nursing personnel on all three shifts.

- *Future budget.* Plan with the budget director to have funds allocated to repaint patients' rooms and replace worn and torn furniture.

- *Current budget.* Implement the classes for expectant parents for which funds have been allocated.

Source: Author.

enabling nurses to understand the desired endpoint and the path toward that end; objectives become the basis and motivation for nursing achievement. They make possible the concentration of human and material resources and of human efforts. Objectives are needed in all areas on which the survival of nursing and healthcare services depends. In nursing, all objectives should be performance objectives that provide for existing nursing services. They should provide for abandonment of unneeded and outmoded nursing services and healthcare products and for new services and products; they should provide for existing patient populations, for new populations of patients, for the distributive organization, and for standards of nursing service. Last but not least, objectives should exist for research and development of best practices within the nursing arena.

Although concrete, objectives are not written in stone; they should be changed as necessary, particularly when evaluation proves them outmoded, when a change of mission occurs, or when the objectives no longer are functional.[26] Refer to Figure 9-12 for a breakdown of the elements of objectives.

Figures 9-13, 9-14, and 9-15 are examples of objectives for an organization, a nursing division, and a nursing unit, respectively. Figure 9-16 contains standards for evaluating the objectives of an organization.

STRATEGY

The theory of a business lies in its objectives, results, customers, and customer's values. Strategy converts theory into performance. In the 21st century, strategy is based on five certainties[27]:

1. Collapsing birthrate in the developed world
2. Shifts in the distribution of disposable income
3. Defining performance
4. Global competitiveness
5. Growing incongruence between economic globalization and political splintering

Planning is the strategy of an organization and is essential to all businesses, including those providing health care. Planning techniques used in business and industry are increasingly being adopted by

---

FIGURE 9-12 ELEMENTS OF OBJECTIVES

- *A performance objective:* The patient receives individualized care in a safe environment to meet total therapeutic nursing needs—physical, emotional, spiritual, environmental, social, economic, and rehabilitative (also illustrates next provision).

- *Existing nursing services for existing patients:* Nurse consultants have been made available from medical nursing, surgical nursing, mental health nursing, and maternal and child health nursing. Their services can be requested by any professional nurse or physician.

- *Abandonment of outmoded nursing services and products:* Universal precautions have been implemented and the old handwashing basins have been discarded.

- *New nursing services for new groups of patients:* Plans are being made to offer consultative nursing services from the general hospital to nursing homes in the area. In the future this will be extended to retirement homes. Both actions are the result of market surveys.

- *Organization for new nursing services:* The nurse manager has evaluated the necessity of restructuring the organization of the division of nursing to provide new nursing services.

- *Standards of nursing service and performance:* The nurse manager has decided to use the Standards of Nursing Practice developed by the ANA Congress for Nursing Practice for all nurses within the division.

Source: Author.

FIGURE 9-13 **GOALS OF THE METROPOLITAN MEDICAL CENTER**

GLOBAL GOALS

Increase patient population

Seek grants to provide funds for indigent population

Market hospital services to community

Create new markets

Expand upon services presently offered

Improve access to the hospital

Contract with medical schools for resident training

Contract with nursing schools for nursing clinicals

Capture maximum reimbursement

Initiate research

Improve efficiency

DEFINITIVE GOALS

A. Increase patient population
   1. Use incentives for MDs on staff
   2. Investigate joint ventures for specialized services
   3. Survey MDs within community
   4. Market HMO

B. Seek grants to provide funds for the indigent
   1. Division Administrators to write for grants
   2. Community-based volunteer funding

C. Market hospital services
   1. Public relations plan
   2. Increased effort for auxiliary volunteer base

3. "Health awareness" presence at community events
4. Management people in civic organizations
5. Create user-friendly website

D. Expand services
   1. What new products can we sell?
   2. Private vendors for new equipment/training
   3. Feasibility study for clinics: prenatal, diabetes

E. Improve access to hospital
   1. New emergency room ramp
   2. Separate parking for emergency room clientele
   3. New main entrance
   4. Acquisition of adjoining land for increased parking

F. Contract with schools for professional training
   1. Contact University Medical school/incentives to students
   2. Contact University School of Nursing/stipends
   3. Contact Allied School of Health/stipends

G. Capture maximum reimbursement
   1. Training: Social Service Dept. Medicare/Medicaid
   2. Case Management: Facilitate client flow
   3. Audit bills with charts

H. Initiate research
   1. Contact graduate schools/nursing organizations
   2. Contract with private industry/pharmaceutical companies
   3. Create Web site to publicize results

Source: Author.

---

healthcare organizations. Strategy is the process by which an organization achieves success in a changing environment. Beckham states that "real strategy is a plan for getting from a point in the present to some point in the future in the face of uncertainty and resistance."[29] Nursing has only tapped the surface of a business strategy.[30] A myriad of services are available that can be offered to potential clients, such as telephone and e-mail access to information on drug prices, durable medical equipment prices, educational services, research and best practice briefs, and a host of therapeutic nursing products. A nursing strategy outlines how the firm achieves its strategic goals and objectives in a competitive marketplace.

> *To create a future worth experiencing for nurses, strategic thinking and strategic planning are required of all nursing leaders. Strategy is the solution.[28]*

Top management has to answer planning questions like these:

- Where do we go and what do we want to become? Such questions seek to define the organization's mission and objectives.
- What and where are we now? The purpose here is to examine and define the organization's philosophy and objectives.

FIGURE 9-14   OBJECTIVES OF THE DIVISION OF NURSING

SUBJECT: OBJECTIVES OF THE DIVISION OF NURSING

The goals of the Division of Nursing are to provide the patient:

1. Physical, emotional, and spiritual individualized care within a safe environment.
2. Patient education to allow for optimal healthcare choices and participation in that health care.
3. Nursing staff who will act as patient advocates, coordinating care among all disciplines for the highest provision of services.
4. Benefits of a nursing staff supported by the Division of Nursing in educational endeavors meant to promote increased knowledge and skill.
5. Benefits of a positive working milieu in which nursing staff's job satisfaction is achieved.
6. Maximum nursing care presence at the bedside by providing ancillary staff to handle nonnursing functions.
7. Benefits from a supervisory staff able to monitor and evaluate care provided by nursing staff.
8. Benefits from implementation of nursing research results.

Source: Author.

FIGURE 9-15   OBJECTIVES OF A NURSING UNIT

SUBJECT: OBJECTIVES OF THE ACUTE CARE UNIT

The Objectives of the Acute Care Unit are to provide the patient, family, and/or significant others:

1. Individualized care through assessment of the physical, emotional, and spiritual needs in a therapeutic, positive environment.
2. Care based upon the nursing process, with an adequate number of staff.
3. Cost-effective, quality care, with coordination of services by the primary nurse.
4. Adequate information to make the healthcare choices necessary to the attainment of an optimal level of functioning.
5. Nursing staff held to the highest standard of care, per hospital policy and procedure, with a framework for ongoing evaluation of performance.

Source: Author.

- How can we best get there? The answer to this question will take the form of ongoing plans that include organizing, directions and controlling concepts.

Such activities constitute the strategy of top management. They are developed into the strategy of the nursing division and subsequently into the strategy of nursing and other business units of the organization. Planning is neither a top-down nor bottom-up proposition. Each level must harmonize its strategies with those below and above.[31]

A focus on development and use of planning strategies gives direction, cohesion, and thrust to the nursing division. Nurse employees involved in achieving objectives and goals are motivated. These goals should be clearly defined and focus on the future without losing sight of the present. Successful implementation of management plans to achieve mission objectives and goals while sustaining philosophy results in productivity, profitability, and achievement. This process is managing, and managers perform it.[32]

FIGURE 9-16	**STANDARDS FOR EVALUATION OF STATEMENTS OF OBJECTIVES FOR A NURSING DIVISION, DEPARTMENT, SERVICE, OR UNIT**

1. The objectives for the nursing division, department, service, or unit should be in written form.
2. The objectives should be developed in collaboration with the nursing personnel who will assist in achieving them.
3. Nursing personnel should share in an annual (or more frequent) review and revision of the written statements of objectives.
4. The written statement of objectives should meet these qualitative and quantitative criteria:
   a. They operationalize the statements of mission and philosophy; they can be translated into actions.
   b. They can be measured or verified.
   c. They exist in a hierarchy or prioritized sequence.
   d. They are clearly stated.
   e. They are realistic in terms of human and physical resources and capabilities.
   f. They direct the use of resources.
   g. They are achievable (practical).
   h. They are specific.
   i. They indicate results expected from nursing efforts and activities; they are the ends of management programs.
   j. They show a network of desired events and results.
   k. They are flexible and allow for adjustment.
   l. They are known to the nursing personnel who will use them.
   m. They are quantified wherever possible.
   n. They exist for all positions.

Source: Author.

Cavanaugh relates strategy to power, indicating that organizational power gives nurse managers the power to do their jobs better. Her suggestions for nurse managers to strategize are summarized as follows[33]:

1. Use the political system to turn personal power into organizational power.
2. Recognize the self-interests of others in the organization and use them in a win–win manner.
3. Diagnose, plan, and execute an effective political campaign to achieve a thoughtful, purposeful goal.
4. Define ways to achieve objectives while helping others. Know people and their goals.
5. Disengage from losing issues and from issues in which you have to defend yourself on someone else's turf. A technique for doing this is placing the issue at the end of an agenda or omitting it from the minutes.
6. Defend your territory.
7. Plan and carry out an offense on issues of your own choosing and commitment.
8. Build coalitions.
9. Exploit opportunities, using situations to your advantage. Go after winning issues.
10. Set up situations to benefit persons who can benefit you. Then deliver the goods at a cost-effective price.

A political climate exists in any organization, and its nature requires compromise, trade-offs, favors, and negotiation. Nurse managers must be political to gain their goals and objectives. Ehrat identifies four considerations of political strategy[34]:

1. Structural considerations: The first major political concept is to learn the history of the organization, including its past struggles and their outcomes. Budgets reflect one of these political outcomes. What is valued by the organization? The successful nurse manager identifies these valued data and operates within their constraints and boundaries.

2. Economic considerations: What are the costs versus the benefits? Give something in return for gaining something better. All departments expect to gain a fair share of an increased budget. To ensure that nursing has equity, nurse managers develop clientele, confidence, a meaningful network, administrative support, and effective platform skills. Nurse managers also exploit their opportunities. In gaining and sustaining this influence, they do not go beyond tolerated limits.

3. Procedural considerations: Timing is important and is learned from managerial experience and maturation. Resolution is needed to prepare for and carry out negotiation and compromise. Impact must be considered with respect to opposition, support, risks, price, and trade-offs, all of which require strategies.

4. Outcome-related considerations: The outcome must meet minimum standards of satisfaction and avoid problems. It must meet some needs of everyone. (Consensus means 70% to 80% approval, agreement, and support.)

The nurse manager moving into a new nursing management position plans strategies for success. From day one, this person arrives early, listens, is polite, and does not criticize his or her predecessor. This nurse manager makes friends with the boss, assumes authority, eliminates nonessentials, trains subordinates, and delegates decision making to them. He or she establishes a psychological distance, avoids gripers, treats all employees respectfully as adults, maintains an open mind, and follows effective communication skills by keeping people informed and encouraging their input.

66Resources in the healthcare field are scarce, causing political conflicts and power struggles. Nurse managers should learn strategies associated with political knowledge and skills.[35] 99

When conflicts occur, the nurse manager does not take sides. This individual attends to actions that produce quick results, impact the organization, are favorable to employees, and require a small investment. Giving a sense of nursing's mission, its importance, its relevance, and the meaningfulness of nursing work provides vision. This is done by listening, sharing, developing mutual ideas, and enlisting the support of informal leaders.

A research study of the relationship between nursing department purpose, philosophy, and objectives and evidence of their implementation examined documents in 35 nursing departments. Specific indicators used were patient classification systems, staffing patterns, standards of patient care, and cost-containment activity. Implementation rates of desired nursing activity varied from 9% to 25%, indicating that a "low rate of implementation negates a causal relationship between references in the documents to desired nursing activity and actual nursing activity." The researchers suggest that purpose statements are sometimes unrealistic and unachievable. The framework for this study should be used to expand the research in this area.[36]

WHAT IS PLANNING?

Planning, a basic function of management, is a principal duty of all managers. It is a systematic process and requires knowledgeable activity based on sound managerial theory. According to Fayol, the first element of management is planning, which he defines as making a plan of action to provide for the foreseeable future. This plan of action must have unity, continuity, flexibility, and precision. Fayol outlines the contents of a plan of action for his business, a large mining and metallurgic firm. The plan included annual and 10-year forecasts, taking advantage of input from others. Planning improves with experience, gives sequence in activity, and protects a business against undesirable changes. Fayol's concept is that planning facilitates wise use of resources and selection of the best approaches to achieving objectives. Planning facilitates the art of handling people. Because planning can fail, it requires moral courage. Effective planning requires continuity of tenure. Good planning is a sign of competence.[37]

Urwick writes that research in administration provides needed information for forecasting. According to Urwick, investigations should be carried out and their results expressed in concrete terms. Planning should be based on objectives framed in terms of making a product or providing a service for the community. Simplification and standardization are basic to sound planning procedures. The product or service should be of the right pattern. Planning provides information to coordinate work effectively and accurately. A good plan should be based on an objective; have standards; be simple, flexible, and balanced; and use available resources first.[38]

66 Planning is a continuous process, beginning with the setting of goals and objectives and then laying out a plan of action to accomplish them, put them into play, review the process and the outcomes, provide feedback to personnel, and modify as needed. As planning is put into action, the management functions of organizing, leading, and evaluating are implemented, making all management functions interdependent. 99

Planning is a mental process of decision making and forecasting. It is future oriented and ensures desirable probable outcomes. Planning involves determining objectives and strategies, programs, procedures, and rules to accomplish the objectives.[39]

In nursing, planning helps to ensure that clients or patients receive the nursing services they want and need and that these services are delivered by satisfied nursing workers.[40]

Knowledge of the following factors relative to successful planning should be used by successful managers:

- Characteristics of planning
- Elements of the planning process
- Strategic or long-term planning process
- Tactical or short-term planning process—functional versus operational planning
- Planning standards

Ackoff describes four orientations to planning[41]:

1. *Reactivism:* Looks to the past and considers technology an enemy. It supports the old organizational forms of an authoritarian, paternalistic hierarchy, and planning efforts are aimed at returning the organization to a previous state. Control operates from the top, with plans submitted from the bottom. Problems are addressed separately, with immediate supervisors adjusting, editing, and adding to plans as they proceed through the hierarchy to the top. Reactive planning is ritualistic; in such systems, planning is considered a prerogative of management. Experience is considered the best teacher, and age gives knowledge, understanding, and wisdom. Technological advances of other organizations replace products and services of organizations oriented to reactive planning. Reactive organizations support the arts and humanities, people and values, a sense of history, feelings of continuity, and preservation of traditions. Reactivists do tactical (short-term or operational) planning.

2. *Inactivism:* As a planning orientation prevents change and maintains conformity; it operates by crisis management, in which the goal is to control discomfort without addressing its cause. Managers are kept busy with red tape and bureaucracy. The effective instrument is the committee, which operates to keep people busy until the work is outdated or success is thwarted by in-

sufficient resources. Knowledge of current events plus connections is more important than is competence. Manners are valued. Inactivists do tactical or operational planning.

3. *Preactivism:* Dominant in U.S. organizations, preactivist managers accelerate change to exploit the future. They believe technology causes change and is therefore a panacea. Values associated with preactivism include management by objectives, inventiveness, growth, permissiveness, decentralization, and informality. Planning is done from the top down, with objectives. The appeal of preactivism is that planning is associated with science, technology, and the future. Because preactivism is based mainly on long-term forecasting, it is often full of errors.

4. *Interactivism:* Interactivists believe the future can be created and therefore design a desirable future and invent ways to achieve it. In this view, technology is valued depending on how it is used, experience reveals problems, and experiment leads to their solutions. The focus is on development, learning, and adaptation. Interactivistic planners may establish a planning period for achieving goals, objectives, and ideals. Goals are considered ends to be attained within the planning period. Objectives are ends desired, with progress expected within the planning period. Ideals are ends that are not entirely attainable but toward which progress is expected within and after the planning period. Interactivists emphasize normative planning.

The healthcare environment does not always support reactive planning by nurse managers. It is too competitive, both for patients and for scarce expert professional nurse providers. Nurse providers also resist authoritarianism and paternalism because they want to actively participate. Inactivism as a planning orientation is prevalent in subsidized government agencies, service departments of corporations, and universities. Nurse managers participate in such planning in these institutions. Nurse managers fall into the technological traps of preactivism. Plans are frequently made; however, many never become operational. Preactivists concentrate on strategic (long-term) planning.

Ackoff's interactive planning–management model is a systems model that can be applied in nursing management to effect change. A planning board does interactive planning–management. In a decentralized organization the planning board is the nurse manager of a unit, his or her boss, and the employees of the unit.[42]

The following are the five phases of Ackoff's interactive planning–management model[43]:

1. *Formulation of the mess:* The "mess" is the future we are now creating. Formulation of the mess includes determination of the problems and opportunities facing the organization, how they interact, and factors that obstruct or constrain one from addressing them. The output of this phase is a scenario of the future of the organization if its behavior and that of its environment do not change significantly.

2. *Ends planning (idealized redesign):* This is the design of the desired future. The output of this phase is the idealized design. This design is focused on the present; it must be technologically feasible, operationally viable, capable of incorporating learning, and adaptable.

3. *Means planning:* This phase invents ways to close the gaps between the idealized present and the mess. It involves identifying potential means, evaluating the alternatives, and selecting the best ones.

4. *Resource planning:* This phase includes determining when, where, and what resources are required and how they will be generated. Resources include facilities, equipment, personnel, information, money, and other inputs.

5. *Implementation and control:* This involves translating the decisions made in the previous phases into a set of assignments and schedules that specify responsible parties and realistic timeframes.

Figure 9-17 illustrates an interactive planning cycle.

Which type of planning is best for a nursing organization? Many nurse managers would opt for interactivism because it is proactive. Some of the characteristics of reactivism, inactivism, and

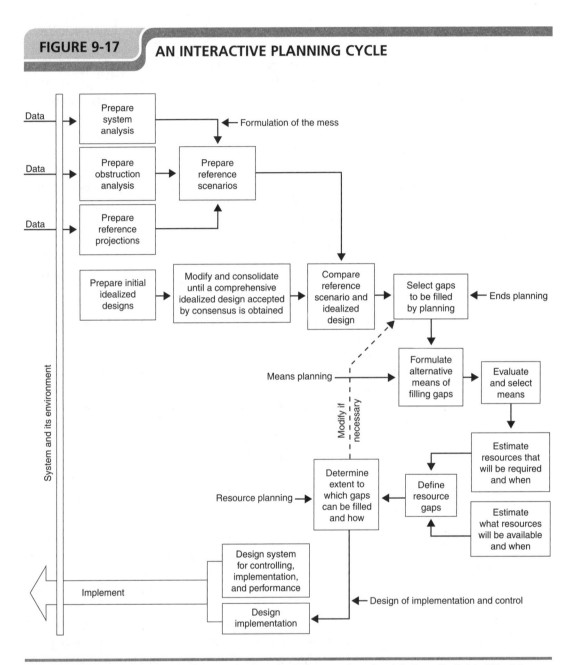

FIGURE 9-17 AN INTERACTIVE PLANNING CYCLE

Source: Ackoff, R. L. (1981). An interactive planning cycle. In *Creating the Corporate Future* (p. 75). Indianapolis, IN: John Wiley & Sons, Inc. Reprinted by permission of John Wiley & Sons, Inc.

preactivism are also useful to nurse managers. One could assess the working environment, decide which orientation to planning is most productive, and attempt to move in that direction. A nurse manager could select a style of planning that blends reactivism, inactivism, preactivism, and interactivism. Ackoff and others opt for the interactive planning–management model.

Purposes

The following are some reasons for planning[44]:

- It increases the chances of success by focusing on results and not on activities.
- It forces analytic thinking and evaluation of alternatives, thereby improving decisions.

- It establishes a framework for decision making that is consistent with top management objectives.
- It orients people to action rather than reaction.
- It includes day-to-day and future-focused managing.
- It helps to avoid crisis management and provides decision-making flexibility.
- It provides a basis for managing organizational and individual performance.
- It increases employee involvement and improves communication.
- It is cost-effective.

Donovan writes that planning has several benefits, among which are satisfactory outcomes of decisions; improved functions in emergencies; assurance of economy of time, space, and materials; and the highest use of personnel. She included decision making, philosophies, and objectives as key elements in planning.[45]

There is no purpose to the planning process unless there is a knowledge of and skill in applying those processes to the work situation; also necessary is skill in bringing the planning process up to the standard set when deficiencies exist.[46]

Characteristics

What is the nature of planning? What is so distinctive about it that it requires a nurse administrator to have specialized knowledge and skills? In an environment of changing technology, mounting costs, and multiple activities, there is a need for the chief nurse administrator and subordinate managers to plan. The forecasting of events and the laying out of a system of activities or actions for accomplishing the work of nursing and of the organization are prerequisites to success. Koontz and Weihrich define planning as "selecting missions and objectives and the actions to achieve them; it requires decision making, that is, choosing future courses of action from among alternatives."[47] They see planning as an elementary function of management. In their view of planning, nurse administrators avoid leaving events to chance; instead, they apply an intellectual process to consciously determine the course of action to take to accomplish the work. Donovan states that the planning process must be deliberate and analytic to produce carefully detailed programs of action that achieve objectives.[48]

The nurse manager plans effectively to create an environment of high-quality practice in which nursing personnel make evidence-based decisions that meet clients' needs. In such an environment, clinical nurses make decisions about the modality of practice, and nurse managers work with nursing personnel to establish and meet their personal objectives while meeting high quality objectives of the organization.

According to Hodgetts, planning forces a firm to forecast the environment, gives direction in the form of objectives, provides the basis for creating effective teams, and helps management learn to live with ambiguity.[49] Planning should be comprehensive, with nurse managers carefully determining objectives and making detailed plans to accomplish them.

Rowland and Rowland state that planning is largely a process of forecasting and decision making. It is future oriented, spanning time beginning in the present. These authors list the following phases of planning: determining objectives, collecting data, developing a plan of action, setting goals, and evaluating.[50]

Planning involves the collection, analysis, and organization of many kinds of data that are used to determine both the nursing care needs of patients and the management plans that provide the resources and processes to meet those needs and keep solutions patient centered. Accepting that nursing is a clinical practice discipline providing a human service, nurse managers plan to nurture the practitioners who provide the service.

> **❝ It has generally been understood that top administrators in nursing focus on long-term or strategic planning, whereas operational nurse managers focus on short-term or tactical planning. This process is outmoded. All managers and representative clinical nurses should have input into strategic planning. There should be strategic plans for every unit. ❞**

The following are examples of data that need to be collected and analyzed for planning purposes:

1. Daily average patient census
2. Bed capacity and percentage of occupancy
3. Average length of stay
4. Number of births
5. Number of operations
6. Trends in patient populations
    a. Diagnoses
    b. Age groups
    c. Acuity of illness
    d. Physical dependency
7. Trends in technology
    a. Diagnostic procedures
    b. Therapeutic procedures
8. Environmental analysis
    a. Internal forces impacting nursing: availability of nurses, turnover, other departments, delivery systems (including nursing modalities), theory-based practice, and physicians
    b. External forces impacting nursing: government, education, accreditation bodies, third-party payers, and others
    c. Trends in health care and in nursing, including changes in characteristics
    d. Threats to the nursing profession
    e. Opportunities for the nursing profession

Figure 9-18 demonstrates examples of data that might be collected and analyzed for planning purposes by nursing managers.

Data on diagnostic and therapeutic procedures are used to plan for new procedures, to revise old procedures, and to make new procedures known to nursing personnel; the preceding list is certainly not exhaustive.

FIGURE 9-18   PLANNING DATA FOR NURSE MANAGERS

- Live births have decreased 30% in the 3 years since the institution of a family planning program.
- Sixty-three percent of live births are discharged within a 24-hour period.
- The number of deliveries with complications has increased from 210 to 257 in 1 year.
- A new cardiac catheterization laboratory has been completed.
- The hospital planning board has decided to coordinate with other hospitals in the area to consolidate specialty services for newborn care, cardiovascular surgery, and neuroscience services.
- Enrollment of students for clinical nursing affiliation has increased from 450 to 792 in 1 year.
- Enrollment of students in the nursing cooperative education program has increased from 102 to 187 students.
- Medicare reimbursement pays $__ per patient for a day of home care.
- Early discharge has decreased average daily census from 381 to 304.
- Patient acuity has increased by 10.6 percentage points overall.

Source: Author.

Planning, a dynamic organizational process, has the characteristics of an open system. Planning does the following:

- Leads to success rather than failure.
- Prevents crisis and panic, which are costly and chaotic, distort achievement, and are dominated by a single person. Planning improves nursing division performance.
- Identifies future opportunities and expectations based on conditions through forecasting techniques that range from simple to complex.

Simple forecasting techniques follow the process of gathering data and analyzing them to determine alternative decisions and the effects each decision will produce. Strengths, weaknesses, opportunities, and threats are part of this analysis, which leads to decision, choice, and implementation. In complex forecasting, computer-based mathematical models are available that are becoming less expensive, require a lot of time and specialized skills, and extend from 3 to 15 years. New simulation models are constantly improving and are essential to modern planning.

Planning rests on logical, reflective thinking that is neither cast in concrete nor all encompassing. If needed, leadership or top management will effect change to undertake effective planning. Leadership should obtain input from all levels to ensure success through format, procedures, time frames, maintenance, and input review.

Through the planning process, nurse managers select and retain the elements of past and present plans that work. They focus on the future, and they implement and evaluate. Thus they successfully manage nursing personnel and material resources to achieve the objectives of the nursing enterprise.

> **"Planning is the key element of nursing that gives it direction, cohesion, and thrust. It causes all nursing personnel to focus on goals and objectives and stimulates their motivation."**

Elements

Although planning is characterized as a conceptual or thinking process, it produces readily identifiable specific elements, including written statements of mission or purpose, philosophy, objectives, and detailed management or operational plans. Operational plans are the blueprints by which the purpose, philosophy, and objectives are put into measurable actions. Management or operational plans include decision-making and problem-solving processes that include strategies, policies, and procedures.

The nursing division's strategic and operational plans are road maps that describe the business by name and location. Nurse managers make them informative by including a summary of the work of the division. The summary describing the nursing division should include enough information to give outsiders a bird's-eye view of its totality, such as the nursing products and services provided (by quantity), admissions, discharges, patient days, number of patients by acuity categories, research and best practice projects, educational programs, students, outpatient visits, and other products and services. The description summarizes marketing activities of the nursing division, including total revenues and expenses, and describes the managerial style of the division and its impact on employees, which is related to the organizational plan of the division of nursing.

Planning is the assessment of the nursing division's strengths and weaknesses, covering factors that affect performance and facilitate or inhibit the achievement of objectives. This assessment process has both long- and short-term objectives of its own. For example, if the clinical promotion ladder is a strength in nurse retention but is weakly applied by selective nurse managers, the problem will be addressed by written objectives.

Planning entails formulation of planning premises by extrapolating assumptions from the information analyzed.[51] If data indicate that nurses will be in increased supply because of increased enrollments in schools of nursing or in short supply as a result of increased opportunities in other fields, these findings should be translated into a premise. Other premises evolve related to increased salaries, benefits, and improved working conditions. These premises lead to further premises for marketing a career in nursing to high-school students and persons changing careers.

Planning entails writing specific, useful, realistic objectives (the why) that reflect both strategic and operational goals for the division of nursing and its personnel. Objectives become the reasons for an operational nursing management plan (the what), which detail the activities to be performed, the time frames for their accomplishment (the when), the persons responsible for accomplishing the activities (the who), and strategies for dealing with technical, economic, social, and political aspects. These operational plans have control systems for monitoring performance and providing feedback. They address the budget.

In addition to the previous elements of planning, Meier indicates that good management begins "with a coordinated purposeful organization of people who collectively on a functional responsibility basis" do the following[52]:

- Plan the organization
- Provide personnel
- Provide facilities
- Provide capital
- Set performance standards
- Develop management information systems
- Activate people

Good management keeps the nursing agency successful, ensuring its growth, success, and direction and a return on investment in the future. It is the responsibility of the nurse manager to prepare a plan carefully. Beyers recommends that nurse executives be involved in the following elements of strategy planning[53]:

- Product/market planning
- Business unit planning
- Shared resource planning
- Shared concern planning
- Corporate-level planning

Nursing in all areas, clinical and managerial, must consider competition. The patient will go where there is higher quality nursing care, which results from effectively planned and managed change. Nurse educators should perform market surveys to determine the nursing products and services that consumers want.[54] This activity itself constitutes change and results in patient-centered changes.

Considering the theory of the business of the healthcare organization and of nursing, what practices or people need to be abandoned? This may include products, services, markets, distribution channels, and every end user who does not fit the theory of the business. End users do not need many organizations to get information; they use the Internet to obtain information on providers and services. Nursing's goal is to improve this information and these services in the interest of survival and progress; the opportunity is with maintaining physical and mental functioning of individuals and populations. Drucker suggests managers look at windows of opportunity[55]:

- The organization's own unexpected successes and failures, as well as the unexpected successes and failures of the organization's competitors
- Incongruities, especially in the process, whether of production or distribution, or in customer behavior
- Process needs

- Changes in industry and market structures
- Changes in demographics
- Changes in meaning and perception
- New knowledge

Strategic Planning

Drucker defines strategic planning as "a continuous, systematic process of making risk-taking decisions today with the greatest possible knowledge of their effects on the future; organizing efforts necessary to carry out these decisions and evaluating results of these decisions against expected outcome through reliable feedback mechanisms."[56]

Nursing administrators can increase effectiveness through strategic planning, which can promote professional nursing practice and the long-term goals of the organization and the division of nursing. Clear, complete plans are developed in seven areas of key results, designed to include standards of performance that challenge and inspire[57]:

1. Client satisfaction
2. Productivity
3. Innovation
4. Staff development
5. Budget goals
6. Quality
7. Organizational climate

Strategic planning in nursing is concerned with what nursing should be doing. Its purpose is to improve allocation of scarce resources, including time and money, and to manage the agency for performance. Strategic planning provides strategic forecasting from 1 to more than 20 years; organizations that change rapidly may need to engage more frequently in strategic planning. It should involve top nurse managers and representatives of all levels of nursing hierarchy; including input from clinical nursing personnel promotes professional satisfaction throughout the nursing department and increases the likelihood of successful implementation. The process includes analysis of factors such as projected technological advances, the internal and external environments, the nursing and healthcare market and industry, the economics of nursing and health care, availability of human and material resources, and judgments of top management.[58]

The strategic planning process is used to acquire and develop new healthcare services and product lines, including new nursing services and products. Strategic planning is also used to divest outdated services and products. Both activities present moral and ethical dilemmas for the managers and practitioners of nursing. Strategic planning can foster better goals, better corporate values, and better communication about corporate direction. It can lead to changes in operation, management, and organization. Strategic planning can produce better management strategy and analysis and can forecast and mute external threats.

"Environmental scans" are tools of the strategic planning process. These scans include identification of future trends, risks, and opportunities. Environmental scans also identify projected governmental, demographic, and social changes that will affect nursing strategic planning in an era of healthcare reform, aging population, single parenthood, drug use, crime and violence, and problems in the education system.[60]

> **"The process of strategic planning is more important than the plan itself. The process serves to give planners a sense of direction, involves everyone, and enables unexpected opportunities to be seized and unexpected crises to be dealt with.[59]"**

Odiorne recommends the following process for crafting strategic plans[61]:

1. Identify the major problems of your organization to determine where you are headed and where you want to be. This process is called *gap analysis*. This technique examines markets, products, customers, employees, finances, technology, and community relations. Cabinets or task forces from each area may be helpful in performing gap analysis and identifying major problems.
2. Examine outside influences that relate to the key problems of your organization. Focus on the few major issues.
3. List the critical issues, that is, those that affect the entire organization, have long-term impact, and are based on irrefutable evidence rather than media hype.
4. Rank the critical issues according to their importance to your organization, and plan accordingly: "must do," "to do," and "important, but not urgent." Then divide these critical issues into "success producers" and "failure preventers."
5. Decide the issues critical to all organization managers.
6. Include time in the budget.

Figure 9-19 lists ways in which strategic planning can be used to improve management. The process of strategic planning has several phases, as summarized in Figure 9-20.

Strategic planning includes both planning of the process and strategy for implementing the plan. During the strategic planning process, analysis of the business environment and the internal capabilities of the organization for producing a product or service suited to success in the business environment are analyzed. Goals and strategies are also set during the planning process.[62]

Peters believes that strategic planning should be a line exercise rather than a staff one. The focus should be on building a work force that is well trained, flexible, and quality conscious.[63] Strategic plans

---

FIGURE 9-19 | **HOW STRATEGIC PLANNING CAN BE USED TO IMPROVE NURSING MANAGEMENT**

- To provide accountability and monitoring of performance; to tie merit to performance.
- To set up more formal planning programs and require divisional and unit planning.
- To integrate strategic plans with operational and financial plans.
- To think and concentrate more on strategic issues.
- To improve knowledge of and training in strategic planning.
- To increase top management involvement and commitment.
- To improve focus on competition, market segments, and external factors.
- To improve communication from top administration and nursing management.
- To allow better execution of plans.
- To be more realistic and rationalize and vacillate less.
- To improve the development of nursing management strategies.
- To improve the development and communication of nursing management goals.
- To put less emphasis on raw numbers.
- To anticipate the future and plan for it.
- To develop the annual budget.
- To focus on quality outputs that will improve nurse performance and productivity, decrease losses, and increase return on equity.

Source: Author.

| FIGURE 9-20 | SUMMARY OF PHASES OF STRATEGIC PLANNING PROCESS |

Phase 1: The Mission and the Creed

Develop statements that define the work, the aims, and the character of the division of nursing. These include idea statements of shared values and beliefs. They are called mission (or purpose) and creed (or philosophy) statements and relate to personnel, patients, community, and all other potential customers.

Phase 2: Data Collection and Analysis

Collect and analyze data about the healthcare industry and nursing. Such data should include internal forces that define the work and affect employees, clients, stockholders, and creditors; technological advances; threats; opportunities to improve growth and productivity; external forces such as competition, communities, governmental and political issues, and legal requirements; marketing and public relations or image; trends in the physical and social work environments; and communication. Use simple and complex forecasting techniques, including trend lines, group consensus, nominal group process, and a qualitative decision matrix that uses probabilities based on conditions of certainty, risk, and uncertainty.

Phase 3: Assess Strengths and Weaknesses

Define those factors from the data analysis that influence management of the division of nursing. List them as strengths/opportunities that facilitate effectiveness and achievement of goals and objectives or as weaknesses/threats that impede achieving goals and objectives. Define the current position and strength of the unit.

Phase 4: Goals and Objectives

Write realistic and general statements of goals. Break the goals down into concrete written statements of objectives the division of nursing intends to accomplish in the next 3 to 5 years.

Phase 5: Strategies

Identify untoward conditions that could develop in achieving each objective. Note administrative actions to avoid or manage them. Use this information to modify goals and objectives, making contingency plans for alternative actions. Define the organization needed for implementing strategic plans. It should be interactive if cross-functional activities are involved—a matrix organization.

Phase 6: Timetable

Develop a timetable for accomplishing each objective. Identify by geographic units as well. This phase produces or becomes part of the plans.

Phase 7: Operational and Functional Plans

Provide guidelines or general instructions that lead functional and operational nurse managers to develop action plans to implement the goals and objectives. These include detailed actions, policies, practices, communication and feedback, controlling and evaluation plans, budgets, timetables, and persons to be held accountable.

Phase 8: Implementation

Put the plans to work.

Phase 9: Evaluation

Provide for formative evaluation reports before, during, and after the implementation of operational plan. Provide for summative evaluation that is quantified. Report actual vs. expected results. Evaluate the strategic mission, and plan frequently. Provide continuous feedback that can be used to modify and update the plan. Use people who implement the plan to evaluate it.

Source: Author.

should be developed from the bottom up, the front line where business occurs. The written plan should be shared with everyone and should not be slavishly followed because it is constantly affected by change and should be modified every year.[64]

Obviously, with constant, quick changes in markets and operations, time management is vital to strategic planning. Strategic plans should be capable of being quickly made and changed.

Implementation of strategic plans includes strategies related to proper activities, organizational structure, company resources, and support systems. The various strategic plans of the organization should be linked to avoid internal conflicts. These links include operations, finance, human relations, marketing, budgeting, and personal action. All the elements of a strategic plan make up a system, and these elements of a system need constant monitoring for their success.[65]

Strategic, or long-term, planning came into vogue after World War II and is widely used in business and industry. It is becoming prevalent in the healthcare world because of technological change, modernization of the industry, increased government roles, and increased complexity of nursing management. In strategic planning, nurse managers are required to manage in the future tense by defining the future of nursing in areas such as setting objectives, developing an organization to achieve those objectives, allocating resources, and implementing objectives through specific best practice policies and plans. Nurse managers must continually evaluate and provide feedback for accomplishing these objectives and developing new strategic plans with new objectives that include planning for research use in nursing practice.[66]

A strategic plan is coldly objective in evaluating what the nursing business is and what it will be. It does not leave success to chance, and it prevents the status quo from paralyzing nursing progress. Strategic planning leads to strategic management and becomes an integral part of thinking in all management operations, including budgeting, information, compensation, organization, leadership development, patient education, and decision support systems.[67]

One of the benefits of strategic planning is that it gives a sense of direction to the managers and practitioners of nursing within the organization. The strategic plan becomes a flexible control mechanism that can be modified to deal with variables, conserve resources, and provide professional satisfaction. The strategic plan deals concretely with complex projects or programs in multistage time sequences.[68]

Conclusions About the Strategic Planning Process

Strategic planning is often considered to be a goal-setting process that is largely carried out by top management. There are many instances of long-term plans being made but fewer instances of their having been put to use. Operating nurse managers need to be trained in the strategic planning process; include techniques to involve operational managers and thereby commit them to decisions. Development of global goals and strategies broadens the identification and solution of problems, reducing threats to and unveiling opportunities for the organization.

"A cyclic model of strategic planning provides for continuous assessment of an organization's mission, values, vision, and primary strategies. This assessment is based on feedback from benchmark analysis, shareholder impact, and progress in implementation of strategies.[70]"

The demonstrated usefulness of scientific planning influences the behavior of operating managers. Rewards, in the form of both pay and praise, motivate these operating managers.

Strategic planning has many benefits. It provides for objective consideration of strategic choices or options that are better matched with organizational goals and objectives. With strategic planning, the outlook becomes future oriented, resources are allocated systematically, and rapid change is accommodated.[69] Strategic plans must be dynamic to take advantage of these benefits, projecting trends and directions. These plans are the blueprints that are to be updated as the environment changes the phases and stages in the process of strategic planning (summarized in Figure 9-20).

If they are to survive, urban healthcare organizations have to do strategic planning similar to that done by many rural hospitals[71]:

- Involvement of outside organizations in fostering community change
- A high degree of community commitment and investment in all stages of the process
- Comprehensive identification of problems in the healthcare system by outside consultants
- The use of periodic meetings of communities confronting similar issues
- Identification and development of local leadership
- Enhancing teamwork among local healthcare providers
- Development of conflict-resolution mechanisms within healthcare organizations

"Healthcare institutions have to make global competitiveness a strategic goal. With the world awash in "virtual money" in portfolios of investments, healthcare leaders have responsibility for institutional investments of endowment funds. For-profit institutions are a part of people's investment portfolios.[72] Nurse leaders should take advantage of this situation through the strategic planning process. "

Functional and Operational Planning

Objectives must be converted into actions, that is, activities, assignments, and deadlines, all with clear accountability. The action level is where nurse managers eliminate the old and plan for the new. It is where time is put into perspective and new and different methods can be tried. The action level is where nurse managers answer these questions over and over again: What is it? What will it be? What should it be?

An operational plan is the written blueprint for achieving objectives; it is the organization and direction of the delivery of nursing care. It includes planning to create a budget, to create an effective organizational structure that encompasses a quality monitoring process, and to direct nurse leaders, an administrative staff, and new programs.[73]

The operational plan does the following:

- Specifies the activities and procedures used
- Sets timetables for the achievement of objectives
- Tells who the responsible persons are for each activity and procedure
- Describes ways of preparing personnel for jobs and procedures for evaluating patient care
- Specifies the records kept and the policies needed
- Gives individual mangers freedom to accomplish their objectives and those of the institution, division, department, or unit

The operational plan is sometimes called a management plan (Figures 9-21 and 9-22).

Nursing planning performed at a service or departmental level is referred to as functional planning. It generally relates to a specialty service within a nursing division. For example, the staff development director would be included in development of the strategic plan but would develop operational plans for staff development as a whole and for specific services or units. Likewise, the director of a home healthcare agency would assist in developing the strategic plan for the company but would develop agency mission, philosophy, goals, objectives, and operational plans. With decentralization each nurse manager would develop a strategic plan for his or her unit to be integrated into the organization's strategic plan.

Operational plans are everyday working management plans developed from both long-term objectives and the strategic planning process and short-term or tactical plans. In development of operational objectives, new strategic objectives can emerge or old ones can be modified or discarded. Strategic and tactical plans are made into operational plans and carried out at all levels of nursing management.

FIGURE 9-21 | OPERATIONAL PLAN

Objective

The clients receive skilled nursing services to meet their total individual needs as diagnosed by professional nurses. This process is systematic, beginning with the gathering of base data, and it is planned, implemented, evaluated, and revised on a continual basis. It covers physical, emotional, spiritual, environmental, social, economic, and rehabilitation needs and includes health teaching involved in the planning of total client care. Its ultimate goal is to assist clients to, or return them to, optimal health status and independence as quickly as possible.

Actions	Target Dates	Accomplishments
Institute primary care nursing	January 1–June 30	Assigned to Ms. Scott. Decision made to attempt to use self-care concepts of Orem: (1) definition and (2) nursing systems.
1. Assign problem of overall development of a plan	January 31	
2. Assign development of a self-care concept for application using Orem[15] and Kinlein[16] as references	February 15	January 19: Assigned to Ms. Longez. In a discussion with Ms. Scott and Ms. Longez, the decision was made to investigate application of self-care using the nursing process as described by Kinlein. The nursing staff were particularly interested in the nursing history process described by Kinlein. Ms. Longez has added this dimension to her assignment. She has requested Mr. Jarmann be assigned to assist her, and he has agreed.
3. Organize resources	February 28	February 5: Ms. Scott has just updated me on the project. A good portion of her plan has been developed. They are now making a staffing plan, including job descriptions and job standards.
		February 27: The plan is completed and has been discussed with me. A few minor adjustments are being made.
4. Coordinate plan (a) Nursing personnel (b) Administrator (c) Public relations (d) Physicians (e) Other as needed	March 31	Done. All want to participate. Done. Announcements made to community through news media. Done and well received. Presented to board per request of administrator. They want progress reports.
5. Select and train staff	April 30	Assigned to Ms. Finch for training. Will be assisted by Ms. Scott and Ms. Longez. I will select staff with their recommendation.
6. Implement	June 30	Ms. Scott wants to direct implementation and I have concurred.

Source: Author.

Operational managers develop goals, objectives, strategies, and targets to set the strategic plan in motion. They match each unit goal or objective to a strategic goal or objective; their objectives can be much more detailed and specific than the strategic objectives. Numerous operational objectives can support one strategic objective.

All aspects of an operational plan are based on goals and on their achievement. The individual leadership style determines whether goal setting will be top-down or bottom-up. Bottom-up goal setting is

FIGURE 9-22	STANDARDS FOR EVALUATION OF MANAGEMENT PLAN OF NURSING DIVISION, DEPARTMENT, SERVICE, OR UNIT

1. The written management plan should operationalize the strategic goals of the organization as well as the objectives of the nursing division, department, service, or unit. It should specify activities or actions, persons responsible for accomplishing them, and target dates or time frames, as well as providing for evaluation of progress. Each activity or action should be listed in problem-solving or decision-making format, as appropriate.

2. The management plan is personal to the incumbent, who should select the standards for developing, maintaining, and evaluating it. The nurse manager should solicit desired input from appropriate nursing persons and others.

3. The actions listed should reflect planning for the following:

    a. Nursing care programs to ensure safe and competent nursing services to clients

        i. The nursing process, including data gathering, assessment, diagnosis, goal setting and prescription, intervention and application, evaluation, feedback, change, and accountability to the consumer

        ii. A process and outcome audit

        iii. Promotion of self-care practices

    b. Establishment of policies and procedures for using competent nursing personnel: recruitment, selection, assignment, retention, and promotion based on individual qualifications and capabilities without regard to race, national origin, creed, color, sex, or age

    c. Integration of nursing care programs into the total program of the health care organization and community through committee participation in professional and service activities, and credentialing of individuals in organizations, including nursing organizations

    d. A budget that is evaluated and revised as necessary

    e. Job descriptions that include standards stated as objectives, outcomes, or results and that are known to the incumbents

    f. Specific utilization of personnel. This part of the plan should:

        i. Conform to a staffing plan that is based on timing nursing activities and rating of patients

        ii. Match competencies of people to total job requirements

        iii. Place prepared people in practice

        iv. Place prepared people in administration

        v. Place prepared people in education

        vi. Place prepared people in research

        vii. Foster identification of non-nursing tasks and their assignment to appropriate other departments or non-nursing personnel

        viii. Recognize excellence in all fields: administration, education, research, and practice

    g. Provision of needed supplies and equipment for nursing activities

    h. Provision of input into remodeling and establishing required physical facilities

    i. Orientation and continuing education of all nursing personnel

    j. Education of students in the healthcare field according to a written agreement and collaborative implementation between faculty of the educational institutions and personnel of the service organization

    k. Development of nursing research staff, research activities, and application of the research findings of others

    l. Evaluation of all objectives—organizational, divisional, departmental, and at the service and unit level, as well as those stated in the individual's job description and standards

4. The management plans should have mileposts that are reasonable and attainable, with deadlines included.

5. Management plans should be based on complete information.

Source: Author.

participatory, using guidelines from the operational manager.[74] Participatory goal setting is believed to increase workers' commitment and achievement. Increased participation leads to greater group cohesiveness, which in turn fosters increased morale, increased motivation, and increased achievement and productivity. Individuals, including nurse managers, can ensure greater relative success in achievement of goals by building additional resources and time into their plans. Nurse managers who reject the goals of participating staff should explain reasons for rejection. Participation in goal setting alone will not ensure success. Figure 9-23 suggests a timetable for strategic and operational planning. Like the plan itself, such planning should be flexible.

The concept of goals as global in nature and objectives as detailed is sometimes confusing to some participants in the planning process, particularly nurse managers. In nursing, written organizational goals have seldom been used and probably did not exist in many agencies. More attention is now being given to this aspect of management. External influences create the demand for a strategic plan, and more nurse managers have had management education and training.[75]

Some organizations do not develop separate goals and objectives. Instead, they develop objectives and from them create management plans. In actual practice, as organizational objectives are developed into operational plans, specific goals and objectives are written for each major activity. The goal is to plan, assess progress toward goals and objectives at all levels, and provide feedback to all levels of management.

FIGURE 9-23   **TIMETABLE FOR STRATEGIC AND OPERATIONAL PLANNING**

1. Organization

   Mondays 7–9 A.M. Conference room. Breakfast.

   Attendees: Chief executive officer (CEO), assistants (including for division of nursing), and understudies

   Agenda: CEO, with input from all others, relates each item to strategic plan. CEO updates and develops written operational plans at meeting or immediately following, then reviews them for next agenda for progress and for strategic plan development.

   Minutes: Prepared and distributed to attendees

2. Division of Nursing

   Monday 3–4 P.M. Nursing conference room.

   Attendees: Chief nurse executive (CNE), associates, department heads, chairs of clinical consultants, nursing management, and staff nurse committees

   Agenda: Chairs, with input from CNE and all others, relate each item to strategic plan of division of nursing. These goals and objectives have already been coordinated with the organizational strategic plan. CNE and others update operational plans of division and departments during meeting or immediately following, then review them for next agenda for progress and nursing strategic plan development.

   Minutes: Prepared and distributed to attendees, to CEO, and to selected others

3. Service and Unit

   CNE and/or associates meet with their nurse managers and representative clinical nurses at mutually determined times and places. The groups have agendas, keep minutes, update written operational plans, and provide feedback to top nurse managers and clinical nurse staff.

Source: Author.

Planning New Ventures

In an era of competitiveness, every nurse manager may be called on to develop ideas for new ventures (nursing products or services). For example, continuing education courses can be packaged, marketed, and presented within the organization or taken on the road. Hospitals have moved into home health care, durable medical goods, wellness and fitness programs, and many other ventures. The basic rule for undertaking new ventures is to do sound planning.

Any new venture should have a separate marketing plan. The nurse manager consults with marketing department personnel and develops a marketing operation plan to do the following[76]:

- Define problems and opportunities that may confront the new enterprise and product
- Define the competitive position of the product and set objectives to meet anticipated problems and opportunities
- Detail work steps, schedules, assignment of responsibility, budgets, and other elements of implementation
- Describe the monitoring (control) plan

The marketing plan should be separate from a primary operational plan and should include gathering and analysis of data related to the product or service as it already exists in the area. For example, if the product is continuing education, who are the customers? They could be nurse managers, nurse educators, registered nurses, licensed practical nurses, or members of other healthcare disciplines. What is the competition in the market area? Is it local or imported from educational institutions and for-profit companies? Who pays for the course—employers and/or individuals?

In addition, the operational plan gathers and analyzes data that pinpoint possible strengths, weaknesses, problems, and opportunities. It identifies strategies for taking competitive advantages. Each opportunity, problem, strength, and weakness should be addressed by definitive objectives developed into operational plans for advertising, product development, and even personal selling.

Before any new venture is launched, a control plan is made. This plan includes measures of performance, such as numbers or amounts of products or services to be sold within specific time frames. Managers are assigned responsibility for comparing expected results with actual results and for making corrections in all elements of the plan and its implementation. This plan can be achieved with marketing and operational plan checklists.[77] Figure 9-24 illustrates an operational plan for the development of an intermediate cardiac rehabilitation program.

Nursing service planning supports the mission and objectives of the institution. For this reason, the nurse administrator needs to know the plans and programs of the health facility administrator and of other departments in which personnel contribute to the joint effort of providing healthcare services. The nurse administrator should be a participatory, voting member of all important committees of the institution including those dealing with budgets, planning, credentialing, auditing, utilization, infection control, patient care improvement, the library, or any other committees concerned in any way with nursing service, nursing activities, and nursing personnel.

The nurse administrator who participates in institutional committee work achieves an overall view of agency problems and activities and is in a position to interpret problems, policies, and plans of the agency to nursing personnel. He or she can also interpret nursing needs and problems to personnel of other departments. This planning integrates the nursing care program into the total program of the healthcare institution.

Business Plans

Business plans are detailed descriptions of the process for ensuring launching of a new product or product line, project, unit, or service. Business plans meet many of the standards for strategic planning as they

FIGURE 9-24	DIVISION OF NURSING—CARDIAC REHABILITATION PROGRAM

Strategic Objective

The patient is provided with an effective patient and patient–family teaching program, which includes guidance and assistance in the use of medical center resources and community agencies that can contribute support to the patient's total needs.

Operational Objectives	Actions	Target Dates and Persons Responsible	Accomplishments
Determine cardiologist's perception of the program: goals, resources to be used, breadth of services to be provided, etc.	1. Prepare an agenda for meeting with cardiologist.	Do by July 1, 200x. Swansburg (S) and Perry (P)	The following agenda was developed: • Need for new services. • What will they be? • What will they cost? • What will be charged? • Who will pay? • Where will they be done? • Who will do them? • How many patients? • What equipment and supplies are needed?
	2. Make appointment with cardiologist.	May 3, 200x, at 11 A.M. in Dr. C's office; S and P	May 3, 200x: Had a meeting with Dr. C, the cardiologist. The purpose of this program is to rehabilitate patients following open-heart surgery, angioplasty, and post–myocardial infarction. It is the intermediate phase between acute care and when they enter "bounce back." The following decision evolved from the meeting: 1. This program will be limited because no other such services are available. 2. Services will include physical exercises, monitoring, progress report by patient, counseling as indicated. 3. Only patients with insurance or ability to pay will be accepted. 4. It will be done in PT on Mon., Wed., and Fri. from 7 to 9 A.M. 5. Equipment and supplies will be in-house. 6. The CV clinical nurse specialist will be the project director.
Meet with the CV clinical nurse specialist and plan the program.	3. Make appointment with nurse D to plan the program.	May 4, 200x, 8 A.M.; S and P with D	Plan: 1. D will coordinate with PT director. 2. P will figure cost of program by the hour and set charges with accounting office.

Operational Objectives	Actions	Target Dates and Persons Responsible	Accomplishments
			3. D will borrow equipment to run the program until the next capital budget.
			4. Accomplish this by May 12, 200x.
Have plan completed by May 31, 200x.	4. Set up a control chart to identify when each phase of project will be completed.	May 12, 200x; P	May 10, 200x: Done. Posted.
	5. Write policy and procedure for the program. Include admission and discharge procedures and emergency plan.	May 31, 200x; D	May 29, 200x: Draft presented; minor changes needed.
			May 31, 200x: Done.
	6. Obtain equipment and supplies.	May 31, 200x; D	May 17, 200x: Done.
	7. Coordinate with PT director.	May 12, 200x; D	May 17, 200x: Done.
	8. Meet with cardiologist when all this is done.	June 1, 200x; P, S, and D	June 2, 200x: Met with cardiologist. Dr. C is happy with plan and will be ready to start on July 1, 200x.
Provide for third-party reimbursement. Develop marketing plan. Develop evaluation plan.	9. Discuss with insurance companies.	June 15, 200x; P	June 15, 200x: Insurance reps will visit the program and make decision. Appointment made. Marketing plan is already in operation with announcements mailed to all area cardiologists. D has a good evaluation plan.
	10. Prepare detailed marketing plan.	June 30, 200x; P and D	
	11. Prepare evaluation plan.		
	12. Implement program.	July 1, 200x; D	July 1, 200x: Had our first patient today. Cardiologist was there as required by insurance companies. All went well.
	13. Evaluate the program weekly until stabilized.	D, beginning July 8, 200x.	

Source: Author.

are projected over an extended time period of months or years. Their purpose is to provide sources of information for investors and decision makers, motivation, and measurement of performance.[78] Business plans are the blueprints for ventures. A clinical nurse specialist who decides to enter private practice as a consultant should write a business plan to solidify ideas and prepare for the unexpected.[79]

The following are key elements of a business plan as described by Johnson and others[80]:

- Introduction: The nature, goals, objectives, and desired outcomes of the proposed business
- Description of the business: The goals, nature, and history of the sponsoring institution, nature and history of the product, and industry trends
- Market and competition analyses: The target audience, pricing, promotion, placement, and positioning; data from solid market research are used

- Product development: Product description, resources, time frames for development, and quality control plan
- Operational plan: The location, facilities, labor force, and equipment
- Marketing plan: To market services or products, the mission, marketing research, measurable goals, strategies, and staffing and financial plans
- Organizational plan: To recruit qualified employees, an organizational chart and job descriptions
- Developmental schedule: To include planning for growth
- Financial plan: To secure capital
- Executive summary

Business plans are often categorized as strategic plans. Many of the key elements are the same, although a business plan is more detailed than a strategic plan. Actually, a business plan is developed for each new venture emerging from a strategic plan. This is essentially making the business case for any new project or programs. Developing a business plan is not unlike outlining strategies for a project plan. Using a project management methodology, the business plan has a beginning and an end, designed to specify the need (needs assessment), evidence to support changes, and outcomes to measure to determine efficacy.

Figure 9-25 is a modified business plan/operational plan for accomplishing objectives related to management improvement and resource management for an intensive care unit.

Practical Planning Actions

Practical day-to-day planning actions of value to the nurse administrator include the following exercises:

1. At the beginning of each day, make a list of actions to be accomplished for the day. Cross off the actions as they are accomplished or at the end of the day. At the beginning of the next workday, carry over actions not accomplished. Either do them first or decide if they are actions that really need to be done. Do not hold tasks over from one day to the next indefinitely.
2. Plan ahead for meetings. If the meeting is a nursing responsibility, prepare and distribute the agenda in advance. Have a secretary call members for their items to be listed on the agenda. Have a secretary forward nursing items for the agenda of organizational meetings to the appropriate chair in advance. Prepare for the presentation.
3. Identify developing problems and put them in the appropriate portion of the division's operational or management plans.
4. Review the operational or management plan on a scheduled basis. Do this with key managers so that each knows his or her responsibilities for accomplishment of activities.
5. Review the appropriate portions of the division operational or management plan with other nurse managers when counseling them.
6. Plan for discussion of ideas gleaned from professional publications. This activity can be part of a job standard, with different managers assigned specific topics or journals. Doing so may help integrate best practice solutions from the best available evidence.
7. Suggest similar practical planning actions to other nurse managers.

Planning is also necessary to provide programs for orientation and continuing education for nursing personnel so that all will be current in applying evidence-based practice principles. Sustained improvement at the point of care and with other administrative and hospital services necessitates initiation and utilization of and participation in studies or research projects in the healthcare field. Two additional important areas for planning are educational programs that include student experience in the division of nursing and evaluation of clinical and administrative practices to determine whether the objectives of the division are being achieved.

FIGURE 9-25   **OPERATIONAL PLAN—INTENSIVE CARE UNIT**

Management Improvement: Unit Objectives, February 1, 200x

1. Precipitate imaginative thinking to improve existing procedures, capitalize on time expenditure, and introduce modern concepts and materials that directly enhance unit accomplishment.
2. Promote creativity in improving the existing patient environment.
3. Provide more modern concepts of total patient care by constant review and revision of unit administrative/managerial policies.

Plans for Achievement of Objectives	Actions	Target Dates	Accomplishments
Plan and implement a continuing unit improvement program.	1. Conduct a continuous review and analysis of unit improvement efforts through	February	Reviewed and found current for following reasons: Turnover in personnel is fast. Not all objectives were adequately met; need to establish a better way of accomplishing them.
	a. Monthly unit conferences to review and update philosophy and objectives. Strive to accomplish more in each objective area.	February–July	
	b. Patient suggestions	Review each month	Done.
	c. Suggestions of superiors	Daily	Done. In addition, all nurses were counseled by the charge nurse. Nursing technicians are presently receiving counseling, and all is being documented. Counseling had not been documented in 6 years, except for remarks such as "Things went well and we did our job, so no counseling was needed."
	d. Revision of unit procedures	April	
	e. Briefing of all personnel. Discuss philosophy, objectives, job descriptions, performance standards, hospital and nursing service policies and procedures, and unit procedures.	February	
	2. Review equipment and supplies for improvement by addition or deletion.		Disapproved. Disposable tubing was approved, ordered, and in use by June.
	a. Submit work order to alter a locker as a drying cabinet for respirator parts, because moisture provides a growth medium for *Pseudomonas* bacteria.		New floor to be done by August 1. Compressed air started by March 15. Cardiac monitors arrived April 3. Patient units 1, 3, and 4 were equipped. Unit 4 was designated the maximum monitoring site and is to be used to monitor patients with Swan-Ganz arterial lines and questionable cardiac conditions.
	b. Check on status of new floor, piped-in compressed air system, and cardiac monitors.	February–April	
Review standardized policies and procedures for implementation of more current concepts of improved care accomplishments.	3. Evaluate all areas of management for current standardized efficiency.		This was done, and cleaning procedures were looked at and improved when they appeared poor. HEPA filters were replaced in February. Wall suction valves were replaced. Pipelines were found to be clogged with secretions, and system had to be purged. Shelves were mounted on wall by four units to replace bedside stands.
	a. Check all areas of infection sources.		
	i. Air exchange and pressure checked quarterly.	February	
	ii. HEPA filters changed quarterly.	February	

continues

FIGURE 9-25	OPERATIONAL PLAN—INTENSIVE CARE UNIT (CONTINUED)

Plans for Achievement of Objectives	Actions	Target Dates	Accomplishments
	iii. Check wall suction, because filters do not appear to be doing the job.	February	Respirators, nebulizers, and blenders were mounted on wall above each patient unit. Suction bottles were relocated and outlets changed in an effort to isolate them from the oxygen nebulization units. Swan-Ganz catheters were standardized, and requisitioning was transferred from the unit to central supply. Ambu bags were equipped with corrugated tubing to serve as an oxygen reservoir and deliver a maximum concentration of 99% to 100%. The disposable Aqua-pack nebulizer was deleted, resulting in a $40 per case saving.
	iv. Eliminate messy bedside stands.	February	
	b. Improve safety.		
	i. Secure equipment.	April	
	ii. Isolate oxygen nebulization units from suction.	April	
	iii. Send all equipment to central supply for processing.	April	
	iv. Improve efficiency of Ambu resuscitators.	April	
	4. Projected: An anesthesiologist will be assigned to the intensive care unit. All bronchoscopies will be done here. Open heart surgery is still an open and current topic.		

Resource Management
1. Provide, secure, and maintain the appropriate and economical use of supplies and equipment that permit unit personnel to devote maximum time and care to patient activities.
2. Provide the unit with adequate tools for safe and effective patient care.
3. Provide the unit with conservative utilization and centralization of unit supplies and equipment, thus promoting peak efficiency in meeting patients' needs.

Plans for Achievement of Objectives	Actions	Target Dates	Accomplishments
Plan, evaluate, and project needed supplies and equipment that enhance effective and safe nursing care.	Identify projected needs with unit manager through review of 1. Unit inventories of equipment and budgetary estimate 2. Standards for supplies 3. Availability of supplies and equipment 4. Economical use of supplies and equipment	February	Items ordered (projected replacements for 200x–200x): 1 electronic thermometer 1 IV pump 5 transducers 1 ventilator 1 sphygmomanometer 1 Wright respirometer 4 metal storage cabinets 4 Ambu bags 1 blood gas analyzer New cubicle curtains
Plan and execute appropriate utilization of materials.	1. Economical use of expendable supplies and adequate safeguards to prevent misuse and loss 2. Knowledge of principles of operation of appropriate mechanical equipment and procedures for effecting prompt servicing and repairs		Items replaced: ECG and defibrillator portable ECG machine spirometers suction regulators Items deleted: 1 electronic thermometer 1 internal/external defibrillator (to dog lab) 2 compressor units

Plans for Achievement of Objectives	Actions	Target Dates	Accomplishments
			Miscellaneous:
			file card supply system revamped
			shelving obtained for lower
			doors
			Personnel turnover:
			Projected losses:
			Ms. Speich, RN, June
			Ms. Ullman, RN, August
			Ms. Urbom, RN, May
			Ms. Malloy, RN, June
			Mr. Falco, ward clerk, April
			Projected gains:
			Ms. Tishoff, RN, May
			Mr. Robertshaw, RN, May
			Mr. Angelus, RN, April
			Mrs. Figuera, unit secretary,
			April
			Myra C. Breck, RN
			Nurse Manager, ICU

Source: Author.

Divisional Planning

There are many important reasons for planning, and avoiding duplicated efforts is one of them. Planning also improves communication throughout the division and the institution and reduces fragmentation by helping to keep functional units headed in the same direction. Planning is vital management training for all nurse managers. During its initial phases, planning uses an objective analysis of the division to determine its current status. The mission, strengths, weaknesses, and environment are analyzed, and a survey is performed of how all employees feel about the division. The analysis also assesses the future of the division and the major threats and opportunities it faces during the next year and the next 5 to 10 years. Planning engineers a design for monitoring and evaluating divisional performance. This design involves as many people as possible in planning and managing their areas of responsibility.

Once managers and employees have agreed on objectives, programs and projects, and schedules, employees can control their own jobs and report only when things turn out better or worse than planned.

All planning requires discipline and organization on the part of managers. Planning should be approached logically and calmly; it may threaten the insecure and may even threaten the nurse administrator, who must provide total support in terms of giving or obtaining the resources to accomplish divisional planning. Strategies are developed to address these problems and to ensure that representative nurse managers participate on all planning teams.

66 Planning is such a primary and essential element of management that managers cannot be effective without it. 99

66 Provision of nursing care to patients is the purpose of a division of nursing. Nursing standards require qualified nursing personnel who collect data and make nursing diagnoses based on patients' needs and according to patient care standards. Nursing standards further indicate that cooperation among disciplines is expected. 99

Unit Planning

Planning extends to the operational units of any healthcare agency; the processes involved are the same. It is in the units that the work for which nursing exists takes place. Planning should be done on a daily, weekly, and long-term basis. Daily planning is related to patient care and includes history taking, assessment, and nursing diagnosis and intervention. It involves matching people to jobs, developing policies and procedures specific to the patient population, identifying educational needs, preparing and conducting educational programs, coordinating patient care activities, supervising personnel, and evaluating the planning process and its results as summarized in Figure 9-26. Also included in unit planning are the implementation of theories of nursing care into the management and practice of nursing, an effective and efficient nursing care delivery system, and a system of statistical process control. Unit objectives should be clearly defined and a sound management or operational plan made to achieve them.

EVIDENCE-BASED STRATEGIC PLANNING

Kaplan and Norton describe a balanced scorecard as a strategic planning and management system used in business and industry, government, and nonprofit organizations to align business activities to the vision, mission, values, and strategy of the organization. The authors note this method of measuring performances as a means of giving managers and executives a more "balanced" view of organizational performance. The phrase "balanced scorecard" was defined in the early 1990s; however, this type of approach was included in the beginning work of General Electric on performance measurement in the 1950s and in the work of French process engineers (who created the *Tableau de Bord*—literally, a "dashboard" of performance measures) in the early part of the 20th century.[81]

The balanced scorecard can improve internal and external communications and serve as a means to evaluate an organization's performance against strategic goals. Kaplan and Norton developed this

FIGURE 9-26	STANDARDS FOR PLANNING PROCESS		
		Yes	No
1. The plan is written.		_____	_____
2. It defines the nursing business.		_____	_____
3. It contains objectives (general and specific goals).		_____	_____
4. It defines strategies.		_____	_____
5. It supports the mission.		_____	_____
6. It details forecasted activities for 1 year.		_____	_____
7. It details forecasted activities for longer than 1 year.		_____	_____
8. It has been developed with input from clinical nurses and line managers.		_____	_____
9. It addresses resources (personnel and facilities).		_____	_____
10. Changes are evident.		_____	_____
11. Financial plans are included.		_____	_____
12. Needs are identified and supported.		_____	_____
13. Priorities are listed.		_____	_____
14. Timetables are listed.		_____	_____
15. It is based on current data analysis.		_____	_____
16. It assesses both strengths and weaknesses.		_____	_____
17. It derives from a good nursing management information plan.		_____	_____
18. It is used and modified consistently.		_____	_____

Source: Author.

performance measurement framework, adding strategic nonfinancial performance measures to more traditional financial indicators. Kaplan and Norton describe the importance of the managing process and identify four aspects to consider[82]:

1. Translating the vision and strategy: Clarifying the vision, gaining consensus
2. Communicating and linking: Communicating and educating, setting goals, linking rewards to performance
3. Business planning: Setting targets, aligning strategic initiatives, allocating resources, establishing milestones
4. Feedback and learning: Articulating the shared vision, supplying strategic feedback, facilitating strategy review and learning.

Using the balanced scorecard from the four aspects described, four perspectives are outlined with each perspective identifying objectives, measures, targets, and initiatives. The four perspectives are[83]:

1. Financial
2. Internal business processes
3. Learning and growth
4. Customer

Considering each perspective and the objectives, measures, targets, and initiative in each area, a manager has a more comprehensive approach to their organizational business plan. Specifically, the balanced scorecard aids in aligning unit and individual goals with the strategy, linking strategic objectives to long-term targets and annual budgets, and identifying and aligning strategic initiatives. Using this framework, periodic evaluations can become a more systematic and methodical approach to planning.[84]

Successful Planning

Keeping the responsibility for planning as a line management function is better than creating a separate planning staff of nurses, because nurses who use plans make them effective and productive, and they should be the ones to write the plans. Nurse managers ensure the plans are based on data from all sections and not biased by a few. Some people see planning as a management style; planning is a tool as well. Plan for what the health care of the future will be; with inflation and recession, the impact of the local economy on healthcare needs will always be an issue. Economics is forcing us to teach people to do more for themselves and their families. Nurse managers will certainly have to plan for changes in value systems.

Nurse managers should make decisions about the kind of planning to be undertaken and which management level should perform specific aspects of the planning. Involve personnel in planning activities they will carry out. Teach and combine the elements of planning with other management functions; ensure that all managers are involved. Accept outcomes that are different from those originally planned, as activities may quickly become outdated and require modified plans.

Research studies show that 20% of small businesses that did not perform strategic planning failed, whereas only 8% of small businesses that performed strategic planning failed.[85] Figure 9-26 outlines standards for the planning process.

Evidence-Based Practice 9-1

Clancy describes planning as predicting the future state of a system after a change has been introduced. Currently, descriptions of a system are important to predicting and may be challenging given the complex nature of healthcare systems. Clancy provides examples of three applications and their usefulness in planning: phase plots, system dynamics, and social network analysis. Phase plots have their roots in physics,

continues

engineering, and dynamic systems. "The shape of trajectories in phase plots can identify subtle, underlying structures in a complex system." System dynamics involve experts gathering data interviews of key staff, surveys, management reports, and other forms of data. Using systems dynamics, the goal is to understand how entities flow through the system and identify feedback loops. Flowcharts are used extensively. Social networks are defined as the pattern of relationships that exist between entities and the information that flows between them. Using this application includes combining theories from sociology and information science (network theory). Terms such as "nodes" and "ties" are used. Surveys are used to determine the relationship between ties and nodes and fed into social network analysis software. Clancy purports that understanding the "factors underlying systems attractors provide new insights into existing processes and powerful tools to predict system behavior."[86]

SUMMARY

The basic tools of planning are statements of mission or purpose, vision and values, philosophy or beliefs, and objectives and an active operational or management plan. All managers use such documents to accomplish the work of nursing.

Statements of mission, philosophy, and objectives support each other at different agency levels, from the unit to the service or department, and then to the division and finally to the organization.

The statement of mission or purpose gives the reasons an entity exists, whether it is an organization, division, department, or unit. The nursing mission statement pertains to the clinical best practice of nursing supported by research, education, and management.

The statement of philosophy reflects the values and beliefs of the organizational entity. It is translated into patient-centered action by nursing personnel.

Objectives are concrete statements describing the major accomplishments nurses desire to achieve. Major categorical areas for objectives include the following:

- Organization and use of all resources: human, financial and physical
- Social responsibility
- Staffing
- Requisition of supplies and equipment
- Planning of educational programs
- Innovation
- Marketing
- Evaluation of patient care
- Evaluation of personnel performance

Major strategies of an organization are the planning process; the formulation and use of statements of mission, philosophy, and objectives; and the formulation of organizational plans developed with the broadest possible input.

Planning is the mental process by which nurse managers use valid and reliable data to develop objectives, determine the resources needed, and create a blueprint for achieving the objectives. The major purpose of planning is to make the best possible use of personnel, supplies, and equipment.

Strategic planning sets objectives for long-term nursing activities of 1 to 5 years or longer. Although traditionally done by top managers, strategic planning is an important skill for all nurse managers to develop. It ensures survival. Human resource planning ensures effective use of a scarce commodity, the professional nurse. Strategic planning has a mission, collects and analyzes data, assesses strengths and weaknesses, sets goals and objectives, uses strategies, operates on a timetable, gives operational and functional guidance to nurse managers, and includes evaluation.

Tactical planning is short-term planning. Operational or management plans convert objectives into action and include activities, assignments, deadlines, and provision for accountability. They include goals, objectives, strategies, actions, a timetable, identification of responsible persons, and note of accomplishments. Operational planning is daily, weekly, and monthly planning and can provide data for further strategic and tactical planning.

Planning within the nursing organization is intended to assist in fulfilling the mission of the healthcare facility. Planning supports the organization's objectives, meshes with the plans of all other departments contributing to provision of total healthcare needs, and ultimately provides for optimum support of the nursing agency.

APPLICATION EXERCISES

Exercise 9-1

Interview a nurse manager on a nursing unit. Describe the understanding the nurse manager has of the overall planning process of the organization and their particular unit. Can the nurse manager articulate a vision, mission, philosophy, and objectives? What are the core values of the organization? Are they operationalized? How did you determine?

Exercise 9-2

Use Figure 9-5, Standards for the Evaluation of Mission Statements of the Nursing Division and Its Departments, Services, and Units, to

1. Evaluate a mission statement.
2. Develop a mission statement.

Exercise 9-3

Use Figure 9-9, Standards for Evaluation of Philosophy Statements of the Nursing Division, Department, Service, or Unit, to

1. Evaluate a philosophy statement.
2. Develop a philosophy statement.

Exercise 9-4

Use Figure 9-16, Standards for Evaluation of Statements of Objectives for a Nursing Division, Department, Service, or Unit, to

1. Evaluate objectives.
2. Develop objectives.

Exercise 9-5

Use Figure 9-22, Standards for Evaluation of Management Plan of Nursing Division, Department, Service, or Unit, to

1. Evaluate management plans.
2. Develop a management plan.

Exercise 9-6

Identify and develop a statement of the planning strategy for a nursing organization or unit.

Exercise 9-7

Explore the idea of creating an evidence-based practice council; write its mission, vision, philosophy, and objectives. Create a strategic plan for the present and 2 years and 5 years in future projections.

APPLICATION EXERCISES

Exercise 9-8

Write a summary of a nursing unit, service, department, or division that describes its work, the volume of products and services, marketing activities, trends, financial summary, and impact on employees.

Exercise 9-9

Interview a chief executive officer and a chief nurse executive officer of an organization. Determine their orientation to strategic planning. Compare the results. Prepare a list of questions to ask from figures in this chapter before doing the interview.

Exercise 9-10

Make a management plan for your work for a day; include planning data pertinent to that manager's area(s) of responsibility.

Exercise 9-11

List opportunities and threats to nursing, their severity, and the probability that they will occur. Consider technological, economic, demographic, politicolegal, and sociocultural forecasting.

Notes

1. For a classic article on purpose, philosophy, and objectives, refer to Moore, M. A. (1971). Philosophy, purpose, and objectives: Why do we have them? *Journal of Nursing Administration, 1*(3), 9–14.
2. Calfee, D. L. (1993). Get your mission statement working! *Management Review, 1,* 54–57.
3. Crosby, P. (1989). *Running things: The art of making things happen.* New York: NAL-Dutton.
4. Ireland, R. D., & Hitt, M. A. (1992). Mission statements: Importance, challenge, and recommendations for development. *Business Horizons, 1,* 34–42.
5. Truskie, S. D. (1984). The driving force of successful organizations. *Business Horizons, 1,* 43–48.
6. Beyers, M. (1984). Getting on top of organizational change: Part 1, process and development. *Journal of Nursing Administration, 14*(3), 32–39; Gillen, D. J. (1986). Harvesting the energy from change anxiety. *Supervisory Management,* 40–43.
7. Reyes, J. R., & Kleiner, B. H. (1990). How to establish an organizational purpose. *Management Decision: Quarterly Review of Management Technology, 28,* 51–54.
8. Ibid.
9. Spragins, E. E. (1992). Resource-Constructing a vision statement. *Inc.,* 33.
10. Campbell, A. (1992). The power of mission: Aligning strategy and culture. *Planning Review, 1,* 10–12, 63.
11. Farnham, A. (1993, April 19). State your values, hold the hot air. *Fortune,* 117–124.
12. Henderson, V. (1966). *The nature of nursing* (p. 15). New York: Macmillan.
13. Yura, H., & Walsh, M. B. (1988). *The nursing process* (5th ed., p. 1). New York: Appleton-Century-Crofts.
14. King, I. M. (1968). A conceptual frame of reference in nursing. *Nursing Research,* 27–31.
15. Orem, D. E. (1995). *Nursing: Concepts of practice* (5th ed., p. 7). New York: McGraw-Hill.
16. Kinlein, M. L. (1977). *Independent nursing practice with clients* (p. 23). Philadelphia: J. B. Lippincott.
17. Sussman, G. E. (1985). CEO perspectives on mission, healthcare systems, and the environment. *Hospital & Health Services Administration, 6,* 21–34.
18. Farnham, 1993; Reyes & Kleiner, 1990.
19. Hodgetts, R. M. (1990). Management: Theory, process, and practice (5th ed., pp. 73–74). Orlando, FL: Harcourt, Brace, Jovanovich.
20. Coile, R. C. (2001). Magnet hospitals use culture, not wages, to solve nursing shortage. *Journal of Healthcare Management,* 224–227.

21. Poteet, G. W., & Hill, A. S. (1988). Identifying the components of a nursing service philosophy. *Journal of Nursing Administration, 18*(9), 29–33.

22. Corporate philosophies. (1988). *Compressed Air Magazine,* 31–34.

23. Ibid.

24. Moore, 1971, p. 13; Calfee, 1993.

25. Drucker, P. F. (1978). *Management: Tasks, responsibilities, practice* (pp. 99–102). New York: Harper & Row.

26. Canadian Nurses Association. (1966). *Report on the Project for the Evaluation of the Quality of Nursing Service* (pp. 47–48). Ottawa, Ontario: Canadian Nurses Association.

27. Drucker, P. F. (1999). *Management challenges for the 21st century* (pp. 43–44). New York: HarperCollins.

28. Drenkard, K. N. (2001). Creating a future worth experiencing: Nursing strategic planning in an integrated healthcare delivery system. *Journal of Nursing Administration, 31*(7/8), 362–376.

29. Beckham, J. D. (2004). Strategy: What it is, how it works, why it fails. *Health Forum Journal, 2,* 55–59.

30. Morris, D. E., & Rau, S. E. (1985). Strategic competition: The application of business planning techniques to the hospital marketplace. *Health Care Strategic Management,* 17–20.

31. Cushman, R. (1979). Norton's top-down, bottom-up planning process. *Planning Review, 3–8,* 48.

32. Meier, A. P. (1974). The planning process. *Managerial Planning, 1–5,* 9.

33. Cavanaugh, D. E. (1985). Gamesmanship: The art of strategizing. *Journal of Nursing Administration,* 38–41.

34. Ehrat, K. S. (1983). A model for politically astute planning and decision making. *Journal of Nursing Administration, 15*(10), 29–35.

35. Ibid.

36. Trexler, B. J. (1987). Nursing department purpose, philosophy, and objectives: Their use and effectiveness. *Journal of Nursing Administration, 17*(4), 8–12.

37. Fayol, H. (1949). *General and industrial management* (C. Storrs, Trans.) (pp. 43–50). London: Isaac Pitman & Sons.

38. Urwick, L. (1944). *The elements of administration* (pp. 26–34). New York: Harper & Row.

39. Rowland, H. S., & Rowland, B. L. (1997). *Nursing administration handbook* (4th ed., pp. 13, 32–36). Gaithersburg, MD: Aspen.

40. Beyers, M., & Phillips, C. (1979). *Nursing management for patient care* (2nd ed., pp. 41–48). Boston: Little, Brown.

41. Ackoff, R. L. (1986). Our changing concept of planning. *Journal of Nursing Administration, 16*(4), 35–40.

42. Schmeling, W. H., Futch, J. R., Moore, D., & MacDonald, J. W. (1991). The interactive planning/management model. *Nursing Administration Quarterly, 14,* 31.

43. Ibid.

44. Curtin, L. (1994). Learning for the future. *Nursing Management, 25,* 7–9.

45. Donovan, H. M. (1975). *Nursing service administration: Managing the enterprise* (pp. 50–64). St. Louis, MO: Mosby.

46. Drucker, 1978, pp. 121–129.

47. Koontz, H., & Weihrich, H. (1988). Management (9th ed., p. 16). New York: McGraw-Hill.

48. Donovan, 1975, pp. 63–64.

49. Hodgetts, 1990, pp. 123–124.

50. Rowland & Rowland, 1997.

51. Reif, W. E., & Webster, J. L. (1976). The strategic planning process. *Arizona Business,* 14–20.

52. Meier, A. P. (1974). The planning process. *Managerial Planning, 1–5,* 9.

53. Beyers, M. (1984). Getting on top of organizational change: Part 2. Trends in nursing service. *Journal of Nursing Administration, 14*(3), 31–37.

54. Ibid.

55. Drucker, 1999, pp. 81–85.

56. Ibid., p. 125.

57. Sherman, V. C. (1982). Taking over: Notes to the new executive. *Journal of Nursing Administration, 12*(2), 21–23.

58. Fox, D. H., & Fox, R. T. (1983). Strategic planning for nursing. *Journal of Nursing Administration, 13*(4), 11–16; Paul, R. N., & Taylor, J. W. (1986). The state of strategic planning. *Business,* 37–43.

59. Osborne, D., & Gaebler, T. (1992). *Reinventing government* (pp. 233–234). New York: Plume.

60. Odiorne, G. S. (1987). The art of crafting strategic plans. *Training,* 94–96, 98.

61. Ibid.

62. Baldwin, S. R., & McConnell, M. (1988). Strategic planning: Process and plan go hand in hand. *Management Solutions,* 29–36.

63. Peters, T. (1987). *Thriving on chaos* (p. 477). New York: Harper & Row; Sull, D. N. (1999). Why good companies go bad. *Harvard Business Review,* 42–48, 50–52, 183; Campbell, A. (1999). Tailored, not benchmarked: A fresh look at corporate planning. *Harvard Business Review,* 41–48, 50, 189.

64. Peters, 1987, pp. 615–617.

65. Baldwin & McConnell, 1988.

66. Mercer, Z. C. (1980). Personal planning: An overlooked application of the corporate planning process. *Managerial Planning,* 32–35; Van Mullem, C., Burke, L. J., Dohmeyer, K., Farrell, M., Harvey, S., John, L., Kraly, C., Rowley, F., Sebern, M., Twite, K., Zapp, R. (1999). Strategic planning for research use in nursing practice. *Journal of Nursing Administration, 29*(12), 38–45.

67. Ibid.; Mercy Health Services Nurses Council. (1991). Mercy Health Services: Systemwide redesign of patient care services. *Nursing Administration Quarterly,* 38–45.

68. Fox & Fox, 1983.

69. Jones, D., & Crane, V. (1990). Development of an organizational strategic planning process for a hospital department. *Health Care Supervisor, 9,* 1–20.

70. Begun, J., & Heatwole, K. B. (1999). Strategic cycling: Shaking complacency in healthcare strategic planning. *Journal of Healthcare Management,* 339–352.

71. Amudson, B. A., & Rosenblatt, R. A. (1991). The WAMI Rural Hospital Project. Part 6: Overview and Conclusions. *Journal of Rural Health,* 560–574.

72. Drucker, 1999.

73. Johnson, L. J. (1990). Strategic management: A new dimension of the nurse executive's role. *Journal of Nursing Administration,* 7–10.

74. Cushman, 1979.

75. Newhouse, R. P., Dearholt, S., Poe, S., Pugh, L. C., & White, K. M. (2007). Organizational Change Strategies for Evidence-Based Practice. *Journal of Nursing Administration, 37*(2), 552–557.

76. Nylen, D. W. (1985). Making your business plan an action plan. *Business,* 12–16.

77. Singleton, E. K., & Nail, F. C. (1985). Guidelines for establishing a new service. *Journal of Nursing Administration,* 22–26.

78. Vestal, K. W. (1988). Writing a business plan. *Nursing Economics,* 121–124.

79. Schulmeister, L. (1999). Starting a nursing consultation practice. *Clinical Nurse Specialist, 2,* 94–100.

80. Johnson, J. E. (1990). Developing an effective business plan. *Nursing Economics, 4,* 152–154; Johnson, J. E., Sparks, D. G., & Humphreys, C. (1988). Writing a winning business plan. *Journal of Nursing Administration,* 15–19; Reiboldt, J. M. (1999). Writing a group practice business plan. *Healthcare Financial Management, 1,* 58–61.

81. Kaplan, R. S., & Norton, D. P. (2004). Measuring the strategic readiness of intangible assets. *Harvard Business Review,* February, 1–14.

82. Kaplan, R. S., & Norton, D. P. (2000). Having trouble with your strategy? Then map it. *Harvard Business Review.*

83. Kaplan, R. S., & Norton, D. P. (2000). Putting the balanced scorecard to work. *Harvard Business Review.*

84. Kaplan, R. S., & Norton, D. P. (1996). Using the balanced scorecard as a strategic management system. *Harvard Business Review.*

85. Ireland & Hitt, 1992.

86. Clancy, T. R. (2007). Planning: What we can learn from complex systems science. *Journal of Nursing Administration, 17,* 436–439.

References

Anderson, M., Cosby, J., Swan, B., Moore, H., & Broekhoven, M. (1999). The use of research in local health service agencies. *Social Science Medicine,* 1007–1019.

"Balanced scorecard" helps fix Overlake strategic plan. (1999). *Healthcare Benchmarks,* 103–105.

Brendtro, M., & Hegge, M. (2000). Nursing faculty: One generation away from extinction. *Journal of Professional Nursing,* 97–103.

Cohen, M. (2000). Tools for the practice manager. *New England Journal of Medicine,* 49–50.

Development of an organizational strategic planning process for a hospital department. *Health Care Supervisor,* 1–20.

Edsel, W. M. (1999). How to develop a business plan for your medical group. *Medical Group Management Journal,* 36–39.

Glen, S. (1999). Educating for interprofessional collaboration: Teaching about values. *Nursing Ethics,* 202–213.

Hansen, R. D. (1999). Strategic planning: The basics and benefits. *Medical Group Management Journal,* 28–35.

Kramer, M., Maguire, P., Schmalenberg, C. E., Andrews, B., Burke, R., Chmielewski, L., et al. (2007). Excellence through evidence: Structures enabling clinical autonomy. *JONA, 36,* 41–52.

Matthews, P. (2000). Planning for successful outcomes in the new millennium. *Topics in Health Information Management,* 55–64.

McNeese-Smith, D. K. (2000). Job stages of entry, mastery, and disengagement among nurses. *Journal of Nursing Administration,* 140–147.

Mendes, I. A., Trevizan, M. A., Nogueira, M. S., & Sawada, N. O. (1999). Humanizing nurse–patient communication: A challenge and a commitment. *Medical Law, 18,* 639–644.

Moller-Tiger, D. (1999). Long-range strategic planning: A case study. *Healthcare Financial Management,* 33–35.

Molloy, J., & Cribb, A. (1999). Changing values for nursing and health promotion: Exploring the policy context of professional ethics. *Nursing Ethics,* 411–422.

O'Rourke, M. W. (2006). Beyond rhetoric to role accountability: A practical and professional model of practice. *Nurse Leader, 4,* 28–33, 44.

O'Rourke, M. W. (2007). Role-based nurse managers: A linchpin to practice excellence. *Nurse Leader,* 44–48, 53.

Pender, N. J. (1992). The NIH Strategic Plan. How will it affect the future of nursing science and practice? *Nursing Outlook,* 55–56.

Sabatino, C. J. (1999). Reflections on the meaning of care. *Nursing Ethics,* 374–382.

Schmieding, N. J. (1999). Reflective inquiry framework for nurse administrators. *Journal of Advanced Nursing,* 631–639.

Sechrist, K. R., Lewis, E. M., & Rutledge, D. N. (1999). Data collection for nursing work force strategic planning in California. *Journal of Nursing Administration,* 9–11, 29.

Siwicki, B. (1999). What's the CEO's role? Why more chief executives are playing pivotal roles in I.T. strategic planning. *Health Data Management,* 76–78, 80–82, 84–85.

Sorrells-Jones, J., & Weaver, D. (1999). Knowledge workers and knowledge-intense organizations: Part 3. Implications for preparing healthcare professionals. *Journal of Nursing Administration,* 14–21.

Thunhurst, C., & Barker, C. (1999). Using problem structuring methods in strategic planning. *Health Policy Planning,* 127–134.

Weaver, H. N. (1999). Transcultural nursing with Native Americans: Critical knowledge, skills, and attitudes. *Journal of Transcultural Nursing,* 197–202.

Zuckerman, A. M. (2005). *Healthcare strategic planning* (2nd ed.). Chicago: Health Administration Press.

10 STAFFING AND SCHEDULING

Beth Anderson, RN, MSN
Elizabeth Simms, RN, MSN

LEARNING OBJECTIVES AND ACTIVITIES

- Relate staff and scheduling to business skills of the nurse executive.
- Describe the components of the staffing process.
- Do a work-sampling study covering a specific period of time.
- Recognize factors influencing planning for staffing.
- Prepare a staffing plan for a nursing unit.
- Determine the modified approaches to nurse staffing and scheduling used by a healthcare organization.
- Describe the components of a patient classification system.
- Use a patient classification system to classify patients on a nursing unit.
- Define and recognize elements of a nursing management information system.
- Identify methods for improving productivity in a healthcare agency.
- Measure the productivity of the nursing staff on a nursing unit.

CONCEPTS

Staffing philosophy, staffing process, staffing activities, work contract, staffing modules, cyclic staffing, self-scheduling, patient classification systems, productivity.

NURSE MANAGER BEHAVIORS

Uses input from employees to develop and implement a staffing philosophy and staffing policies that inspire personnel to work to their maximum level of productivity; is responsible for staffing and scheduling staff with assignments that illustrate appropriate staffing mix based on scope of practice, competencies, client/resident needs, and acuity of care.

NURSE EXECUTIVE BEHAVIORS

Oversees staffing activities through human resource management that includes use of a patient classification system and provision of qualified nursing personnel in adequate numbers to meet patient care needs; evaluates and revises staffing systems and processes of nursing services to facilitate nurse-sensitive patient/client/family-centered outcomes; oversees measurement of patient/client/resident need for nursing care.

Introduction

Staffing is one of the most important issues in the delivery of health care. It is widely recognized that there is a crisis in nursing. In a survey performed by the American Nurses Association (ANA) in 2001, 7,000 nurses reported compromise in the care of patients because of a lack of qualified staff. Up to 20% of nurses are expected to leave the field within 5 years.[1] There is no correlation in increased nursing school enrollments to fill the need created by these exits.[2]

The nursing shortage of this decade is rooted in the following factors:

- The average age of nurses currently employed is 46.
- After age 50, many nurses work part time or retire.
- Nursing salaries "plateau" unless nurses make the transition to upper management.
- The plateau offers little financial compensation for nurses wishing to remain at the bedside.
- It is increasingly difficult to recruit faculty for nursing schools.[3]

There is strong evidence that an adequate number of nursing staff available to care for and coordinate care among the disciplines has an impact on patient outcomes.[4] In a study conducted in 589 hospitals encompassing 10 states, inverse relationships were recognized between nursing staff levels and negative outcomes for postsurgical patients.[5] In a separate study, the proportion of hours of care provided by nursing staff was inversely related to such adverse events as medication errors, decubiti, and patient complaints.[6]

It is well documented throughout nursing literature that staffing levels can and do affect the clinical outcomes of patients. Job dissatisfaction within the profession, a nursing shortage, and financial pressures contribute to the complexities of these issues.[7]

STAFFING PHILOSOPHY

Staffing is one of the major problems of any nursing organization, whether that organization is a hospital, nursing home, home healthcare agency, ambulatory care agency, or another type of facility. Aydelotte[8] stated the following:

> Nurse staffing methodology should be an orderly, systematic process, based upon sound rationale, applied to determine the number and kind of nursing personnel required to provide nursing care of a predetermined standard to a group of patients in a particular setting. The end result is prediction of the kind and number of staff required to give care to patients.

Components of the staffing process as a control system include a staffing study, a master staffing plan, a scheduling plan, and a nursing management information system (NMIS) (Figure 10-1). West adds a position control plan and a budgeting plan that integrates all aspects of staffing needs.[9]

Nurse staffing must meet certain regulatory requirements, among which are legal requirements of the Centers for Medicare & Medicaid Services. This legal standard is further supported by the standards of the Joint Commission on Accreditation of Healthcare Organizations. Other standards include the ANA *Scope and Standards for Nurse Administrators*, the ANA *Standards of Clinical Nursing Practice*, state legislation and state licensing requirements, state mandated ratios, and boards of nursing.

From all these standards and from the expectations of the community, of nurses, and of physicians, the nurse administrator develops a staffing philosophy as a basis for a staffing methodology. Community expectations will be related to economic status, local value and belief systems, and local standards of culture. Nurses' expectations will be related to the same community standards, their own perceptions of the practice of nursing, and its components, desired results, and tolerated work load.

Nurse managers can discern various values related to staffing from the nursing division's existing statements of purpose, philosophy, and objectives. A staffing philosophy may encompass beliefs about using a patient classification system (PCS) for identifying patient care needs.[10] A successful nursing leader's personal philosophy should include allowing nursing staff some degree of control within their work environment. Nurses who believe their work environment offers them a higher level of control are more likely to work for improvements rather than leave the organization.[11]

Objectives of nurse staffing are excellent care, positive patient outcomes, and high productivity. Professional nurses can develop a statement of purpose that is comprehensive in stating the quality and quantity of performance it is intended to motivate. Purpose statements should be quantified.[12]

FIGURE 10-1	COMPONENTS OF A STAFFING PLAN

- Staffing study
- Master staffing plan
- Scheduling plan
- Nursing management information system (NMIS)
- Position control
- Budgeting plan

Source: Author.

Staffing Study

A staffing study should gather data about internal and external environmental factors affecting the staffing requirements of an organization. Aydelotte listed four techniques drawn from engineering to measure the work of nurses, all of which involve the concept of time required for performance[13]:

1. Time study and task frequency
   a. Tasks and task elements (procedures)
   b. Point and time started and ended
   c. Sample size
   d. The measurement of standard time, which is the sum of average time, plus allowance for fatigue, personal variations, and unavoidable standby
   e. The measurement of nursing activity, which is the frequency of task × standard time
   f. The volume of nursing work, which is the total of all tasks × standard time
2. Work sampling (variation of task frequency and time)
   a. Identify major and minor categories of nursing activities
   b. Determine number of observations to be made
   c. Observe random sample of nursing personnel performing activities
   d. Analyze observations. Frequency occurring in a specific category = percentage of total time spent in that activity. Most work sampling studies direct care and indirect care to determine ratio.
3. Continuous sampling (variation of task frequency and time). The technique is the same as for work sampling, except that
   a. The observer follows one individual in the performance of a task.
   b. The observer may observe work performed for one or more patients if these tasks can be observed concurrently.
4. Self-reporting (variation of task frequency and time)
   a. The individual records the work sampling or continuous sampling on himself or herself.
   b. Tasks are logged using time intervals or time tasks start and end.
   c. Logs are analyzed.

Many work-sampling studies focus on procedures, ignore standards, and are lacking in objectivity, reliability, and accuracy. The techniques themselves, however, are sound.[14]

According to West, three "cardinal rules" exist for forecasting staffing requirements.[15] The first is to base staffing projections on past staffing history. A data sheet that includes types of task and procedure, average time to complete, measurement of nursing activity, and volume of nursing work is one aspect of such a model. The data can be collected from the PCS reports and census reports. Such data are readily available in most hospitals. Some NMISs, such as Medicus, provide numbers of personnel required, including the mix of registered nurses (RNs), licensed practical nurses (LPNs), and nursing assistants. Other data needed are sick time, overtime, holidays, and vacation time; the attrition rate is also important. In some PCSs, these data are built into the staffing formula. A second rule for staffing is to review current staffing levels (Figure 10-2). Review of future plans for the institution is the third cardinal rule.[16] Clinical nurses involved in staffing plans have confidence in the plans.

Staffing requires much planning on the part of the nurse administrator. Data must be collected and analyzed. These data include facts about the following:

- The product, that is, the needs of patient care.
- Diagnostic and therapeutic procedures performed by physicians and nurses.
- The knowledge elements of professional nursing translated into the skills of taking a medical history, performing an assessment, providing a nursing diagnosis and prescription, applying care,

---

FIGURE 10-2 **FORECASTING STAFFING REQUIREMENTS**

1. Staffing projections on past staffing history
   a. Type of task and procedure
   b. Average time to complete
   c. Measurement of nursing activity
   d. Volume of nursing work

2. Review current staffing levels
   a. Involve clinical nurses
   b. Collect pertinent information (patient acuity, skill level of nurses, case mix)
   c. Hours per patient day

Source: Author.

evaluating, keeping records, communicating, and taking all other actions related to primary health care of patients.

Changing, expanding knowledge and technology in the physical and social sciences, medicine, and economics influence planning for staffing. Healthcare institutions are treating more clients on an outpatient basis than ever before. New drugs, improved diagnostic and therapeutic procedures, and reimbursement changes have decreased the lengths of hospitalization. The result of decreased length of stay is often increased inpatient acuity. Standards of the Joint Commission on Accreditation of Healthcare Organizations, ANA, and other professional and governmental organizations have required the upgrade of health care.

66 Basic to planning for staffing of a division of nursing is the fact that qualified nursing personnel must be provided in sufficient numbers to ensure adequate, safe nursing care for all patients 24 hours a day, 7 days a week, 52 weeks a year. Each staffing plan must be tailored to the needs of the agency and cannot be determined with a simple worker-to-patient ratio or formula. 99

Planning for staffing requires judgment, experience, and thorough knowledge of the requirements of the organization in which the individual nurse administrator is employed. It requires the support of hospital administration, physicians in charge of clinical services, and nursing staff. The basic requirement for staffing is unchanging, regardless of the type or size of the institution: Plan for the kinds and numbers of nursing personnel that give safe, adequate care to all patients and ensure that the work of nursing is productive and satisfying.

The following influence planning for staffing[17] (Figure 10-3):

- Changing concepts of nursing roles for clinical nursing practitioners, clinical nurse specialists, and clinical nurse leaders

---

FIGURE 10-3 **PLANNING FOR STAFFING**

- Changing nursing roles
- Changing patient population with birthrate declines and longevity
- Institutional mission and objectives
- Personnel policies and practices
- Polices and procedures related to patient processes
- Support services, including non-nursing support services

- Composition of medical staff and medical services
- Physical plant and environmental issues
- Organization of nursing services; structure, processes
- Data analysis of indicators such as admissions, discharges, patient acuity, staff mix

---

Source: Author.

- Patient populations that are changing as birth rates decline and longevity increases
- Institutional missions and objectives related to research, training, and many specialties
- Personnel policies and practices
- Policies and practices related to admission and discharge times of patients, assignment of patients to units, and intensive and progressive care practices
- The degree to which other departments carry out their supporting services. Plans should be made to furnish staffing requirements for nursing personnel to perform non-nursing duties such as dietary functions, clerical work, messenger and escort activities, and housekeeping. Whether these services should or should not be carried out by nursing personnel is not the point; the relevance is that the degree to which the situation exists must be considered in any planning. Nurse managers should evaluate carefully assuming responsibility for non-nursing services and should encourage the appropriate departments to perform such services.
- The number and composition of the medical staff and the medical services offered. Nursing requirements are affected by characteristics of patient populations determined by the size and capability of the medical staff. Several factors affect the quality and quantity of nursing personnel required and influence their placement: special requirements of individual physicians; the time and length of physicians' rounds; the time, complexity, and number of tests, medications, and treatments; and the kind and amount of surgical procedures.
- Arrangement of the physical plant has a large impact on staffing requirements. Fewer personnel are needed for a modern, compact facility equipped with labor-saving devices and efficient working arrangements than for one that is spread out and has few or no labor-saving devices. Different staffing is required for a facility that is arranged functionally than for one that is not. If, for example, the surgical suite is not next to the birthing rooms, recovery room, and intensive care units, more staff is needed to meet acceptable standards of quality and safety. Many other architectural features must be considered, such as the location of specialized units; the location of patient rooms in relation to nursing stations, work rooms, and storage space; and the time required to transport patients to other sections of the hospital for diagnostic or therapeutic services, such as radiography and nuclear medicine.
- The organization of the division of nursing. Plans should be reviewed and revised to organize the department to operate efficiently and economically with written statements of mission, philosophy, and objectives; sound organizational structure; clearly defined functions and responsibilities; written policies and procedures; effective staff development programs; and planned periodic systems evaluation.
- Data to be analyzed include number of admissions, discharges, and transfers; outpatient activity; patient acuity; amount of supervision needed for ancillary personnel; patient teaching; emergency responses; mode of care delivery; and staff mix.

Staffing Activities

Numerous staffing activities have been identified by Price; he suggests that the nurse administrator assign and identify by name the persons responsible for each activity. Among his suggestions are the following[18]:

- One person ultimately responsible for each activity should be identified.
- The category and position of the person who should be responsible for each activity should be identified.
- The activity should be specified as requiring nursing or non-nursing personnel.
- The review should be performed for the day, evening, night, weekend, and holiday shifts.

A modified format by Price for gathering data and analyzing responsibility for staffing activities covers the following:

- Recruiting, interviewing, screening, and hiring RNs, LPNs, and nursing assistants
- Assigning personnel to clinical units and shifts
- Preparing work schedules in advance
- Maintaining daily schedules, adjusting for staff absences and patients' needs
- Calculating turnover and hours of care
- Checking time cards and payroll
- Developing policy
- Handling telephone communication
- Ensuring contract compliance

Orientation Plan

The orientation plan offered to new employees can impact both recruitment and retention; orientation is a time when a sense of belonging can be instilled. A main purpose of orientation is to help the nursing employee adjust; it should be a planned program overseen by the education department or a unit-based clinical coordinator, with a one-on-one preceptor. Experienced nurses can ease the discomfort of a new work situation by[19]:

- Encouraging new nurses in the work unit as well as throughout the organization
- Readily sharing information, and being willing to learn from both new graduates and experienced nurses accustomed to different systems
- Modeling positive and professional behaviors and attitudes
- Allowing new employees to establish their own practice patterns
- Encouraging continuing education in the field
- Practicing patience

Figure 10-4 gives an example of a nursing orientation.

Policies and procedures should be introduced to the new employee in this phase. Because there are too many policies and procedures to be absorbed at once, empower the new employees by enabling them to refer to appropriate sources for reference.

Internship Programs

Many nursing departments are developing internship programs for new graduate nurses to expand the orientation process to include critical thinking skills development, clinical reasoning, and clinical skills while in a supportive and protected environment. These programs can last from months to a year with structured educational experiences based on the needs of the hospital's patient environment. The cost of an internship could be paid back in lower turnover rates, improved nursing outcomes, and increased nursing satisfaction.

Staffing Policies

Staffing policies are best derived through consultation with clinical nurses. Written staffing policies should be readily available for at least the following areas:

- Vacations, holidays, and sick leave
- Emergency leave
- Weekend shifts: number worked, days considered as "weekend"

FIGURE 10-4	NURSING ORIENTATION—WEEK 1

Monday	Tuesday	Wednesday	Thursday	Friday
8:00–4:30	8:00–10:00	8:00–8:15	8:00–4:30	8:00–8:45
Personnel	Introduction	Computer class	RN IV Therapy	XYZ Eye Center
Orientation	Philosophy	assignment		8:45–9:30
Benefits	Dress code	8:15–12:00		XYZ Organ Center
Performance im-	Staffing	Code 1		9:30–9:45
provement	Time/attendance	CPR		Break
Employee health	Skills assessment	12:00–1:00		9:45–10:00
Infection control	10:00–10:15	Lunch		Nutrition Service
Fire and safety	Break	1:00–4:30		10:00–11:00
	10:15–12:15	Clinical skills		Telephone system
	Documentation	RN/LPN		11:00–12:00
	12:15–1:15	BGM		Lunch
	Lunch	Emergency trach		12:00–4:30
	1:15–4:30	R.		Team building
	*MAR	**TPN dressing C.		
	Medical policies	CNA		
	Medical exam	Vital signs		
		Body mecha-		
		nisms		
		Infection control		
		Legal		

Source: Author.
*Medication Administration Record
**Total Parental Nutrition

- Shift rotation
- Overtime
- Part-time and temporary personnel
- Use of float personnel
- Schedule changes
- Use of educational time
- Requests of personnel and management
- Work week

A work contract can be set up between each employee and the organization. The contract should state the date employment is to commence, job classification, job description, work hours, pay rate, full-time or part-time designation, and all other specific points agreed on between the employee and organizational representative.

Staffing the Units

❝According to the Joint Commission on Accreditation of Healthcare Organizations, staffing effectiveness is defined as "the number, competency, and skill mix of staff as related to the provision of needed services.❞[20]

Each patient care unit should have a master staffing plan that includes the basic staff needed to cover the unit for each shift. Basic staff is the minimum or lowest number of personnel needed to staff a unit and includes fully oriented full- and part-time employees. The number may be based on examination of previous staff records and expert opinion of nurse managers. Basic staff includes all categories: RNs,

LPNs, and ancillary personnel for each shift. Figure 10-5 shows a formula for determining a core staff per shift. Figures 10-6 and 10-7 provide other tools that can be used to assist with staffing. For example, a staffing board showing the number of personnel needed for a period of time, along with a self-scheduling form, can be useful in meeting staffing challenges.

The number of complementary personnel is determined next. Complementary personnel are scheduled as additions to the basic group. Financial resources and the availability of personnel control the total number in both groups. Not ensured a permanent pattern of staffing, complementary personnel provide the flexibility needed to meet short-term and unexpected changes.

Float personnel are not permanently assigned to a station. Managed by a centralized staffing office, they provide flexibility to meet increased patient loads and unexpected personnel absences. They may be cross-trained to a number of different medical milieus or may specialize in one field. The number and kinds of float personnel can be accurately determined from general monthly records that show absence rates, personnel turnover, and fluctuations in patient care work loads.

Part-time nursing personnel may be an economic or cost-control factor in staffing, because they receive fewer benefits than full-time personnel. Part-time personnel are better motivated if they receive some benefits, such as a number of paid holidays and vacation days proportionate to days worked and pay increases when they complete the aggregate days worked by full-time personnel. Their total hours worked can be controlled to fill actual shortfalls.

FIGURE 10-5	FORMULA FOR ESTIMATING A CORE STAFF PER SHIFT

The average daily census for a 25-bed medical–surgical unit over a 6-month period is 19 patients. The basic average daily hours of care to be provided are 5 hours per patient per 24 hours. How many total hours of care will be needed on the average day to meet these standards? $19 \times 5 = 95$ hours. If the workday is 8 hours, this means $95 \div 8 = 11.9$ or 12 full-time-equivalent (FTE) staff are needed to staff the unit for 24 hours. An FTE is one person working full time (40 hours a week) or several persons who together work a total of 40 hours a week. A total of 12 FTE $\times$ 7 days per week = 84 shifts per week, if the staffing is to be the same each day. If each employee works five 8-hour shifts per week, $84 \div 5 = 16.8$ is the number of FTEs needed as basic staff for this unit.

The number of nursing personnel to cover sick leave, vacations, and holidays or other absences can also be determined and added to the basic staff. This information is determined from a study of personnel policies and use. It is frequently included in PCS formulas. Such additional staff may be provided from a float pool.

The next determination to be made is the ratio of RNs to other nursing personnel. If the ratio is determined to be 1:1, how much of the basic staff of 16.8 should be RNs? One half of the total, which would be 8.4 RNs and 8.4 others (LPNs, nurses' aides, orderlies, or nursing assistants). A study of staffing patterns in 80 medical–surgical, pediatrics, and post-partum units in 12 Salt Lake City community hospitals recommends a mix of 58% RNs, 26% LPNs, and 16% aides.[21]

The final determination is how many personnel are needed for each shift. Warstler recommends the following proportions: day, 47%; evening, 35%; and night, 17%.[22] This means that for a total staff of 16.8 personnel, 8 would be assigned to days, 6 to evenings, and 2.8 to nights. Obviously, this is an approximation; other patterns could also be chosen by the nurse administrator.

The number of complementary nursing personnel would be added to this basic staff. They could be a group of one RN, one LPN, and one other, assigned accordingly. The staff is entered into the following table as numbers in parenthesis added to the figure for basic staff.

In an environment that emphasizes reimbursement, complementary personnel may be budgeted as a pool and may exist as only a portion of basic personnel assigned to a pool.

Basic Staffing Plan for a 25-Bed Medical–Surgical Unit

Category	Day	Evening	Night	Total
RNs	4 + (1)	3	1.4	8.4 + (1)
LPNs	2	2 + (1)	1.4	5.4 + (1)
Others	2	1	0 + (1)	3 + (1)
Totals	8 + (1)	6 + (1)	2.8 + (1)	16.8 + (3)

Source: Author.

FIGURE 10-6 — STAFFING BOARD SHOWING THE NUMBER OF PERSONNEL NEEDED FOR 6 WEEKS

The left row of pegs is coded by category of personnel: RN, LPN, and NA (nursing assistant). There are peg holes on the board for 29 persons for 7 weeks. Larger boards can be used. Pegs for scheduling would be color-coded for shifts: day, evening, night, weekend, off, etc.

⊘ = Days   ⊗ = Evenings   ● = Nights

Source: Author.

Staffing Modules

Many different approaches to nurse staffing and scheduling are being explored in an effort to satisfy the needs of employees and meet work load demands for patient care (Figure 10-8). These include modified work weeks (10- or 12-hour shifts), team rotation, "premium day" weekend nurse staffing, and "premium vacation" night staffing. Such approaches should support the underlying purpose, mission, philosophy, and objectives of the organization and the division of nursing and should be well defined

FIGURE 10-7 — SELF-SCHEDULING FORMAT

	S	INITIALS	M	INITIALS	T	INITIALS	W	INITIALS	TH	INITIALS	F	INITIALS	S	INITIALS
Week Jan 15 11 A.M.	3RNs 1LPN 1NA	JH	5RNs 2LPNs 1NA		4RNs 3LPNs 1NA		4RNs 3LPNs 1NA		4RNs 2LPNs 1NA		5RNs 2LPNs 1NA		3RNs 1LPN 1NA	
3 P.M.	3RNs 1LPN 1NA	JH	5RNs 2LPNs 1NA		4RNs 3LPNs 1NA		4RNs 3LPNs 1NA		4RNs 2LPNs 1NA		5RNs 2LPNs 1NA		3RNs 1LPN 1NA	
7 P.M.	2RNs 1LPN 1NA		4RNs 3LPNs 1NA		3RNs 2LPNs 1NA		3RNs 2LPNs 1NA		4RNs 3LPNs 1NA		3RNs 2LPNs 1NA		2RNs 1LPN 1NA	
11 P.M.	2RNs 1LPN 1NA		4RNs 3LPNs 1NA		3RNs 2LPNs 1NA		3RNs 2LPNs 1NA		4RNs 3LPNs 1NA		3RNs 2LPNs 1NA		2RNs 1LPN 1NA	
3 A.M.	1RN 1LPN 1NA		2RNs 2LPNs 1NA	JH	2RN 2LPN 1NA	JH	1RN 1LPN 1NA	JH	2RNs 2LPNs 1NA	JH	1RN 1LPN 1NA		1RN 1LPN 1NA	
7 A.M.	1RN 1LPN 1NA		2RNs 2LPNs 1NA	JH	2RN 2LPN 1NA	JH	1RN 1LPN 1NA	JH	2RNs 2LPNs 1NA	JH	1RN 1LPN 1NA		1RN 1LPN 1NA	
Week 11 A.M.														
3 P.M.														
7 P.M.														
11 P.M.														
3 A.M.														
7 A.M.														

Each block represents 4 hours of staffing.
Names and Initials:

RN Jane Hatfield   JH   _____   _____   _____   _____

_____   _____   _____   _____   _____

_____   _____   _____   _____   _____

_____   _____   _____   _____   _____

_____   _____   _____   _____   _____

Source: Author.

FIGURE 10-8 — STAFFING THE UNIT: STAFFING MODELS

- Cyclic scheduling
- Self-scheduling
- Modified work week
- 10-hour shifts
- 12-hour shifts
- Weekend alternatives
- Flextime

Source: Author.

in a staffing philosophy statement and policies. Nurses are like other employees in one respect: They want to live as normal a home life as possible. In addition, shifts must be staffed and patient care needs met. The successful nurse executive will try to accommodate both by using the best available administrative staffing methodology, which must be considered from the economic or cost–benefit viewpoint, and in conjunction with and out of concern for the nursing staff.

Staffing and scheduling are reasons for both turnover and job retention. Understaffing has a negative effect on staff morale, delivery of quality care, and the nursing practice modality. Insufficient staffing can contribute to closure of beds. It causes absenteeism from staff fatigue, burnout, and professional dissatisfaction. Conversely, nurse managers must receive value for their money. Economic constraints exist that are further limited by the costs of recruiting, hiring, and orienting new nurses and for overtime and temporary personnel when the environment creates turnover and absenteeism. Overstaffing is expensive and has a negative effect on staff morale and productivity. Staffing and scheduling must balance the personal needs of nurses with the economic and productivity needs of the organization.[23]

Patterns of staffing should be reviewed periodically to determine whether they are meeting the purpose, philosophy, and objectives of the organization and the division of nursing and whether they are practical regarding the numbers and qualifications of personnel. The ultimate objective of staffing patterns is to ensure that patients' needs are being met.

Cyclic Scheduling

Team rotation is a method of cyclic staffing in which a nursing team is scheduled as a unit. It is used in the team nursing modality.[24]

Cyclic scheduling is one way of staffing to meet the requirements of equitable distribution of hours of work and time off. A basic time pattern for a certain number of weeks is established and then repeated in cycles. There are several advantages to cyclic scheduling:

- Once developed, it is a relatively permanent schedule, requiring only temporary adjustments.
- Nurses no longer have to live in anticipation of their time off-duty, because it may be scheduled for as long as 6 months in advance.
- Personal plans may be made in advance with a reasonable degree of reliability.
- Requests for special time off are kept to a minimum.
- It can be used with rotating, permanent, or mixed shifts and can be modified to allow fixed days off and uneven work periods, based on personnel needs and work period preferences.
- It can be modified to fit known or anticipated periods of heavy work loads and can be temporarily adjusted to meet emergencies or unexpected shortages of personnel.

Because cyclic scheduling is relatively inflexible, it works only with a staff that rotates by policy and personal choice. Personnel who need flexible staffing to meet their personal needs, such as those related to family and educational pursuits, do not generally accept it.

An infinite number of basic cyclic patterns can be developed and tailored to suit the needs of each unit. Patterns should reflect policy, work load factors, and staff preferences. Nursing personnel may use a staffing board (Figure 10-6) to develop a pattern and cycle satisfactory to them. A staffing board may be used to show the number of nursing personnel required for each day of the week for 6 weeks.

Self-Scheduling

Self-scheduling is an activity that may make a staff happier, more cohesive, and more committed. It should be planned carefully on a unit (cost center) basis with a written policy in place as a guideline. Planning may use either a self-directed work team or a quality circle technique approach. Personnel are scheduled to work

"A nurse manager who had 12 RNs with absentee problems asked a nurse administrator how she could reduce these absences. A discussion followed about self-scheduling and the procedures necessary to implement. Several months later, the nurse manager reported to the nurse administrator that self-scheduling and absenteeism had decreased with only one employee still posing a problem. The problems were solved with self-scheduling. The nurse manager then successfully proceeded to use self-scheduling with all other employees who requested it."

their preferred shift as much as possible, as long as their preferred shifts meet the needs of the unit and balance with the needs of their coworkers. Self-scheduling has been found to shorten scheduling time; increase retention and satisfaction; and reduce conflicts, illness time, voluntary absenteeism, and turnover.

Self-scheduling leads to more responsible employees. It meets personal goals such as family, social life, education, child care, and commuting. It is an example of participatory management with decentralized decision making. The planning must include the givens, or rules, to be followed. These rules should be minimal to meet legal and professional standards.[25] Figure 10-7 gives an example that can be used to assist with self-scheduling.

Modified Work Week

Modified work week schedules using 10- and 12-hour shifts and other methods are commonplace. A nurse administrator should be sure work schedules are fulfilling the staffing philosophy and policies, particularly with regard to efficiency. Such schedules should not be imposed on the nursing staff but should show a mutual benefit to employer, employees, and clients.

The 10-Hour Shift One modification of the work week is the creation of four 10-hour shifts per week in organized time increments. One potential problem with this model is time overlaps of 6 hours per 24-hour day. The overlaps can be used for patient-centered conferences, nursing care assessment and planning, and staff development. The overlap can also be scheduled to cover peak work load demands, which can be identified by observation, consensus, or self-recording by professional nurses. It can be done by hour or by a block of 3 to 4 hours. Starting and ending times for the 10-hour shifts can be modified to provide minimal overlaps, with the 4-hour gap staffed by part-time or temporary workers.

The 4-day, 10-hour work schedule for night nurses was studied in a hospital that had difficulty recruiting qualified nurses for the night shift. It was found that 10-hour shifts had stabilized staffing in intensive care, with increased productivity and decreased turnover. Turnover on the night shift had been 70% for an 8-month period. Positions stayed vacant longer than for other shifts, and sick time was higher, which increased recruitment and orientation time. Nurses were involved in planning the 4-day, 10-hour night shift schedule. Night nurses agreed to use overlapping hours to assist with day shift care, and the day shift

Evidence-Based Practice 10-1

Vik and MacKay report a study of the quality of care by nurses who worked 12-hour shifts versus those who worked 8-hour shifts. It was a matched study of three units each. The Quality Patient-Care Scale was the measuring instrument. Results indicated that patients perceived a significantly higher quality of care from nurses working 8-hour versus 12-hour shifts. Shift patterns worked by nurses do affect the care received by patients. Recruitment and retention of nurses, however, can balance out reduced quality of care when vacancies are high. This study was limited and needs to be replicated.[28]

A research study was done to measure the effect of fatigue from 12-hour shifts on critical thinking. The study found "no significant differences between levels of fatigue and critical thinking ability in nurses working 8 and 12 hours."[29]

The break-even point for costs is the point at which recruiting, absenteeism, retention, and overtime cost savings equal the shift losses from 12-hour scheduling.[30]

agreed to reduce staff by one full-time equivalent (FTE). Plans were discussed with and accepted by the union. Personnel assignments and meeting schedules were addressed and resolved through participatory management. The results of these changes included reduced sick time on the 10-hour shift, reduced turnover, increased incentive, increased requests for night shift, and decreased labor hours.[26]

The 12-Hour Shift   A second scheduling modification is the 12-hour shift; in this system, nurses work seven shifts in 2 weeks. They work a total of 84 hours and are paid 4 to 8 hours of overtime. Twelve-hour shifts and flexible staffing have been reported to improve care and save money because nurses can better manage their home and personal lives.[27] Another commonly used pattern is of the use of six 12-hour shifts with one 8-hour shift for a total of 80 hours, with no "forced" overtime.

Weekend Alternative

"Weekend specials" have long been an attractive alternative form of scheduling. Not only do they afford the nurse weekdays with which to pursue educational opportunities or to spend time with family, they free "regular" staff from the perceived burden of working every other weekend to balance staffing. At one time, those nurses working two 12-hour shifts on the weekend were paid for a full 40-hour work week with benefits; that pay mode is rarely an option with today's budgetary constraints. There are, however, part-time packages modeled after this weekend schedule that afford greater pay than hours worked, with benefits attached.

"Premium day weekend" nurse staffing is a scheduling pattern that gives a nurse an extra day off-duty, called a premium day, when he or she volunteers to work one additional weekend within a 4-week scheduling block. This staffing technique could be modified to give the nurse a premium day off for every additional weekend worked beyond those required by nurse staffing policy. This technique does not add directly to hospital costs.[31]

"Premium vacation night" staffing follows the same principle as does premium day weekend staffing. An example is the policy of giving 5 extra working days of vacation to every nurse who works a permanent night shift for a specific period of time.

Flextime

Nurses often want flexible scheduling to better accommodate their personal lives. Such scheduling options have, in fact, become an essential component of job satisfaction.[32] Flexible time (frequently called "flextime") schedules have become an increasingly important aspect of employment practices since 1980, when 11.9% of all nonfarm wage and salary workers were reported to be on flextime schedules. These schedules have resulted in improved attitudes and increased productivity as employees have gained more control over their work environment. Employees have been able to adjust to their own biological clocks. Transportation has become more efficient and flexible. Employees have better control of work activities.[33]

To control for weaknesses of previous studies, the New York State government conducted a study of staggered work hours compared with fixed work hours. The study showed the following results[34]:

1. The greatest level of satisfaction and the lowest level of dissatisfaction with the workday were expressed by employees in agencies with the greatest flexibility in scheduling.
2. Those in agencies with fixed schedules expressed the strongest dissatisfaction and lowest level of satisfaction.
3. Decreased commuting time may improve satisfaction with flextime.

"Flexible scheduling improves recruiting, reduces absenteeism, and increases retention by boosting morale."

There are multiple scheduling options open for nurse managers to explore. In the case of a staff working 80 hours in a unit (six 12-hour shifts and one 8-hour shift), a need was found between the 7 A.M. to

> ## Evidence-Based Practice 10-2
>
> A study by Imig, Powell, and Thorman indicates that flexible staffing filled vacant positions but did not increase payroll costs, hours per patient day, or overtime. It did decrease absenteeism by 60%. The hospital in this study returned to 8-hour shifts because primary nursing was threatened. In this particular study, there was no change in incidence of medication errors, patient and staff injuries, quality of care plans, complaints, recruitment, or staff attitudes from before to 6 months after flexible staffing. Also, the use of agency nurses was not reduced.[35]

3 P.M. shift and the 11 P.M. to 7 A.M. shift. One RN volunteered to work a straight shift 5 days a week from 3 P.M. to 11 P.M.; her "bonus" was working straight weekdays, with no weekends and holidays off. It is up to the nurse manager and the staff involved to find innovative solutions suitable to their own workplace.

Flexible Role: Resource Acuity Nurse

At West Virginia University Hospital, top nurse executives established a resource acuity nurse position to provide greater flexibility and ensure adequate staffing during peak work load periods. The executives envisioned having nurses in the position available to provide immediate relief to units when the greatest care needs arose. The resource acuity nurse would stay at the agency for as long as needed.

The nurse managers developed guidelines for undertaking the resource acuity nurse responsibilities:

- Assisting with special procedures, such as central line placement and extensive dressing changes
- Supporting nursing staff whenever an increased number of patients return from the operating room
- Assisting in cardiac arrests or other emergencies
- Transferring unstable patients to the intensive care units

This program has enabled the hospital to better meet the staffing needs of units when work load increases. Since the establishment of the resource acuity nurse position in this organization, nurses' morale has improved, because they know short-term help is more readily available and will be more equitably distributed among units.[36]

Cross-Training

Cross-training of nursing personnel can improve flexible scheduling (as in the example of the resource nurse role). Nurses can be prepared through cross-training to function effectively in more than one area of expertise. They can be kept in similar clinical specialties (such as an intensive care unit cluster) or in families of clinical specialties. To prevent errors and increase job satisfaction during cross-training, nurses assigned to units and in pools require complete orientation and ongoing staff development. Nurses should be provided with policies, job descriptions, and performance evaluations.

Temporary Workers

Nurses have been temporary agency employees for several decades. They have turned to staffing agencies because they wanted control over their lives, personal and professional. Agency work was the only way they could gain such control until nurse managers and hospital administrators realized the need to apply the science of behavioral technology, including human resources management, to nursing. Many organizations are downsizing to be more productive by decreasing overhead, and one result of downsizing is the use of agency or external workers. They are required to meet standards and competencies of the agencies that use them.

The number of temporary jobs, professional and nonprofessional, has increased annually and is now in the millions. In many instances temporary employment has caused workers to experience downward mobility. The lesson for nursing personnel is to gain a reputation for competence in more than one clinical area or in more than one of the areas of clinical practice, teaching, research, and management.

Workforces in today's organizations are leaner. Temporary employees prevent hiring mistakes by employers and employees. An increased number of hospitals continue to use temporary personnel.

Potential temporary employees should become informed about the temporary agency they will use. They can ask other nurses who have used it about it, screen the agency by telephone to determine customer treatment, visit the agency on a busy Monday morning, and then interview with the agency.[37]

Strategic Staffing

Accounting firms have developed strategic staffing as an approach to downsizing. Strategic staffing analyzes a unit's staffing needs, based on long-term objectives for the unit and organization, to find a combination of permanent and temporary employees with the best skills to meet these needs. Temporary staffing may protect the jobs of permanent or core employees when the temporary employee is used to cover a vacancy while the position or job is analyzed.

Temporary staff may want to sample the work. A variety of professional occupations are represented in the temporary workforce. Temporary workers provide relief for overworked permanent employees; many do one-time projects, including internal audits and forensic accounting. They work as trainers of permanent employees. Using temporary employees controls personnel expenses related to benefits, rehiring, and training. To make strategic staffing work, managers should study staffing once annually, analyzing work load peaks and valleys, looking at the financial blueprint, and communicating with providers and staff.

The warning signs that strategic staffing is required include excessive overtime, high turnover, excessive absenteeism, employees whose skills do not match job requirements, absence of regular staffing planning, missed deadlines, last-minute staffing using temporary employees, lack of a budget line for temporary employees, absence of communication with the human resources department, and low employee morale. Obtaining the best temporary workers may require consultation with specialized temporary employment firms.[38]

Temporary staff members are cost-effective for small businesses, because they eliminate the expense of a human resources department. For large businesses, temporary workers are cost-effective for the flexibility needed for seasonal and short-term work. Using temporary employees also enables employers to evaluate those employees for permanent jobs.[39]

Travel Nursing

A step beyond the nurses who work for local agencies, travel nursing is an increasingly popular career choice. The mobility of society at large has increased the willingness of nursing workers to relocate for weeks- or months-long assignments. Nurses engaged in travel nursing run the gamut from young single professionals with a taste for adventure to older "empty-nesters," free from family ties and ready to experience more than their local healthcare systems can offer.

"The rapidly growing nursing shortage was the impetus for the development of the travel nursing industry years ago and, as it continues, the shortage will likely fuel the demand for travel nurses in the future."[40] The offer of benefits (401(k)s, health and dental insurance) and a high rate of pay attract many applicants; it has become difficult for organizations to match the travel packages available, and many organizations have lost nurses to such enticing offers.

Travel nurses give organizations the benefit of a fresh outlook, a variety of experiences, and a willingness to work within a new system. To their new coworkers, they give a glimpse of another culture and perhaps share their willingness to learn.

Transfer Fair

In an effort to minimize the negative repercussions of downsizing, one hospital used a "transfer fair" to place staff quickly and fairly. The key participants were as follows:

- Managers with vacancies
- Recruitment staff with a list of vacancies
- Employee relations staff to answer personnel policy questions
- Staff affected by downsizing

Each affected staff member made three choices. Seniority then determined placement, and decisions were made within 48 to 72 hours.

The atmosphere and tone of a transfer fair is gracious, welcoming, professional, relaxed, and supportive. Planners prepare well and make the fair convenient for all shifts. Refreshments are served and top nursing administrators attend.[41]

Magnet Hospitals

In 1982 a groundbreaking study by the American Academy of Nursing identified 41 facilities as "magnet" hospitals, which consistently attracted and retained good nurses and provided excellent nursing care. In response, the Magnet Recognition Program was developed 9 years later by the American Nurses Credentialing Center.[42] In a study of staff nurses working in 14 magnet hospitals, those attributes identified as essential to delivering quality care were as follows:

- Organizational support for education
- A workforce of clinically competent nurses
- Positive relationships between nurses and physicians
- Autonomy in nursing practice
- A client-centered culture
- Control of nursing practice
- Perception of adequate staffing
- Support of nursing administration

In the face of chronic understaffing, many hospitals use competitive wages and benefits to attract nurses. Competitive wages are important, but they are not the ultimate tool for attraction and retention of nurses. "Current health care concerns mandate innovative, culture-based approaches to recruiting and retaining staff."[43]

Patient Classification Systems

The component of a traditional system of nurse staffing that is essential to all facets of the total system is patient classification. A PCS, which quantifies the quality of nursing care, is essential to staffing nursing units of hospitals and nursing homes. In selecting or implementing a PCS, a representative committee of hospital administration, nurse managers, and clinical nurses should be used. Skill mix index data may be used rather than a PCS for determining staffing needs. Because of increased length of stay, most patients require total patient care with self-care limited to observation patients.

> *"The primary aim of patient classification is to be able to respond to the constant variation in the care needs of patients."[44]*

Classification systems originated in the 1960s, when R. J. Connor's doctoral research work resulted in the development of a classification tool for hospitals to better use nursing staff. Three categories of patient acuity, with guidelines describing typical characteristics, were identified[45]:

1. Category I: Self-care
2. Category II: Intermediate care
3. Category III: Total care

Connor's guidelines described the time necessary for the care of a patient in each category. He created a staffing algorithm using a patient index,

$$I = \frac{0.5N}{1} + \frac{1.0N}{2} + \frac{2.5N}{3}$$

in which I represents the patient care index and N the number of patients in each category. The constant (0.5, 1.0, 2.5) represents the amount of direct care in hours and the subscripts (1, 2, 3) represent the specific classification level.[45]

Purposes   The committee identifies the purposes of the PCS to be purchased or developed (Figure 10-9). Among such purposes are the following[46]:

- *Staffing:* The system establishes a unit of measure for nursing, that is, time, that will be used to determine numbers and kinds of staff needed. Perceived patient needs can be matched with available nursing resources.
- *Program costing and formulation of the nursing budget:* A prescribed unit of time is used to determine the actual costs of nursing services. Profits and losses of nursing can then be determined.
- *Tracking changes in patient care needs:* A PCS gives nurse managers the ability to moderate and control delivery of care services, adjusting intensity and cost.
- *Determining values for the productivity equation: output divided by input:* Reducing input costs reduces the cost of each output (time unit). In the prospective payment system, this output measure has been the discharged patient. Outputs become the criteria for measuring nursing productivity, regardless of quality. PCSs provide work load indices as productivity measures.
- *Determining quality:* Once a standard time element has been established, staffing is adjusted to meet the aggregate times. A nurse manager can elect to staff below the standard time to reduce costs, making a decision to reduce quality by reducing times and costs. It is best to do this in collaboration with clinical nurses. These nurses can assist with developing and applying more efficient procedures and protocols, which can involve rearrangement of the physical setting and the assembling of equipment and supplies. Involvement by clinical nurses will increase their trust and respect, improve their attendance and work habits, improve workforce stability, and reduce errors.

Desired Characteristics   A PCS should do the following[47]:

1. Differentiate intensity of care among definitive classes.
2. Measure and quantify care to develop a management engineering standard.

FIGURE 10-9   **PURPOSES OF PATIENT CLASSIFICATION SYSTEM**

- Staffing
- Program costing and formation of the nursing budget
- Tracking changes in patient care needs
- Determining values for productivity equation output
- Determining quality

Source: Author.

3. Match nursing resources to patient care requirements.
4. Relate to time and effort spent on the associated activity.
5. Be economical and convenient to report and use.
6. Be mutually exclusive, counting no item under more than one work unit.
7. Be open to audit.
8. Be understood by those who plan, schedule, and control the work.
9. Be individually standardized as to the procedures needed for accomplishment.
10. Separate requirements for RNs from those of other staff.

Components The first component of a PCS is a method for grouping patients or patient categories. Johnson describes two methods of categorizing patients. Through factor evaluation, each patient is rated on independent elements of care, each element is scored (weighted), scores are summarized, and the patient is placed in a category based on the total numerical value obtained. In prototype evaluation, each patient is categorized to a broad description of care requirements.[48]

Johnson describes a prototype evaluation with four basic categories (self-care, minimal, moderate care, extensive care) and one category for a typical patient requiring one-on-one care. Each category addresses activities of daily living, general health, teaching and emotional support, and treatments and medications. Data are collected on average time spent on direct and indirect care. For example, under activities of daily living, aspects of eating, grooming, excretion, and comfort are identified. At a minimal care level, the patient requires help in preparing food and positioning or encouragement to eat but can feed him- or herself.

A second component of a PCS is a set of guidelines describing the way in which patients will be classified, the frequency of classification, and the method of reporting the data. The third component of a PCS is the average amount of time required for care of a patient in each category. The fourth component is finding a method for calculating required staffing and required nursing care hours. The sum of the standard times for each category multiplied by the number of patients in that category plus the indirect care time equals required hours of patient care. Dividing this value by the number of hours staff actually works each shift results in the number of staff required to work each shift.[49]

The Commission for Administration Services in Hospitals (CASH) system of patient classification is an example of the prototype evaluation type. CASH rates patients by intensity of care and establishes a category relating to nursing hours required based on patients' ability to feed and bathe themselves with supervision; mobility status; special procedures and treatments; and observational, institutional, and emotional needs. The CASH design is quantified by determining the nursing care time associated with the critical indicators.

The GRASP® PCS uses a work load measurement design to evaluate the categories of tasks that nurses perform in providing patient care and identifies how much nursing time is required for each task. The time is then totaled.[50] GRASP® is a factor evaluation design, as is Medicus.

General agreement exists that three to five categories of patient acuity are sufficient for a PCS. Alward argues that four categories are best to reduce variance and statistical probability of error. She also states that the factor evaluation instrument is better than the prototype system because the former prevents ambiguity and overlap among the categories.[51] Research has indicated that different PCSs can generate different hours of work load and related nursing work load.[52]

Nursing Models PCSs based on a model of nursing are rare. Dee and Auger describe one based on the Johnson Behavioral System Model, which has eight behavioral subsystems: ingestive, eliminative, affiliative, dependency, sexual, aggressive-protective, achievement, and restorative. Patient behaviors and nursing interventions were rank ordered for four categories of patient acuity, with category 1 identified as reinforcing independent behaviors in adaptive areas and providing supervision. Category 4 denotes care provided on a one-to-one basis for 8 hours per shift, as, for example, in suicide observations. In this model, specifically in the eliminative subsystem, patients' behaviors that might be noted include absence of bowel and bladder control and excessive diaphoresis. Nursing interventions would include implementing a behavioral program for toilet training, bedwetting, and encopresis. Other systems would be assessed with nursing interventions identified to address the behaviors.

Dee and Auger list four advantages to relating nursing models to PCSs[53]:

1. Providing a frame of reference for the systematic assessment of patient behaviors and the development of nursing intervention
2. Providing a frame of reference for all practitioners in the clinical setting
3. Providing a theoretical framework of knowledge and behavior
4. Providing for consistency and continuity of care

Dee and Auger emphasize orientation and teaching of all new personnel so the system is used effectively. This is true of all PCSs and of their use to make decisions about admissions.

In-House Versus Purchased Purchased PCSs are very expensive and must be modified for specific hospitals. An in-house PCS can be developed using work analysis techniques. Methods for developing such systems are described in several references; most use observation or self-reporting techniques. In the self-reporting techniques, personnel are trained to list activities they perform at timed intervals. Observation on a continuous or internal basis can be costly in time and money. Self-reporting is cheaper, but employees must be trained.[54]

Alward states that it is more realistic to use the budget to determine staffing. She suggests selecting a prototype or factor-evaluation classification instrument and revising it to conform to the division's nursing practice.[55]

Nyberg and Wolff describe a PCS that calculates the total time, direct and indirect, needed to care for each patient by unit, shift, and job classification. The required time is compared with actual and budgeted nursing care hours per patient. This system has been found to identify patient care trends, improve efficiency of staffing, and justify budgeting changes. It has been used for utilization review, using access to admitting and working diagnoses, surgical procedures, physician-consultants, patient classification categories, and a list of all daily nursing care activities. When hospitalization is not justified, a chart review is done. This computerized system determines nursing costs per patient by unit, Medicare patients and non-Medicare patients by diagnosis, and average and total costs of Medicare and non-Medicare patients. In one 2-week period, Medicare patients required 10% more nursing resources per day and 40% more nursing time for their entire hospitalization.[56]

Computer Models There are also personal computer models of PCSs. One of these, described by Grazman, has modules for planning nursing care and dealing with the budget. This system projects the number of hours of care, for each of four patient levels, that will meet budgetary and program delivery constraints of the staffing parameters. It is a staffing system that addresses the "demand" function based on planning and the "management" function based on a blending of planning and actual situations. Thus the input variables can be changed and the budget renegotiated. This model plans nursing time and resource allocation daily, based on patient case mix and census. It gives the nurse manager control over resource use.[57]

Adams and Duchene describe a PCS that includes nursing diagnosis with related cause, nursing care goals, and potential patient outcomes. It is an in-house system, the advantages of which include the following[58]:

- Knowledge of the data tool
- Ability to alter the system to accommodate changes in procedural time standards
- Ability to make changes in staffing levels
- Ability to make percentage alterations of time given to indirect care activities

This PCS produces a plan of care, with acuity used as the basis of determining staffing needs.

Problems One of the major problems of PCSs is maintaining reliability and validity. This can be addressed through continuing education and quality checks. A calendar can be established to have external personnel from staff development or another nursing department or unit perform a classification after one is done by unit personnel (interacter reliability). This classification can be done monthly or more or less often, depending on the results. Patients can be monitored on different days and different shifts, with a stratified random sample of 15% or 20% of the patient census. Simple percentage agreement of 90% or higher indicates satisfactory reliability. If agreement is below 80%, the system should be reviewed and adjusted.

A calendar can also be established to take a unit rotation work sample to determine whether procedures or tasks change with time and technology. The calendar can be used as an annual spot-check. Validation of PCSs varies. A questionnaire can be used to evaluate nursing staff's satisfaction with hours of care. Validity can also be tested by an expert panel of nurses. Patient category descriptions or critical indicators of nursing intervention and patient requirement lists should be reviewed annually according to standards. The PCSs must be altered when results of quality checks or work samples so indicate.

Orientation and continuing education are the best methods of ensuring reliability and validity. The nursing staff must find the PCS credible. If nurses believe that the classifications are accurate and useful, they will try to rate patients accurately. They need periodic classes to be updated, and they must be kept well informed. Managers must support the use of a valid and reliable PCS, because it indicates the institution's commitment to quality patient care.

> ❝ *Practicing nurses want the PCS to provide more staff. Managing nurses want to use it to validate staffing and scheduling and to permit variable staffing. These objectives must be kept in harmony.* ❞

Nursing should orient other department heads and physicians to the use of PCSs. Admission and placement of patients are related to PCS outcomes.[59]

Fixed-Ratio Staffing: The California Experience

Another method of determining the level of staffing necessary to deliver patient care is a fixed-ratio pattern, predetermined by nursing administrators and frequently based on historical data from PCSs, productivity reports, and admit/discharge data. Its major negative aspects include its disregard for the type of patient and for the education and experience level of the nursing staff.

The ANA of California lobbied for and facilitated the creation of the nation's first law mandating nurse-staffing ratios for acute care hospitals. AB 394, authored by Assemblywoman Sheila Kuehl, was signed into law by Governor Gray Davis (CA) on October 10, 1999. Despite a tentative agreement for implementation by January 2002, it was not until January 2004 that the regulations stipulated within the law were implemented. Those regulations are as follows[60]:

- Nurse staffing is determined based on the severity of illness and the need for specialized equipment.
- RNs must receive an orientation to the area assigned; orientation and competency validation is required for temporary personnel.
- Nursing positions are mandated; ancillary positions are not.
- Both the education and experience levels of the nurse are to be factored in with acuity levels when determining staffing patterns.

Nursing Management Information Systems

Hanson defines a management information system as "an array of components designed to transform a collective set of data into knowledge that is directly useful and applicable in the process of directing and controlling resources and their application to the achievement of specific objectives."[61]

The NMIS includes these five elements[62]:

1. Quality of patient care to be delivered and its measurement
2. Characteristics and care requirements of patients
3. Prediction of the supply of nurse power required for components 1 and 2
4. Logistics of the staffing program pattern and its control
5. Evaluation of the quality of care desired, thereby measuring the success of the staffing itself

A management information system is basic to a sound system of staffing, of scheduling, and of classification of patients. It provides shift reports of personnel by type needed and assigned, staffing and productivity data by unit and area, average data on the intensity of care needed by class of patient, and the cost per time unit of patient care.[63]

Staffing is a major reason to have an NMIS. A personal computer can be used to show, via menus and printouts, the number of nurses required by time slot, restrictions, off-duty policy, continuous or other than intermittent days off, cyclical schedules, and single rotations.[64]

Information stimulates action through management decision making. Data do not; they must be processed to be useful. Information must be timely to be useful. The following is the process for establishing any management information system[65]:

1. State the management objective clearly.
2. Identify the actions required to meet the objective.
3. Identify the responsible position in the organization.
4. Identify the information required to meet the objective.
5. Determine the data required to produce the needed information.
6. Determine the system's requirement for processing the data.
7. Develop a flowchart.

Productivity

"The most valuable asset of the twenty-first century institution, whether business or non-business, will be its knowledge workers and their productivity." Frederick Winslow Taylor set the stage for scientific management in developing a method for job analysis and eliminating un-needed motions. Scientific management makes the worker productive.[66]

Definition

Productivity is commonly defined as output divided by input. Hanson translates this definition into the following equation:

$$\frac{\text{Required staff hours}}{\text{Provided staff hours}} \times 100 = \text{Percent productivity}$$

For example,

$$\frac{380.50 \text{ required staff hours}}{380.50 \text{ required staff hours}} \times 100 = 94.7\% \text{ productivity}$$

Productivity can be increased by decreasing the provided staff hours while keeping the required staff hours constant or increasing them. These data become information when they are related to an objective that indicates variances.[67] Because healthcare resources are limited, the nurse manager is faced with the task of motivating clinical nurses to increase productivity.

Productivity in nursing is related to both efficiency of use of clinical nursing in delivering nursing care and the effectiveness of that care relative to its quality and appropriateness. Brown suggests that U.S.

productivity can decline with increased labor costs without corresponding increases in performance. This decline can be due to factors such as inexperienced workers, technological slowdown from outdated equipment and decreased research and development, government regulations, a diminished work ethic, increased size and bureaucracy in business and industry, and erosion of the managerial ethic.[68]

Measurement

In developing a model for a management information system, Hanson details several formulas for translating data into information. He indicates that in addition to the productivity formula, hours per patient day (HPPD) are a data element that can provide meaningful information when provided for an extended period of time. HPPD is determined by the following formula:

$$\frac{\text{Staff hours}}{\text{Patient days}} = \text{HPPD}$$

For example,

$$\frac{52,000 \text{ staff hours}}{2,883.5 \text{ patient days}} = 18.03 \text{ HPPD}$$

Staff hours are calculated as follows:

$$52,000 \text{ staff hours} = 25 \text{ FTEs} \times 2,080 \text{ work hours per year}$$

$$2,883.5 \text{ patient days} = 7.9 \text{ average daily census} \times 365 \text{ days per year.}$$

No allowance is made for personal time such as coffee breaks, meals, vacations, holidays, sick time, and decreased census time. The figure of 18.03 HPPD may be a high provision of HPPD even for intensive care.

Another useful formula is for budget utilization:

$$\frac{\text{Provided HPPD}}{\text{Budgeted HPPD}} \times 100 = \text{Budget utilization}$$

For example,

$$\frac{18.03 \text{ provided HPPD}}{16.0 \text{ budgeted HPPD}} \times 100 = 112.7\% \text{ budget utilization}$$

The result would have been over budget if the provided hours had been the net of personal time. Because they were not, the HPPD provided may be highly productive. The adequacy of the budget is determined as follows:

$$\frac{\text{Budgeted HPPD}}{\text{Required HPPD}} \times 100 = \text{Budget adequacy}$$

or

$$\frac{16.0 \text{ budgeted HPPD}}{18.03 \text{ required HPPD}} \times 100 = 88.74\% \text{ budget adequacy}$$

Obviously, if the required HPPD are equal to the provided HPPD and exceed the budgeted HPPD, productivity is high because of budget inadequacy. According to Hanson, all data become information when related to the objective.[69] Staffing should be defined in terms of the goal of HPPD to be provided. This goal will relate to productivity, budget utilization, and budget adequacy. Whether it is effective or not depends on measurement of quality of outcomes.

Davis[70] writes that productivity in nursing is the volume and quality of products divided by the cost of producing and delivering them. It is directly related to what nurses do and how they do it. Systems have been developed to determine nursing cost per patient per shift. For example, at University Hospital of Cleveland, the following formula is used:

$$\begin{aligned} \text{Nurse competence rank} &\times \text{hourly salary rate} \\ &\times \text{required nursing hours} \\ &\times \text{care acuity} \\ &= \text{nursing cost per patient} \end{aligned}$$

For example,

$$\begin{aligned} \text{Clinician III} &\times \$25.00 \\ &\times 3 \text{ hr} \\ &\times 5 \\ &= \$1,125.00 \text{ per shift} \end{aligned}$$

One could conclude that the more acutely ill patients are, the more licensed nurse contacts they require.

Smith, Mackey, and Markham developed a productivity monitoring system for the recovery room. The performance ratio was the required FTEs divided by worked FTEs. The data were used to decide whether to fill vacant positions and to develop a budget.[71]

Mailhot reported an analysis of problems in an operating room: poor physical environment, inadequate financial support, poor systems, and low morale. The department was overstaffed by 10 FTEs. Task forces used brainstorming and open forums to solve the problems. They used Lewin's force field analysis, putting complex decision alternatives through an outcome matrix, developing needed evaluation tools, and using pilot projects to test all changes. The task forces made 87 changes in 1 year. In addition, the task forces marketed services to patients and surgeons, provided management training for operating room managers, analyzed operating room procedures, and held an open day between director and staff once every 6 weeks during which each person could see the director. They reduced the staffing by 38 FTE positions and the budget by $1.5 million in 3 years. Job satisfaction surveys indicated improvement.[72]

High input for low output produces low productivity, and high output for low input produces high productivity. Thus the objective of a nursing productivity model is low input for high output.

Productivity Model Differences

Producers of services do not fit the same productivity models as do producers of material goods. Marked discretion exists in determining both expected and actual role performances of nurses who do not produce physical outputs. For this reason, nursing prescriptions such as "emotional support" are difficult to measure. Patient outputs or outcomes can be measured by client satisfaction and client condition on discharge.

Greater emphasis has been placed on the nursing process than on nursing outcome. Haas defines efficiency as the relationship of personnel assigned and time spent to materials expended, as well as capital and management employed, for the greatest economy in use. Productive nurses must balance their personal energies and their institution's resources with their own effectiveness.[73]

Curtin proposes that productivity in nursing is related to the application of knowledge. Professional productivity must be measured by means of efficacy, effectiveness, and efficiency in applying knowledge. Curtin indicates that these processes can be objectively measured by using the following guidelines[74]:

- Objective measures of efficacy: years of formal education, levels of academic achievement, evidence of continuing education and skill development, and years of experience
- Objective measures of effectiveness: demonstrated ability to execute job-related procedures, prioritize activities correctly, perform according to professional and legal standards, record appropriate information clearly and concisely, and cooperate with others
- Objective measures of efficiency: Promptness, attendance, reliability, precision, adaptability, and economical disposition of resources

Curtin and Zurlage acknowledge that human services such as nursing are difficult to test, to return, or to exchange if they are unsatisfactory. These authors propose a system for measuring nursing productivity that includes a nursing productivity equation, an equation relating nursing productivity ratio to hospital revenue, and a nursing productivity index.[75]

Improving Nursing Productivity

The first step toward improving productivity is to study or measure it as it exists. For example, the personnel of an education department decided to improve their productivity. They considered using a time-based method versus a value-based method in developing the productivity system.

A time-based method of productivity considers the length of time required to do each task. The first steps of a time-based method are to review the literature, do a time study, and then compare the results with those in the literature. This is done for activities unique to the unit. Units are then assigned to activities according to the estimated time for completing each. The time-based method does not give priority to activities.

A value-based system considers the value of activities to the institution. Steps for developing a value-based system of productivity include listing activities, grouping them by their value to the institution, and assigning units of productivity. The human resources department should be involved in developing a productivity system.

The McKay-Dee education department at McKay-Dee Hospital Center (Ogden, UT) uses data-collection tools that provide useful methods to better understand productivity from a qualitative and quantitative perspective.[76]

The reported knowledge and skills from improved nursing productivity add to the theory of nursing management. Rabin writes that professionals can impose productivity values on themselves. Managers should develop managerial goals and values. They need a standard of performance for themselves. Professionals must commit themselves to fostering innovative attitudes and technologies, stimulating performance by commitment to constructive action and follow-up, living up to standards of practice, keeping up-to-date, and being receptive to public review. Most professions can develop measurable standards of performance and productivity using online spreadsheets and software programs such as Lotus or Excel.[77]

Employers should measure nursing output objectively and pay for it accordingly in salary, benefits, and promotions. Some progress has been made in nursing in the form of standards of practice, clinical ladders, and models of peer review. These tools, along with respect for the individual dignity of nurses, support for their personal commitment to professional goals, and support for the integrity of their professional judgments, need to be enacted in the workplace.[78]

Productivity can be managed and improved through the following[79]:

- Planning that increases the variations between inputs and outputs by
  - Outputs increasing, inputs decreasing
  - Outputs increasing, inputs remaining constant
  - Outputs increasing faster than inputs
  - Outputs remaining constant, inputs decreasing
  - Outputs decreasing more slowly than inputs
- Involving staff; soliciting staff's ideas and recommendations
- Creating challenges
- Showing interest in the staff's achievement and concerns
- Praising and rewarding good performance; using incentives such as staff development, books and tuition reimbursement, paid meals, bonuses, and vacation days
- Setting the climate for productivity by asking nurses what makes them productive, acting on their suggestions, and measuring the results
- Having a meaningful set or family of easily understood outcome measures for which data are available or easy to gather and over which workers have some control
- Monitoring work load changes in staffing requirements with established standards
- Combining support with employees' understanding, motivation, and recognition
- Increasing the ratio of professional to nonprofessional staff
- Placing admitted patients based on resource availability
- Using approaches such as work simplification and workflow analysis
- Making an organizational diagnosis of problems, resources, and realities
- Stimulating nurse managers and clinical nurses to want to achieve excellence
- Setting targets for increasing output annually without additional capital or employees
- Having personnel keep and analyze time diaries to determine personal improvement actions; setting personal objectives, and measuring performance against them
- Making a commitment to improved productivity, effectiveness (doing the right things), and efficiency (doing things right)
- Seeking new products and services and new methods and ways of producing them; seeking new and useful approaches to old problems
- Maintaining concern about the process and methods of producing nursing care
- Reducing the costs of what nurses do by returning unused budgeted funds
- Improving aesthetics: the quality of work life and the pleasantness and beauty of the environment
- Applying the ethical policy statements of professional nursing organizations
- Improving use of time
- Gaining the confidence of peer
- Recognizing the need to do better

Personnel working in service areas can improve productivity by doing the following[80]:

- Focusing on organizational strategy, customer service, mission, and results rather than on methodology
- Using self-directed work teams to break jobs into observable tasks and responsibilities
- Observing and then making changes or providing training to correct deficiencies
- Watching for problems such as repetition, duplication, recurring delays, and waste of resources
- Observing the outcome of the person's work by splitting the job into four main areas: managing self, resources, and activities and working with others. Suggestions for the key skills required are

analytical thinking, ability to learn, adaptability, positive self-image, emphasis on results, good time management, concern for standards, ability to influence others, and independence.
- Providing feedback that is specific, constructive, and frequent

Case Study

At the Presbyterian Hospital of Dallas, a study revealed that more time was spent on clerical functions, telephone calls, and reporting patient conditions to other caregivers than on direct patient care. Several actions were taken that greatly improved productivity[81]:

- A fax machine network was instituted between nursing units and the pharmacy, reducing the number of telephone calls and medication errors.
- A keyless narcotics system was installed that included personnel pass codes. The main control system was in pharmacy, but nurses could enter their personal pass code at the narcotics cabinet. This reduced time wasted to search for keys and produced an audit trail.
- A unit beeper system with eight beepers was purchased at a local store for $375. Beepers given to every staff member at the beginning of each shift made nursing assistants feel valued.

Decision Making in Planning for Staffing

Planning and decision making in staffing issues takes into account a number of variables, including patient acuity (patient classification), organizational dynamics, geographical issues, experience, and competency of staff. Mandated ratios have posed a number of concerns, particularly considering a one-size-fits-all model. As noted, legislation has occurred related to mandated nurse-to-patient ratios at the state and federal levels. In 1999, California passed Assembly Bill 394, the first comprehensive legislation in the United States to mandate minimum staffing levels for nurses. AB 394 directed the California Department of Health Services to establish minimum, specific, nurse-to-patient ratios by licensed nurse classification and by hospital unit. The legislation became effective on January 1, 2004, and the medical/surgical ratios were tightened effective January 1, 2005.[82]

The benefits and consequences of mandating ratios continue to be debated. The American Organization of Nurse Executives opposes mandated ratios and recommends an increase in evidence-based and outcomes-driven research that includes patient acuity in the development of staffing guidelines.[83] The Society for Health Systems recommends a systematic approach to developing optimal clinical staffing, considering multiple variables to be evaluated, in creating a safe, quality staffing model[84]:

- Matches clinical staffing to the specific needs of patients based on patients' acuity, age, and ability to perform activities of daily living.
- Reflects the dependency of the patient upon nursing assistance, and takes into account the absence or presence of family support during the hospital stay.
- Takes into account hospital variables such as physical layout of the nursing unit, operating rooms, emergency department and support departments, technology available to the staff (such as manual or electronic nursing documentation, electronic medical records, medicine administration procedures, automated supply cabinets, and computerized physician order entry), the degree of turnover of the units (admissions, discharges and transfers), and the role of the hospital as either teaching or nonteaching, level 1 trauma center or not, and any specializations within the hospital.
- Fluctuates staffing by shift and day based on variations in census and patient care requirements.
- Reflects the culture of the hospital with respect to provision of nursing care and skill mix of nursing providers.
- Is objective, repeatable, and tested to be a valid method to set staffing levels.

• Involves the major hospital stakeholders in developing the staffing model, including administrators, nursing leadership and staff, support, and ancillary departments.

The Society for Health Systems reports that these factors cannot be addressed in a static, mandated nurse-to-patient ratio. An efficient, comprehensive staffing plan can only be developed through careful analysis with key stakeholders and devised to adjust staffing requirements on a daily and shift basis.[85]

Evidence-Based Practice 10-3

Mittmann et al. discussed how poorly nursing costs are estimated in economic studies conducted in hospitals. This is primarily due to the lack of data on nursing times for day-to-day activities related to patient care. The researchers describe their study of nursing work load associated with hospital patient care, calculating patient care hours, using the Grace Reynolds Application and Study of PETO (GRASP®) system, extracting these data from patient records. A total of 483 patients with five different indications (acute myocardial infarction [MI], n = 98; diabetes mellitus, n = 93; pneumonia, n = 98; schizophrenia, n = 94; and stroke, n = 100) who were hospitalized in March 2002 at the Sunnybrook Health Sciences Centre, Toronto, Canada were included. The primary objective of the study was to determine standard time values for nursing activities for specific indications of a cohort of hospital patients. The patient care hours were converted into minutes, and the results were stratified by patient diagnosis and evaluated as to the frequency and duration of each nursing task. The researchers noted that nurses reported the greatest amount of time spent providing care for patients with MI (2.50 ± 2.31 hours of care per patient per hospital stay), followed by those with pneumonia (2.35 ± 2.02 hours), diabetes (1.96 ± 1.31 hours), schizophrenia (1.72 ± 1.95 hours), and stroke (1.70 ± 1.47 hours). Cardiovascular assessment was the task most frequently undertaken in patients with MI; in patients with diabetes and pneumonia it was routine teaching/emotional support, in patients with schizophrenia it was ongoing assessment, and in patients with stroke it was administration of medications. Pulmonary artery pressure monitoring took the most time in caring for MI patients (110.83 minutes), whereas one-to-one nurse–patient supervision (i.e., 1:1 sitter) took the most time in patients with diabetes, pneumonia, schizophrenia, and stroke.[87]

Evidence-Based Practice 10-4

Clarke described policy implications of staffing-outcomes research. Results from this work indicated that hospitals and units in study samples with the lowest levels of nurse staffing generally experienced worse patient outcomes than peer units and hospitals at higher levels. "There also appear to be differentials in outcomes at staffing points in between the extremes." Clarke stated that it was not clear which of these inconsistencies were from a lack of sensitivity of some outcomes to nursing staffing, which resulted from circumstances (including a variety of patient, nurse, and institutional factors) that can modify the effects of staffing seen in a particular geographical location or time period, and which negative findings relate to methodological limitations in the research. Additionally, the literature had limited information regarding patient safety, particularly over time. The researcher concluded that more research, particularly addressing patient safety and staffing over time, was necessary, specifically for policy changes in critical nursing shortage areas. [88]

SUMMARY

Staffing and scheduling are major components of nursing management. A nursing division needs a practical and written philosophy that guides all staffing and scheduling activities and that is acceptable to the staff.

Staffing studies can be used to determine staffing needs related to personnel skills, numbers of personnel, and time and work load requirements. There are as many possible approaches to staffing as there are nursing managers and staff to create them. Staffing innovations are key to the satisfaction, and therefore retention, of nurses.

Staffing can be planned with models that calculate work load requirements from patient classification data or at the discretion of nursing administration with fixed-ratio staffing.

Productivity, the unit of output of nursing, is a focus of increasing interest to nurse managers. It must include quality care indicators that can be observed and measured.

Productivity, quality of care, and a safe and healthy workplace are all enhanced when concern for the individual seeking healthcare services is the top priority and when nursing administrators ensure

- Adequate numbers of clinically competent staff
- Positive working relationships among the healthcare team
- Autonomy and accountability for nursing practice, adequate compensation, commensurate with responsibilities, education, and experience
- Access to education and research
- Access to appropriate technologies and promotion of evidence-based practice[86]

APPLICATION EXERCISES

Exercise 10-1

Interview a nurse manager. Identify staff activities that are determined to be most productive and why. Describe nonproductive activities and strategies to improve efficiency and effectiveness of staff.

Exercise 10-2

Based on the information listed below, use Figure 10-5, Formula for Estimating a Core Staff per Shift, to do the following exercise.

1. The average daily census of a unit is 29 patients.
2. The basic average daily hours of care to be provided are 6 hours per patient per 24 hours.
3. The workday is 8 hours. Also, consider the 12-hour workday.
4. Determine the following:
   a. The total hours of care needed on the average day to meet these standards
   b. The total number of FTEs needed to staff the unit for 24 hours
   c. The number of 8-hour shifts needed per week
   d. The number of FTEs needed as basic staff for this unit
5. Using the Salt Lake City Community Hospital recommendation of staff mix, determine the mix of RNs, LPNs, and aides.
6. Using Warstler's proportion for staffing shifts, determine the number of FTEs for days, evenings, and nights.
7. Create a table for basic staffing for this unit. Do not add complementary staff without a specific reason for doing so.

Exercise 10-3

Use cyclic scheduling and then self-scheduling to schedule a staff of six RNs and one nursing assistant for a period of 1 month. In the self-scheduling section, you may use any combination of schedules effective for unit coverage and satisfactory to the staff.

Exercise 10-4

Identify at least 12 activities that can be done to improve productivity in a division or department of nursing in which you work.

Notes

1. Rewick, D., & Gaffey, E. (2001). Nursing system makes a difference. *Health Management Technology, 1,* 24–26.
2. Materra, M. D. (2001). Nurses' problems are yours. *Medical Economics, 4,* 32–39.
3. Coile, R. C., Jr. (2001). Magnet hospitals use culture, not wages, to solve nursing shortage. *Journal of Healthcare Management,* 224–227.
4. Page, A. (Ed.). (2004). *Keeping patients safe: Transforming the work environment of nurses.* Washington, DC: The National Academies Press.
5. Kovner, C., & Gergen, P. J. (1998). Nurse staffing levels and adverse events following surgery in US hospitals. *Image: Journal of Nursing Scholarship,* 315.
6. Blegen, M. A., Goode, C. J., & Reed, L. (1998). Nurse staffing and patient outcomes. *Nursing Research,* 43–49.
7. White, K. (2003). Effective staffing as a guardian. *Nursing Management,* 20–24.
8. Aydelotte, M. K. (1973). *Nurse staffing methodology: A review and critique of selected literature* (p. 3). Washington, DC: US Government Printing Office.
9. West, M. E. (1980). Implementing effective nurse staffing systems in the managed hospital. *Topics in Health Care Financing,* 11–25.
10. Althaus, J. N., Hardyck, N. M., Pierce, P. B., & Rodgers, M. S. (1982). Nurse staffing in a decentralized organization: Part I. *Journal of Nursing Administration, 12*(12), 34–39.
11. Parker, L. (1993). When to fix it and when to leave: Relationships among perceived control, self-efficacy, dissent, and exit. *Journal of Applied Psychology, 78,* 949–959.
12. Minetti, R. C. (1983). Computerized nurse staffing. *Hospitals,* 90, 92; Shaheen, P. P. (1985). Staffing and scheduling: Reconcile practical means with the real goal. *Nursing Management,* 64–69.
13. Aydelotte, 1973, pp. 26–31.
14. Bell, H. M., McElnay, J. C., & Hughes, C. M. (1999). A self-reported work sampling study in community pharmacy practice. *Pharmacy World Science,* 210–216; Upenieks, V. V. (1998). Work sampling: Assessing nursing efficiency. *Nursing Management,* 27–29; Urden, L. D., & Roode, J. I. (1997). Work sampling: A decision-making tool for determining resources and work redesign. *Journal of Nursing Administration, 27*(9), 34–41; Cardona, P., Tappen, R. M., Terrill, M., Acosta, M., & Eusebe, M. I. (1997). Nursing staff time allocation in long-term care: A work sampling study. *Journal of Nursing Administration, 27*(4), 28–36; Miller, M. E., James, M. K., Langefeld, C. D., Espeland, M. A., Freedman, J. A., Martin, D. M. (1996). Some techniques for the analysis of work sampling data. *Statistical Medicine,* 607–618.
15. West, 1980, p. 16.
16. Ibid., p. 17.
17. Schroder, P. J., & McKeon, K. L. (1990). What is a safe staffing pattern for locked long-term and acute care units for adults? *Journal of Psychosocial Nursing, 28,* 36–37.
18. Price, E. M. (1970). *Staffing for patient care* (p. 12). New York: Springer.
19. Steed, C. K. (2004). Eating our young isn't practiced here. *Nursing 2004,* 43.
20. Joint Commission in Accreditation of Healthcare Organizations. (2001). *Accreditation process improvement: Introduction to staffing effectiveness presentation.* Retrieved September 3, 2004 from http://www.amda.com/caring/april2002/staffing.htm
21. Study questions all-RN staffing. (1983). *RN,* 15–16.

22. Warstler, M. E. (1972). Some management techniques for nursing service administrators. *Journal of Nursing Administration,* 25–34.

23. American Hospital Association (AHA). (1985). *Strategies: Flexible scheduling.* Washington, DC: Author.

24. Froebe, D. (1975). Scheduling: By team or individually. *Staffing: A Journal of Nursing Administration Reader.* 5(4), 22–35.

25. Rondeau, K. V. (1990). Self-Scheduling can increase job satisfaction. *Medical Laboratory Observer,* 22–24; Teahan, B. (1998). Implementation of a self-scheduling system: A solution to more than just schedules. *Journal of Nursing Management,* 361–368; Irvin, S. A., & Brown, H. N. (1999). Self-scheduling with Microsoft Excel. *Nursing Economics,* 201–206.

26. Ricci, J. A. (1984). 10 Hour Night Shift: Cost vs. Savings. *Nursing Management,* 34–35, 38–42.

27. Fagin, C. M. (1982). The economic value of nursing research. *American Journal of Nursing,* 1844–1849.

28. Vik, A. G., & MacKay, R. C. (1982). How does the 12-hour shift affect patient care? *Journal of Nursing Administration,* 12.

29. Washburn, M. S. (1991). Fatigue and critical thinking on eight- and twelve-hour shifts. *Nursing Management,* 80A–CC, 80D–CC, 80 F–H–CC.

30. Lant, T. W., & Gregory, D. (1984). The impact of 12-hour shift: An analysis. *Nursing Management,* 38A–38B, 38D–38F, 38H.

31. Fisher, D. W., & Thomas, E. (1975). A "premium day" approach to weekend nurse staffing. *Staffing: A Journal of Nursing Administration Reader.*

32. Robb, E. A., Determan, A. C., Lampat, L. R., Scherbring, M. J., Slifka, R. M., & Smith, N. A. (2003). Self scheduling: Satisfaction guaranteed? *Nursing Management,* 16–18.

33. McGuire, J. B., & Liro, J. R. (1986). Flexible work schedules, work attitudes, and perceptions of productivity. *Public Personnel Management,* 65–73.

34. Ibid.

35. Imig, S. I., Powell, J. A., & Thorman, K. (1984). Primary nursing and flexi-staffing: Do they mix? *Nursing Management,* 39–42.

36. O'Donnell, K. (1992). A flexible role: Resource acuity nurse. *Nursing Management,* 75–76.

37. Bruzzese, A. (1994, April 19). Companies turning to temps to fill voids in workplace. *San Antonio Express-News,* pp. 1C, 7C.

38. Messmer, M. (1992). Strategic staffing. *Management Accounting,* 28–30.

39. Hicks, L. (1993, December 12). The rise in temps. *San Antonio Express-News,* pp. 1–H, 6–H.

40. Randolph, L. (2003). Tracking travel trends. *Nursing Management Supplement,* 4, 9–11.

41. Tuttle, D. M. (1992). A "transfer fair" approach to staffing. *Nursing Management,* 72–74.

42. Kramer, M., & Schmalenberg, C. (2004). Essentials of a magnetic work environment: Part 1. *Nursing 2004,* 50–54.

43. Kramer, M., & Schmalenberg, C. (2002). Essentials of magnetism. In M. McClure & A. Hinshaw (Eds.), *Magnet hospitals revisited: Attraction and retention of professional nurses.* Kansas City, MO: American Nurses Publishing.

44. Fagerstrom, L., & Rainio, A. K. (1999). Professional assessment of optimal nursing care intensity level: A new method of assessing personnel resources for nursing care. *Journal of Clinical Nursing,* 369–379.

45. Connor, R. J. (1961). A work sampling study of variations in nursing workload. *Hospitals, 35,* 40–41.

46. Herzog, T. P. (1985). Productivity: Fighting the battle of the budget. *Nursing Management,* 30–34; Porter-O'Grady, T. (1985). Strategic planning: Nursing practice in the PPS. *Nursing Management,* 53–56; Johnson, K. (1984). A practical approach to patient classification. *Nursing Management,* 39–41, 44, 46; Schroeder, R. E., Rhodes, A. M., & Shields, R. E. (1984). Nurse acuity systems: CASH vs. GRASP. *Nursing Forum,* 72–77; Alward, R. R. (1983). Patient classification systems: The ideal vs. reality. *Journal of Nursing Administration,* 14–18; Nyberg, J., & Wolff, N. (1984). DRG panic. *Journal of Nursing Administration,* 17–21.

47. Schroeder et al., 1984.

48. Johnson, 1984.

49. Ibid., p. 41.

50. Schroeder et al., 1984.

51. Alward, 1983.

52. O'Brien-Pallas, L., Leatt, P., Deber, R., & Till, J. (1989). A comparison of workload estimates using three methods of patient classification. *Canadian Journal of Nursing Administration*, 16–23.

53. Dee, V., & Auger, J. A. (1983). A patient classification system based on the behavioral system model of nursing: Part 2. *Journal of Nursing Administration*, 18–23.

54. Alward, 1983.

55. Ibid.

56. Nyberg & Wolff, 1984.

57. Grazman, T. E. (1983). Managing unit human resources: A microcomputer model. *Nursing Management*, 18–22.

58. Adams, R., & Duchene, P. (1985). Computerization of patient acuity and nursing care planning. *Journal of Nursing Administration*, 11–17.

59. Giovannetti, P., & Mayer, G. G. (1984). Building confidence in patient classification systems. *Nursing Management*, 31–34; Alward, 1983.

60. American Nurses Association (ANA). (1999, October 13). *Press Release*. Retrieved September 1, 2004 from http://www.nursingworld.org/pressrel/1999/pr1013.htm

61. Hanson, R. L. (1982a). Applying management information systems to staffing. *Journal of Nursing Administration*, 5–9.

62. Aydelotte, 1973, p. 26.

63. Halloran, E. J., & Kiley, M. (1984). Case mix management. *Nursing Management*, 39–41, 44–45.

64. Moores, B., & Murphy, A. (1984, July 4). Planning the duty rota, one, computerized duty rotas. *Nursing Times*, 47–48; Canter, D. (1984, July 4). Planning the duty rota, two, back to basics. *Nursing Times*, 49–50.

65. Hanson, 1982a.

66. Drucker, P. F. (1999). *Management challenges for the 21st century*. New York: HarperCollins, 135–140.

67. Hanson, R. L. (1982b). Staffing statistics: Their use and usefulness. *Journal of Nursing Administration*, 29–35.

68. Brown, D. S. (1983). The managerial ethic and productivity improvement. *Public Productivity Review*, 223–250.

69. Hanson, 1982b. The formulas are Hanson's; applications are the author's.

70. Davis, D. L. (1984). Assessing and improving productivity in the operating room. *AORN Journal*, 630, 632, 634.

71. Smith, J. L., Mackey, M. K. V., & Markham, J. (1985). Productivity monitoring: A recovery room system for economizing operations. *Nursing Management*, 34A–D, K–M.

72. Mailhot, C. B. (1985). Setting OR's course toward greater productivity. *Nursing Management*, 42I, J, L, M, P.

73. Haas, S. A. W. (1984). Sorting out nursing productivity. *Nursing Management*, 37–40.

74. Curtin, L. (1984). Reconciling pay with productivity. *Nursing Management*, 7–8.

75. Curtin, L. L., & Zurlage, C. L. (1986). Nursing productivity: From data to definition. *Nursing Management*, 32–34, 38–41.

76. Waterstradt, C. R., & Phillips, T. L. (1990). A productivity system for a hospital education department. *Journal of Nursing Staff Development*, 139–144.

77. Rabin, J. (1983). Professionalism and productivity. *Public Productivity Review*, 217–222; DiJerome, L., Dunham-Taylor, J., Ash, D., & Brown, R. (1999). Evaluating cost center productivity. *Nursing Economics*, 334–340.

78. Curtin, 1984.

79. Fralic, M. F. (1982). The modern professional and productivity. Annual Meeting of the Alabama Society for Nursing Service Administrators, Huntsville, Ala.; Hanson, R. L. (1982c). Managing human resources. *Journal of Nursing Administration*, 17–23; Kaye, G. H., & Utenner, J. (1985). Productivity: Managing for the long term. *Nursing Management, 1*, 12–13, 15; Haas, 1984; Davis, 1984; Brown, 1983.

80. Ancona, P. (1993, July 24). How to measure productivity and improve effectiveness among workers. *San Antonio Express-News*, p. 1B.

81. Gilliland, M., Crane, V. S., & Jones, D. G. (1991). Productivity: Electronics saves steps-and builds networks. *Nursing Management, 1*, 56–59.

82. UC Davis Center for Health Services Research in Primary Care and UC Davis Center for Nursing Research, Hospital nursing staff ratios and quality of care: Final report on evidence, administrative data, an expert panel process, and a hospital staffing survey. May 2002.

83. Policy statement on mandated staffing ratios. American Organization of Nurse Executives, December 2003.

84. Society for Health Systems, Position statement on mandated nursing ratios. Approved by the SHS Board of Directors, August 2005.

85. Ibid.

86. American Nurses Association (ANA). (2004). *Scope and standards for nurse administrators* (2nd ed., p. 4). ANA Press, Silver Spring, MD.

87. Mittmann, N., Seung, S., Pisterzi, L., Isogai, P., & Michaels, D. (2008). Nursing workload associated with hospital patient care. *Disease Management & Health Outcomes, 16,* 53–61.

88. Clarke, S. P. (2004). The policy implications of staffing-outcomes research. *Journal of Nursing Administration, 35*(2), 17–19.

References

Advisory Committee on Health Human Resources. (2003). *The nursing strategy for Canada, report of the Advisory Committee on Health Human Resources.* Retrieved April 14, 2003, from www.hc-sc.gc.ca/english/pdf/nursing.pdf

Aiken, L. H., Sloane, D., Lake, E. Y., Sochalski, J., & Weber, A. (1999). Organization and outcomes of inpatient AIDS care. *Medical Care, 37,* 760–772.

American Nurses Association. (1999). *Principles for nurse staffing.* Washington, DC: Author.

Baumann, A., O'Brien-Pallas, L., Armstrong-Stassen, M., Blythe, J., Bourbonnais, R., Cameron, S., et al. (2001). *Commitment and care: The benefits of a healthy workplace for nurses, their patients, and the system.* Ottawa: Canadian Health Services Research Foundation.

Blakeman Hodge, M., Romano, P. S., Harvey, D., Samuels, S. J., Olson, V. A., Sauvé, M. J., et al. (2004). Licensed caregiver characteristics and staffing in California acute care hospital units. *Journal of Nursing Administration, 34,* 125–133.

Blegen, M. A., Goode, C. J., & Reed, L. (1998). Nurse staffing and patient outcomes. *Nursing Research, 47,* 43–50.

Boehm, C. (2005). Staffing ratios smashing success down under. *Revolution: The Journal for RNs and Patient Advocacy, 6,* 9–9.

Buchan, J., & Calman, L. (2005). *Summary: The international shortage of registered nurses.* Geneva, Switzerland: International Council of Nurses.

Canadian Federation of Nurses Unions. (2005). *Enhancement of patient safety through formal nurse-patient ratios: A discussion paper.* Retrieved February 3, 2006, from www.nursesunions.ca/en/Docs/2005-10-03-Nurse-Patient-Ratio-EN.pdf

Canadian Nurses Association. (2004a). *Nursing staff mix: A literature review.* Ottawa, Canada: Author.

Canadian Nurses Association. (2004b). *Patient safety: Developing the right staff mix. Report of think tank.* Ottawa, Canada: Author.

Canadian Nurses Association. (2005). *Evaluation framework to determine the impact of nursing staff mix decisions.* Ottawa, Canada: Author.

Donaldson, N., Burnes Bolton, L., Aydin, C., Brown, D., Elashoff, J. D., & Sandhu, M. (2005). Impact of California's licensed nurse-patient ratios on unit-level nurse staffing and patient outcomes. *Policy, Politics, & Nursing Practice, 6*, 198–210.

Ellis, J., Priest, A., MacPhee, M., & Sanchez McCutcheon, A. (2006). *Staffing for safety: A synthesis of the evidence on nurse staffing and patient safety.* Ottawa: Canadian Health Services Research Foundation.

Hall, L. M. (2005). *Quality work environments for nurse and patient safety.* Sudbury, MA: Jones and Bartlett.

International Council of Nurses. (n.d.). *The Global Nursing Review Initiative: Policy options and solutions.* Retrieved November 16, 2006, from www.icn.ch/global/

Joint Commission on Accreditation of Healthcare Organizations. (2004). *2004 comprehensive accreditation manual for hospitals.* Chicago: Author.

Kovner, C., & Gergen, P. J. (1998). Nurse staffing levels and adverse events following surgery in U.S. hospitals. *Image: Journal of Nursing Scholarship, 30*, 315–321.

Lankshear, A. J., Sheldon, T. A., & Maynard, A. (2005). Nurse staffing and healthcare outcomes. A systematic review of the international research evidence. *Advances in Nursing Science, 28*, 163–174.

Lichtig, L. K., Knauf, R. A., & Milholland, D. K. (1999). Some impacts of nursing on acute care hospital outcomes. *Journal of Nursing Administration, 29*, 25–33.

McGillis Hall, L., Doran, D., Baker, G. R., Pink, G., Sidani, S., O'Brien Pallas, L., et al. (2003). Nurse staffing models as predictors of patient outcomes. *Medical Care, 41*, 1096–1109.

McGillis Hall, L., Doran, D., & Pink, G. H. (2004). Nurse staffing models, nursing hours, and patient safety outcomes. *Journal of Nursing Administration, 34*, 41–45.

McGillis Hall, L., Pink, L., Lalonde, M., Murphy, G., O'Brien-Pallas, L., Laschinger, H., et al. (2006). *Evaluation of nursing staff mix and staff ratio tools and models. Final report.* Ottawa: Canadian Nurses Association and Health Canada.

Needleman, J., Buerhaus, P. L., Mattke, S., Stewart, M., & Zelevinsky, K. (2001). *Nurse staffing and patient outcomes in hospitals.* Boston: U.S. Department of Health and Human Services, Health Resources and Services Administration.

Nursing Sector Study. (2005, May). *Building the future: An integrated strategy for nursing human resources in Canada. Phase 1 final report.* Ottawa, Canada: Nursing Sector Study Corporation.

Ritter-Teitel, J. (2002). The impact of restructuring on professional nursing practice. *Journal of Nursing Administration, 32*, 31–38.

Ritter-Teitel, J. (2004). Registered nurse hours worked per patient day. *Journal of Nursing Administration, 34*, 167–169.

Seago, J. A., Spetz, J., Coffman, J., Rosenoff, E., & O'Neil, E. (2003). Minimum staffing ratios: The California Workforce Initiative Survey. *Nursing Economics, 21*, 65–70.

Seago, J. A., Spetz, J., & Mitchell, S. (2004). Nurse staffing and hospital ownership in California. *Journal of Nursing Administration, 34*, 228–237.

11

BUDGETING PRINCIPLES FOR NURSE MANAGERS

Beth Anderson, RN, MSN
Denise Danna, RN, DNS, NEA, BC, FACHE

LEARNING OBJECTIVES AND ACTIVITIES

- Discuss concepts of budgeting.
- Identify budget-planning steps.
- Identify stages of the budget.
- Examine elements of cost accounting in a healthcare organization.
- Define selected terms related to budgeting.
- Differentiate between direct and indirect costs.
- Differentiate among fixed, variable, and sunk costs.
- Describe various budgets: operating or cash budget, personnel budget, supplies and equipment budget, and capital budget.
- Discuss the budget as a controlling process.
- Discuss monitoring of the budget.
- Discuss motivational aspects of the budget.
- Discuss cutting the budget.
- Observe preparation of the budget for an agency or a cost center.
- Describe the elements of managed care and their impact on patients.
- Explain the effects of managed care relative to managers, nurses, physicians, healthcare organizations, and other providers.

CONCEPTS

Budget, budgeting, cost center, budget stages (calendar), cost accounting, fixed costs, variable costs, sunk costs, direct costs, indirect costs, activity-based costing, revenue budgeting, expense budgeting, operating budget, cost-to-charge ratio, zero-base budgeting, cost-benefit analysis, negative cash flow, service units, chart of accounts, inventory, financial standards, performance budgeting, personnel budget, supplies and equipment budget, capital budget, managed care, fee-for-service reimbursement, indemnity insurance plans, health maintenance organization, capitation, preferred provider organization, contracting.

NURSE MANAGER BEHAVIORS	NURSE EXECUTIVE BEHAVIORS
Is involved in the development of personnel, supplies, equipment, and capital budgets, with expenditures projected. Solves problems resulting from managed care, and promotes interests of patients and personnel.	Decentralizes budget development for personnel, supplies, equipment, and capital expenditures and for projected revenues to cost-center managers. Provides budget guidance through budget stages and provides cost-center managers with current reports of expenditures and revenues while they manage all aspects of their budgets. Assists personnel in maximum understanding of their healthcare benefits. Empowers professional nurses to produce quality outcomes for patients, personnel, and insurers within an environment heavily influenced by managed care.

Introduction

Budgeting is an ongoing activity in which revenues and expenses are managed to maintain fiscal responsibility and fiscal health. The nurse manager has financial responsibility, is accountable for managing the nursing budget, and makes all of the decisions about how to adjust the nursing budget to manage programs and costs, including those related to adding and dropping programs, expanding and contracting programs, and modifying revenues and expenses within the nursing unit.

With limited resources and in a competitive market, healthcare organizations must use personnel and material resources wisely and efficiently. The enlightened nurse knows that the person who controls the budget is the person who controls nursing services. Because the amount and quality of nursing services depend on budgetary plans, nurses should become proficient in budgeting procedures. This proficiency provides the resources necessary for safe and effective nursing care. The costs of nursing services have been identified for many years, but the income earned from nursing services has been included in "bed and board" on the budget sheets. Achieving reimbursement for nursing services means that many government regulations and third-party payer policies must change to allow for direct payment to nursing providers, based on the amount of care given and the skills of the persons giving it.

BASIC PLANNING

In most organizations, planning yields forecasts for 1 year and for several years. The budget is an annual plan, intended to guide effective use of human and material resources, products, or services and to manage the environment to improve productivity. Budgetary planning ensures that the best methods are used to achieve financial objectives. It should be based on valid objectives to provide a product or service that the community needs and for which it will pay. In nursing, budgetary planning helps ensure that clients or patients receive the nursing services they want and need from satisfied nursing workers. A good budget is based on objectives; is simple, flexible, and balanced; has standards; and uses available resources first to avoid increasing costs.

There is no formula for the form, detail, or periods covered by budgets. Each budget system is designed for the situation at hand and must take into consideration the character of the company, the company's position, and the nature of the plans involved. Ordinarily, the budget system is most detailed in aspects of operations most important to the firm's success. Furthermore, the period covered by the budget varies with the nature of the plans and with the degree of accuracy possible in the preparation of estimates.[1]

A nursing budget is a systematic plan that is an informed best estimate by nurse administrators of revenues and nursing expenses. It projects how revenues will meet expenses, and it projects a return on equity, that is, profit. The budget should be stated in terms of attainable objectives to maintain the motivation of nurses at the unit or cost-center level. The nursing budget serves three purposes:

1. To plan the objectives, programs, and activities of nursing services and the fiscal resources needed to accomplish them
2. To motivate nursing workers through analysis of actual experiences
3. To serve as a standard to evaluate the performance of nurse administrators and managers and to increase awareness of costs

These purposes should include the organization's mission, strategic plans, new programs or projects, and goals. Managing the financial end of nursing through an operational budget obviously can create a new sense of involvement for nurses. The budget can be a strong support for developing written objectives for the nursing division and for each of its units. It can provide motivation for effective planning and standards by which to evaluate the performance of nurse managers.[2] Effective planning provides for contingencies by indicating which programs or activities can be reduced or eliminated if budget goals are not met.

Procedures

Decentralized budgeting involves the nursing unit managers and their staff in the process. Nursing service is labor intensive, which is reflected in the fact that the first six budget-planning steps pertain to labor. Note that only steps 7 and 8 are concerned with nonlabor expenses. The steps are as follows[3]:

1. Determine the productivity goal. The chief nursing officer (CNO) and the nurse manager determine the unit's productivity goal for the coming fiscal year. Changes to the organization's service line and patient outcome measure results all must be considered when planning the unit and overall nursing services budget.
2. Forecast the work load. The number of patient days expected on each nursing unit for the coming fiscal year is calculated.
3. Budget patient care hours. The expected number of hours devoted to patient care for the forecasted patient days is calculated.
4. Budget patient care hours and staffing schedules. The budgeted patient care hours are reflected in recommended staffing schedules by shift and by day of the week.
5. Plan nonproductive hours. Vacation, holiday, education leave, sick leave, and similar hours are budgeted for the coming year.
6. Chart productive and nonproductive time. To aid in the planning process, a graph is used to show nurses how the level of forecasted patient days, and therefore the staffing requirements, are

expected to increase and decrease during the year. Productive time is the time spent on the job in patient care, administration of the unit, conferences, educational activities, and orientation.

7. Estimate costs of supplies and services. Consideration should be given to any new services or changes in patient mix. The supplies and services to be purchased for the year are budgeted.

8. Anticipate capital expenses. The expected capital investments for the coming year are included in the budget.

These eight steps result in a proposed budget that goes to the CNO for review. After preliminary acceptance, this budget is sent to the accounting department, where the forecasted patient days are translated into expected revenue. The budgeted productive and nonproductive times are converted into dollars, as are the costs for supplies, services, and other operating expenses that will be allocated to a given nursing unit for the coming year. A pro forma operating statement is then returned to the director of nursing for review with the nurse manager. Once the CNO and the nurse manager accept the budget, it is returned to the accounting department and forwarded with the rest of the agency manager's budgets to administration and the board of directors.[4]

People who pay high prices for health care want accountability of both costs and quality of service. The nursing budget can be a shared responsibility, with unit budgets being prepared with staff involvement at the clinical level. The planning and controlling processes are ongoing. Through their participation, clinical nurses enhance their professional stature. A budget prepared and executed as a shared experience becomes an object of ownership to a staff that puts forth effort to work within its framework.

Managing Cost Centers

A cost center is a given area of assigned accountability for both direct and indirect expenditures. A department of nursing is a cost center, as are each of its units, each clinic, in-service education, surgical suites, long-term care, home health care, and any other section with a nursing mission in which nurses provide services to clients. Each cost center is assigned a code. A uniform accounting and reporting system for hospitals is available (Seawell, 1994). An organization may use this coding system, usually referred to as the patient care system. Work load measurements, sometimes referred to as performance classifications or units of measure, are necessary. The unit of measure for each cost center is identified as a specific, quantitative statistic, such as inpatient days or number of tests. Each cost center has a manager, called the cost-center manager, who is responsible for identifying needs for equipment and programs to maintain progress at the current level of technology in the unit.

Each cost center is an internal department dealing with distribution of services and products. The cost-center manager is responsible for determining the cost of such services or products and how they are distributed within the organization. Two types of cost centers are mission, or revenue producing, and service. Examples of mission centers are radiology and laboratory departments. These centers have monetary income related to the purpose of the organization. A service center is a support center that provides a service to other units and charges for that service; no exchange of revenue takes place. The unit served adds the costs of these support services to its costs of output.[5] Examples of support centers are food service, purchasing, and laundry.

Budgeted costs within the cost center are broken down into subcodes. This promotes better budgetary planning and control because items are specifically identified during the budget planning process. Also, each item purchased is charged to (deleted from) the balance shown for that specific subcode.

Relationship of Budget and Objectives

One of the chief planning activities is to identify the objectives of the nursing division and each of its units, including developing a management plan with a budget for each objective. One of the first sources of budgetary information is the nursing objectives. By using these objectives, nurse managers see the benefit of developing pertinent, specific, and practical budgeting objectives. These objectives must align with the organization's financial plan and objectives and third-party payer requirements for reimbursement to the organization and be monitored for changes.

Budget Stages

For practical purposes, the nursing budget follows three stages of development: formulation, review and enactment, and execution. The entire budgeting process is given a specific time frame, and a target date is assigned for each step (Figure 11-1). During the fiscal year of the execution stage of budgeting, the formulation and review and enactment stages for the next fiscal year are carried out. The budget stages are sometimes labeled forecasting, preparation, and control, respectively.[6]

Formulation Stage

The formulation stage is usually a set number of months (6 or 7) before the start of the fiscal year for the budget. During this period, procedures are used to obtain an estimate of the funds needed, funds available, expenses, and revenues. Financial reports of expenses and revenues of the previous fiscal year and the year to date are analyzed by the CNO, department heads, and cost-center managers.

One of the first steps in writing a budget is gathering data for accurate prediction of expenses (costs) and revenues (income). This task can be developed into a system. Primary sources of data are the objectives for the division of nursing and for each cost center. Each program and activity needs to have an estimated cost placed on it. If in-service educators want new audiovisual equipment, they should not walk into the nurse administrator's office and expect to have it next week or next month. Purchasing this equipment should be planned 6 to 7 months before the next fiscal year begins, and it may be budgeted for any quarter or month within that fiscal year. In surveying the objectives, nurse administrators and managers evaluate the previous year, review the philosophy, and rewrite the objectives for the future.

Other data include programs from other departments that require use or expansion of nursing resources, expansion of nursing clinics and client teaching programs, travel costs for attendance at professional and educational meetings, incentive awards, library requirements, clinical and office supplies and equipment, investment equipment and facilities modification on a 5-year plan, and contracts for items such as intravenous pumps and oxygen equipment. Data can be obtained from historical financial records of the organization.

FIGURE 11-1   **THE BUDGET CALENDAR**

Formulation Stage

1. Develop objectives and management plans.
2. Gather all financial, historical, and statistical data and distribute to cost-center managers.
3. Analyze data.

Review and Enactment Stage

4. Prepare unit budgets.
5. Present unit budgets for approval.

6. Revise and combine into organizational budget.
7. Present to budget council.
8. Revise and present to governing board.
9. Revise and distribute to cost-center managers.

Execution Stage

10. Direct and evaluate expenses and receipts.
11. Revise budget if indicated.

Source: Author.

Several cost-center reports may assist the nurse manager:

- Daily staffing reports
- Monthly staffing reports
- Payroll summaries
- Daily lists of financial categories of patients
- Biometric reports of occupancy
- Biometric reports of work load
- Monthly financial summaries of revenues and expenses

Review and Enactment Stage

Review and enactment are budget development processes that put all the pieces together for approval of a final budget. Once the cost-center managers present their budgets to the budget council, the CNO consolidates the nursing budget. The budget officer then further consolidates the budget into an organizational budget. The chief executive officer of the organization and the governing board then give their approval. Throughout this process, conferences are held at which budget adjustments are made. Nurses can sell a budget by using a marketing strategy, anticipating challenges, being persuasive without being emotional, and working toward a win–win situation.[7]

Execution Stage

The formulation stage and the review and enactment stage of the budget are planning activities. Execution of the budget involves directing and evaluating activities. The nurse administrators and managers who planned the budget execute it. Revisions in execution of the budget are scheduled at stated intervals, usually once or twice during the fiscal year. Certain procedures are followed for evaluating the budget at cost-center levels. Budgets are prepared for either fiscal years that coincide with government budgets or calendar (fiscal) years, depending on the policy of the organization.

Cost Factors

Cost is money expended for all resources used, including personnel, supplies, and equipment (Figure 11-2). The acuity and volume of service provided are the greatest factors affecting costs. Others factors

FIGURE 11-2	COST FACTORS IN THE BUDGETING PROCESS

- Patient acuity
- Volume of service
- Length of patient stay
- Salaries
- Price of materials
- Case mix
- Seasonal factors
- Efficiencies (prevention of errors; decreased patient complications)

- Regulation
- Competition for market share
- Third-party payers
- Age and size of agency
- Type and amount of services
- Agency mission
- Relationship of personnel (collaborative)

Source: Author.

include length of patient stays, salaries, price of materials, case mix, seasonal factors, and efficiencies (such as simplification of procedures and quality management to prevent errors that increase patient complications and increase costs). Still other factors that have an impact on costs are regulation and competition for market share, third-party payers, the age and size of the agency, type and amount of services provided, the agency's mission, and relationships among nurses, physicians, and other personnel.

Expenses

Expenses are the costs of providing services to patients. They are frequently called "overhead" and include wages and salaries, fringe benefits, supplies, food service, utilities, and office and medical supplies. As part of the budget, expenses are a collection or summary of forecasts for each cost center's account.

Full costs include both direct and indirect expenses. Although direct costs such as nursing can be traced to the source, indirect costs such as utilities, telephones, or purchasing services are allocated to the source department by a standard formula.

Expense Budgeting

Expense budgeting is the "process of forecasting, recording, and monitoring the manpower, materials and supplies, and monetary needs of an organization in such a manner that the operation of the various components of the organization can be controlled."[8] The components of expense budgeting are cost centers. Purposes of expense budgeting are included (Figure 11-3).

Historical trends are the single best inexpensive indicator available to the institution. They are valid for prediction of present and future trends.

Types of Expenses/Costs

Fixed, Variable, and Sunk Costs

Fixed costs are not related to volume. They remain constant as volume increases and decreases over a period of time. Among fixed costs are depreciation of equipment and buildings, salaries, benefits, utilities, interest on loans or bonds, and taxes.

Variable costs do relate to volume and census (patient days). They include items such as meals and linen. Supplies are usually volume responsive, meaning that total costs increase or decrease according to use. The cost of supplies varies by patient census, physician orders, and diagnosis. For example, the cost of surgical dressings increases when a patient's wound has drainage and dressings must be changed frequently. Also, the cost of supplies increases or decreases with the census. For this reason, every cost center should have an established unit of measure for productivity. This unit may be numbers of tests,

---

FIGURE 11-3 **PURPOSES OF EXPENSE BUDGETING**

- Predict labor hours, material, supplies, and cash flow needs
- Establish procedures for making comparative studies
- Provide mechanism for change management

Source: Author.

procedures, patients of a specific acuity type, hours or minutes of service, or discharges. Most activities include elements of both fixed and variable costs. For example, personnel costs and utility costs can be both fixed and variable because a minimum is required for each.

Sunk costs are fixed expenses that cannot be recovered even if a program is canceled. Advertising is a good example.[9]

Direct and Indirect Costs

Direct costs are the costs of providing the product or service and are often considered to be those directly related to patient care, such as personnel costs and the variable cost of supplies. The definition of direct costs varies by department. In areas not involved in direct patient care, each department incurs its own category of direct costs.

Indirect costs are those incurred in supporting the provision of the product or service, are not directly related to patient care, and include utilities, administration, housekeeping, and building maintenance. As previously mentioned, however, they are direct costs for the source department. Some indirect costs are fixed, such as depreciation and administration. Others, such as laundry and accounting, are variable. All indirect costs are allocated or transferred by a specific method to the departments that use the service.

Every hospital has a method to establish costs, including the Hospital and Hospital Health Care Complex Cost Report Certification and Settlement Summary, commonly known as the Centers for Medicare & Medicaid Services (CMS) Cost Report. In a few agencies the method is more refined. Nurse administrators should become informed about the methods favored by their organizations.

Cost Accounting

A cost-accounting system assigns all costs to cost centers. Periodically, usually monthly, reports of costs are provided to cost-center managers, but they do not reflect all costs. Many indirect costs are allocated only once a year in the CMS Cost Report. Included are costs of items such as utilities, accounting, administration, data processing, and admitting. Informed and influential nurse managers use these cost allocations when preparing budgets. Such allocations are usually hidden in the operational budget under the category of "room costs."

Cost assignments to cost centers are made on the basis of direct costing if they are direct costs of patient care. Otherwise, they are made by transfer costing from a patient care support department or by cost allocation if they are not related to direct patient care or support. Job order sheets are a method used to account for all services to patients. Direct overhead costs that cannot be identified with specific services rendered are allocated based on some other measurement, such as square feet of floor space.

Service Units

Service units are measurable units of productivity or volume for identifying and counting costs. They must be measurable, known to managers, and affected by volume. The number of service units produced measures productivity.

Unit of Service

The unit of service is a measurement of the output of agency services consumed by the patient. In the surgical suite and recovery room it is measured in minutes or hours, in the emergency room it is the number of visits or time and procedures, and in the nursing units it is based on the acuity category of patients and hours per day expressed as a targeted number. Types of measurement include procedures, patient days, patient visits, and cases.

With the increased sophistication of information systems, it is easier for nurse managers to become involved in identifying and costing service units, which can be quantified by hours of nursing care per category of acuity of illness.

Chart of Accounts

A chart of accounts that includes a number and table for each cost center is subdivided into major classifications and subcodes (see Seawell, 1994). Examples are salaries and wages, employee benefits, medical and surgical supplies, professional fees, purchased services, utilities, other direct expenses, depreciation, and rent. These classifications are divided into further subcategories.

To assign items to the correct cost center, one must record all movement of labor and materials between cost centers. All benefits must be charged to the appropriate cost center by some established method, and so must all purchases, including shared ones. This is usually done using allocated shares of service units.

Amortized expenses are deferred charges allocated to units over a specified period of time. They include depreciation charges for aging plant and equipment in addition to prepaid items. Prepaid items usually are charged monthly as service units. Other deferred expenses include unamortized borrowing costs and costs incurred for capital expansion or renovation programs.

Inventory and Cost Transfer

Identifying actual costs of any service unit is improved through an accurate system of inventory control. Based on the number of orders or requisitions for any item, the appropriate proportion of its costs can be transferred to the cost center that ordered the items.

Financial Accountability

In accepting financial accountability, nurses' first duty is to their patients, who have given them their trust. Nurses should be accountable to themselves for their work, to their professional peers, to their employers, and to taxpayers in publicly funded institutions.

In one way or another, patients pay the costs of health care. They may do so through insurance premiums, taxes, or benefits or from their own pockets. Financial accountability means that nurses and others can account for the efficient spending of the money paid for health care.

Nurse managers need information on the costs of all services provided by their own and competing institutions. This information, in turn, can be provided to clinical nurses, who should know what it costs to do their work. Cost consciousness leads to waste reduction and effective cost management.

Some managers mistakenly believe that controlling nursing labor power and expenditures can control overspending. Holding nurses accountable for their budgets, including both revenues and expenses, can rectify this misconception.[10]

Cost of Nursing Care

To determine the cost of nursing care, one must consider several factors. Nursing charges should be quantifiable. A patient acuity system serves this purpose. The patient acuity system usually separates patients into four or five levels of nursing care and enumerates nursing requirements for each level. Charges could be set by level and negotiated with third-party payers. These costs could be separated from the cost of non-nursing requirements. Non-nursing tasks could then be reassigned to ensure that the charges for nursing care reflect the actual cost of providing such care.

A second method of costing nursing services is determining what share of total agency cost is attributable to nursing. This varies by medical severity diagnosis-related group. An industry-wide effort for each region could produce standards for nursing costs and charges. Otherwise, most healthcare institutions in the United States would need to undertake research to determine nursing costs and charges on an agency-specific basis. Multinational corporations, of course, can apply research studies across member institutions.

Activity-Based Costing

Drucker recommends activity-based costing that accounts for the total process of doing business from personnel, supplies, material, and parts to installation and service of products. Healthcare organizations know and manage the costs of the entire economic chain, tying the costs to all sources of payment. To do this requires foundation, productivity, competence, and resource allocation information. Personnel perform to meet specific expectations, and they are evaluated accordingly. Old organizational structures are replaced with new cost centers that support activity-based costing, in which managers turn data into information through analysis and interpretation that lead to action.[11]

Definitions

Budget

According to *Webster's New Twentieth Century Dictionary*, Unabridged (2nd ed.) a budget is "a plan or schedule adjusting expenses during a certain period to the estimated or fixed income for that period." Herkimer states, "An effective budget is the systematic documentation of one or more carefully developed plans for all individually supervised activities, programs, or sections. The budget is a tool which can aid decision makers in evaluating operating performance and projecting what future operations might produce."[12]

A budget is an operational management plan, stated in terms of income and expenses, covering all phases of activity for a future division of time. It is a financial document that expresses an operation's plan of action. In the division of nursing, it sets the limits of financial support, thereby controlling the extent and quality of nursing programs. The budget determines the number of kinds of personnel, materials, and financial resources available for patient care and for achievement of the stated nursing objectives. It is a financial policy statement. Budgeting is the process whereby objectives and plans are translated into financial terms and evaluated using financial and statistical criteria.

Revenue

Revenue is the income from sales of products and services. Nursing revenue traditionally has been included with room charges. It can be unbundled from the room rate as a separate charge per patient acuity category and per visit, day, or procedure.

Revenue can include assets, such as accounts receivable and income-producing endowments. The latter can be restricted to specific purposes. Buildings, land, and other items can be assets if they produce income or are capable of producing income. Total income is frequently termed gross income; the excess of revenues over expenses is known as net income or profit.

Revenues also come from research grants, gift shops, donations, gifts, rentals of cots and televisions, parking fees, telephone charges, and vending machines. Revenues may be elements of product lines such as orthopedic services that include orthopedic nursing, traction equipment, and prostheses. In hospitals, revenue may refer to sources such as Medicare, Medicaid, third-party payers (insurance companies), and patients.[13]

Revenue Budgeting

Revenue budgeting, or rate setting, is the process by which an agency determines revenues required to cover anticipated costs and to establish prices sufficient to generate these revenues. Not all patients (purchasers) pay an equal share of an agency's costs, which complicates the process.

To remain viable, any business must generate sufficient revenues to cover operating costs and make a profit. These revenues include increases in working capital, capital replacements, and inflation adjustments.

Nonprofits use profits to improve plants and services; profits do not go to stockholders or owners. Profit appears as a positive balance on account ledgers. Fundamental to the rate-setting process are adequate statistical data, historical and projected, for implementing the rate-setting method to be used. On a departmental basis, these data include volume of services, current rate, allocated costs, and rate increase constraints. The goal is to obtain the greatest impact from a minimum cumulative rate increase in a cost-management environment. This can be accomplished by increasing rates in high-profit departments while instituting rate reductions in low-profit departments so that they offset each other. Revenues are often budgeted before expenses. This is necessary to determine how much revenue is available.

Patient Days

Patient days are used to project revenues. They are commonly used as units of service to compute staffing. Patient day statistics are usually derived from census reports that are done daily at midnight and summarized monthly for the year to date and annually. A patient admitted on May 2 and discharged May 10 is charged for nine patient days. Figure 11-4 illustrates the number of patient days per unit for 1 month. Midnight census does not fully reflect the nursing resources required to accommodate outpatients that occupy a bed for 23 to 48 hours or swings in census that require nursing work

---

FIGURE 11-4   **SAMPLE OF PATIENT DAY CENSUS**

	Current Year			Year to Date		
	May	**OCC (%)**	**April**	**Current Year**	**OCC (%)**	**Previous Year**
Nursing Station						
3rd Floor	1,014	79.8	833	9,792	78.6	8,650
4th Floor	811	76.9	718	7,834	75.8	7,255
5th Floor N.	526	65.3	524	5,300	67.1	4,838
5th Floor S.	622	77.2	592	5,587	70.7	5,603
6th Floor	792	71.0	866	8,730	79.8	8,176
7th Floor	850	68.5	895	9,086	74.7	8,885
8th Floor N.	376	60.6	383	4,624	76.1	2,393
8th Floor S.	303	69.8	274	3,253	6.4	1,729
9th Floor N.	526	84.8	501	5,332	87.7	2,690
9th Floor S.	481	77.6	506	5,118	84.2	2,617
MINU	104	83.9	89	1,041	85.6	432
SINU	73	58.9	84	964	79.3	471
Burn Unit	173	79.7	188	1,723	81.0	1,912
Labor and Delivery	138	37.1	99	1,228	33.7	1,258
CCU	206	83.1	148	1,848	76.0	1,937
Clinical Research Unit	137	73.7	132	1,342	73.6	1,361
EAU	23	0.0	7	390	0.0	634
MICU	213	85.9	191	2,099	86.3	2,291
PICU	169	54.5	112	1,612	53.0	1,834
SICU	229	92.3	207	2,175	89.4	2,302
NTICU	209	84.3	87	1,891	77.8	2,277
Total	7,975	73.2	7,436	80,969	75.3	79,086

(EAU: Emergency Admit Unit; MICU: Medical Intensive Care Unit; PICU: Pediatric Intensive Care Unit; SICU: Surgical Intensive Care Unit; NTICU: Neurotrauma Intensive Care Unit)

Source: Author.

loads to increase with admissions and discharges. The CNO and nurse manager must track these trends to adequately plan resource needs.

Fiscal Year

The fiscal year is the budgetary or financial year. It may be the calendar year in some organizations, beginning on January 1 and ending on December 31. Many organizations use October 1 to September 30 as the fiscal year. Some use July 1 to June 30 to coincide with budget decisions of state legislatures and the U.S. Congress. In the latter examples, the fiscal year overlaps 2 calendar years.

Year to Date

The term "year to date" describes the accumulated units of service at a particular point in the fiscal year. If the fiscal year begins October 1, the year-to-date patient days for December 31 would be the summary for 92 days.

Average Daily Census

The census is summarized for a specific number of days and divided by that number of days. For example, the average daily census for the month of May is the total patient days for May divided by 31. In Figure 11-4, the number of patient days for May is 7,975. When this is divided by 31, the average daily census is 257.

Hours of Care

Hours of care have traditionally been the number of hours of care allocated per patient per day (24 hours) on a unit. With the use of patient acuity rating systems, hours of care can be determined to the hour or even to the fraction of an hour. Patients usually fall into one of four or five patient acuity categories, each of which is assigned a specific number of hours of care per patient day.

Caregiver

Each nurse who works with patients is called a caregiver. In nursing, the three common types of caregivers are registered nurses (RNs), licensed practical nurses, and nurse aides or extenders. Most personnel budgets have a ratio of RNs to other caregivers and patients. Considerable research supports a high proportion of RN caregiver staff. The current cost-management environment often makes this difficult.

Case-Mix

The patient's acuity of services is known as a case-mix. Case-mix refers to the type of patients cared for by the institution. Some of the variables included in the case-mix are diagnosis, comorbidities, and treatment patterns.

Budgeting Approaches

Zero-Base Budgeting

Zero-base budgeting is a method of budgeting used to control costs. In a zero-base budget, the budgeting process starts from zero, and everything must be justified by each new budget cycle. A previous activity can be included in the budget, but its relation to the current organizational objectives must justify funding for it. In theory, each function in a zero-base budget must stand on its own merits, and the merits of each function are reviewed annually. All labor power and costs are recalculated, and decisions are made about whether to continue the function and at what levels.

Program Budgeting

Program budgeting is a part of budget planning. Items such as continuing education programs, employee benefits fairs, and health promotion programs should be incorporated into the annual budget. The budget for each program should enumerate fixed expenses, such as rent, advertising, fixed speaker fees, and department overhead, and variable expenses, such as for food, handouts, and per-person honorarium speaker fees. Some costs, such as those for advertising, are unrecoverable even if the program is canceled. They are sunk costs and should be in the cost center budget as well as in the individual program's budget.

Program budgets should include a break-even analysis. If the cost of the program is $2,000 and the reasonable charge is $50 per participant, the break-even point is 40 participants. A break-even chart can be made for each program (Figure 11-5). Income above the break-even point is profit; below it is loss.

The point at which the cost to carry out a program is equal to the cost to cancel it is called the least-loss point. If enough people have registered to pay the sunk costs, the net loss is the same whether the program is canceled or held. It may be good public relations to carry out a program at the least-loss point.[13]

Flexible Budgeting

Flexible budgeting takes into account variations or ranges from low to high points.[14] This approach requires a well-prepared and educated nurse manager. It determines a range of volume instead of an actual volume, which is much more difficult to plan and manage.[15]

Fixed Budgeting

A fixed budget is based on a fixed annual level of volume. For example, the annual number of x-rays performed is divided by 12, giving a monthly average of x-rays. This approach to budgeting does not take seasonal or monthly variations into consideration.[16]

FIGURE 11-5 **BREAK-EVEN ANALYSIS**

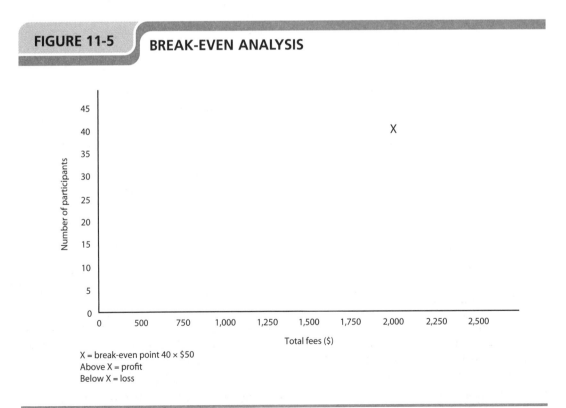

X = break-even point 40 × $50
Above X = profit
Below X = loss

Source: Author.

Types of Budgets

Operating Budget

The operating budget is the overall plan identifying expected revenues and expenses, both fixed and variable, for the forthcoming fiscal year. It is an annual budget that includes the cash budget and the capital budget. In addition, the operating budget identifies the source and nature of expected revenues and expenses. The operating budget determines the per diem and other charges to be made to the patient.

Cost-to-Charge Ratios

Cost-to-charge ratios are convenient tools for computing the cost of providing a service. For example, if the charge to a patient for the endoscopic laboratory services is $1,000, and the cost-to-charge ratio is 0.815626, then the cost to the hospital for these services is approximately $815.63. This cost includes the expense of running the endoscopic laboratory and a portion of the hospital's overhead cost. In some instances, the cost-to-charge ratio is greater than 1, which means the cost of operating these cost centers is greater than the charges.

The hospital has two types of cost centers. The first is the revenue-producing cost center, such as the endoscopic laboratory, which bills patients for services provided. The second type is the overhead cost center, such as the accounting department, which exists to support the revenue-producing centers. The cost of the overhead cost centers is allocated to the revenue-producing centers by various statistical methods. For example, utility costs are allocated to revenue-producing departments based on the square footage of space they occupy. Accounting department costs, however, are allocated based on the size of the operating budget of each revenue-producing cost center. The cost-to-charge ratio is computed by dividing the total cost of the cost center, both direct and overhead, by the total charges for the same department.

Cost–Benefit Analysis

Cost–benefit analysis is a planning technique that answers the following questions[17]: What are the costs of pursuing a goal, an objective, a program, or a specific nursing intervention? How do costs compare with the benefits? Is the project worthwhile? Comparison of different nursing interventions for the same nursing diagnosis or problem results in using the least costly interaction to achieve similar or better results. The intervention used is then cost-effective.

Operating or Cash Budget

The cash budget is the actual operating budget in detail, usually excluding the capital budget. A cash budget indicates whether cash flow will be adequate to meet anticipated payments, such as debt obligations, including replacement and expansion of facilities, unanticipated requirements, payroll, payment for supplies and services, and a prudent investment program. Cash receipts come from third-party payers, tuition, endowment fund earnings, and sales of food, gifts, and services.

The cash budget is the day-to-day budget and represents money coming in and going out. It is advisable to have cash reserves so that cash flow and the money coming in pay the bills. Otherwise, revenues must be sped up or payment of bills slowed down.

Organizations often review their revenue cycle to ensure cash and expenses are kept in the appropriate ratio. Cash reserves should not be excessive; they may represent money that should be working for the organization. Cash budgets show revenues and expenses, whereas operating budgets show plans. They are usually considered integrated entities.[18]

Negative Cash Flow

Five major factors influence negative cash flow:

1. There is a time lag between delivery of services and collection of payments.
2. Timing of cycles between net income and flow of cash is different.

3. Lag occurs by the large up and down cycles of volume during different seasons (cash deficit during a busy census cycle or surplus during a low census cycle).
4. Labor expense (60% to 70% of operating expense) paid out in salary and wages does not cycle concurrently with collections.
5. Service line costs have outpaced reimbursement such as implants for certain cardiac and orthopedic procedures.

To maintain solvency, cash flow must be managed carefully and cycles of cash shortage planned for appropriately. The cash budget should plan for the ability to borrow cash during shortfalls, the investment of excess cash, and the strict monitoring and reporting of lost charges and of the billing and collecting process. The cash budget is a part of the total budget and is apportioned to departments based on individual cost-center activity.[19]

Developing the Operating Budget

Operating budget information supplied to the chief nurse executive, department heads, and cost-center managers includes a budget worksheet (Figure 11-6) and a worksheet that explains budget adjustments (Figure 11-7). The budget worksheet depicts information by the account number and subcode of each cost center and lists prior-year expense, original budget, and annualized expense. This form usually is provided during the new budget formulation stage, and the annualized expense is the projected total expense if current rates continue to the end of the fiscal year. The column headed "Budget Adjustments" is empty so that the cost-center manager can fill in the budget expenses for the projected fiscal year. The column

FIGURE 11-6	BUDGET WORKSHEET

Operating Expenses

Subcode	Description	Prior-Year Expense	Original Budget	Annualized Expense	Budget Adjustments	Approved Budget
6000	Total–Supplies		0.00	1,000	$915	$650
6100	Forms	860	0.00	200		$200
6200	Books	450	0.00	450		$450
6434	Brochures	398	0.00	0.00		
6660	Film rental	100	0.00	0.00		
Total Supplies		**1,808**	**1,000**	**650**		
8000	Total–Repairs & Maintenance		0.00	1,360		
8200	Main., & Repair	100	0.00	800	$900	$1,190
8310	Minor Equip.	675	0.00	100		$100
8524	Telephone	185	0.00	190		$190
Total Repairs & Main.			**960**	**1,360**	**1,090**	
9000	Total–OCE		0.00	1,370		
9200	Travel	1,345	0.00		$685	$1,085
9300	Airfare	800	0.00		200	$400
9600	Entertainment	275	0.00		220	
Total Other Controllable		**2,420**	**1,370**	**420**		
Account Total		**5,188**	**3,730**	**2,160**		
Total $2,925						

Source: Author.

FIGURE 11-7 | ADJUSTMENT EXPLANATION FOR FISCAL YEAR 2004

Emergency Department Budget Unit: Supplies and Minor Equipment, Fiscal Year 2004

Subcode	Description	Budget Adjustment	Justification
8200	Maintenance and repairs	100	Ice machine is breaking more frequently
9200	Travel	685	Two extra conferences for TJC
9300	Airfare	200	As above

Source: Author.

"Approved Budget" is the budget that has been approved by the finance department along with administration after reviewing the requested adjustments. Note in Figure 11-6 that the cost-center manager had projected an increased budget of $1000 for subcode 6000, supplies. This amount was reduced to an annualized projection of $650 (subcodes 6100 and 6200), at the annual budget meeting.

Also in Figure 11-6, note that subcode 8200, maintenance and repairs, was increased by $100 (from $800 to $900). This increase was justified on the adjustment explanation (Figure 11-7). Overall, increases were approved for subcodes 8200 (maintenance and repair), 9200 (travel), and 9300 (airfare). A total budget for supplies and minor equipment for this cost center was approved for $2,925. Figure 11-7 shows the adjustment explanation for subcodes 8200 and 9200.

Osborne and Gaebler refer to the operational budget as the expenditure control budget. It sets up accounts for various major expenditures. These authors recommend shifting among accounts as needed and allowing departments to carry over into the new budget what they do not spend. A recommended formula for establishing an expenditure control budget is the same as previous year plus account for inflation and growth or decline plus any carryover funds. Management should apply additional money for the new initiatives. The strengths of such a mission-driven budget include the following[20]:

- Every employee has an incentive to save money.
- Resources are freed up to test new ideas.
- Managers have the autonomy they need to respond to changing circumstances.
- A predictable environment is created.
- The budget process is enormously simplified.
- Money can be saved on auditors and a budget office.
- Management can focus on other important issues.

Personnel Budget

Most budgets for nursing personnel are based on quantitative work load measurements, such as a patient acuity system. A computer software program usually produces staffing requirements by shift and day. It produces an acuity index for each patient, and the formula indicates needed staff by skill mix (RN), licensed practical nurse, certified nurse aide and by shift. It also compares actual staffing with that required, and a summary can be provided by month and year. Each day either the unit secretary or nurse enters the acuity rating for each patient into a computer.

Figure 11-8 is a nursing personnel budget based on a patient-acuity rating system. The average daily census is obtained from records produced in the admissions office. It is the result of dividing the total patient days for a unit for 1 year by 365 days. Census reports are generated daily, monthly, and annually by a computer.

FIGURE 11-8	NURSING PERSONNEL BUDGET

Nursing Budget

1. The personnel budget is based on total number of hours of care needed which is determined by the acuity levels (1–4).

   Patient Acuity Level HPPD (hours per care per patient day)
   1   4.0 hours
   2   6.4 hours
   3   10.5 hours
   4   16.0 hours

2. The staffing formula is

$$\frac{\text{Average census} \times \text{nursing hours} \times 1.4 \times 1.14}{7.5}$$

3. The total nursing personnel needed for an average daily census (ADC) and specific patient acuity is presented below. The total nursing personnel also includes unit secretaries.

Medical

Unit	ADC	Acuity	HPPD	RN	LPN	CNA	Other	Total
Oncology	17.1	3.0	10.5	24	2	12	4	42
BMT	8.2	4.0	16.0	22	0	6	2	30
Telemetry	22.3	2.0	6.4	18	3	9	6	36
4S	19.4	1.0	4.0	9	2	6	3	20
MICU	8.0	4.0	16.0	27	0	0	3	30
Total				100	7	33	18	158

Surgical

Unit	ADC	Acuity	HPPD	RN	LPN	CNA	Other	Total
Orthopedics	30.0	2.0	6.4	26	5	10	6	47
SICU	8.0	4.0	16.0	27	0	0	4	31
4CW	20.3	2.0	6.4	22	0	6	3	31
5CW	26.7	2.0	6.4	28	1	7	3.5	39.5
Total				103	6	23	16.5	148.5

Women's & Infants

Unit	ADC	Acuity	HPPD	RN	LPN	CNA	Other	Total
NBN	18.4	2.0	6.4	21	0	4	4.0	29
NICU	19.3	4.0	16.0	65	0	0	4.5	69.5
L & D*	28	0				7	3.5	38.5
Women's	24.1	2.0	6.4	25	2	6	2	35
Total				139	2	17	14	172.0

(L & D: Labor and Delivery)

Inpatient Rehabilitation

Unit	ADC	Acuity	HPPD	RN	LPN	CNA	Other	Total
3 East	11.7	2.0	6.4	9	1	6	4	20

* No acuity system.

Source: Author.

Acuity is the sum of all acuities for 1 year divided by 365 days. This figure is also generated daily, monthly, and annually. The nursing hours are generated from the acuity standard listed in item 1 of Figure 11-8.

Application of a staffing formula for preparing the personnel budget for a specific unit is illustrated in Figure 11-9. If the nursing department does not use an acuity system, hours (of care) per patient day (HPPD) can be used. Several organizations benchmark HPPD comparing specific types of units and

FIGURE 11-9   CALCULATING THE NURSING PERSONNEL BUDGET

The staffing formula is

$$\frac{\text{Average census} \times \text{nursing hours} \times 1.4 \times 1.14}{7.5}$$

Example: Oncology Unit

- Average daily census = 17.1
- HHPD = 10.5
- 1.4 is a constant representing 7 days in a week with a full-time employee working 5 days a week: 7 ÷ 5 = 1.4

- 1.14 is a constant which allows for 0.14 FTE for vacation, sickness, etc. for each 1.0 FTE
- 7.5 is one workday

$$\frac{17.1 \times 10.5 \times 1.4 \times 1.14}{7.5} = 38 \text{ FTEs}$$

The budgeted staffing for the Oncology Unit consists of 24 RNs, 2 LPNs, and 12 CNAs. In addition, the unit has 4 unit secretaries.

Source: Author.

types of hospitals that can assist the CNO in determining if these HPPDs need to be adjusted. Changes in the Medicare case-mix index can also be used as a justification for HPPD adjustments.

In planning the personnel budget, the nurse has quantitative information related to staffing and can accurately predict the number of FTEs needed for patient care. Other considerations must be weighed at the same time: Will there be a pay increase next year? If so, it must be calculated and budgeted. Will benefits increase or decrease? They must also be budgeted. If new programs are being implemented, do they require additional labor power? Will this labor power come from cutbacks in other programs, or from added FTEs? Figure 11-10 provides a worksheet for adding new positions to the budget.

Personnel account for the largest portion of the nursing budget. When one is preparing budgets for clinics, emergency departments, recovery rooms, operating rooms, delivery rooms, and home care, one

FIGURE 11-10   NEW POSITION REQUISITION

1. Job Title:
2. Department:
3. FTE Status:
   - Exempt
   - Non-Exempt
4. Expected Starting Date:
5. Hours/Shift:
   - Full time
   - Part time
   - Permanent
   - Temporary: If temporary, provide finishing date
6. Description of Essential Job Duties:

7. Justification for New Position (i.e., new program/increased volume):
8. Requirements essential for position (i.e., licensure, education):
9. Advertising:
10. Preferred publication:
    - Yes
    - No
11. Approvals:

    Supervisor: Date:

    Human Resources: Date:

Source: Author.

must have quantitative data, such as numbers of visits, procedures, and deliveries. Records of length of time required for each activity can be obtained by using management–engineering techniques in which visits, procedures, or other activities are charted over a period of time.

Data should be collected over a representative period to show the actual hours worked by shift and by day. These data indicate fluctuations in the work load by shift and by day of the week. Use a second data sheet to determine the total number of patients in the emergency department area at any one time, including patients in a holding status. Conversion of these data into graphs provides information to compare staffing with work load. These data provide the following information[20]:

- Current nursing hours available per patient visit
- Fluctuations in available hours by shift and by day
- Fluctuations in work load by time of day
- Fluctuations in ratio of staffing levels to patient load

Piper writes that the basic staffing of an emergency room should be calculated to handle a critical mass, the staffing level required to handle an unexpected emergency. In addition to quantitative data, the CNO should collect qualitative data from the staff to assist in containing stress, determining mix of staff, and improving support services. Data can be compared with those from other institutions. The result is then translated into personnel dollars.[21]

In the process of budgeting, the nurse manager knows how much each decision will cost and whether it involves numbers and kinds of personnel or amounts and kinds of supplies and equipment. Few nurse managers have the luxury of a budget that provides all the resources that can be used. Hard decisions must be made. These decisions are easier to substantiate when work loads are quantified. If the patient dependency or acuity system is reliable and valid and has quality checks on the raters, it will provide data that justify the personnel budget. When the number of adult patients of the highest acuity level increases from 24 to 32 per shift and day, the budget must be adjusted. Comparisons must be made to determine whether other levels have decreased. Estimates must be made as to whether the increases and decreases are permanent or temporary. Then the budget decisions are made.

Nurse managers study fluctuation trends in patient census and use these data for minimum staffing requirements to determine the percentage of time to staff one nurse less and the percentage of time to staff one nurse more per shift. The salary expense for the one time that one nurse less per shift is needed should be subtracted from the budget. The salary expense for the one time that one nurse more per shift is needed should be added to the budget. The result is an improved salary expense budget result.

The following strategies can reduce budget overages[22]:

- Maintain good staff retention.
- Use nurse extenders to perform non-RN functions.
- Monitor and control unscheduled absenteeism.
- Implement an effective on-call system.
- Institute a "flex-team" in related clinical areas to avoid overtime and agency nurse expenses.
- Create a large pool of part-time nurses.
- Budget according to trends.
- Negotiate for a reasonable budget that considers turnover and orientation.

Nonproductive Full-Time Equivalents

Nonproductive FTEs are hours for which an employee is paid but does not work, such as vacation days, holidays, sick days, education and training time, jury duty, leave for funerals, and military leave. These nonproductive hours must be determined and added to personnel expenditures as replacement FTEs. An FTE is based on 2,080 hours per year. If the nonproductive FTE average is to be used for personnel budgeting, the human resource department payroll section will provide it. For example,

Average vacation FTE	12.5 days
Average holiday FTE	7.0 days
Average sick days FTE	3.5 days
Average training and education FTE	3.0 days
Average other leave FTE	1.5 days
Total	27.5 days, or 220.0 hours

The total work time is 2,080 hours less 220 hours; the actual work time is 1,860 hours. The percentage of nonworked to total hours paid is 10.6%. The percentage of nonworked to worked hours is 11.8%.

A cost-center manager prepares the budget according to management rules. The budget should include a line item for replacement FTEs to cover nonproductive FTEs by assigning a fixed amount to each person's paid time off. An option is to determine percentage of nonproductive FTEs and add this total to the budget. This information is then used for staffing determination, as are seasonal fluctuations for vacations, census, and other pertinent factors.[23]

Supplies and Equipment Budget

The supplies and equipment budget is part of the operating or cash budget. It includes all supplies and equipment used in provision of services, except capital equipment and supplies charged directly to patients. Minor equipment, such as sphygmomanometers, otoscopes, and ophthalmoscopes, costs less than the base amount set for capital equipment. If the base amount is $500, all equipment under $500 appears as minor equipment in the supplies and equipment budget.

Generally, the director of materials management furnishes the total cost of supplies and equipment per cost center to the accounting office, which generates a cost per patient day. This cost is used for budgeting purposes and increases for inflation are a decision of top management. Based on projected patient days and revenues, decisions can be made to increase or decrease the supplies and equipment budget. Controlling the amounts of supplies can decrease costs and equipment kept in inventory. Nurse managers should look at the inventories they control and reduce them according to usage.

Factors that might influence the supply and equipment aspects of the budget include new program development in the institution, new physicians, and product upgrades. A product evaluation committee may be very cost-effective.

Product Evaluation

Product Evaluation Committee

A product evaluation committee usually has as its members representatives of nursing, central supply, infection control, finance, purchasing, administration, and education. The committee is usually chaired by the materials manager. This committee is responsible for evaluation and purchase of supplies and equipment. The following are among its goals:

- Standardization, with all units using the same products
- Lower prices through higher volumes
- Providing a clinical perspective in focusing on the quality of the product for improved patient care
- Minimizing inventory levels wherever possible
- Decreasing the cost of education and training by standardization

Thus systematic control of the introduction of patient care products into the institution is achieved. Figure 11-11 presents a product evaluation checklist used to justify the product under consideration.

FIGURE 11-11	PRODUCT EVALUATION CHECKLIST

The purpose of product evaluation is to provide a mechanism to ensure that the evaluation of products emphasize quality of care and cost containment. A checklist will be completed for products that have been selected for evaluation. The checklist will be submitted to the Director of Material Management for consideration by the Product Evaluation Committee. The checklist must be reviewed by your Department Director before submitting it to the Director of Material Management. An example of the questions needed for the committee are provided below:

1. Name and purpose of the product.

2. Is this product new, a replacement, or an upgrade?

3. What is the price and cost of this product? (purchase price, installation, training, staff, facility, service agreement)

4. How dependable is this product?

5. What type of service and vendor support will be provided?

6. What is the patient benefit from this product?

7. What resources are required to support this product? (staff, education, plant/environmental requirements)

8. How do the financials look? Where will the funds to pay for this product come from?

9. Are revenues generated by this product?

10. How and what is the reimbursement potential?

11. What is the anticipated utilization of this product? If it is a replacement or upgrade, what is the utilization of the current product?

12. Can the facility potentially hold or increase market share with this product?

Source: Author.

The following is a suggested process for product evaluation by a committee[24]:

1. Determine objectives of product evaluation.
2. Define use of the product with input from potential users.
3. Define objectives for each evaluation project.
4. Do initial review of various products: features, techniques for use, and prices.
5. Select products for evaluation and evaluate techniques for use, staff acceptance, and problems.
6. Conduct in-service tests to use products.
7. Use simple closed-ended questions, open-ended questions, and rating scales to evaluate the product.
8. Compile and analyze data, including costs, cost savings, conversion cost, and reimbursement potential. (See Chapter 17 for Deming's theory of working with one supplier to improve products.)
9. Make a decision for purchase.
10. Evaluate products that are not functioning as intended and determine if replacement is needed.

Capital Budget

A capital budget is usually separate from the operating budget (Figure 11-12). A capital budget projects the planned costs of major purchases. Each capital budget item is defined in terms of dollar value and

CAPITAL BUDGET REQUESTED FISCAL YEAR 200X–200X: METROPOLITAN MEMORIAL HOSPITAL

Dept.	Item	Quantity	Amount
66h & 7th	Beds & misc. pat. furn.	85	$200,000.00
Admin	Pneumatic tube system	1	75,000.00
Anest	Capnograph-portable	1	4,200.00
Anest	Trans. Mon.–inc NIPB & O_2 Sat	1	9,200.00
Anest	Ventilators	2	5,050.00
ER Med	Pro Pac 106	1	13,790.00
Bio Med	Safety tester	1	1,695.00
Blood Bk	Table top centrifuge	1	2,000.00
Blood Bk	Automated cell washer	1	6,250.00
Cath Lab	Pulse oximetry	1	2,600.00
Cath Lab	Dynamap	1	3,800.00
Clin Lab	Miscellaneous equipment	1	250,000.00
Dialysis	Dialysis machine	1	25,000.00
Dietary	Refrigerator-bakery	1	3,500.00
Dietary	Refrigerator-bakery	1	6,950.00
Dietary	Refrigerator-cook area	1	3,500.00
Dietary	Refrigerator-PFS	1	3,100.00
Dietary	Meat slicer	1	3,500.00
ER	New monitoring system	1	160,000.00
ER	Propak monitor	1	3,500.00
Envir	High-speed burnisher	4	8,000.00
Envir	Slow-speed buffers	2	1,600.00
GI Lab	Video processor CV-100	1	20,000.00
CVStation	Blood pressure monitor	1	4,500.00
CVStation	Stress test system	1	20,000.00
CVStation	ECG management system	1	70,000.00
MICU/CCU	Faceplates-central monitors	12	4,920.00
Nursing	Medication carts	17	25,000.00
Nutri	Computer & printer	1	2,011.00
OR	Laparoscopic video system	1	30,165.00
OR	Electrosurgical cautery	2	17,200.00
PACU	RR stretchers	10	20,000.00
Plant Op	4000-watt portable generator	1	1,495.00
Plant Op	8 ch. OPS card for telephone switch	1	1,337.00
Radio	Rebuilt film processor	1	12,000.00
Res Th	Sterile pass-through drier	1	12,567.00
SPD	Washer decontaminator	1	75,000.00
Staff Dev	Overhead projector	1	700.00
Staff Dev	CPR manikin	1	5,641.00
Total requested Metropolitan Memorial Center			$1,114,771.00

Source: Author.

is an item of equipment that is used over a period of time. The budget provides for depreciation of each item in the capital budget, sets aside the amount of depreciation in an escrow account, and uses this account to finance new capital budgets. Depreciation records the declining value of a physical asset. In addition, department heads are required to justify and set priorities on capital budget items (Figure 11-13). The exact definition of what constitutes a capital budget item with regard to dollar amount and life expectancy varies among hospitals.

Capital budgets also deal with maintenance, renovations, remodeling, improvements, expansion, land acquisition, and new buildings. The financial manager for nursing is the nurse manager, who should evaluate past decisions and advise the nurse administrator whether they were good or bad.

FIGURE 11-13	CAPITAL EQUIPMENT REQUISITION FORM

1. Project description: _____   2. Date: _____

3. Submitted by: _____   4. Department: _____

5. Equipment requested: _____   6. Useful life: _____

7. Justification for equipment: 8. How often will equipment be requested/utilized?
   - Regulatory
   - New service
   - Replacement
   - Upgrade

9. Equipment description: _____

10. Impact to other departments: _____
    - Plant operations (renovation, installation)
    - Bio-Med
    - ISD
    - Education department
    - Other

11. Costs:
    - Equipment Costs:_____
    - Renovation/installation:_____
    - Service agreement: _____
    - Personnel: _____
    - Education/training: _____
    - Shipping: _____
    - Storage: _____

12. For any equipment $5,000 or over, an equipment evaluation must be completed.
    _____Yes   _____ No (attach evaluation form)

13. For any equipment $25,000 or over, a financial pro forma must be completed.
    _____Yes   _____ No (attach pro forma)

14. Approvals:
    Department Director: Date:
    Administrator: Date:

Source: Author.

All proposals for capital equipment must be fully evaluated for amount of use, method of payment, safety, replacement, duplication of service, and every other conceivable factor, including the need for space, personnel, and facility renovation. The needs and desires of the medical staff should be considered. Staff involvement in planning helps ensure wise purchases of capital equipment.

A strategic capital-budgeting method based on principles of decision analysis can help health care organizations allocate capital effectively when meeting requests for capital expenditures. There are eight steps of the strategic capital-budgeting method:

1. Establishing evaluation criteria
2. Classifying proposals by area of investment
3. Ensuring that proposals are complete and easy to understand
4. Determining costs of proposals
5. Rating proposals with respect to individual criteria
6. Setting priority weights for criteria

7. Calculating weighted value scores for each proposal
8. Ranking proposals by cost–benefit ratios

The results provide a reliable basis for optimal capital allocation.[25]

The capital budget must address increased forms of competition, dwindling financial resources, and regulatory constraints. Management should enhance conditions under which effective planning and capital budgeting increase the agency's chance of long-term survival. Capital budgeting is a part of the overall budget-planning process for the organization and not an entity unto itself. When each entry or item in the capital budget list has been analyzed and reduced to the amount available, the budget is again tabulated. It is now ready to present to the board of directors. With the board's approval, the list is distributed to cost-center managers, who prepare requisitions for purchase. The purchasing department prepares bid specifications, with input from cost-center managers. Purchases are finalized based on results of bids submitted by vendors who meet the required specifications. Finally, purchases are entered into the depreciation budget schedule. The latter is published by American Hospital Publishing and is considered the standard for the industry. The following are a few examples of the composite estimated useful lives of depreciable hospital assets: boiler house (30 years); masonry building, wood/metal frame (25 years); bed, electric (12 years); and otoscope (7 years). For budgetary purposes, the nurse manager should have access to the entire publication.[26]

When evaluating capital equipment, one should evaluate similar products one at a time. When purchasing capital equipment, one should determine whether it can be upgraded or must be replaced when the technology improves. One should consider construction, durability, modularity, warranty, availability of parts, and service agreements as part of the total cost of equipment. One should also consider leasing rather than buying.[27] There are companies who, for an annual subscription fee, assist an organization in evaluating a potential capital purchase and maintain a database that compares features, cost to own, average purchase price, and annual maintenance costs of several different manufacturers of equipment. This information can assist a department manager and the purchasing department to determine if they are getting the best value for the purchase price.

Part of the capital equipment budgeting process includes estimating the use of each item. For revenue budgeting purposes, a price or charge should be assigned to the use of each item. The cost-center manager can then determine the break-even point at which the item will be paid for.

Performance Budgeting

Performance budgeting focuses on the activities of a cost center such as indirect care, direct care, and quality monitoring. Each activity has objectives with specific financial resources, and the focus is on what is expected to be accomplished. Performance is evaluated based on a variety of outputs. Flexible budgeting that evaluates actual costs based on actual work load is an improvement over traditional budgeting but is a limited evaluation of nursing performance. Performance budgeting is an improvement over flexible budgeting because it ties performance to financial resource consumption. The steps involved are as follows[28]:

1. Define the performance activities or area of accomplishment for the cost center, which may include direct care, improved quality of care, nursing staff satisfaction, patient satisfaction, productivity, and innovation.
2. Identify the line-item operating-budget costs for the cost center being evaluated. These costs will be manager and clinical salaries, education costs, supplies, and overhead.
3. Define how much of the resources represented by each line item are to be devoted to each of the performance areas.
4. Choose measures of performance for each performance area, budget an amount of work for each area, and determine the budgeted cost per unit of work based on these measures.

The performance budget evolves or is converted from the operating budget. Potential output measures are proxies and consist of both process and outcome measures. These output measures may include the following[29]:

- Compliance with patient care plan procedures, with the goal of a percentage reduction in errors
- Compliance with evidence based medical practices such as CMS Core Measures
- Improved compliance costs (the fix, which is usually additional resources of some kind)
- Staffing decisions using reduced management time
- Cost reduction
- Increased productivity
- Increased patient and staff satisfaction
- Innovation and planning
- Direct care
- Indirect care

Multiple measures can be developed for each performance area.

Revenues

The sources of nursing revenue or for securing a financial base for nursing include grants, continuing education, private practice, community visibility, health care for students and staff, health maintenance organizations, city health departments, professional corporations, and nurse-managed centers.

Operating room nursing is an example of a cost that can be billed as a source of revenue. Determining the level of care needed for different procedures and the room charges, based on use of supplies and equipment, and billing the services separately may be considered revenue. In computing the nursing charges, the cost of nursing personnel per case can be determined from the records. To this can be added the cost of preparation time for assembling supplies and equipment and setting up the room, preoperative and postoperative patient visits, nursing administration, and staff development. Room costs include environmental services and maintenance.[30] Using product-line strategy, nursing divisions can sell a number of product lines, such as staff development programs, consultation services, home health services, wellness programs, and computer software.

Controlling Process

Now that we have seen the nursing budget from its planning and directing aspects, we can turn to its controlling or evaluating aspects. The budget establishes financial standards for the division of nursing and through the division's cost center for each nursing unit. Daily, weekly, monthly, and quarterly feedback provide information to compare managerial performance with the established standards. The results are used to make adjustments. What kind of feedback do nurses need relative to their budgets and cost control? Nurses need information to determine whether their goals are being met. Are they exceeding the budget? Is the excess both for costs and for revenues? Are the supplies and expenses of the quantity and quality planned? Is the equipment being purchased and installed as scheduled? Are employees being recruited and used effectively to produce the expected quality and quantity of nursing services? Is employee morale good? What adjustments need to be made? Where are the problems, and who is responsible for them?

Budget processes should be flexible to allow for increased and decreased volume of business. The hospital's finance department provides cost-center managers with needed biometric information to make adjustments in staffing and in use of supplies. The colossal mistakes of budgeting are made in the control area. Variations in budget should be used as a tool for decision making, not as an instance or reactionary intervention to make arbitrary cuts that result in unrealistic operating budgets for line managers.[31]

Monitoring the Budget

Various techniques have been described for monitoring the budget; however, all budget objectives should contain procedures for quality review, including identification of a team to perform such a review. If a program is not successful—that is, if it is not meeting objectives or is running above predicted costs and below predicted revenues—then a decision should be made about whether to rework or cancel it. Although very difficult, making this decision is essential to good control. The technique of canceling budgeted programs is sometimes referred to as "sun setting." A nurse manager should accept the responsibility for "sun setting" programs that are costly and unprofitable.

In developing the nursing budget, it is necessary that the unit structures for nursing administration are comparable in type and quantity of work load. Developing and providing financial policies and guidelines is most successful when the top administrative team works with the budget monitor. The CNO is part of this team and brings to its meetings standards of service that are defensible (such as data on work load, including numbers and types of procedures, patients, surgical operations, and visits). These policies should reflect the long-term plans of the governing board.

Part of the information furnished to CNO and managers is in the form of reports, which include statistical reports of revenues and expenditures for the current year. Figure 11-14 illustrates financial information needed by the cost-center manager and the CNO.

Note that the account number at the head of the table in Figure 11-14 is 2-7010. The prefix 2 denotes that the account balance does not turn over at the end of the fiscal year. The cost center or department is 7010. Financial transactions, including purchase orders for supplies and minor equipment, and payroll are identified with this cost-center number and are charged by the purchasing and accounting departments to this number and to the appropriate subcodes 1000 through 5000. Table columns indicate the operational budget, the actual expenditures for the current month and for the fiscal or budget year, open encumbrances, and the balance available. Because 83% of the fiscal year (which begins January 1) has elapsed, these figures have some relationship to the Percent Used column. Although 103% of the budgeted salary has been used, only 70% of employee benefits have been used, which indicates a use of overtime plus part-time employees working less than the 20 hours per week required to qualify for benefits. Zero percent of the budgeted money for minor equipment has been spent to date. Total budget expenses were 97%, indicating a variance of 10% overspending. This report serves as a control for nurse managers, but the expenditure of budgeted money for any one subcode could cause the total expenses to date to be greater than the percentage of fiscal year elapsed without creating an alarm. In this instance, overspending should be related to increased census and revenue.

Figure 11-15 informs the nurse managers of the specific financial transactions that took place during the month of October. These transactions can be checked against Figure 11-14. Information on revenues is reported in a similar manner. Figure 11-16 illustrates the inpatient revenue for the Medical-Surgical Unit, which includes nursing and hotel services. All the revenue is credited to nursing. The revenue account is 2-40815, and the cost center is the same as for expenses, 7010. The budgeted revenues for the year are listed, as are the revenues for the month and for the fiscal year. Note that although 83% of the fiscal year has elapsed, only 76% of the budgeted revenues have been charged, a variance of 7%. Also, Figure 11-17 indicates that 76% of budgeted equipment revenues have been billed.

Because the amount billed (i.e., the unit's revenues), 76%, is less than the 83% of fiscal year elapsed, the nurse managers can note that revenues are currently lower than expenses, which is a negative financial report. The manager's goal is to improve this financial status by the end of the fiscal year.

Additional financial information can be furnished to each nurse manager, including summary reports in whole dollars and for all cost centers supervised. This can be done by subcode, by subcode and cost center, or by any unit or department.

FIGURE 11-14	ACCOUNTING SYSTEM REPORT

Account: 2-7010
Department: 7010

Fiscal Year Ending 200x
January–October (83% fiscal year elapsed)
Medical-Surgical Unit—Expense

Subcode	Description	Actual Budget Approved	Current Month	YTD	Open Encumbrances	Remaining Budget	Percent Used
1000	Pool–Salary & Wages	901,053				901,053	0
1100	Professional Salary	72,533	775,790	775,790-			$
1200	Nursing Asst Salary	4,085	50,947	50,947-			$
1300	Secretary Salary	4,347	53,168	53,168-			$
1400	Orderly Salary	3,936	52,195	52,195-			$
1500	Students	14,898	1,518	14,898			100
1600	Accrued Salaries	32,791	11,462	32,791			100
	Salaries	**$948,742**	**97,881**	**979,789**		**31,047-** **55,722**	**103**
2000	Pool–Empl Benefits	55,722					0
2100	FICA	112	112				100
2200	Health Insurance	59,973	5,887	59,973			100
2300	Retirement	62,158	5,591	62,158			100
2400	Disability	4,869	526	4,869			100
2500	Life Insurance	2,569	264	2,569			100
	Employee Benefits	**185,403**	**12,268**	**129,681**		**55,722**	**70**
3000	Pool–Med/Surg	10,000	10,000				0
3100	Med & Surg Supplies	185,000	22,000	185,000			100
3110	Drugs	2,317	1,100	2,317			100
3114	Solutions	44,000	10,000	44,000			100
	Med/Surg Supplies	**241,317**	**33,100**	**231,317**		**10,000**	**96**
4000	Pool–General Supply						0
4010	Office Supplies	1,010	220	1,009			100
4120	Forms	1,490	1,090	400			100
4134	Copying	35	30	36			100
4260	Dietary	620	50	620			100
4330	Linen Bedding	215	215				100
4440	Housekeeping Supply	2,880	350	2,880			100
	General Supplies	**6,250**	**650**			**5,850**	**100**
5000	Minor Equipment	450				450	0
	Total Expenses	**1,382,212**	**143,899**	**1,346,637**	**400**	**35,725**	**97**
	Account Total	**1,382,212**	**143,899**	**1,346,637**	**400**	**35,725**	**97**

OPEN ENCUMBRANCE STATUS

P.O. Account	P.O. Number	Date	Original Description	Liquidating Encum.	Current Expenditures	Last Act Adjusts Encum.	Date
2-7010-4120	D3333	4/10/04	Print-All	400.00	400.00		10/4/04

Source: Author.

Rollover funds are also included in the financial reports that can be provided to the chief nurse executive and nurse managers. Balances in these funds are carried over into the next fiscal year to be spent at any future date. The chief nurse executive, a department head, or a cost-center manager can manage rollover funds.

FIGURE 11-15   ACCOUNTING SYSTEM REPORT

Report of transactions for fiscal year ending 200x

Acct: 2-7010
Dept: 7010

Distribution code = 600
Medical–Surgical Unit—Expense

Subcode	Description	Date	Ref.	J.E. Offset Account	Current Rev/Exp	Encumbrances	Batch Ref	Batch Date
1100	Payroll Expense	10/07	60001	0-11181-128CR	35,017.03		TTS584	10/7
1100	Payroll Expense	10/21	60001	0-11181-128CR	37,516.33		TTS588	10/21
1100	Total Profess. Salary				72,533.36			
1200	Payroll Expense	10/07	60001	0-11181-128CR	2,115.98		TTS584	10/07
1200	Payroll Expense	10/21	60001	0-11181-128CR	1,969.04		TTS588	10/21
1200	Total Asst. Salary				4,085.00			
1300	Payroll Expense	10/07	60001	0-11181-128CR	2,012.56		TTS584	10/07
1300	Payroll Expense	10/21	60001	0-11181-128CR	2,334.44		TTS588	10/21
1300	Total Secretary Salary				4,347.00			
1400	Payroll Expense	10/07	60001	0-11181-128CR	1,936.22		TTS584	10/07
1400	Payroll Expense	10/21	60001	0-11181-128CR	1,999.78		TTS588	10/21
1400	Total Orderly Salary				3,936.00			
1500	Payroll Expense	10/07	60001	0-11181-128CR	751.56		TTS584	10/07
1500	Payroll Expense	10/21	60001	0-11181-128CR	766.44		TTS588	10/21
1500	Total Student Salary				1,518.00			
	Susp Corr/Accr Sal	9/30	R3490	0-12000-140CR	35.00		JJV002	10/10
	Susp Corr/Accr Sal	9/30	R3490	0-12000-140CR	55.00		JJV002	10/10
	RVS Acc Sal & Wage	10/01	06510	0-14300-110DP	21,462.00–		JJV001	10/10
	RVS Acc Sal & Wage	10/01	06510	0-14300-110DP	35.00–		JJV001	10/1
	RVS Acc Sal & Wage	10/01	06510	0-14300-110DP	65.00–		JJV001	10/10
	Accrued Sal & Wgs	10/31	06500	0-14300-128CR	32,924.00		JJV019	10/31
1600	Total Accrued Salaries				11,462.00			
2200	Payroll Expense	10/07	60001	2-66000-170CR	65.81		TTS588	10/07
2200	Payroll Expense	10/21	60001	2-66000-170CR	5,821.12		TTS588	10/21
2200	Total Health Ins.				5,886.93			
2300	Payroll Expense	10/07	60001	2-66000-170CR	2,659.96		TTS588	10/07
2300	Payroll Expense	10/21	60001	2-66000-170CR	2,930.66		TTS588	10/21
2300	Total Retirement				5,590.62			
2400	Payroll Expense	10/21	60001	2-66000-170CR	526.48		TTS588	10/21
2400	Total Disability				526.48			
2500	Payroll Expense	10/21	60001	2-66000-170CR	264.04		TTS588	10/21
2500	Total Life Insurance				264.04			
3100	Inventory Exp Alloc	10/31	06526	0-14100-130CR	22,000.00		JJV027	10/31
3100	Total Med/Surg Supplies				22,000.00			
3110	Pharmacy Distrib–Oct	10/31	07500	4-50730-214CR	1,100.00		JJV033	10/31
3110	Total Drugs				1,100.00			
3114	Inventory Exp Alloc	10/31	07524	0-121000-120CR	10,000.00		JJV027	10/31
3114	Total Solutions				10,000.00			
4010	Inventory Exp Alloc	10/31	07526	0-12100-T40CR	220.00		JJVO27	10/31
4010	Total Office Supplies				220.00			
4120	Inventory Exp Alloc	10/31	07508	4-69669-965CR	400.00		JJVO26	10/31
4120	Total Forms				400.00			
4134	Xerox Expense	10/31	07501	4-60960-960CR	30.00		JJVO28	10/31
4134	Total Copying				30.00			
4260	Inventory Exp Alloc	10/31	07506	0-12100-144CR	50.00		JJVO27	10/31
4260	Total Food Expense				50.00			
4440	Inventory Exp Alloc	10/31	07564	0-12100-140CR	350.00		JJV028	10/31
4440	Total Housekeeping Sup.				350.00			
	Account total				143,899.00	400.00		

Source: Author.

FIGURE 11-16

ACCOUNTING SYSTEM REPORT

Fiscal Year Ending 200x
January–October (83% of fiscal year elapsed)
Distribution Code = 600
Medical–Surgical Unit—Revenue

Acct: 2-40815
Dept: 7010

			Actual				
Code	Description	Approved Budget	Current Month	Fiscal Year	Open Encumbrances	Remaining Budget	Percent Used
030	Inpatient Revenue	2,345,200–	225,800–	1,782,352–		562,848–	76
0/0	Total Revenues	2,345,200–	225,800–	1,782,352–		562,848–	76
	Account Total	2,345,200–	225,800–	1,782,352–		562,848–	76

Source: Author.

FIGURE 11-17

ACCOUNTING SYSTEM REPORT

Fiscal Year Ending 200x
January–October (83% of fiscal year elapsed)
Distribution Code = 600
Medical–Surgical Unit—SP & D—Revenue

Acct: 2-40818
Dept: 7010

			Actual				
Code	Description	Approved Budget	Current Month	Fiscal Year	Open Encumbrances	Remaining Budget	Percent Used
030	Inpatient Revenue	1,895,000–	201,647–	1,440,200–		454,800–	76
	Total Revenues	1,895,000–	201,647–	1,440,220–		454,800–	76
	Account Total	1,895,000–	201,647–	1,440,220–		454,800	76

Source: Author.

Motivational Aspects of Budgeting

Budgeting can be a motivating force for personnel if current programs must increase in effectiveness and efficiency to remain, if decentralization and staff involvement provide an increased sense of responsibility and satisfaction, and if merit increases, promotions, and bonuses are tied or linked to budgetary performance.

Cutting the Budget

When the budget must be cut, planning is a vital aspect of the process. Budget cuts happen as hospital admissions and stays decrease and reimbursement changes. The form and the process of nursing management can determine the course of events when the budget has to be cut.

A nursing administration that delegates decision making to the lowest level and encourages partic
ipative management is an effective administration. When clinical nurses are informed at the unit level
and invited to give their input, they can help with suggestions for cutting costs. They gladly implement
and support the activities they recognize as resulting partly from their input. A nursing organization
that promotes self-direction at the levels of clinical nurse, nurse manager, clinical consultant, and executive nurse supports direction to reduce costs and to increase productivity and profits. For example,
when a hospital chief executive officer discovered that self-pay patient care was the only category not
reviewed for use of resources, a clinical nurse established a review process. Physicians and other healthcare professionals supported this process.

Nursing budgets are enormous, and budgets for a single unit can run into hundreds of thousands of dollars per year. Pay awards or increases must be met by budget cuts (personnel cutbacks), use of less expensive supplies and techniques, or increased productivity. The latter requires more paying patients, shorter
stays, and increased sales of all paying services. When personnel cuts are to be made, nursing is vulnerable.
Some cuts can come from all services, but nursing has greater numbers. The nurse manager who controls
these numbers daily, weekly, and yearly has greater credibility. Many sources indicate that turnover is costly.
The cost of turnover of personnel low on the salary scale is sometimes weighed against the higher cost of
employees who are at the top of the salary scale. An assumption is made that long-time employees are better satisfied with their jobs and do better work. This assumption needs to be validated through research.

As work load data indicate shifts from one unit to another, resources also must be shifted. Asking for
volunteers, moving vacated positions, and using as needed pools can do this. Inpatient procedures in hospitals have shifted to outpatient procedures either in hospitals or at ambulatory surgery centers. New reimbursement rates, which are part of a system of ambulatory patient classifications, have been issued by
CMS and affect revenues from ambulatory services. Many more diagnostic procedures are now being
done on an outpatient basis; as a result, inpatients are often a sicker group, requiring more nursing care.

Because CNOs control multi–million-dollar budgets, they are powerful people. They are also vulnerable to personnel cuts. Much of this vulnerability stems from external controls imposed by state and
federal governments and health insurance companies. Power comes from the ability of CNOs to use
knowledge and skills in defending, directing, and controlling their budgets. They learn to hold the line
on staffing and overtime and monitor for the appropriate use of supplies and equipment.

Legitimate Budget Activities

Healthcare organizations should be managed like other businesses. Charges should be determined from
costs and should include allowance for profits or return on equity and for bad debts. The practice of
cost shifting to make certain services revenue producers should be stopped.

Oszustowicz suggests the following seven-step system by which total financial requirements eventually determine the gross patient revenue equal to meet the financial needs of a department[32]:

1. Detail demand for nursing services and equipment needs.
2. Detail direct expenses.
3. Detail indirect expenses.
4. Detail working capital requirements.
5. Detail capital requirements.
6. Detail earnings (profit) requirements.
7. Detail deductions from patient revenues.

Reimbursement

With the continued escalation of healthcare costs, the healthcare system has evolved to emphasize patient outcomes, controlling costs, and rewarding those organizations that can do both. Basically, there are four major sources of revenue for healthcare providers: charges, retrospective reimbursement, prospective reimbursement/medical severity diagnosis-related groups, and managed care.[33] The following gives a brief overview of how quality in the form of pay for performance has evolved.

Reimbursement Based on Clinical Performance

It is important for the CNO and nurse managers to beware of the changing environment of reimbursement based on clinical quality. Although traditional forms of reimbursement are still maintained, the amount reimbursed to the organization or their ability to be a hospital of choice for covered lives depends on required reporting and performance of evidenced-based criteria, better known as pay for performance. Driven by the Institute of Medicine report, *To Err is Human: Building a Safer Health System*, which outlined the cost of poor quality in the form of medical errors, hospital acquired infections, and medical errors resulting in patient harm,[34] CMS and other payers are focusing on improving patient safety and outcomes through financial penalties for lack of participation or poor performance compared with peer hospitals. This information is currently available on the CMS website, www.hospital compare.hhs.gov. The public can review and draw conclusions on a hospital's performance. It is important in the budgeting process for the CNO to understand how these performance requirements affect the nursing department budget and the overall bottom line of their organization. Additional resources could be needed to monitor and meet these performance requirements.

U.S. Health Care System

The U.S. healthcare system has many components: patients, insurers, and employers; providers such as hospitals, ambulatory care services, home health services, long-term care facilities, physicians, nurses, allied health personnel, pharmacists and pharmacies, and providers of durable medical equipment; and federal, state, and local public health services. As costs have increased, physicians who have been reimbursed based on fees for services are increasingly being reimbursed by capitation through contracts with managed care insurers, or they have themselves become employees of the managed care insurers. Employees have switched from indemnity insurance plans to managed care plans. Figure 11-18 outlines the sequential development of healthcare insurance in the United States.

Indemnity insurance plans cover bills from most providers and pay most health care bills by charges or costs, with some deductibles or copayments. Indemnity plans are fast disappearing as employers and governments switch to managed care plans. As healthcare costs have soared, employers have increased employees' share of indemnity insurance premiums. Indemnity insurance plans do not keep costs down. Indemnity insurers are changing to become organizers and administrators of managed care networks and subsequently deliverers of health care. This transformation is reducing the number of insurers.[34]

In the new managed care environment, many providers are integrated into insurance plan services through individual contracts and subcontracts. Clients accept the providers of these contract services, thus limiting their choices regarding most healthcare provider services. Clients receive a total package of health care dictated by the contracts between employers and insurers.

Managed Care

Managed care is a patient care system that includes insurance companies, employers, providers, and clients. Most enrollees of managed care plans are employees of businesses that contract for health insurance as a benefit. Many plans accept individual enrollees, particularly plans that enroll Medicare beneficiaries. Managed care is also the process by which healthcare benefits are monitored for purposes of cost management, resulting in limitation of benefit coverage and access to healthcare benefits. Managed care organizations manage the distribution of healthcare dollars, use of services, and access to benefits.

FIGURE 11-18 HISTORICAL DEVELOPMENT OF HEALTH CARE INSURANCE

1929	Blue Cross	1986	Gramm–Rudman Deficit Reduction Amendment and Omnibus Budget Reconciliation Act
1935	Social Security Act		
1946	Hospital Survey and Construction Act (Hill–Burton)	1987, 1988	Omnibus Budget Reconciliation Act (OBRA)
1964	Hill–Harris Hospital and Medical Facilities Amendments	1989	Physician Payment Review Commission
1965	Public Law 89-97, Medicare and Medicaid	1994	Medicare Choice Act
1982	Public Law 97-248, Tax Equity and Fiscal Responsibility Act (TEFRA)	1996	Health Insurance and Accountability Act
		1997	Balanced Budget Act
1983	Public Law, 98-21, Social Security Amendments Prospective Payment System	2003	Medicare Prescription Drug, Improvement, and Modernization Act
1985	Consolidated Omnibus Budget Reconciliation Act (COBRA)	2005	Deficit Reduction Act
		2006	Tax Relief and Healthcare Act

Source: Author.

Organizations and Alternative Delivery Systems

Patients now accept healthcare plans that limit their freedom of choice. The following sections discuss some of these plans.

Health Maintenance Organizations   Financing of health maintenance organizations (HMOs) is done by capitation, in which there is a predetermined payment per patient or per service. Managed care is designed to cut costs.

The HMO is defined as

> [A] prepaid health plan delivering comprehensive care to members through designated providers, having a fixed periodic payment for healthcare services, and requiring members to be in a plan for a specified period of time (usually 1 year). A group HMO delivers health services through a physician group that is controlled by the HMO unit or contracts with one or more independent group practices to provide health services. An individual practice association (IPA) HMO contracts directly with physicians in independent practice, and/or contracts with one or more associations of physicians in independent practice, and/or contracts with one or more multispecialty group practices. Data are based on a consensus of HMOs.[35]

HMOs have the following characteristics:

- Utilization risks are shifted from payer to provider.
- Competition draws consumers to less costly services when they have a choice of plans.
- Use of preventive care and ambulatory facilities decreases hospital admission rates, lowering insurance costs by 10% to 40%.
- Use of primary care physicians and nurse practitioners at fixed salaries decreases the use of expensive surgeons and specialists.
- HMOs eliminate unneeded facilities such as hospitals, operating rooms, and radiation therapy units.
- Paperwork and overhead are reduced.

- HMOs provide organized, cooperative care for individuals and families.
- Enrollees make appointments with gatekeeper physicians or nurses, mostly family practice physicians, internists, and pediatricians.
- Gatekeepers control all referrals to specialists.
- Enrollees pay a small fee per visit and for medications.
- Gatekeepers control un-needed procedures, both diagnostic and therapeutic.
- HMO plans contract for discounted prices with various providers, such as hospitals, laboratories, radiologists, physician specialists, and pharmacists.
- HMO plans emphasize complete patient care, management of chronic illnesses, education, disease prevention, and wellness. Oxford Health Plans hired 20 nurse practitioners because they are trained to provide services for disease prevention and health promotion. These RN practitioners perform more preventive care and are reimbursed at the same rate as physicians.
- HMOs make physicians business-oriented practitioners.
- HMO plans do mass customization to give each of a mass of customers what the customer desires.
- HMOs offer capitated payments, one price per enrollee.
- HMOs reduce the risks of un-needed procedures, such as cesarean sections and hysterectomies.
- Half of HMO physicians are paid flat fees that are incentives to reduce care.

Although HMOs are the most common type of managed care organization, many more millions of people belong to other types, which are discussed in the following sections.

Preferred Provider Organizations   In a preferred provider organization (PPO), a group of providers acts as healthcare brokers, providing services to a group of patients at reduced fees. PPOs have the following characteristics:

- PPOs contract with consumers through employers and insurers and with providers, including physicians, hospitals, and allied services.
- PPO services are discounted, and patients have no out-of-pocket expenses.
- In PPOs, patients are limited to using the listed providers or paying larger fees for out-of-network providers.
- PPOs are intermediaries between payer and subscriber groups, furnishing marketing and administrative services.
- PPOs set their own size, number of staff specialists, geographical availability, time limits for claims and payments, and other features.
- PPOs place hospitals but not physicians at risk. Physicians are paid discounted rates for a steady flow of patients.

Arguments that the traditional physician–patient relationship will be destroyed are inconsequential because these relationships will soon disappear. Working people want efficiency; they do not want to sit in a physician's office waiting for hours past their appointed time. Given adequate information, they will make choices about their care, and they should. The old concept of withholding information is outmoded and dangerous and in some cases illegal (i.e., informed consent). The objective of all competitive healthcare plans is to provide quality care less expensively. There are approximately 1,036 PPOs in the United States and more than 50.2 million enrollees.[36]

Health Care Cost Coalitions   Health care cost coalitions are organizations of employers, and sometimes unions, that effectively bargain for better rates and parity with Medicare, Medicaid, and other insurers. They work to develop PPOs and utilization review programs.

Prudent Buyer Systems Prudent buyer systems are characterized by joint purchasing arrangements, purchasing consortia composed of multiple providers, and competitive bidding for exclusive contracts.

Health Promotion and Wellness Programs Increased education and awareness enable these programs to emphasize illness prevention.

Hospital Physician Organizations The hospital physician organization is a relatively new entity. Its objective is to combine and reduce overhead, which can be done by sharing services such as billing.

Provider-Sponsored Organizations Provider-sponsored organizations (PSOs) are networks of physicians and hospitals that are their owners. Approximately 84 PSOs exist in the United States. Supporters of PSOs say they are health providers engaged in treating patients, whereas HMOs are insurance companies that invest in stocks, bonds, and other liquid assets. PSOs offer less risk to providers than do HMOs because providers receive only part of their income from the PSO.[37,38]

Management Implications

Managers of all healthcare provider organizations face the need to maintain financial stability. To do this, they become experts in negotiating contracts, planning new ventures, and reorganizing their organizations to make maximum use of human resources. Successful managers provide leadership that empowers employees to provide maximum quality outcomes for their patients. As managers pursue these functions, they oversee evaluation techniques that are simple to administer and lead to quality improvement.[39,40]

Evidence-Based Practice 11-1

Spetz, Jacobs and Hatler reported the results of a small trial of a patient vigilance system in a postneurosurgery unit of a large acute care hospital. The system included two components: (1) passive sensor array placed under the patient in a hospital bed and (2) a bedside unit that connected to the nurse call system already in place at the hospital. The researchers found that the trial demonstrated the overall effectiveness of the vigilance system in reducing the rate of patient falls. Additionally, the cost-effectiveness analysis revealed that use of this system was associated with somewhat higher measured costs. The researchers noted that the higher costs may not be entirely accurate given that the trials did not take into account unmeasured costs, such as costs associated with pain and suffering, lost revenue due to decreased competitiveness, and the cost of lawsuits after falls. Additionally, the researchers' report that they were unable to assess the cost savings associated with the patients with other problems and issues, such as patients identified with cardiac and respiratory issues. The researchers cautioned readers to consider the results of their work as suggestive rather than definitive given the small trial size.[41]

SUMMARY

It is important for nurses to have a working knowledge of the objectives of budgeting and of component costs. Every activity that takes place in a healthcare agency costs money. A standard must exist for assigning costs to user departments. The nursing department should pay its user share, and no more. Knowledge of the cost-accounting system provides accurate information for budgeting and for cost management.

Efficient nurse managers use a budget calendar that covers formulation, review and enactment, and execution stages of the total budget process.

The major elements of nursing budgets are personnel, supplies and equipment (minor), and capital equipment. Generally, equipment that costs less than a fixed dollar amount is included in the supplies and equipment budget. A product evaluation committee is useful for ensuring that supplies and equipment promote effective and efficient patient care. The capital equipment budget includes equipment that costs more than a fixed dollar amount; it is prepared separately from the supplies and equipment budget.

Evaluation is an administrative aspect of budgeting that in itself serves as a controlling process. Decentralization vests control at the lowest competent level of decision making. Good budget feedback is essential if the budget is to be an effective controlling process. Good feedback includes information about revenues and expenses as well as internal comparisons of projected and actual budgets. The budget can motivate professional nurses to facilitate their development of innovations.

The belief that budgets are beyond comprehension can sabotage a nurse's effectiveness. Spiraling healthcare costs, cost-management efforts, and increasing accountability from individual cost centers should serve as an impetus for nurses to learn at least the fundamentals of budgets and the budgeting process. Assuming the responsibility for budget work increases the nurse's potential realm of planning, predicting, and reviewing programs within the nurse's jurisdiction.

Like a nursing care plan, the budget is an activity guidance tool. It is a plan expressed in monetary terms and carried out within a time frame. To be an effective caregiver, the nurse must know how to develop and use a nursing care plan. Similarly, to be most effective as a manager, the nurse manager must know how to develop and use a budget.

One main competency the nurse manager must possess is understanding financial information and evolving payment for performance processes and measures. The objectives of this transformation are reduced costs, improved clinical quality, and increased efficiency. Although pay for performance continues its development, it is here to stay and the nursing department must understand the implications of this reimbursement plan to play an active role in the organization's overall performance.

APPLICATION EXERCISES

Exercise 11-1
Develop a performance budget for a cost center to be used as a model for a healthcare organization.

Exercise 11-2
Every hospital prepares the Hospital and Hospital Health Care Complex Cost Report Certification and Settlement Summary, commonly known as the Center for Medicare and Medicaid (CMS) Cost Report. Obtain the latest one for your employing or clinical experience hospital. Select a nursing cost center and complete Figure 11-19, Preparing a Budget for a Unit or Project.

This exercise has acquainted you with the Medicare Cost Report. You can use projected medical inflation rates to prepare a budget for the following year. For instance, if the inflation rates are projected to be 8%, multiply all costs by 1.08 to project and budget costs. Note that intensive care units are budgeted separately. All other inpatient units are grouped as Adults and Pediatrics (General and Routine Care). To separate these units for revenue and expenditures, make the following calculations:

1. Select a patient care unit of a hospital:
2. Determine the number of patient days of occupancy for this unit (from the biometric records):

FIGURE 11-19   PREPARING A BUDGET FOR A UNIT OR PROJECT

Unit _____ Revenue Center Number _____

Direct Expenses (Directly Assigned)

Salaries (attach position questionnaire for new ones)	$_____.___
Employee benefits	$_____.___
Personnel services	$_____.___
Supplies	$_____.___
Other	$_____.___
Total Direct	$_____.___

Indirect Expenses

Depreciation of capital buildings and fixtures	$_____.___
Capital equipment (movable)	$_____.___
(attach requests for new items)	$_____.___
Worker's compensation	$_____.___
Life insurance	$_____.___
Communications	$_____.___
Data processing	$_____.___
Purchasing	$_____.___
Admitting	$_____.___
Patient accounts	$_____.___
General administration	$_____.___
Plant operations	$_____.___
Biomedical	$_____.___
Laundry	$_____.___
Housekeeping	$_____.___
Nursing administration	$_____.___
Patient transport	$_____.___
Preparation	$_____.___
Central supply	$_____.___
Pharmacy	$_____.___
College of nursing (or other college)	$_____.___
Interns and residents	$_____.___
Other	$_____.___
Total Indirect	$_____.___
Total Costs (Direct + Indirect)	$_____.___
Total Charges or Revenues	$_____.___

Cost-to-Charge Ratio (Divide total costs by total charges or revenues.) $_____.___
                                                      divided by $_____.___
                                                         minus $_____.___

or _____%

Source: Author.

3. From the Medicare Cost Report determine:

   3.1. Total direct and indirect costs: $ _____

   3.2. Total patient days:

   3.3. Divide the total direct and indirect costs $ _____ by total patient days _____ = $_____ cost per patient day.

   3.4. Patient days for unit (from 3.2) _____ ×3 cost per patient day (from 3.3) _____ = $_____, or approximate expenses for the nursing unit for this year.

For help, refer to Swansburg, R. C., & Sowell, R. L. (1992). A model for costing and pricing nursing service. *Nursing Management,* 33–36; Swansburg, R. C. (1997). *Budgeting and financial management for nurse managers.* Sudbury, MA: Jones and Bartlett.

Exercise 11-3

A 16-bed intensive care unit needs to replace the patient beds. Research intensive care unit beds on the market and develop a capital budget for the project. Prepare justifications for the replacement and the projected depreciation of the equipment.

Exercise 11-4

Attend a marketing session given by an insurance company offering healthcare products. Analyze the presentation. What are the advantages and disadvantages for the patient?

Exercise 11-5

Locate and read five recent articles on pay for performance published in nursing journals. Summarize the implications for the nursing profession.

Exercise 11-6

Determine if there is a cost difference between 8- and 12-hour shifts for a nursing unit using the example in Figure 11-9.

Notes

1. Johnson, R. W., & Melicher, R. W. (1982). *Financial planning.* Boston: Allyn & Bacon.
2. Baker, J. D. (1991). The operating expense budget, one part of a manager's arsenal. *AORN Journal, 54,* 837–841; Klann, S. (1989). Mastering the OR budgeting process is key to success. *OR Manager, 13*(3), 10–11.
3. Althaus, J. N., Hardyck, N. M., Pierce, P. B., & Rodgers, M. S. (1981). *Nursing decentralization: The El Camino experience.* Gaithersburg, MD: Aspen.
4. Whitman, G. R. (1991). Analyzing and forecasting budgets. In C. Birdsall (Ed.), *Management issues in critical care* (pp. 287–307). St. Louis, MO: Mosby.
5. Ibid.
6. Anthony, R. N., & Young, D. W. (1988). *Management control in nonprofit organizations* (4th ed.). Chicago: Irwin.
7. Klann, 1989.
8. Huttman, B. (1964). Taking charge: Selling your budget. *RN, 1,* 25–26.
9. Covert, R. P. (1982). Expense budgeting. In W. O. Cleverly (Ed.), *Handbook of health care accounting and finance* (pp. 261–278). Rockville, MD: Aspen.
10. Talbot, G. J. (1983). Key for successful program budgeting. *Journal of Continuing Education in Nursing, 14,* 8–10.
11. Drucker, P. F. (1999). *Management challenges for the 21st century* (pp. 111–129). New York: HarperCollins.
12. Herkimer, A. G., Jr. (1978). *Understanding hospital financial management* (p. 132). Rockville, MD: Aspen.
13. Hoffman, F. M. (1984). *Financial management for nurse managers* (p. 9). East Norwalk, CT: Appleton-Century-Crofts.
14. Talbot, 1983.
15. Rowland, H. S., & Rowland, B. L. (1992). *Nursing administration handbook* (3rd ed., p. 174) Gaithersburg, MD: Aspen.
16. Ibid., p. 175.
17. Ibid., p. 174.
18. Buchan, J. (1992). Cost-effective caring. *International Nursing Review, 39,* 117–120.
19. Campbell, R. K. (1989). Understanding the management process and financial and managerial accounting: Part IV. Cash flow analysis and budgeting. *Diabetes Education,* 126–127, 129.

20. Osborne, D., & Gaebler, T. (1992). *Reinventing government* (119–124). New York: Plume.
21. Piper, L. R. (1982). Basic budgeting for ED nursing personnel. *Journal of Emergency Nursing,* 285–287.
22. Ibid.
23. Tzividies, E., Waterstraat, V., & Chamberlin, W. (1991). Managing the budget with a fluctuating census. *Nursing Management,* 80B, 80F, 80H.
24. Meyers-Levyand, J., Tybout, A. M. (1989). Schema congruity as a basis for product evaluation. *Journal of Consumer Research, 16,* 39–54.
25. Dickerson, M. (1988). Product evaluation: A strategy for controlling a supply and equipment budget. In H. C. Scherubel (Ed.), *Patients and purse strings* (pp. 2, 465–468). New York: National League for Nursing.
26. Kleinmuntz, C. E., & Kleinmuntz, D. N. (1999). A strategic approach to allocating capital in healthcare organizations. *Healthcare Financial Management, 52–58.*
27. Arges, G. S. (1998). *Estimated useful lives of depreciable hospital assets.* Chicago: American Hospital Publishing.
28. Aronsohn, B., & Deal, N. (1992). Navigating the maze of capital equipment acquisition. *Nursing Management,* 46–48.
29. Finkler, S. A. (1991). Performance budgeting. *Nursing Economics,* 404–408.
30. Ibid.
31. Palmer, P. N. (1984). Why hide the revenue produced by perioperative nursing care? *AORN Journal,* 1122–1123.
32. Oszustowicz, R. J. (1979). *Financial management of department of nursing services* (pp. 1–10). New York: National League for Nursing.
33. McGrail, G. R. (1988). Budgets: An underused resource. *Journal of Nursing Administration,* 25–31.
34. Kohn, L. T., Corrigan, J. M., & Donaldson, M. S. (Eds.). (1999). *To err is human: Building a safer health system.* Committee on Quality of Health in America, Institute of Medicine. Washington, DC: National Academies Press.
35. Westmoreland, D. (1995). Managing costs and budgets. In P. Yoder-Wise (Ed.), *Leading and managing in nursing* (p. 256). St. Louis, MO: Mosby.
36. Loomis, C. J. (1994, July 11). The real action in health care. *Fortune,* 149–153, 155–157.
37. U.S. Census Bureau. (1999). *Statistical abstract of the United States 1999* (118th ed., p. 149). Washington, DC: Author.
38. Westmoreland, D. (1995). Managing costs and budgets. In P. Yoder-Wise (Ed.), *Leading and managing in nursing* (p. 256). St. Louis, MO: Mosby.
39. Driscoll, K. (1997, April 13). Hospitals take lesson in quality improvements from GM. *San Antonio Express-News,* p. 3H.
40. May, D. (2007). By the numbers. *Modern Healthcare,* December, 1–96.
41. Spetz, R., Jacobs, J., & Hatler, C. (2007). Cost effectiveness of a medical vigilance system to reduce patient falls. *Nursing Economics, 25,* 333–352.

References

Geyman, J. P. (2003). The corporate transformation of medicine and its impact on costs and access to care. *Journal of the American Board of Family Medicine, 16,* 443–454.

Kilty, G. L. (1999). Baseline budgeting for continuous improvement. *Hospitals Materials Management Quarterly,* 29–32.

Lin, H. C., Xirasagar, S., & Tang, C. H. (2004). Costs per discharge and hospital ownership under prospective payment and cost-based reimbursement systems in Taiwan. *Health Policy and Planning, 19,* 166–176.

Page, A. (2004). *Keeping patients safe: Transforming the work environments of nurses.* Washington, DC: National Academies Press.

Potter, L. (1999). The managed care contract: Survival or closure. *Nursing Administration Quarterly,* 58–62.

Schirm, V., Albanese, T., & Garland, T. N. (1999). Understanding nursing home quality of care: Incorporating caregivers' perceptions through structure, process, and outcome. *Quality Management Health Care,* 55–63.

Seawell, V. L. (1994). *Chart of account for hospitals: An accounting and reporting reference guide.* Burr Ridge, IL: Probus.

Shmueli, A., & Glazer, J. (1999). Addressing the inequity of capitation by variable soft contracts. *Health Economics,* 335–343.

12 MANAGING THE PROCESS OF CARE DELIVERY

Robert W. Koch, DNS, RN
Marylane Wade Koch, RN, MSN, CNA

LEARNING OBJECTIVES AND ACTIVITIES

- Define directing.
- Describe the nature of the directing function of nursing management with relation to the physical acts of directing.
- Make a plan for delegating duties, tasks, and responsibilities.
- Make a plan for using management by objectives.
- Differentiate between content (exogenous) theories of motivation and process (endogenous) theories of motivation.
- Describe Maslow's hierarchy of needs.
- Describe nurse dissatisfaction as it relates to productivity and the nurse's role as a knowledge worker.
- Describe nurse satisfaction as it relates to applications of behavioral science.
- List examples that indicate the value of career planning, communication, self-esteem, and self-actualization as management strategies.

CONCEPTS

Directing (leading), delegating, management by objectives, organizational development, benchmarking, Six Sigma, motivation, content theories of motivation, process theories of motivation, self-esteem, and self-actualization.

> (Q U O T E)
>
> ***Motivation is the art of getting people to do what you want them to do because they want to do it.***
>
> —President Dwight Eisenhower

Introduction

The nurse administrator faces growing challenges in directing and leading healthcare organizations. The American Organization of Nurse Executives states that leadership is necessary to create work environments that will attract and retain nurses. One priority established by this organization is that nurse leaders should create positive and healthy work environments in nursing and health care. The nurse administrator is responsible for directing (Figure 12-1) and leading organizations that promote professional growth and continuous learning.[1]

DIRECTING AND NURSING ADMINISTRATION

Directing is the interpersonal process by which nursing personnel accomplish objectives. As part of the directing process, the nurse manager must examine functions of planning and organizing. From the mission, purpose, beliefs, and the vision statement to the written objectives of the organization, the nurse manager develops management plans; this process includes the methods and techniques selected and used to accomplish the work of the nursing unit. Directing should inspire and motivate nursing personnel to accomplish work. Three of the major elements of directing are embodied in supervision of nursing personnel: motivation, leadership, and communication.[2]

Nursing associates must be hired and managed as total human beings who respond to many institutions within society, such as church, school, government, family, service organizations, and professional societies. Similarities and differences exist between managers and staff members, who both need

FIGURE 12-1	ACTIVITIES RELATED TO DIRECTING

1. Implementing the theory (knowledge) base of nursing.
2. Making and using strategic and tactical plans with input from nursing personnel.
3. Facilitating the achievement of the organizational mission, vision, goals, and objectives.
4. Providing and maintaining resources: people, supplies, and equipment.
5. Maintaining morale.
6. Providing education and training programs to maintain competence.
7. Maintaining standards in the form of policies, procedures, rules, and regulations.
8. Facilitating maximum communication.
9. Providing leadership.
10. Facilitating and maintaining intrapersonal relationships.
11. Counseling and coaching.
12. Facilitating trust, teamwork, and cooperation.
13. Resolving conflict.
14. Evaluating processes that increase and maintain quality and productivity.
15. Organizing human resources.
16. Facilitating nursing research and evidence-based practice.

Source: Author.

physiological well-being, safety, achievement, and human associations. Most individuals place their own concerns before those of others. They enjoy work when the benefits exceed the costs, and they take a job that meets their established priorities for income and other life goals.

The nursing leader must create a positive environment that inspires others to work at the full levels of their capabilities. A positive work environment has the following properties:

- Group identity and group purpose
- Pleasant surroundings and coworkers
- Interesting work
- Employee recognition
- Opportunity and challenge
- Fair and equitable compensation
- Congruence between organizational and individual goals

A nurse leader who is also a nurse manager must persuade the group to work to achieve organizational objectives. The nurse leader knows organizational policies, goals, new programs, and plans for change. The leader has good judgment based on breadth of experience and directs the careers of employees. The nurse leader has a socially acceptable manner, exhibits acceptable personal qualities, and demonstrates skill in leadership, communication, and motivation.

Effective directing increases employee contributions to achieve nursing management goals and creates harmony between nursing management's goals and the workers' goals. The nurse manager acts as a facilitator and coach by providing educational needs for primary nurses and case managers, which helps them become leaders and managers of care. Nurse managers teach nursing personnel to work in self-managed teams. Personnel should learn to plan, self-schedule, manage personnel, budget, make decisions, and solve problems.

Delegating

Delegating is a major element of the directing function by which the manager accomplishes the work done through their employees. Delegation requires professional management training and development.

As nurse managers learn delegation, they become more productive. They learn to delegate by critically thinking about the delegation process, carefully planning, gaining knowledge of clinical nurses' capabilities, implementing effective interpersonal communications, and tasking risk. Delegation frees the nurse manager of daily pressures and time-consuming chores. Hansten and Jackson[3] outline the following priorities for delegation:

- Know your world (practice, organization)
- Know your organization (communication channels, collaboration, and resolution)
- Know your practice (professional scope of practice based on expected outcomes)
- Know yourself (barriers, benefits)
- Know your delegate (competency, motivation)

Delegation fosters a greater sense of responsibility, general understanding, and job satisfaction of employees. Authority should be commensurate with assigned responsibility. As professional nurses gain individual self-esteem, organizational self-esteem follows. Through effective delegation, employees actively participate in decision making and gain satisfaction with their jobs and the organization. Delegation can promote an environment that bolsters cohesiveness and trust.

Skills of Delegation

Nurse managers must consider what authority to delegate to clinical nurses. Generally speaking, nurse managers should not delegate the power to discipline, responsibility for maintaining morale, overall control, "hot potato," jobs that are too technical, or duties involving a trust or confidence.[4] These complicated areas of nursing management require specialized knowledge and skills. Nurse managers who handle these responsibilities should be well educated in the sciences of management. Furthermore, the nurse manager should avoid delegating tasks that can be accomplished by nonlicensed personnel to the clinical staff.

Barriers to the delegation process vary by level of personnel and environment. For example, the manager's preference for operating by oneself, insecurity, fear of being disliked, lack of confidence in associates, and refusal to allow mistakes result in ineffective delegation. Personnel barriers may include lack of experience or competence, avoidance of responsibility, disorganization, and overload of work. The work environment may provide barriers such as intolerance for mistakes, understaffing, criticism of decisions, and confusion in responsibilities and authority.

Management by Objectives

Management by objectives (MBO) was first advocated by Peter Drucker and made famous by George Odiorne, who defined it as "a process whereby the superior and subordinate managers of an organization jointly identify its common goals, define each individual's major areas of responsibility in terms of the results expected of him [sic], and use these measures as guides for operating the unit and assessing the contribution of each of its members."[5]

MBO allows the individual staff nurse to contribute to the common goal of the enterprise while nurse managers focus on the business goals. MBO promotes high standards, focusing on the job and not on the manager or the worker. Nurse managers know what to expect of employees. Furthermore, nursing staff should know their areas of accountability.

MBO spells out the results expected of the clinical nursing unit itself in relation to other units. MBO emphasizes teamwork and team results and includes short- and long-term objectives. MBO allows people to control their own performance and measure themselves. Through MBO, clinical nurses make demands of themselves. With this model, nurse managers assume that clinical nurses will be responsible, want to contribute, and will achieve goals.

According to Drucker,[6]

> What the business enterprise needs is a principle of management that will give full scope to individual strength and responsibility, as well as common direction to vision and effort, establish team work, and harmonize the goals of the individual with the commonwealth. MBO and self-control make[s] the commonwealth the aim of every manager. It substitutes for control from outside the stricter, more exacting, and more effective control from inside. It motivates the manager to action, not because somebody tells him [sic] to do something or talks him into doing it, but because the objective task demands it. He acts not because somebody wants him to but because he himself decides that he has to—he acts, in other words, as a free man.
>
> I do not use the word "philosophy" lightly; indeed I prefer not to use it at all; it's much too big a word. But MBO and self-control may properly be called a philosophy of management. It rests on a concept of the job of management. It rests on an analysis of the specific needs of the management group and the obstacles it faces. It rests on a concept of human action, behavior, and motivation. Finally it applies to every manager, whatever his level and function, and to any organization whether large or small. It ensures performance by converting objective needs into personal goals. And this is genuine freedom.

The MBO Process

Several steps are necessary to implement the MBO process. These include learning the process, discussing specific goals, taking action, and evaluating results.

Learning the Process Understanding the MBO process should begin with the nurse managers. Managers learn the characteristics of the process, the objectives of initiating an MBO program, the procedures to be used, and the methods for evaluating the program's effectiveness. Once nurse managers learn MBO, all nursing employees are oriented to MBO. Employees define and work toward their personal objectives as they support organizational objectives. They learn the value of synergy of personal and organizational objectives.

Discussing the Goals: First Meeting The first MBO meeting with the employees should be held in quiet surroundings with sufficient time for discussion. The nurse manager should put the employee at ease. As the clinical nurse presents each personal objective, the nurse manager relates it to an objective of the organization. In this way, the manager can assess the methods for meeting the nurse's needs, including the removal of obstacles, encouragement of growth, and provision of guidance.

During this first meeting, the nurse manager and clinical nurse set specific measurable goals that are attainable and promote teamwork. Goals should involve enough risk to challenge but not defeat. They should include objectives that are routine, solve problems, are creative or innovative, and result in personal development.[7] Formulating goals is not an easy task for employees, and most people do not master goal setting immediately.

At the end of the first meeting, both the nurse manager and clinical nurse should be satisfied with the written objectives. Each will have a copy of these objectives. The nurse manager and the clinical nurse conclude with an understanding of mutual expectations on how future meetings will progress. A time for the next meeting will be established to evaluate the outcomes.

Taking Action   Employees must have sufficient time to implement established goals. Between meetings, employees perform work that meets personal and organizational objectives. An important factor in an MBO process is its emphasis on the results achieved by employees rather than the activities performed in their jobs. The employee will periodically review these objectives and summarize their accomplishments.

Evaluating Results: Second Meeting   The second MBO meeting provides a time for evaluation of results, review, appraisal, and setting additional goals. The employee is encouraged to relate gratifying experiences, perform self-evaluation, and communicate his or her thoughts about work. The nurse manager should listen with a nonjudgmental attitude to support the employee–organization fit. Managers examine their own reactions without criticizing the employees to build trust and confidence. Together managers and employees can establish the climate for personal and organizational achievement.[8]

MBO should include the staff's appraisal of the manager regarding how well the manager helps employees do their jobs, supports them, assists with problems, and demonstrates proficiency and visibility. Both nurse managers and employees should exit the second meeting with a sense of accomplishment. Deficiencies and shortcomings are recognized in the form of needed additions or changes, increased progress, and even deletions. All relate to patient care and organizational development. The process tells the employee what is expected and provides constructive feedback when an error has been made.

The MBO process is repeated at intervals. At the end of an appraisal period, a performance results contract is signed by both the employee and the manager. The performance appraisal can be used to identify promotion potential and to determine merit pay increases.

Problems with MBO

MBO must be viewed as genuine and fair by all employees. It must allow for errors and for adjustments that result from work constraints and individual capabilities. The following are some specific problems of MBO:

1. Top management is not supportive.
2. Inconsistency exists among managers.
3. Goals are too easy or are unattainable.
4. Conflicts between goals and policies exist.
5. Accountability is beyond the control of employees.
6. Employees lack commitment.

MBO is a superb tool if the objectives are (1) simple, (2) focused on what's important, (3) genuinely created from the bottom up (the objectives are drafted by the person who must accomplish them, with no constraining guides), and (4) a "living" contract, not a form-driven exercise. MBO should promote flexibility.[9]

Some leaders recommend management by results rather than MBO. When using management by results, managers should ensure that key results include quantity, quality, and cost of outcomes. Subjectivity and favoritism should be avoided to prevent resentment and distrust. Workers should be rewarded for results. When possible, work groups should be rewarded so that people share information and work together.

When using management by results, follow these principles:

1. Employees are capable of crafting solutions to problems because they know the system and its problems.
2. Use budget systems that fund outcomes rather than inputs.

3. Outcomes are measures of the volume of something produced and of quality.
4. Two-thirds of workers today work more with their minds than with their bodies.
5. The work force comes from a society with great cultural diversity.[10]

Organizational Development

Organizational development advances the internal capacity of the agency to effectively and efficiently accomplish its mission and sustain itself over time. Organizational development allows the organization to be evaluated by goals and results. Organizational development occurs as management skills and organizational processes are applied to shape and develop the conditions for human effectiveness. These conditions include the following[11]:

- Interpersonal competence. The individual has high expectations, respect for others, honest relationships, freedom to act, and a team orientation.
- Meaningful goals. The goals are understandable, desirable, attainable, and synergistic. The individual influences the goals.
- Helpful systems. Users understand and control systems because systems are goal-oriented and provide feedback. Users adapt to and adopt systems.
- Achievement and self-actualization. As the organization grows, the individual grows. People are committed to goals, are highly motivated, and have high trust and minimal dissatisfaction.

The management philosophy should support these conditions for human effectiveness. Management practices emphasize meaningful work, delegated decision making with defined limits, and accountability met by evaluating results.

Benchmarking and Six Sigma Strategies

MBO provides a mechanism in which an organization can compare goal setting to goal attainment. Another method of comparison is benchmarking. "Benchmarking is simply comparison of one's own activity or results with the level of activity or results of another department or organization."[12] External benchmarking sources include Joint Commission on Accreditation of Healthcare Organizations, the American Society for Testing and Materials, and American Health Information Management Association, which provide best practice models within their respective industries. Benchmarks prescribe measures to direct a quality organization and work force. Six Sigma is an approach to quality management and continuous improvement. This strategy is based on measurement and statistical analysis that incorporates process improvement teams to minimize variation from the desired norms. Teams work together through a process described as DMAIC[13]:

- <u>D</u>efine (project goals and customers/clients, both internal and external)
- <u>M</u>easure (processes to determine performance)
- <u>A</u>nalyze (determine root cause(s) of defect)
- <u>I</u>mprove (eliminate defect)
- <u>C</u>ontrol (future process performance)

Figure 12-2 lists the standards for evaluating the directing function.

Theories of Motivation

Motivation is a concept used to describe both the extrinsic conditions that stimulate certain behavior and the intrinsic responses that demonstrate that behavior. The intrinsic response is sustained by sources of energy, termed motives—often described as needs, wants, or drives. All people have motives.

FIGURE 12-2 | **STANDARDS FOR EVALUATING THE DIRECTING FUNCTION**

1. Managers have established a medium by which nursing workers feel free to ask for advice, counsel, and consultation.

2. Necessary written directions are available in the form of policies, procedures, standards of care, job analyses, job descriptions, job standards, and nursing care plans. They are clearly stated and current and are kept to a minimal number.

3. A training program is in effect that meets nursing employees' needs as they perceive them. They participate.

4. Supervisors are competent in needed knowledge and skills of administration and clinical specialization.

5. Nurse managers periodically work evening, night, weekend, and holiday shifts to keep abreast of clinical and administrative behaviors peculiar to these shifts.

6. The nurse administrator has operationalized the American Nurses Association (ANA) *Scope and Standards for Nurse Administrators*.

7. The nurse managers have operationalized the ANA *Standards of Clinical Nursing Practice*.

8. Nurse managers are knowledgeable about and apply the appropriate standards of the Joint Commission on Accreditation of Healthcare Organizations, National League for Nursing, Medicare, and Medicaid.

9. The nurse administrator uses techniques of operations analysis. (This service is available at no charge to member hospitals of the American Hospital Association and its state affiliates.)

10. Nurse managers use a system of management by objectives or results.

11. The nurse administrator works with the consent and knowledge of patients and solicits input from consumers regarding nursing services desired.

12. Nursing unit personnel are organized into and working as direct care personnel and clerical personnel.

13. Nurse managers use the physical plant to the best advantage for patients and personnel.

Source: Author.

Motivation is measured by observable and recorded behaviors. Deficiencies in needs stimulate people to seek and achieve goals to satisfy these needs. Consider the following questions:

- What motivates registered nurses to pursue areas of specialization?
- What motivates a nurse to go the extra mile with a patient and family?
- Why are some nurses goal oriented and others not?
- Why are some nurses dedicated to improving the quality of people's lives, whereas others merely exert minimal effort to maintain it?

The answer to the preceding questions is motivation. Some nurses are motivated to excel and be creative; others put forth just enough effort to do the job. Managers' beliefs about motivation are reflected in their personal management styles. Theories of motivation have been classified into various categories such as content theories and process theories. Key theories for consideration are presented.

Content Theories

Content theories of motivation focus on factors or needs within a person that energizes, direct, sustain, and stop behavior. The most widely recognized work in motivation theory is that of Maslow. Although not universally accepted because of its lack of scientific evidence or research base, Maslow's work is universally known.

Nursing includes human motives and goals that are created, renewed, and maintained. Nurses are motivated by physiological needs, social needs, ego needs, and self-fulfillment or self-actualization needs. Many nurses are motivated by cognitive needs for knowledge and understanding. Nurses are motivated by aesthetic needs for beauty, symmetry, simplicity, and order and by their need to express themselves. How many of these needs are related to a nurse's desire to keep learning and applying new knowledge and skills? What can the nurse manager do to motivate a nurse? The motivation may be a feeling of identification with people in general, love for human beings, a desire to help people, the need to earn a living or express oneself, or a combination of all these needs working together. An individual's needs are diverse and unique.[14]

Alderfer, who reduced Maslow's hierarchy of needs from five to three, developed a second content theory of motivation: existence (E), relatedness (R), and growth (G) (the term ERG theory). To compare Alderfer's scheme with Maslow's, existence needs to correspond to physiological and safety needs; relatedness needs to belongingness, social, and love needs; and growth needs to self-esteem and self-actualization.

Whereas Maslow's theory proposes that the next level of needs emerges when the predominant (satisfaction–progression) ones have been fulfilled, Alderfer's theory adds a frustration–regression process. When higher level needs are frustrated, people regress to the satisfaction of lower level needs.[15]

Limited research is available to support or sustain the ERG theory. As with other theories of motivation, nurse leaders should become familiar with ERG. Herzberg's research on a third content theory labeled a two-factor theory of motivation. One set of factors—dissatisfiers—is extrinsic conditions or hygiene factors. These factors include salary, job security, working conditions, status, company policy, quality of technical supervision, and quality of interpersonal relations among peers, with supervisors, and with employees. These factors must be maintained in quantity and quality to prevent dissatisfaction. These conditions become dissatisfiers when not equitably administered, causing low performance and negative attitudes. The other set of factors—satisfiers—are intrinsic conditions or motivators, which include achievement, recognition, responsibility, advancement, the work itself, and the possibility of growth. They create opportunities for high satisfaction, high motivation, and high performance. The individual must be free to attain intrinsic conditions. Both factors, hygiene and motivation, must be implemented simultaneously.

McClelland proposed and researched a fourth content theory of motivation closely associated with learning concepts, the learned needs theory. The three primary groups of learned needs acquired from the culture are the need for achievement, the need for affiliation, and the need for power. McClelland used the Thematic Apperception Test (TAT) to measure the need for achievement. He contended that needs can be learned through organizational and nonorganizational meetings. Persons high in the need for achievement want to set their own performance goals, which they prefer to be moderate and achievable. They want immediate feedback, and they like responsibility for solving problems.[15]

Many nursing personnel enjoy working together and are motivated by these affiliations. In some situations, such as in nursing homes, nurses do not get the recognition they need from clients, so they look for it from colleagues. Some nurses want to socialize on the job. They enjoy and prefer group-centered work activities, teamwork, interdependence, dependability, and predictability. The nurse manager works with these nurses to maintain this affiliation need at a mutually acceptable level.

Process Theories

Process theories deal with variables such as expectancies and attitudes "that are amenable to modification only indirectly in response to variation in one or more exogenous variables." Four endogenous theories are as follows[16]:

1. Arousal–activation theory, which focuses on internal processes that mediate the effects of conditions of work on performance

2. Expectancy–valence theory, which focuses on people's expectations that their efforts will result in good performance and on valued outcomes

3. Equity theory, which focuses on fair treatment; inputs from the employee will result in equal inputs from the employer

4. Intention–goal theory, which focuses on performance as determined by commitment to goals

Most behavior within organizations is learned behavior: perceptions, attitudes, goals, emotional reactions, and skills. Practice that occurs during the learning process can result in enduring change in behavior. Skinner advanced a process theory of motivation called operant conditioning, or behavior modification. Learning occurs as a consequence of behavior. Behaviors are the operants, controlled by altering the consequences with reinforcers or punishments.

Desired behaviors should be rewarded or reinforced, increasing the strength of a response or inducing its repetition. Continuous reinforcement speeds up early performance. Intermittent reinforcement at fixed or variable ratios sustains performance. Reinforcers tend to weaken over time, and new ones have to be developed.

Undesirable organizational behavior should not be rewarded. Although frequently used, punishment creates negative attitudes and can decrease employee morale. Behaviorists believe that people repeat behavior when consequences are positive.

Behavior modification is used by large companies, resulting in improved attendance, productivity, efficiency, and cost savings. Reinforcers center on praise, recognition, and feedback. The problem-solving method below is used to apply behavior modification[17]:

1. Identify and define (observe and measure) the specific behavior.
2. Measure or count the occurrences.
3. Analyze the antecedents, behaviors, and consequences of the behavior.
4. Perform positive reinforcement, negative reinforcement/punishment, or extinguish the behavior. Positive reinforcement is best because people repeat behavior that is rewarded and avoid behavior that is punished.
5. Evaluate changes. Provide feedback for reinforcement or correction. Follow-up reinforcement motivates people to put plans into effect because of the attention generated.

A second process theory of motivation is Vroom's expectancy theory, which postulates that a person voluntarily controls most behaviors. The effort–performance expectancy is a person's belief that a chance exists for a certain effort to lead to a particular level of performance. The performance–outcome expectancy is the belief that this person will have certain outcomes. Given choices, the individual selects the one with the best expected outcome. Research on expectancy theory is increasing although not systematic or refined. [18]

Equity theory is a third process theory. Persons believe they are being treated with equity when the ratio of their efforts to rewards equals those of others. Equity can be achieved or restored by changing outputs, attitudes, the reference person, inputs or outputs of the reference person, or the situation. Research on equity theory has focused on pay.[19]

A fourth process theory of motivation is the goal-setting theory of Locke. This theory is based on goals as determinants of behavior. The more specific the goals, the better the results produced. Research indicates that goals are a powerful force. Goals must be achievable; their difficulty level should be increased only to the level to which the person commits. Goal clarity and accurate feedback increase security.[20]

Maslow

Maslow's theory of motivation is based on a holistic–dynamic theory. At the base of a needs system are the physiologic needs, based on homeostasis, a condition of constancy of body fluids, functions, and states. The constancy is maintained automatically by uniform interaction of counteracting processes. Human beings do not just eat; they eat selectively to maintain homeostasis. The same is probably true of other physiological needs, although not all physiological needs are homeostatic. Some are relatively independent of each other while at the same time interdependent. For example, smoking may satisfy the hunger need in some persons. Some needs are in opposition to each other, such as the tendency to be lazy and the desire to be industrious.

Maslow proposed that human needs are organized in a hierarchy of prepotency: Higher needs emerge as lower ones are satisfied. When the physiological needs are satisfied, they no longer motivate the human being. However, a person tolerates deprivation of a long-satisfied need better than one that has been long or previously deprived.

When unsatisfied, physiological needs are the most potent, the strongest, of human needs. A starving person will steal food and perform other acts that threaten his or her safety. The dominance of a physiological need changes the individual's philosophy for the future.

Safety needs are the second group in the hierarchy. Among these are security, protection, dependency, and stability; freedom from anxiety, chaos, and fear; need for order, limits, structure, and law; and strength in the protector. Satisfaction of these needs influences a person's values and philosophy of life. What threatens the safety of nursing? Are nurses threatened by increased consumer interest in their shortcomings, which may lead to consumer control of practice? What motivates people? Is it a fear of the high cost of extended illnesses and results of poor care? The average person likes law, order, predictability, and organization, which may be one reason that people resist change. Insurance programs, job tenure, and savings accounts are expressions of safety needs. People prefer familiar to unknown things. Today's managers are often threatened by the new generation of personnel who question regulations and use the law to achieve their goals.

Once the physiological and safety needs have been satisfied, the needs for love, affection, and belonging emerge. Most nurses in practice today have had their physiological and safety needs satisfied. Now they want to be part of a group or family with love, acceptance, friendliness, and a feeling of belonging. Are these needs thwarted by frequent moves? How are the needs of the individual, as well as those of the organization, satisfied? A society that wants to survive and be healthy will work to satisfy these needs. Otherwise, people will be maladjusted and exhibit severe emotional and behavioral pathology.

Two categories emerge under the fourth set of needs, the esteem needs. All people share these needs. First, they desire strength, achievement, adequacy, mastery and competence, confidence before the world, independence, and freedom. Second, they desire reputation or prestige, status, fame and glory, dominance, recognition, attention, importance, dignity, or appreciation. A person whose self-esteem is satisfied has feelings of self-confidence, worth, strength, capability, adequacy, usefulness, and being needed in society. For self-esteem to be stable and healthy, it must be based on known or deserved respect. The reason for self-esteem must be known and recognized by its recipient.

Finally, at the pinnacle of the hierarchy of needs is the emotional gold—the need for self-actualization, the effort of people to be what they can be. Nurses want to become everything that they are capable of becoming, to achieve their potential, to be effective nurses, to be creative, and to meet personal standards of performance.

Certain conditions are prerequisites to satisfying basic needs. When basic needs are thwarted, the individual feels threatened. These necessary conditions include the following:

- Freedom to speak (communication)
- Freedom to do what one wishes to do without harming others (choice of jobs, friends, and entertainment)
- Freedom to express oneself (creativity)
- Freedom to investigate and seek information
- Freedom to defend oneself (justice, fairness, honesty, and orderliness in the group)

The hierarchy of needs is not a simple classification. Individuals order their needs differently. Some place self-esteem before love; others place creativity before all else. Certain people have low levels of aspiration.

A long-satisfied need may become undervalued. A person who has never been deprived of a particular need does not regard the need as important. If two needs emerge, a person will probably want the more basic one satisfied first. People who have loved and been well loved and who have had many deep friendships can hold out against hatred, rejection, or persecution.

Most normal persons in our society have partially satisfied and partially dissatisfied basic needs at the same time. They may have more satisfied physiological needs and correspondingly fewer satisfied self-actualization needs. New needs emerge gradually and are more often unconscious than conscious. Basic needs are common throughout different cultures. Most behavior is multidetermined: All the basic needs are involved. A single act of an individual could be analyzed to show how it addresses physiological needs, safety needs, love needs, esteem needs, and self-actualization needs. Not all behavior is internally motivated; some is stimulated externally. Some is highly motivated, some weakly, and some not at all. Some is expressive and some rote. A gratified or satisfied need is not a motivator of behavior. Healthy persons are primarily motivated by the need to develop and actualize their fullest potential and capabilities.

Usefulness to Nurse Managers

Motivational theory has been used in a number of studies of behavior modification for smoking cessation, weight control, exercise, and general reduction of cardiovascular risk factors. To date, modifying risk-taking behavior has had limited positive results.

Although much has been written about motivation, there is no easy way to motivate employees. Human motivation is diverse, subtle, and complex. Some theories of motivation are contradictory. Nurse managers who apply motivation theory may help alleviate dissatisfactions of nurses. To use motivation theory effectively, the nurse manager selects and uses those elements that appear to be practical and workable.

Nurse as Knowledge Worker

Knowledge worker comprises those individuals who work for their living by developing or using knowledge in contrast with persons who work for their living by manual labor. Nurses are knowledge workers. Peter Drucker defined this term in 1959, suggesting that knowledge workers are productive only with self-motivation, self-direction, and achievement. The nurse as knowledge worker is self-directed and assumes responsibility. Rewarding and reaffirming self-direction and responsibility produces learning.

Nurses perform work of equal difficulty and want economic rewards of equal value to those of other knowledge workers. Economic rewards that are mismanaged can create dissatisfaction with work, becoming deterrents to job satisfaction and productivity.[21] Pay is part of the social or psychological need of nurses. They also want rank, power, and status commensurate with those of other knowledge workers.

More formal education and skills translate into higher incomes and increased living standards. Money invested in education is an investment in the economic health and future of the United States. Educated people are mobile. Nurses can move to jobs in other organizations. Highly skilled workers can switch jobs more easily, and therefore spend less time unemployed, than can unskilled workers.

When used inappropriately, discipline can cause resentment and resistance, becoming a demotivator. Direction and control are useless in meeting ego needs. Unsatisfied needs lead to negative behavior. To focus on needs already satisfied is ineffective; however, employers should consider the self-esteem and self-actualization need of employees. Otherwise, money becomes the only means used to try to satisfy needs. At some point, money and material rewards fail as incentives or managerial tools.

Nurses are independent adults who want to be treated with dignity and respect. The organization should recognize that practicing clinical nurses achieve healthcare productivity gains, not capital spending and automation. Nurses may believe they are competent and able to do good work. They are dissatisfied because organizational resources do not allow them to meet the standard of care they consider appropriate. Nurses want to provide high quality care for their patients.

Science of Human Behavior

An entire branch of science has tried to determine why people act the way they do. Finding the answers to this question is not easy, and there have been no hard-and-fast answers. People behave the way they do for a reason, although the reason may be not be clear, logical, or rational. Douglas McGregor, in his book *The Human Side of Enterprise*, published in 1966, examined theories of behavior of individuals at work. He formulated two models, known as Theory X and Theory Y.

Theory X and Theory Y

Douglas McGregor's theories of leadership and motivation remain influential. The following concepts summarize Theory X[22]:

1. Management is responsible for organizing the elements of productive enterprise—money, materials, equipment, people—in the interest of economic ends.
2. With respect to people, this is a process of directing their efforts, motivating them, controlling their actions, and modifying their behavior to fit the needs of the organization.
3. Without this active intervention by management, people would be passive—even resistant—to organizational needs. They must therefore be persuaded, rewarded, punished, and controlled; their activities must be directed. This is management's task—in managing subordinate managers or workers. We often sum it up by saying that management consists of getting things done through other people.
4. The average person is by nature indolent—he or she works as little as possible.
5. He or she lacks ambition, dislikes responsibility, and prefers to be led.
6. He or she is inherently self-centered, indifferent to organizational needs.
7. He or she is by nature resistant to change.
8. He or she is gullible, not very bright, the ready dupe of the charlatan and the demagogue.

The following precepts summarize Theory Y:

1. Management is responsible for organizing the elements of productive enterprise—money, materials, equipment, people—in the interest of economic ends.
2. People are not by nature passive or resistant to organizational needs. They have become so as a result of experience in organizations.
3. The motivation, the potential for development, the capacity for assuming responsibility, and the readiness to direct behavior toward organizational goals are all present in people. Management does not put them there. It is the responsibility of management to make it possible for people to recognize and develop these characteristics for themselves.
4. The essential task of management is to arrange organizational conditions and methods of operation so that people can achieve their own goals best by directing their own efforts toward organizational objectives.

Based on this theory, McGregor suggests that managers subscribe to one of these viewpoints. Managers who subscribe to Theory X typically maintain tight control over workers, provide almost constant supervision, try to motivate through fear, and make decisions in an autocratic fashion, eliciting little or no input from their subordinates. However, this creates a dilemma in that Theory X managers do not take into account people's needs for companionship, esteem, and personal growth.

Theory Y subscribers, in contrast, assume that workers like to work and that under proper conditions seek out responsibility in an attempt to satisfy their social, esteem, and self-actualization needs. Theory Y managers maintain less control and supervision, do not use fear as the primary motivator, and are more democratic in decision making, allowing subordinates to participate in the process.

Nurse Managers as the Motivator

Nurse managers should apply techniques, skills, and knowledge, such as motivational theory, to help nursing staff obtain their personal and professional goals. At the same time these efforts should support the mission of the institution and the division of nursing.

To persuade people to achieve nursing and organizational goals requires many abilities in the nurse manager: sensitivity to people, energy and negotiating skills, and capability to facilitate mutual goal setting among the leader, the profession, and the organization. To successfully lead today's nurses, nurse managers should be aware of the findings of motivational research and apply them to personnel management.

Some authors say that one person cannot motivate another and that motivation lies within the individual. The manager should use motivation and incentives that are meaningful to the nurse; the nurse selects his or her course of action. A successful contract depends on the employer's authority to give or withhold rewards and the employee's level of aspiration.

Motivation is a psychological process. The nurse leader should help the nurse to use available tools to achieve their goals. These motivators include associations with people on the job, using their skills at work, and recognition for a satisfactory performance. Motivational patterns are learned early and followed for years. Often, no conscious selection, judgment, or decision making is involved in chosen actions. Each individual is unique, with personally defined behaviors. Within each individual, motivating needs differ from time to time. The key is to determine which need is currently predominant.

Motivational theory asserts that when people no longer struggle with the necessities of life and reach a level of security, they pursue goals associated with higher level needs. These needs include control over their fate, self-respect, using and increasing their talents, responsibility, and achievement. They seek ways to satisfy their physical needs for recreation, relaxation, and play.

Practical Approaches to Enhance Motivation

Nurse leaders can enhance staff motivation in various ways. Some of these include assistance with career planning, effective communication, and promotion of self-actualization.

Career Planning

Career planning is a continuous process of self-assessment and goal setting. Career planning is an organized system with short- and long-term career goals fitted to those of the organization. Career planning includes examination of needs, motivators, and job satisfiers. Most nurses benefit from participation in a career development program, even if it improves only the quality of their working lives.

Effective Communication

Nurse leaders can motivate nurses by sharing information about the organization. Nurse leaders consult with nurses on problems, solutions, and decisions, and they share information about results. Open and nonjudgmental communication fosters motivation.

Endorsing Teamwork

Nurse leaders can motivate practicing nurses by encouraging teamwork. Teams can discuss and resolve work-related issues. Teams should have identifiable output, inclusive membership, agreement on purpose, and measurable goals, resources, and feedback. Teams are successful because they pool interpersonal skills, knowledge, and the expertise needed to accomplish goals effectively and efficiently.

Teamwork helps workers achieve personal recognition, raise self-esteem, and increase motivation and commitment. It is stimulated by trust, support, completion, acknowledgment, communication, and agreement.[23]

Building Self-Esteem

The manager must understand the importance of self-esteem to motivation. Being held in esteem by others because of personal accomplishments and reputation provides status and recognition, leading to appreciation and respect. Self-esteem is gained through achievement of goals, adequacy, mastery, confidence, and independence. Self-esteem comes from satisfaction as a person in society and as a worker. Individuals must be free to express themselves, to seek information, and to defend themselves. They must be treated with justice, fairness, and honesty.

People meet their esteem needs in different ways. They are influenced by culture, including the culture of the organization in which they work. The results of achieving self-esteem are more important than the roads taken to achieve those ends. All human beings want to be esteemed. Meeting the self-esteem needs of employees is of great significance to managers in nursing.

Managers can set the conditions under which professional nurses become committed to organizational goals and exercise self-control and self-direction, which leads to creativity. Strategic planning by top management can involve professional clinical nurse participation. The strategic plan can then be submitted to the department level for input by clinical nurses and other professionals. They critique the plan, strengthen it, and make it one to which nurses can commit. This management process gives professional nurses new knowledge and skills, opportunity for creativity, and recognition and prestige in the eyes of others, meeting the need for self-esteem.

Encouraging Self-Actualization

Self-actualization is defined by Maslow as an ego need at the top of the needs hierarchy. Self-actualization does not exist in isolation. Self-actualized persons have the following characteristics:

- Ability to see reality more clearly than do others.
- Comfort with and attraction to the unknown.
- Creativity in whatever they do and perceive.
- Less defensiveness; acceptance of and adjustment to their own shortcomings.
- Discomfort when they are not doing something to improve their shortcomings, prejudices, jealousies, envy, and other faults.
- Autonomous codes of ethics.
- Ability to conform easily when no great issues are involved.
- Acceptance of their own nature, human nature, the realities of social life, and the constraints of physical reality.
- Problem-centered, not ego-centered.
- Broad and universal values.
- Deeply democratic, as opposed to authoritarian, natures; thus they respect others.
- A strong sense of right and wrong, of good and evil.
- Not interested in hostile humor. Their humor is of a philosophical bent, stated only to produce a laugh.

- Self-movers.
- Detachment and objectivity in conditions of turmoil.

The self-actualized person achieves a highly satisfactory quality of life that extends from the gratified self into society. The social environment of work can positively influence gratification or satisfaction of the higher level needs.

The nurse leader should selectively apply knowledge and skills of the social and behavioral sciences to create an environment or climate in which practicing nurses can become self-actualized. In doing so, nurse managers themselves become self-actualized. The products and services of nursing increase in quantity and quality.

Other Activities to Stimulate Motivation

Motivation is stimulated by activities such as job enrichment, praise, empowerment, promotions, inclusion, and focus on vision, values, and strategy. Managers should recognize the value of people by trusting, respecting, and encouraging them. They should tie rewards to values of teamwork, innovation, safety, growth, and profitability and provide employees with financial and nonfinancial rewards.

Managers can motivate employees by offering various work options:

- Paternity leave or work-at-home policies.
- Reduced work week schedules, job sharing, unpaid leaves of absence, and early retirement.
- Rearranged workdays to allow parents to attend children's school functions or meet other personal and family needs.
- Child or elder care assistance.

Evidence-Based Practice 12-1

McGuire et al. describes their work in the implementation and evaluation of the critical care assistant (CCA) role within a large teaching trust. Pilot work was undertaken with nine CCAs employed across six critical care units. To establish the influence of the new role on the critical care time and this role's contribution to patient care, a multiple stakeholder evaluation was performed. The evaluation was a questionnaire format and focus group interviews. This was undertaken over a 6-month period. Mixed results were observed, with some improvements noted especially within high-dependency care. This was particularly noticeable where the introduction of the role eased some of the work load pressures on qualified staff and allowed nurses to focus on the more dependent patients. As part of the study, a structured education and training program was implemented and supported by the National Vocational Qualification, Level 3. This program helped to prepare the CCAs theoretically for the extension in their role. Difficulties were experienced with the appropriate allocation of tasks and general communication with nursing staff. Patients and relatives feedback were sought and positively evaluated as they were satisfied with the standard of care received. There was a noted comfort level with a CCA providing their care, supporting the future development of the role.[24]

SUMMARY

Effective directing results in greater harmony in the actions of managers and employees as they achieve mutual objectives. Directing that encourages leadership, motivation, and communication and emphasizes the human aspects of managing individuals is most desirable. Personal and motivational goals are met as the nurse becomes responsible, shows initiative, supports fellow nurses and the employing institution, welcomes change, and demonstrates individual abilities.

Effective leadership can be fostered by nursing administrators who desire to improve their directing or leading activities. The following rule leads to successful leadership in nursing: Find out where nurses want to go and what they want to accomplish, then mesh these goals with those of the organization. In this way, nurses accomplish organizational goals as they achieve their own.

APPLICATION EXERCISES

Exercise 12-1
Look at the statements of mission, philosophy, vision, and objectives of a division of nursing in which you work as a student or an employee.

1. What is the work of the unit or division?
2. What is the implication for the directing function of the unit or division?

Exercise 12-2
Scenario: As a nurse manager, Ms. Pressley, RN, believes that clinical nurses do not really have careers. However, a clinical ladder is nonexistent within this healthcare facility. Ms. Pressley plans to counsel her clinical nurses regularly and to advocate for a clinical promotion ladder that recognizes advanced competence, education, and certification. This activity falls within the directing category of management. Compare Ms. Pressley's actions with those of several other nurse managers you know or have known. Summarize your findings.

Exercise 12-3
Select one or more goals you would like to accomplish in the unit in which you work as a student or employee. Make a management plan to accomplish them.

1. State your individual objectives.
2. Have a plan for achieving each objective.
3. Discuss and adjust your plan with your supervisor.
4. Set a time to evaluate accomplishments with your supervisor.

Exercise 12-4
Use Figure 12-2, Standards for Evaluating the Directing Function, to evaluate one of the entities in the organization where you work as a student or employee. Identify one concrete example for each standard. Summarize your results. If the directing function does not meet the standards, use a problem-solving approach and implement a plan of improvement.

Exercise 12-5
Use Figure 12-3, Future Goals Worksheet, to develop a list of goals. Once you have them written down, you can evaluate them using Figure 12-4, Goal Evaluation Checklist.

Exercise 12-6
Small Group Session

1. Write a statement that provides a vision of what you want to accomplish in stimulating the motivation of your peers or employees. (20 minutes)
2. Outline a process for accomplishing this vision. (20 minutes)
3. Report.

Exercise 12-7
Scenario: Ms. Sanchez has been director of nursing of a 250-bed hospital for 8 years. Although her management operation has followed traditional patterns, she has read extensively on the subject and has

FIGURE 12-3 FUTURE GOALS WORKSHEET

You should set goals in at least three areas:

1. Personal goals. What would you really like to do with your life? Write down the personal goals you want to accomplish. Examples are "Become a role model for the profession," "Achieve as a writer in the field of staff development," or "Serve people who need but lack the means to buy health care."

2. Family goals. Do you want to save money to travel? To put yourself and your family through school? To supplement a primary income? To buy something special? You may want to discuss these goals with your spouse and children, but write down your family goals.

3. Professional goals. Do you want to become a professor, a director of nursing, a consultant in nursing care of cancer patients, or a clinical researcher? Something outside of nursing altogether? Write down your professional goals.

Source: Author.

FIGURE 12-4 GOAL EVALUATION CHECKLIST

Standards for Evaluating Goals	Yes	No
1. I have reviewed my short-term goals within the past 3 months.		
2. I have reviewed my long-term goals within the past year.		
3. My goals reflect my personal beliefs and the purpose or reason I want to achieve them.		
4. My goals can be measured or verified as being achieved.		
5. I have set my goals in the priority or sequence in which I want to accomplish them.		
6. My goals are clear to me. They are specific and indicate actions to take to achieve them.		
7. My goals are flexible and realistic so that I will have as many opportunities as possible.		
8. I have the resources to accomplish my goals.		
9. My goals are stated for a specific job.		

Source: Author.

been taking business administration courses in the evenings at the state university. Ms. Sanchez has decided to make some management changes in her department.

Although meetings with members of the nursing staff had been held on a scheduled basis, they were never productive and served mainly as a medium for information to flow from management downward. Ms. Sanchez carefully planned an agenda for her next staff development faculty meeting and distributed it a week in advance. An item of new business on the agenda was to write specific objectives for these meetings that would benefit the members and ultimately the nursing employees throughout the institution. At the same time, Ms. Sanchez would present a working draft of an operational plan for accomplishing the objectives of the department of nursing. The staff development nurse group would be asked to discuss the departmental mission, philosophy, objectives, and operational plan to determine whether the statements express a vision that would motivate nursing personnel.

At the meeting, Ms. Sanchez was pleased with the active participation by the members. They had many suggestions for changes and for additional activities that would be helpful in achieving the mission, philosophy, objectives, and operational plan. During the discussion Ms. Sanchez learned about much major dissatisfaction of the personnel. For example, they did not understand the personnel rating system and wanted to know how she arrived at decisions for promotions. One of the suggested activities for accomplishment of objectives was that job standards be written and that they use the American Nurses Association standards for nursing practice as a basis for them. The members appointed an ad-hoc committee to do this, without the prodding of Ms. Sanchez, and they set a target date for completion. It was their intent to help Ms. Sanchez strengthen the objectivity of the rating system, thereby giving them input into the promotion process. The members also made plans to expand the project through inclusion of representatives of the entire nursing staff.

Next, Ms. Sanchez asked if the statements of the department's mission, philosophy, objectives, and operational plan should be presented to all the nursing staff, and a large majority of members agreed that they should. They also recommended that Ms. Sanchez do this, because the staff would be impressed with being able to discuss these important statements with the boss. A suggestion was made that Ms. Sanchez meet with the staff of each unit; the ad-hoc committee members wrote a schedule that was acceptable to her. The committee then decided to assist unit personnel with developing or revising statements of mission, philosophy, and objectives, and operational plans for each of the units and to have them done by a specific date.

Ms. Sanchez discussed means of encouraging the nursing staff to be more productive and better satisfied with their working conditions. Several suggestions were made by the staff development nurse group. These included modifications in policies related to the uniform, staffing, and time schedules. The nurses also stated that many nursing personnel had expressed the desire to become more involved in unit in-service education and other nursing activities but had not been encouraged to do so. Ms. Sanchez said she would welcome all suggestions for change but that she could not guarantee that all would take place immediately, because some would have to be approved by the hospital administrator. If Ms. Sanchez did not agree with any of the recommendations she would tell the people involved the reasons why. They agreed that this was acceptable to them, and the meeting was adjourned. From this scenario,

1. Identify a factor that encourages or discourages freedom to speak, that is, communication.
2. Identify a factor that encourages or discourages freedom to do what one wishes to do without harming others, that is, choice of jobs, friends, or entertainment.
3. Identify a factor that encourages or discourages freedom to express oneself, that is, creativity.
4. Identify a factor that encourages or discourages freedom to defend oneself, justice, fairness, honesty, or orderliness in the group.
5. Identify a factor that encourages or discourages freedom to investigate and seek information.

Exercise 12-8

Scenario: Ms. Rather is in charge of pediatric unit and encourages employees to discuss their families and their off-duty activities. They tell her of their hopes and dreams and even of confidential personal happenings.

Scenario: Mr. Pottinger is in charge of in-service education on an intensive care unit. He gives personnel needed supervision and training and supports them well while on duty. He lets it be known that he does not want to know anything about employees' personal lives unless it relates to their work.

1. Which nurse exhibits the best understanding of motivational theory? Explain your answer
2. Identify how each style affects staff motivation. List advantages and disadvantages of each.

Exercise 12-9

Using Herzberg's two-factor theory of motivation and the items in Figure 12-5, Checklist for Assessing Job Satisfaction, do the following:

1. Summarize the results of the extrinsic conditions, hygiene factors, or dissatisfiers related to yourself and your job.
2. Summarize the results of the intrinsic conditions, motivators, or satisfiers related to yourself and your job.

| FIGURE 12-5 | CHECKLIST FOR ASSESSING JOB SATISFACTION |

In my current job I am	No or Yes	Insufficient
Happy with being able to help others.		
Intellectually stimulated and challenged.		
Given opportunity to progress educationally.		
Learning new skills.		
Sharpening old skills.		
Learning a new discipline.		
Qualifying for more responsibility.		
Qualifying for more respect.		
Given opportunities to attend staff meetings, patient care conferences, and staff-development programs.		
Rewarded for doing my job well.		
Adequately paid.		
Given opportunity for advancement.		
Given opportunity to innovate and be creative.		
Given opportunity to choose shifts and hours of work.		
Given opportunity to be a leader.		
Given opportunity to grow as a bedside nurse.		
Able to trust my supervisors and peers.		
Supported by administration.		
Communicated with by administration.		
Being paid for my total knowledge and experience.		
Confident of job security.		
Working with adequate staffing.		
Feeling satisfied with my accomplishments.		
Supported by nursing management in resolving physician–nurse conflict.		
Able to resolve peer conflict.		

Adequately paid for overtime. _____

Given opportunity to schedule extra time off above and
   beyond holidays and vacation. _____

Given opportunity to schedule my working hours. _____

Prepared to function as a team leader or charge nurse. _____

Supported by competent professional nurses who assist and teach me. _____

My job satisfaction could be increased by: _____

_____

Identify specific steps to gather the information or make the changes that will help you reach your goal.

One of my job satisfaction goals is:

_____

_____

As a step toward reaching this goal I will talk to: _____

about: _____

And I will undertake the following activities myself: _____

Source: Author.

Exercise 12-10

The following is a list of matched pairs of personal characteristics. Complete the list by circling the characteristic in each pair that you think applies to you, and write a statement summarizing your personal characteristics. Make a plan to change any personal characteristics you believe should be changed to improve your self-esteem.

Personal Characteristics

A	B	A	B
Vivacious	Languid	Honest	Dishonest
Intelligent	Stupid	Truthful	False
Bright	Dull	Accurate	Deceptive
Clever	Clumsy	Confident	Pessimistic
Funny	Solemn	Respectful	Rude
Courteous	Rude	Pleasant	Obnoxious
Prompt	Late	Candid	Deceitful
Tolerant	Prejudiced	Courageous	Fearful
Gracious	Surly	Decent	Gross
Unpretentious	Complacent	Unselfish	Egotistic
Sincere	Devious	Having integrity	Fraudulent
Friendly	Antagonistic	Sincere	Sly
Humble	Arrogant		

Source: Swansburg, R. C., & Swansburg, P. W. (1984). *Strategic career planning and development for nurses* (p. 76). Rockville, MD: Aspen.

Notes

1. American Organization of Nurse Executives (AONE). (2004). *2004–2006 strategic plan.* Washington, DC: Author.
2. Koontz, H., O'Donnell, C., & Weihrich, H. (1990). *Essentials of management* (5th ed., p. 300). New York: McGraw-Hill.
3. Hansten, R. I., & Jackson, M. (2004). *Clinical delegation skills: A handbook for professional practice* (3rd ed., pp. 3–4). Sudbury, MA: Jones and Bartlett.
4. Rowland, H. S., & Rowland, B. L. (Eds.). (1992). *Nursing administration handbook* (3rd ed., p. 10). Gaithersburg, MD: Aspen.
5. Odiorne, G. S. (1965). *Management by objectives* (pp. 55–56). New York: Pitman.
6. Drucker, P. F. (1973). *Management: Tasks, responsibilities, practices* (pp. 430–442). New York: Harper & Row.
7. Bell, M. L. (1980). Management by objectives. *Journal of Nursing Administration, 10*(2), 19–26.
8. Levinson, H. (1970). Management by whose objectives? *Harvard Business Review,* 125–134.
9. Peters, T. (1987). *Thriving on chaos* (pp. 603–604). New York: Harper & Row.
10. Osborne, D., & Gaebler, T. (1992). *Reinventing government* (pp. 156–158). New York: Plume.
11. Beck, A. C., Jr., & Hillman, E. D. (1975). OD to MBO or MBO to OD: Does it make a difference? In A. T. Hollingsworth & R. M. Hodgetts (Eds.), *Readings in basic management* (pp. 190–196). Philadelphia: W. B. Saunders.
12. Liebler, J. G., & McConnell, C. R. (2004). *Management principles for health professionals* (4th ed., p. 270). Sudbury, MA: Jones and Bartlett.
13. Breyfogle, F., Cupello, J., & Meadows, B. (2000). *Managing six sigma: A practical guide to understanding, assessing and implementing the strategy that yields bottom-line success.* Indianapolis: John Wiley and Sons.
14. Maslow, A. H. (1970). *Motivation and personality* (2nd ed.). New York: Harper & Row; http://www.accel-team.com/motivation/theory
15. Gibson, J. L., Ivancevich, J. M., & Donnelly, J. M., Jr. (1994). *Organizations: Behavior, structure, processes* (8th ed., pp. 151–193). Burr Ridge, IL: Richard D. Irwin.
16. Katzell, R. A., & Thompson, D. E. (1990). Work motivation. *American Psychologist,* 144–153.
17. Gibson et al., 1994, pp. 168–193; Roach, K. L. (1984). Production builds on mutual respect. *Nursing Management,* 54–56; Youker, R. B. (1985). Ten benefits of participant action planning. *Training, 52,* 54–56.
18. Gibson et al., 1994; www.accel-team.com/motivation/theory
19. Ibid.
20. Ibid.
21. Drucker, 1973, pp. 176, 195–196.
22. McGregor, D. (1966). *The human side of enterprise* (pp. 5–6). New York: McGraw-Hill.
23. Allender, M. C. (1984). Productivity enhancement: A new teamwork approach. *National Productivity Review, 1*(1), 181–189.
24. McGuire, A., Richardson, A., Coghill, E., Platt, A., Wimpenny, S., & Eglon, P. (2007). Implementation and evaluation of the critical care assistant role. *Nursing in Critical Care, 12,* 242–249.

References

Carrigan, M. D., & Kujawa, D. (2006). Six Sigma in healthcare management and strategy. *Health Care Manager, 25,* 133–141.

de Konig, H., Verver, J. P. S., van den Heuvel, J., & Bisgaard, S. (2006). Lean six sigma in healthcare. *Journal for Healthcare Quality: Promoting Excellence in Healthcare, 28,* 4–11.

Fairbanks, C. B. (2007). Using six sigma and lean methodology to improve inputs and throughputs. *AORN Journal, 86,* 73–82.

Glower, M. M. (2006). Six sigma: bringing it to your team. *Nurse Leader, 2,* 44–46.

MacPhee, M. (2007). Strategies and tools for managing change. *Journal of Nursing Administration, 37,* 405–413.

McConnell, C. R. (2005). Motivating your employees and yourself—how different is manager from the staff? *Health Care Manager, 24,* 284–292.

Pearce, C. (2007). Leadership resource—ten steps to staff motivation. *Nursing Management, 13,* 21.

Toofany, S. (2007). Applied leadership: Team building and leadership—the key to recruitment and retention. *Nursing Management, 14,* 24–27.

13

INFORMATION MANAGEMENT AND TECHNOLOGY

Donna Faye McHaney, DNP, BSCS, RN, ARNP-C

LEARNING OBJECTIVES AND ACTIVITIES

- Document how technology has changed in the workplace and at home.
- Discuss data management and the difference between data mining and data cleansing in health care.
- Discuss computer networking and identify ways the Internet can support nursing.
- Identify personal skills and skills necessary for high-tech environments.
- Identify and discuss the purpose of various information systems.
- Illustrate uses of application software.
- Define concepts such as confidentiality, security, and privacy.

CONCEPTS

Confidentiality, data, database, information, Internet, intranet, multimedia, network, security, spreadsheet, technology, word processing, informatics, information systems.

QUOTE

The hardest thing is not to get people to accept new ideas; it is to get them to forget old ones.

—John Maynard Keynes

Introduction

The information and technology revolution is thought to be one of three fundamental changes that have taken place in society. In the classic work, *The Third Wave*, Toffler observed those three fundamental changes to be the agricultural revolution, the industrial revolution, and the information and technology revolution.[1] The information and technology revolution has redefined how we live and work, what values we place on health care and education, and our family structure.[1] Technology has made rapid progress throughout the past two centuries, revolutionizing and redefining many aspects of human life: steam engines, electricity, printing machines, vaccines, automobiles, airplanes, telephones, radio, weapons of mass destruction, satellites, television, computers, genetic engineering, cloning, and so on. The impact of technology continues with technological innovations daily. Computers are the major technological breakthrough of the past 25 to 30 years. Computers, once thought to be for business use only, now exist in many households, becoming a common part of life. Nearly every aspect of our lives has become automated with computers enhancing the process.

Although technical tools, especially computers, continue to be invented and rapidly placed in industry, the ability of organizations to accept, accommodate, and even embrace technology is moving at a varied pace. The healthcare industry has been one of the slowest businesses to embrace the computer revolution in regards to patient care even though many healthcare organizations have had their business departments functioning on computers for years. With technology creating constant transition from old to new, the healthcare industry will need to advocate education and training. "As the business world changes at an ever increasing rate, many of us are finding that our jobs require us to constantly enhance our skills and develop new ones—possibly some we never thought we'd need. Today, staying in place means falling behind, and no one can afford to do that in our technology-driven world."[2] Nursing, being one of the slowest to embrace technology to its fullest, must meet the challenges of using new technology in all aspects of information management. New skills need to be taught and learned to assimilate and use the technology involved in information management. Nurse leaders need to embrace technology, advocating and supporting its use in all nursing operations to meet the demand for high-quality care.

Health care involves the use and management of an abundance of information that must be collected, managed, reviewed, processed, and mined. High-quality patient care relies on careful documentation of every patient's medical and family history, health status, current medical conditions, and treatment plans. A clinical decision based on information that has been efficiently managed and processed lends itself to quality care outcomes. Specialty roles for nurses have developed over the past 10 to 15 years, and many nurses have found themselves in nursing informatics roles. In 1992, the American Nurses Association declared nursing informatics a specialty, and, currently, master level–prepared nurses with a certification in informatics may sit for the national exam.[3] Nursing informatics is a specialty area that integrates nursing science, computer science, and information science. This specialty area provides expertise in developing and implementing information management systems that can be used by nursing to enhance daily tasks and integrate various aspects of patient care.

Today, there are abundant resources available for healthcare environments. Multimedia that interacts with the user through text, sight, sound, and voice are commonly used. These techniques are used to seamlessly integrate technology and information that may be located within a geographical area or even across international boundaries. The use of the Internet has tooled the healthcare industry with an avenue to provide continuity of care. With advancement of technology and integration across boundaries, concerns of security and privacy continue to loom over the healthcare industry. Management must continue addressing ethical and legal issues with regard to control of information.

NURSING INFORMATICS ROLE IN HEALTH CARE

Healthcare informatics is a board term involving the application of computer and information science in all basic and biomedical sciences. Medical informatics refers to the application of informatics to all healthcare disciplines as well as to the practice of medicine.[4] Nursing informatics is the use of information and computer technology to support all aspects of nursing practice. This may include direct delivery of care, education, research, and management. Nursing informatics facilitates the integration of data, information, and knowledge to support patients, nurses, and other providers involved in the decision-making process.[4]

Managers need to collaborate with the Information Systems (IS) department in design, development, and implementation of management and clinical applications. Nurses filling roles as nursing informaticists will act as a liaison between management, staff, and the IS department. Although informatics nurses may be removed from bedside care, they remain focused on patient care while working toward improved clinical outcomes and quality care. These nurses can communicate how tasks are completed each day providing an understanding of the work flow for IS staff. Often, nurse managers may fill this role as well. The informatics nurse may fill a variety of roles. Figure 13-1 lists various roles of an informatics nurse.

DATA MANAGEMENT IN HEALTH CARE

Nurses and nursing management handle large amounts of data and information during any given day. Data are a collection of numbers, characters, or facts. These are usually gathered because they are needed for analysis or some other action at a later time. Information is a set of data that has been in-

FIGURE 13-1	ROLES OF INFORMATICS NURSES

Project manager	Informatics nurses analyze, design, develop, select, test, implement, and evaluate new or modified informatics projects that support optimal data and delivery of quality patient care.
Consultant	Consultants may take on a variety of roles, including project manager, market research, planning conferences, strategic information technology planning, reviewing clinical software, redesigning the workplace, and others. They may work for an organization or with a consulting firm.
Educator	Informatics nurses may educate staff nurses, managers, and others in using the healthcare information system. Their role would include educating all staff on confidentiality and security matters as well.
Researcher	As a researcher, the informatics nurse may research clinical situations that arise, help implement evidence-based practice, evaluate the current system for improved outcomes, and conduct research to improve clinical information systems and clinical outcomes.
Product developer	The informatics nurse may develop software applications for clinical and nonclinical healthcare environments.
Decision support/ outcomes manager	Nurses in this role use technology and other systems tools to maintain data integrity and reliability, identify outcomes, and develop performance measurements. Aggregate data are used by these nurses.
Policy developer	Nurses in this role help to develop policies for clinical and administrative health care information systems.
Chief information officer (CIO)	This role provides leadership and management at the executive level for both the organization and vendors.
Entrepreneurs/Innovator	Entrepreneurs emerge every day and informatics nurses may fit here by managing their own practice, developing applications, or owning their own healthcare information systems business.
Other	Many other roles exist and will emerge as health care continues to embrace the technology that expands.

Source: Author.
American Nurses Association (2006). *Scope and standards of nursing informatics practice.* Nursesbooks.org.: Silver Spring, MD.
Hebda, T., Czar, P., & Mascara, C. (2005). *Handbook of informatics for nurses & health care professionals.* Pearson Education, Inc.: Upper Saddle River, New Jersey.

terpreted covering some aspect of time, such as over the course of a day. Figure 13-2 shows examples of data and information.

Knowledge can be defined as applying facts or ideas acquired by study, investigation, observation, or experience.[5] It is the synthesis of information that may have been derived from several sources producing a concept or idea. Nurses acquire knowledge over time and use it extensively in their daily task of direct patient care. Data collection, with the aid of computer and information technology, helps to provide evidence of best practices supported by research. This collection of evidence-based information provides a substantial database of knowledge that can be applied to everyday practice situations. See Evidence-Based Practice 13-1 for an evidence-based practice example.

Data Integrity

It is not enough to collect data, interpret it, and build a database of knowledge. Data that make up the database of information must be maintained with optimal assurance that quality data exist. Data

FIGURE 13-2	EXAMPLES OF DATA AND INFORMATION

Time	Temperature	Pulse	Respirations
0730	99.2 F	66	18
1130	99.8 F	69	20
0400	101.4 F	74	22
0800	102.2 F	82	24

Source: Author.

Each single value in the table represents data, and the entire table represents a collection of data over a course of a day. The trend of the data represents information. Trends are more useful than single data to the healthcare provider.

Fictitious data, for illustration purposes only.

Evidence-Based Practice 13-1

Knowledge can be seen when nurses use the most effective nursing interventions for the prevention of skin breakdown. Quality care aimed at preventing skin breakdown has been identified as a nursing priority and evidence-based research drives the interventions when appropriately implemented. Studies such as that of Harrison, Logan, Joseph, and Graham[6] provide interventions that address prevention of skin breakdown.

integrity must be maintained so that current data are available when needed. If data integrity is less than optimal, it could result in inappropriate decisions that could possibly harm a patient. Quality data have characteristics that can be identified. Data must be timely, accurate, rapidly and easily available, precise, clear, comprehensive, reliable regardless of whom collects it, easy to interpret, current, and appropriate for the user's needs.[4,7] Following policies that identify procedures for collection, validation, storage, management, and retrieval of data results in quality data. Quality data are needed for nurses to make sound clinical decisions and potentially impacts patient care.

Several techniques exist to help alleviate erroneous data. These techniques include educating staff, system prompts, various verification techniques, data mining, and data cleansing.

Educating Staff

Today, most nurses lack skills that enable them to integrate information technology into practice. The Institute of Medicine has strongly emphasized that informatics is a core competency required of healthcare professions, including nursing. It is time for nursing to embrace technology with care and become a part of the information and technology revolution. Educating staff is vital to having quality data and reducing erroneous data. Nurses should have a general understanding of how to use software, enter data, extract data, print reports, and evaluate data to make good clinical decisions. Nurses need to be taught for the future. They need to know how to find information and procedures rather than know, they need to learn to question rather than answer, they need to achieve rather than accomplish, and they need to inspire rather than inform.[9]

"On any given day, documenting care consumes from 13% to 28% of a nurse's time."[10]

System Prompts

Managers, staff, and informatics nurses can work with the IS department to develop system prompts that alert the user to recheck the data, enter data in a field that has been left blank, check that the data fall in a specific range, or confirm that data have been entered correctly. These system prompts are embedded in the application software that is developed by the IS department or a vendor of the information systems software. For example, a system prompt may display on the screen to inform the nurse that the allergy field on the assessment screen has been left blank. This display would prompt the nurse to fill in the allergy field.

Verification Techniques

Verifying data is very crucial to having quality data that can be utilized for clinical decision making. System prompts certainly help, but other techniques may be used to check and recheck data that are being entered at the point of care. Many verification techniques may exist, including verbal questioning and visual verification. Both techniques are very effective in the right environment. However, there are some things to think about when applying these techniques to verify data. It is important to be sure that patients understand what is being asked of them and understand what they are reading. Consideration should be given to hearing, language barriers, reading, and comprehension of the material. If a patient presents with any of the mentioned issues, then the nurse must accommodate, whether by getting an interpreter, a family member to help, or explaining the material in a simpler form, so that the patient understands what is being asked.

Data Mining

Technology has aided in rapid advances in data capture and storage, resulting in large databases of data. These data are stored internally in what is called "relational databases" that consist of rows and columns of data. Relational databases provide an easy method for internal storage, retrieval, and analysis.

The traditional method of analyzing data manually is no longer feasible. Extracting data from these databases is known as data mining. The process of data mining has become known as knowledge discovery and data mining or data to knowledge.[8] Data to knowledge usually begins by answering questions that are being asked. Assessing the question gives managers and others an advantage toward filtering through numerous large databases. Without a clear objective of what is being asked or needed, data overload may occur instead of gaining knowledge. Once the data are gathered, then the data must be prepared for data mining by selecting and formatting the data for use. Clinical data must be defined appropriately to identify like items when data mining. For example, "CABG" and "coronary artery bypass graft" must be identified as the same.

Data-mining processes may begin after the formatting has been completed by evaluating and analyzing for trends and predictive attributes. Trends that may be identified can then be interpreted and finally used within nursing environments. For data mining to be successful, nurse managers as well as staff nurses must be proficient in understanding current issues in managing data. Nurse managers, especially, should be aware of the uses of techniques such as data mining that allows them to extract, predict, evaluate, and apply knowledge to daily task.

Data Cleansing

Data cleansing is another technique used to clean up erroneous data that have been captured and stored in databases. Software is used that flags the erroneous data and generates a report. After reviewing the report, the files or records that have been flagged may be deleted or corrected. This process should be conducted on a routine basis to keep electronic records free from errors.

COMPUTER NETWORKING

Networks have become the infrastructure of today's electronic world and are the media for transfer of information from one location to another. Networks can be any computer devices that are attached, providing a conduit for information to be passed. There are two main types of computer networks: local area networks (LANs) and wide area networks (WANs). LANs are just what their name implies. All the computers in this type of network are local, meaning they all exist in a common geographical location and have a common owner. A WAN is two or more computers that are remote, meaning they are over a large geographical area from each other and they are connected by leased telecommunications equipment. LANs and WANs have largely given way to intranets and extranets, discussed below.

Designing networks is a crucial part of the design, development, and implementation of any healthcare information system. Organization size, needs, and willingness to spend money need to be considered and may range from very simple to very complex. Unfortunately, many organizations spend less money and end up with less than desirable systems.

Networks require management from the time the process starts, to the planning and design phase, and continues as an ongoing process. IS department staff may be involved in the management process, especially when troubleshooting network problems. Routine monitoring to evaluate capacity and performance should be done. A network administrator manages the server and users. Server administration includes the maintenance of daily backups and any shared resources. Management of users includes the maintenance of user identification and passwords and security-related issues between users.

When considering networks and design of systems, organizations should take into account budget and spending expenses, growth of the company and future needs, the healthcare information systems to be implemented, number of employees using the system, and the amount of data to be stored, retrieved, and transferred, among other things. One of the most important things is to plan for the future. Nursing leaders should become involved in planning, designing, developing, implementing, and evaluating networks that will be used by nurses.

Intranets, Extranets, and Virtual Private Networks

Examples of networks include intranets, extranets, and virtual private networks. Each of these forms of networks is used widely today by many organizations. These networks use Internet/World Wide Web technologies for information transfer and distribution.

Intranets are used by organizations for internal use and use a variety of communication technologies. Intranets usually are not geographically limited but do have a common owner. Employees generally have access to intranets for organizational information and applications that are easily accessible when using web browsers. Portals into the site are developed and maintained providing centralized access by employees. Because information can be kept more current and accurate, organizations use this method of network to aid in reduction of errors and improve quality health care.

Extranets extend beyond intranets and an organization's information providing access to anywhere in the world. They generally use multiple types of communication technologies and are not geographically limited just as intranets. Extranets are used to connect different parties that have common interests. With extranets, staff has access to information from almost anywhere, including patients' homes, their own homes, while at conferences, or even on vacation. Nurse leaders have access to this information for evaluating staffing conditions, monitoring staff ratios, and patient care. Those outside the organizations may also have access through some portal or gateway that allows them to provide or obtain information to or from the organization.

Virtual private networks are just what the name implies: They are private networks that provide stronger security with flexible remote access. Well-designed virtual private networks are secure, reliable, and easy to administer. For organizations to have these networks, software may need to be purchased and installed so connection to the organization's intranet can occur. This software interacts with software on the organization's intranet to manage authentication and encryption.[10]

Wireless Networking

Wireless networking has rapidly become the norm for most computer users. Wireless access points are available in most areas such as academic areas, shopping malls, coffee shops, and neighborhoods. There are some cities that are connecting their entire city with a network.

Wireless technology is suited for the healthcare environment where providers are mobile and dependent on current data generated and captured continuously during daily tasks and activities. Many technologies used today include wireless technology. Handheld wireless devices continuously download data, including laboratory, pharmacy, and radiographic data, saving many hours of time specially dedicated to searching for this information. Bedside infusion pumps, blood glucose machines, blood pressure machines, ultrasound machines, EEG and ECG machines, and other equipment can store and download information into the electronic records, saving valuable time in patient care.

This technology is rapidly changing, as are other technologies: Radiofrequency identification tags, monitoring devices to locate staff, and voice-over technology are being used. As wireless capabilities increase, technology will continue to enhance the way nursing performs task, providing quality care at the bedside.

Internet

The largest wide area global network is the Internet. The Internet allows us the ability to connect and communicate with any computer. When connected, the user can function on the Internet with simple point-and-click techniques, creating an interactive environment. The Internet has provided an opportunity for health care to reinvent the way medicine and health care is delivered. This transformation of health care has great potential to provide access to health care to many individuals that once had none.

> *The arrival of the Internet offers the opportunity to fundamentally reinvent medicine and healthcare delivery.... Internet technology may rank with antibiotics, genetics, and computers as among the most important changes for medical care delivery.* [11]

Patients have access to vast amounts of information that provides education related to their diagnosis and care. However, patients should be told to beware of information found on the Internet. There have been systematic evaluations of medical content on the web that have been found to be inconsistent or the reading level too high for the average consumer. There are several key points to remember when searching for information on the Internet:

- Reading level of material found on the Internet may be too high for the average consumer to understand.
- Medical information may be inaccurate or inconsistent.
- Internet medical information can come from reputable, other providers, drug companies, practitioners looking to sell their "product," or even from other groups.
- It is crucial to evaluate the credentials of the content providers to determine their qualifications and if the information on the site might be biased.[12]

More and more physician's offices, hospitals, clinics, and other healthcare provider organizations are creating Web sites that patients can access for information that is current and accurate concerning various diseases and treatment options. Many nurses have begun to work in areas such as creating and maintaining Web sites, consulting over the Internet, and reviewing cases, and some nurse practitioners are even providing care across the Internet via telemedicine.

As healthcare organizations continue to transition into the electronic world, many changes are occurring. Electronic medical records are mandated to be completed by 2014, and many organizations are working toward this goal. Data can be captured and stored, providing access to information that is readily available. As this movement continues, patients will be able to access their electronic records, complete medical forms before admissions or appointments, list their medications and allergies themselves, fill out their medical history, and provide insurance information and select payment options. Self-scheduling is beginning to be used, and patients will soon have the opportunity to schedule appointments as needed over the Internet.

Patients are already being assessed, diagnosed, and treated via the Internet, and as telemedicine continues to grow this effort will continue and expand. Opportunities for consultations, primary visits, and research are growing as expansion of health care to the Internet grows. Capturing data in real-time or point-of-care environments creates large databases of data for research, providing evidence-based data that can be translated into practice fairly quickly. Video conferencing is being used to consult with colleagues concerning evaluation of diagnoses and treatments. Available resources are being used as well to improve the clinical decision-making process.

Evidence-Based Practice 13-2

More than 75% of the patients who participated in an online-based communication system with their doctors said the service was easy, convenient to use, and better than a phone call or actual office visit.[13] Physicians were satisfied with the service, and over half of the physicians preferred it to an actual visit from the patient.[14]

The Internet has changed the way education is provided to nurses, patients, and students and has become the ideal vehicle for multimedia instruction and education on demand. Continuing and higher education for nurses is available online, providing convenient times for learning. Continuing education programs are available over the Internet, and many organizations use the Internet for yearly education requirements and updating skills information. Even policy and procedures are found on organizations' intranets today. Higher education programs can be found online, and many institutions are using technology to enhance traditional classrooms. There are many programs available that are completely offered online. These programs provide classroom environments on demand and offer convenient education for individuals needing flexibility.

The Internet has changed the way healthcare organizations are doing business with many aspects of business involving electronic transfer of information between parties. Healthcare organizations market their products and services, their facilities, and recruit for employees and patients via the Internet. Current employees can access personnel records and communicate with others through e-mail over the Internet.

Finally, privacy and security are concerns when using the Internet. As Internet and technology use increase and change, privacy and security issues will continue to be a concern. The Health Insurance Portability and Accountability Act (HIPAA) addressed many issues related to privacy and security. However, the ever-increasing demand for technology implementation in health care will create new issues as this ranks as one of the top issues related to technology.

HEALTHCARE INFORMATION SYSTEMS

There are several types of healthcare information systems. Some of these systems help to manage the daily operations of general healthcare organizations and others are classified as hospital information systems. For the purposes of this text, hospital information systems are discussed.

Hospital information systems consist of two types, administrative information systems and clinical information systems. Each of these systems plays a major role in the operations of an organization providing health care to consumers such as hospitals. As the demand for automation and data management increases in nursing, nurses will become more involved with evaluating, selecting, designing, and implementing information systems. They are becoming the norm for the clinical areas and have been used in administrative activities for years.

Hospital Information Systems

Hospital information systems are large complex computer systems designed to help manage information needs of a hospital. Hospital information systems are tools that can be used interdepartmentally or intradepartmentally. These large systems are composed of smaller systems that are used for the daily operations of a hospital. Figure 13-3 lists some examples of administrative and clinical information systems that may be found in a hospital.

Implementing Hospital Information Systems

Nurse leaders need to become more and more involved in implementing hospital information systems, both in the administrative and clinical areas. Implementing information systems requires more than just installing and using the systems. A management plan should be devised by the nurse leader that incorporates input for selection, design and development, implementation, and evaluation of the information system being considered (Figure 13-4). Nurse leaders should work closely with the IS department or the nursing informatics nurse in obtaining the optimal system that will enhance the delivery of quality care.

FIGURE 13-3   **HOSPITAL INFORMATION SYSTEMS**

Administrative Systems	Clinical Systems
Nursing administrative systems	Nursing information systems
Payroll / human resource systems	Order entry systems
Patient registration systems	Radiology systems
Quality improvement and assurance systems	Laboratory systems
Scheduling systems	Pharmacy systems
Billing and payment systems	Dietary systems
Financial systems	Surgical and other department specific systems
Other business operations systems	Other ancillary department systems

---

Source: Author.

FIGURE 13-4	EXAMPLE OF A PROJECT IMPLEMENTATION PLAN[10]

ID	Activity	Duration	Start	Finish
1	UNIVERSITY HOSPITALS RESULTS REPOSITORY PROJECT STARTUP	2.5d	9/11/00	9/13/00
4	ADMINISTRATIVE	120d	9/13/00	2/28/01
5	Project Status Meetings	115.25d	9/15/00	2/23/01
13	Project Steering Committee Meetings	95.25d	9/20/00	1/31/01
19	Quality Assurance Review Visit	2d	9/13/00	9/15/00
20	Project Supervision	120d	9/13/00	2/28/01
21	PROJECT INITIATION	10d	9/14/00	9/27/00
22	Pre-Implementation Planning	1d	9/14/00	9/14/00
24	Project Planning	2d	9/15/00	9/18/00
28	Adapt Network	5d	9/18/00	9/22/00
30	Project Kickoff	7d	9/19/00	9/27/00
35	HARDWARE AND SOFTWARE	12.5d	9/13/00	9/29/00
36	Hardware/Software Installation	12.5d	9/13/00	9/29/00
39	Software Delivery Validation	9d	9/13/00	9/26/00
43	ANALYSIS	58d	9/28/00	12/18/00
44	Results Repository Surveys/Process Flow/Tables	15d	9/28/00	10/18/00
48	Results Repository Interfaces	20d	10/19/00	11/15/00
51	Results Repository Profiles/Procedures	11d	11/16/00	11/30/00
59	Nursing Assessment Surveys/Process Flow/Procedures	11d	11/27/00	12/11/00
63	Nursing Assessment Master Files	3d	12/12/00	12/14/00
65	Nursing Assessment Reports/Project Scope	2d	12/15/00	12/18/00
68	TRAINING	42d	12/18/00	2/13/01
69	Training Preparation	12d	12/18/00	1/2/01
73	Educate Users	30d	1/3/01	2/13/01
77	LIVE EVENT	28d	1/22/01	2/28/01
78	Live Event Preparation	22d	1/22/01	2/20/01
83	Results Repository Live Event	4d	2/23/01	2/28/01
86	Nursing Assessment Live Event	5d	2/22/01	2/28/01
88	Live Event Support	5d	2/22/01	2/28/01
90	POST-LIVE	10d	3/1/01	3/14/01
91	Evaluation and Feedback to Management	10d	3/01/01	3/14/01
92	Monitor Production System			
95				

Source: Author.

Several processes must be completed when an organization has committed to implementing technologies. Nurse leaders and other appointed or volunteer staff nurses along with multidisciplinary team members should determine the needs of the unit, department, or division within the organization. First, a thorough assessment should be conducted that involves looking at the current system for capturing and analyzing data for delivery of care. Determining weakness and strengths of the current system provides insight into what works and does not work for daily operations. The needs of the organization are determined during the assessment phase. Nurse leaders should evaluate what is needed currently and what will be needed in the future.

Second, nurse leaders along with IS staff and administrative personnel need to evaluate and select a hospital information system that meets the needs found. Several information systems should be evaluated for the closest fit to the organization's budgetary guidelines, goals, and the needs that were determined earlier.

Third, the implementation phase begins once the selection has been made. This phase involves intensive training of employees, both administrative and staff, over some period of time. Timelines need to be developed for completing training, installation of equipment and software, and testing of the new system. Once training and installation have been completed, the systems are brought online for the users to use. Multiple support personnel should be available the day the system is started to help with problems that may arise or to guide employees through the process of computerized daily tasks.

Finally, the systems should be evaluated. Mechanisms should be developed during the planning phases that provide methods for support and evaluation of the system. These methods may include but are not limited to a call-in help desk, support technicians that are available on demand as questions and problems arise, request for help forms that can be submitted online, and suggestion boxes.

Administrative Information Systems

Administrative information systems include a wide variety of systems that work to maintain information used in the daily operations of an organization. These include financial systems, human resource systems, nonclinical patient systems such as registration and scheduling systems, and even nursing administrative systems that nurse leaders use.

Information systems that are classified as administrative systems involve any operation that is not directly linked to hands-on patient care. Operations may include nonclinical patient activities, medical records activities, business and accounting activities, and some nursing management tasks. Nonclinical patient activities may involve such tasks as patient scheduling, admissions, discharges, transfers, census functions, bed assignments, and other nonclinical activities association with the patient. Medical records procedures include master patient index functions, abstracting (diagnosis/procedure/and coding), transcription, and correspondence. Business and accounting functions may include patient insurance verification, billing, accounts payable, accounts receivable, cash processing, maintenance activities, and other business operations. Nursing management tasks may involve budget projections, employee records (annual skills and educational updates, evaluations, staffing), and other management activities required for daily operations by nurse leaders.

Clinical Information Systems

Clinical information systems involve any system that is used in patient care and may not be nursing information systems. However, these systems are generally associated with the nursing information system in hospitals, such as a laboratory or medication administration system. Refer back to Figure 13-3 for a list of examples of clinical information systems. Each of the systems shown provides support to the care of patients. They may be general support systems or explicit to a specific nursing area. Many nursing areas benefit from unique information systems. Some of these areas include surgery, infection control, labor and delivery, enterostomal therapy, oncology, mental health, orthopedics, neonatology, and intensive care. Clinical information systems can be used to improve the quality of care while enhancing the environment and reducing cost long term.

Many clinical information systems are designed in modular form, providing flexibility to the organization. General nursing information systems have multiple programs comprising a module that is used to perform various clinical tasks, educational, and management functions. The modules may vary between vendors and software developers but may include medical history, patient assessment documentation, nursing care plan, medication administration, dietary information, patient education, ongoing daily care, vital signs and graphic sheet information, reports, nursing progress notes, discharge planning, and other tasks that nurses perform on a daily basis.

Clinical nurses can use clinical information systems to provide quality patient care. These systems provide a mechanism for capturing data that can be used to formulate treatment plans and evaluate trends. Technology along with clinical information systems continues to change the work environment and improve the quality of work life for nursing.

GENERAL APPLICATIONS SOFTWARE FOR THE NURSE LEADER

General applications software includes such software as communications, database management, word processing and desktop publishing, spreadsheet, personal information managers, graphics programs, and other software information nurse leaders may need on a daily basis. Nurses use computers to perform many aspects of their daily jobs in areas such as budgeting, documentation, policy and procedures, research, inventory, scheduling, patient and staff education, maintaining personnel records, and other tasks as needed. Because of this, nurse leaders should be prepared to encourage and support the increased use of technology in clinical and nonclinical areas of nursing. Fundamental concepts related to computers and the use of applications software is important to the nurse manager and other nurses. Computer literacy is important and will be required more and more as computers continue to be a tool of the profession.

Communications

Communications software is what provides a link for access between computers. Links may be dedicated or nondedicated. Dedicated links remain open even when not in use. Nondedicated links are open only when being used. Organizations tend to use dedicated links to have direct access to the organization's information resources typically through a LAN connection. Small business or home environments tend to use nondedicated links and access information only when needed. However, dedicated links have become the norm with integrated services digital network and digital subscriber lines.

Nurse leaders are not normally involved in communications software selection and installation. The IS department personnel should take care of this portion of implementation. Communications software to support LANs is generally taken for granted and is provided as part of the operating system that comes installed on the equipment. At work, most employees have a dedicated connection, and at home, they can dial in or connect through a portal to the remote access server and perform as if they are at work.

Database Management

Computer databases are much like filing cabinets, only electronic. There are files and contents in those files. Databases are used to store data and can be manipulated to view information based on query options. Database management systems virtually take the place of a filing cabinet to handle many information and record-keeping needs.

Typically, relational tables are used in databases. These tables contain rows and columns where data can be stored that relate to each other. A table is considered a collection of records where one row is a record. The rows and columns consist of cells, and these cells are given data field names. Data fields are defined with length and type of data that will be placed in the field. The fields are defined in a table definition. A database may consist of several relational tables that data can be pulled from to form reports. Reports may be printed or displayed on the computer screen for review. This process of storing and retrieving data provides ease of information management, the timely retrieval of information, and the concurrent access of information to individuals from different locations.

Word Processing and Desktop Publishing

Word processing software is used to produce documents such as memos, letters, signs, books, and resumes. Desktop publishing software generally incorporates graphics into the text and is used for newsletters, posters and signs, books, and other documents that require graphics. Today, both types of software have incorporated aspect of each other, enabling a variety of documents to be produced from either type. Figure 13-6 shows an example of a poster/sign produced with desktop publishing software.

The arrival of the Internet offers the opportunity to fundamentally reinvent medicine and healthcare delivery. . . . Internet technology may rank with antibiotics, genetics, and computers as among the most important changes for medical care delivery. [11]

Word processing and desktop publishing software applications have tools that help to manage the information placed in the document. There are various styles of formatting and, depending on the software, unique styles may exist. Styles can establish the following in a document[15]:

- Font type, size, and style
- Spacing (between lines and paragraphs)
- Page headers and footers and page numbering
- Orientation of the page (portrait or landscape)
- Margins, tabs, and text alignment
- Outline formats (bullets with symbols or numbering)

Many other tools are available in word processing and desktop publishing software. Some of these include but are not limited to spell checkers, thesaurus, word counts, and translators. You can add footnotes, endnotes, change the writing style of the paper, insert objects and captions, and edit, replace, and

---

FIGURE 13-5   **KEY POINTS TO REMEMBER**

Key Points to Remember:

Reading level of material found on the Internet may be too high for the average consumer to understand.

Medical information may be inaccurate or inconsistent.

Internet medical information can come from reputable, other providers, drug companies, practitioners looking to sell their "product" or even from other groups.

It is crucial to evaluate the credentials of the content providers to determine their qualifications and if the information on the site might be biased.[12]

Source: Author.

FIGURE 13-6	EXAMPLE OF A BROCHURE CREATED WITH DESKTOP PUBLISHING

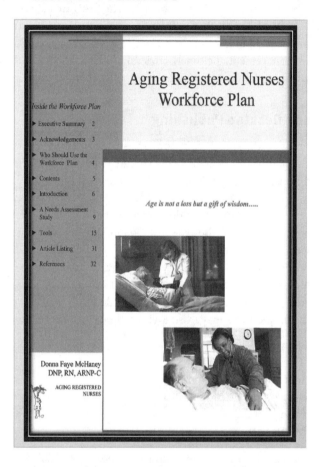

Source: Courtesy of Donna Faye McHaney, DNP, BSCS, RN, ARNP-C; University of South Alabama, Mobile, AL.

add or delete. Standard templates can be used or templates can be defined for use. Both word processing and desktop publishing software provide nurse leaders with software to aid them in producing a variety of documents.

Spreadsheets

Spreadsheets are computer software applications that can be used to manipulate data. Spreadsheets contain multiple cells and rows that make up a grid-type form. The cells may contain alphanumeric text, numeric values, or formulas that define the contents of the cell. Calculations can be performed, graphs can be produced, and statistical abilities are built in most spreadsheets. They have the ability to recalculate an entire spreadsheet automatically after changing a single cell. Spreadsheets can contain large numbers of rows and columns and make handling data easy.[15] Often, spreadsheets are used for creating budgets and handling numerous amounts of data.

Nurse leaders can use spreadsheets for developing budgets, maintaining staff records, calculating and tracking, and creating graphs on statistics pertaining to staffing and patient data. Items can be imported and exported to and from other software applications as well.

Personal Information Manager

Personal information manager (PIM) applications are electronic versions of an appointment book or day planner. It contains an address book, a calendar, e-mail, a journal, notes, and tasks. Today, PIMs work with desktop computers, laptop computers, and personal digital assistants (PDAs). Even cellular phones have some capabilities to support PIM applications. A PDA is a small computing device that offers the same PIM capabilities as a PIM does on a desktop computer. Calendar or contact information can be interchanged between these devices through synchronization.

There are many capabilities of these devices. Some are as powerful and have the same applications available as desktop or laptop computers. Today, e-mail services and Internet access are available from PDAs, providing greater flexibility with technology. PDAs are frequently being used in the clinical setting not only by nurse leaders but by staff as well. Advances in this area continue to progress and can only be refined to produce more efficient devices.

NURSING MANAGEMENT APPLICATIONS

Nursing management must be ready for the technology that is being implemented in administrative and clinical areas. Many applications are available for nursing management that can aid in daily tasks. Computer applications for nursing administration may include patient classification systems, acuity systems, staffing and scheduling systems, unit activity reports, utilization review, census, error reports, drug and allergy reactions, incident reports, shift summary reports, budgeting and payroll, and other systems as well. Nurse executives may also use application software for forecasting and planning, hospital expansion, regulatory reporting, risk pooling, surveys, preventive maintenance, and financial planning.

Today's nurse administrator has moved into the role of executive officer with obligations to report to the institution, to society, and to national accrediting agencies. These responsibilities and others come with the professional practice of nursing. Today's nurse administrator needs more than a basic understanding of e-mail and word processing; they need to have sufficient knowledge about computer technology to help improve health care and healthcare costs by better managing nursing information.[8]

The applications for nursing management include the nursing management minimum data set (NMMDS), calendar of events, general application software as discussed earlier in this chapter, and human resource information systems that support nursing management tasks. Calendars are useful for scheduling meetings, conferences, and educational events. Many nurse managers use PDAs or some general application software for this or use an Internet browser-based application available on the organization's intranet. The advantage to using the Internet browser-based application is that employees and managers can schedule appoints and events such as educational opportunities and their names are added to the class role and automatic notifications can be sent to nursing management.

The NMMDS is available from the American Organization of Nurse Executives and is a research-based management data set. It works in conjunction with the nursing minimum data set. The NMMDS contains 17 elements that fall into three board categories: environment, nurse resources, and financial resources. Nurse executives need hard data to make the difficult quality decisions occurring in today's healthcare operating environment.[16] Having quality data to answer difficult questions such as outcomes of critical pathways, retention and turnover rates of personnel, nursing and patient satisfaction rates, personnel ratings, budgets, and productivity are essential to the nurse manager. Having NMMDS provides a tool for nurse managers to answer these difficult questions.[17]

Although most human resources applications support activities required for the human resource departments, nurse managers find themselves in situations where these data are most helpful. Management of human resources is a huge task for most organizations, requiring significant time and personnel. These applications can be very informative and supportive to the nurse manager. Reports can be obtained that supply such things as the number of individuals who apply for available positions, how many employees there are with a breakdown by rank, educational reports that show what educational programs have been completed, retention and turnover rates, information on credentials and special skills, time and attendance, and much more. Figure 13-7 shows an example of an employee termination report that may be used by nursing management.

With appropriate integration of the overall hospital information systems, these data can be exported and imported into other hospital information systems, nursing information systems, and other general applications software.

ETHICAL, LEGAL, AND SECURITY ISSUES

Ethical, legal, and security issues go hand in hand when using technology. These concepts have been the top issues for IS departments and healthcare organizations for many years. *Webster* defines ethics as a system of conduct or behavior.[18] Ethics is conforming to professional standards that are defined by an organization or group of individuals such as nursing. Security can be defined as being safe and free from danger.[18] Terms related to security are privacy and confidentiality. Privacy is defined by Romano as "control over exposure of self or information about oneself and freedom from intrusion. Privacy denotes the right of an individual to decide how much personal information to share. It includes a right to secrecy of information and protection against the misuse or release of this information."[19] Confidentiality means being entrusted with information that is held secret or secure.[18] Each of these concepts shares a relationship with each other when discussing patient information.

Many legal issues can arise from using technology and should be addressed by organizations. HIPAA of 1996 was originally designed to protect workers from losing their right to insurance coverage when leaving a job (portability) and to protect integrity, confidentiality, and availability of electronic health information (accountability). Key components of HIPAA can be found in Figure 13-8. Components that relate to the development of electronic data, security, and privacy standards play a major role in healthcare delivery. HIPAA has placed attention on the implications on computerized electronic records as they relate to patient's rights.[12] The HIPAA privacy component gives patients access to and control over their medical data and who has access to it. Health plans, healthcare clearing-

---

FIGURE 13-7	EXAMPLE OF AN EMPLOYEE TERMINATION REPORT

Employee Termination Report for the Month of September 200X

position	name	title	date	reason
00356	Johnson, Mary J.	Registered nurse	09/26/xx	Q
10234	Armstrong, Helen M.	Licensed practical nurse	09/08/xx	Q
16212	Mims, Janet K.	Registered nurse	09/13/xx	F
17335	Baker, Donald M.	Registered nurse	09/05/xx	Q
17366	Smitherman, Carolyn S.	Registered nurse	09/22/xx	R
18549	Jackson, Melanie J.	Unit secretary	09/01/xx	Q
18675	Hanson, Marcus K.	Respiratory therapist	09/29/xx	Q

Source: Author.

houses, and healthcare providers must obtain prospective approval from a patient before sharing protected health information.

As a result of the privacy act, security issues concerning electronic health information arose. Security provisions must be made and cover policies, procedures, physical safeguards, and technical aspects of the management of protected health information. Security rules ensure the confidentiality, integrity, and availability of electronic protected health information. The current version of HIPAA legislation represents a relatively flexible set of rules that anticipates future changes in technology but remains achievable by healthcare organizations.[12]

Nursing management needs to be aware of the legal issues surrounding patient information and employees. There are guidelines and strategies (Figure 13-9) available from the American Nurses Association, the American Health Information Management Association, and the Canadian Nurses Association that help to minimize legal risk associated with computerized documentation and technology.[20]

FUTURE TRENDS

It is unclear what the future holds for nursing when thinking about technology and what it can do to enhance the daily work flow involved in producing quality care. Transforming care into quality care is the essence of the clinical environment, and nurse leaders need to recognize the importance of emerging technologies. Two such technologies are virtual reality (simulation) and ubiquitous computing. Both these technologies are emerging and being used in education and other areas of health care.

FIGURE 13-8   **KEY COMPONENTS OF HIPAA**

There are three aspects that relate to computerized medical information and patient's rights.

1. Privacy: The requirement for healthcare providers to obtain consent from patients about protected health information

2. Security: Administrative, physical, and technical safeguards used to protect patient data

3. Code sets: Tags and labels used in identification of patient specific data, including definitions, billing codes, and patient identifiers

---

Source: Author.

FIGURE 13-9   **GUIDELINES AND STRATEGIES TO MINIMIZE RISK**

1. Never give out your computer password.

2. Always log off when you leave a computer terminal.

3. Follow procedures for correcting mistakes because computer entries are permanent.

4. Do not leave patient information displayed on a screen; keep track of printed information and dispose of it properly.

5. Follow your institution's confidentiality policies and procedures.

Source: Author.

Virtual reality allows an individual the ability to interact in a computer-stimulated environment. Most virtual reality environments are primarily visual, displayed either on a computer screen or through some special or stereoscopic display, but some offer additional sensory information such as sound. Others offer tactile information forcing feedback in medical and gaming applications. Users can interact with the computer-driven devices, which have become known as simulation technology. It has been used for years in pilot training and combat training. Currently, simulation is being experimented with and used in the medical industry. Nursing schools, medical schools, and other discipline schools are using simulation technology to train students with hands-on computer-simulated scenarios to replace the demand for clinical environments provided by healthcare organizations. It is unclear at this time where future virtual reality technology will lead the healthcare industry.[21,22]

Ubiquitous computing is a model of human computer interaction where information processing has been integrated into everyday objects and activities. Nurse leaders engaging in ubiquitous computing use many computational devices and systems simultaneously in the course of ordinary activities, and most of the time they may not be aware of it. All models of ubiquitous computing share a vision of small, inexpensive, robust networked processing devices. This natural interaction between humans and computers has yet to emerge, although there is recognition in the computer field that we are already living in a ubiquitous computing world.[23]

SUMMARY

New and emerging technologies will continue to have an effect on the healthcare delivery system. Nursing, as a major player in health care, will be part of this ever-growing era of technology. Having access to learning environments that support this new technology will be a challenge for academia and healthcare organizations. Providing learning that simulates these environments requires a commitment from administrators in both areas. As the nursing shortage, improved quality care, and the push for electronic health records continue to drive technology in health care, nurse leaders will need to be more and more involved in information system technology.

Nurse leaders, both managers and executives, need to be conscious of new emerging technologies and how they can enhance clinical and nonclinical areas of nursing. Understanding the fundamental elements of computing is no longer sufficient. Nurse leaders must have learned knowledge to help lead nursing to a new age of electronic processing. Engaging in collaboration with information systems departments to select, design, develop, implement, and evaluation information systems is essential to the success of fully computer-automated environments.

APPLICATION EXERCISES

Exercise 13-1
Think back 5 to 10 years and consider how technology has changed in your workplace. Consider how technology has affected you and your family. Write down the changes you have seen as technology has advanced.

Exercise 13-2
Think about your skills. Do you have the technology skills needed to perform efficiently in a high-tech environment? What training would you benefit from? What skills do you see as necessary for nurses as it relates to technology?

Exercise 13-3

Visit Vital Health Statistics Web site and search the site. Numerous databases of information are available.

1. List some interesting information that you found.
2. List ways nursing uses data, information, and knowledge specific to your job.

Exercise 13-4

How have you used the Internet in your practice? How do you see the Internet being used in the future? List ways the Internet can enhance healthcare delivery that is different from what is going on today.

Exercise 13-5

1. Considering healthcare information systems, what systems have you used?
2. List healthcare information systems you use or have used and categorize them into administrative and clinical healthcare information systems.
3. What systems would benefit nursing leaders the most? List them.
4. Identify and list information technology used by personnel (unit secretary, nurse technicians, nurses, nurse leaders). Include personal computer applications and information systems.

Exercise 13-6

Gain access to a computer and look for the word processing program. Open the program and experiment with the options that the word processing software has available. Experiment with inserting pictures and graphics. Produce a fact sheet with facts about the word processing software listed.

Exercise 13-7

1. Discuss your views on ethical, legal, and security issues.
2. What security measures do you interact with in your environment? List them.
3. What security measures do you see as needing improvements?
4. How can you contribute to confidentiality and privacy efforts?

Exercise 13-8

List examples where simulation technology would be beneficial for nursing in clinical areas. Think of examples of ubiquitous computing in health care.

Notes

1. Toffler, A. (1980). *The third wave.* New York: Morrow.
2. Rutsky, R. L. (1999). Techno-cultural interaction and the fear of information. *Style, 3,* 267.
3. American Nurses Association. (2006). *Scope and standards of nursing informatics practice.* Silver Spring, MD: Nursesbooks.org.
4. Hebda, T., Czar, P., & Mascara, C. (2005). *Handbook of informatics for nurses & health care professionals* (3rd ed.). Upper Saddle River, NJ: Pearson Education, Inc.
5. Merriam-Webster, Incorporated (2005). *Merriam-Webster online dictionary.* Retrieved January 07, 2008, from http://www.m-w.com/cgi-bin/dictionary
6. Harrison, M., Logan, J., Joseph, L., & Graham, I. (1998). Quality improvement, research, and evidence-based practice: 5 years experience with pressure ulcers. *Evidence-Based Nursing, 1,* 108–110.
7. Austin, C. J., & Boxerman, S. B. (2003). *Information systems for healthcare management.* Foundation of the American College of healthcare executives, Washington, DC.

8. Saba, V. K., & McCormick, K. A. (2001). *Essentials of nursing informatics* (4th ed.). New York: McGraw Hill.

9. The Technology Informatics Guiding Education Reform (TIGER) Initiative (2007). Retrieved January 20, 2008 from www.tigersummit.com

10. Roussel, L., Swansburg, R., & Swansburg, R. (2006). *Management and leadership for nurse administrators* (4th ed.). Sudbury, MA: Jones and Bartlett.

11. Coile, R. C. Jr. (2000). The digital transformation of health care. *Physician Executive,* 8–15.

12. Hanson, C. W. (2006). *Healthcare informatics.* New York: McGraw-Hill.

13. Carns, A. (2002). The check up is in the e-mail: A new service lets patients have online consultation with doctors. So why aren't many people using it? *Wall Street Journal,* November 11, 2002, p. R9.

14. Carns, A. (2002). Online doctor-patient consulting shows promise in California study. *Wall Street Journal,* October, 2002, p. D8.

15. Spreadsheets. Wikipedia, the free encyclopedia. Retrieved January 25, 2008, from http://en.wikipedia.org/wiki/Spreadsheet

16. Simpson, R. L. (1997). What good are advanced practitioners if nobody at the top knows their value? *Nursing Administration Quarterly, 91,* 26–37.

17. Huber, D., Schumacher, L., & Delaney, C. (1997). Nursing management minimum data set (NMMDS). *Journal of Nursing Administration,* 42–48.

18. Security. *Webster's collegiate dictionary and thesaurus.* New Lanark, Scotland: Geddes and Grossett, 2004.

19. Romano, C. A. (1987). Privacy, confidentiality, and security of computerized systems. *Computers in Nursing, 2,* 99–104.

20. Iyer, P. (1993). Computer charting: Minimizing legal risks. *Nursing,* 86.

21. Burdea, G., & Coffet, P. (2003). *Virtual reality technology* (2nd ed.). Wiley-IEEE Press. New York.

22. Rheingold, H. (1992). *Virtual reality.* New York: Simon & Schuster.

References

Barrie, J. M., Presti, D. E. Digital plagiarism—the Web giveth and the Web shall taketh. *J Med Internet Res.* 2000 Mar 31;2(1):e6. doi: 10.2196/jmir.2.1.e6. http://www.jmir.org/2000/1/e6/

Boyer, C., Selby, M., Scherrer, J. R., Appel, R. D. The Health On the Net Code of Conduct for medical and health Web sites. *Comput Biol Med.* 1998 Sep;28(5):603–610

Charnock, D., Shepperd, S., Needham, G., Gann, R. DISCERN: an instrument for judging the quality of written consumer health information on treatment choices. *J Epidemiol Community Health.* 1999 Feb;53(2):105–111.

Childress C. A. Ethical issues in providing online psychotherapeutic interventions. *J Med Internet Res.* 2000 Mar 31;2(1):e5. doi: 10.2196/jmir.2.1.e5. http://www.jmir.org/2000/1/e5

Eng T. R., Gustafson, D. H., editors. US Department of Health and Human Services; Science Panel on Interactive Communication and Health, authors. *Wired for health and well-being; the emergence of interactive health communication.* Washington, DC: US Government Printing Office; 1999.

Eysenbach, G. Report of a case of cyberplagiarism—and reflections on detecting and preventing academic misconduct using the Internet. *J Med Internet Res.* 2000 Mar 31;2(1):e4. doi: 10.2196/jmir.2.1.e4. http://www.jmir.org/2000/1/e4/

Eysenbach, G., Diepgen, T. L. Towards quality management of medical information on the Internet: evaluation, labelling, and filtering of information. *BMJ.* 1998 Nov 28;317(7171):1496–500. http://bmj.com/cgi/pmilookup?view=long&pmid=9831581

Eysenbach, G., Diepgen, T. L. Labeling and filtering of medical information on the Internet. *Methods Inf Med.* 1999 Jun;38(2):80–8.99020080

Eysenbach, G. Towards ethical guidelines for dealing with unsolicited patient emails and giving teleadvice in the absence of a pre-existing patient-physician relationship systematic review and expert survey. *J Med Internet Res.* 2000 Feb 24;2(1):e1. doi: 10.2196/jmir.2.1.e1. http://www.jmir.org/2000/1/e1/

Gustafson, D. H., Robinson, T. N., Ansley, D., Adler, L., Brennan, P. F. Consumers and evaluation of interactive health communication applications. The Science Panel on Interactive Communication and Health. *Am J Prev Med.* 1999 Jan;16(1):23–9. doi: 10.1016/S0749-3797(98)00104-4.S0749379798001044

APPENDIX 13-1

Computer Technology Terms

Central processing unit (CPU): The part of the computer that controls all other parts. It consists of a control unit, an arithmetic and logic unit, and memory (registers and cache).

Character: A letter, digit, or other symbol that is used as part of the representation of data. A byte.

Compact disc (CD): A type of disk storage that uses magneto-optical recording and lasers.

Data: A representation of numbers or characters in the form suitable for processing by a computer.

Database: A collection of files or tables.

Database management system: A specialized type of software used for the organization, storage, and retrieval of data in a database.

Disk (or disc): Round, flat magnetic media used for the storage of data.

Downtime: The elapsed time when a computer is not available for use. It may be scheduled for maintenance or unscheduled because of machine or program problems.

Expert system: An application that contains a knowledge base and a set of algorithms or rules that have been derived from human expertise to provide assistance in decision making.

Extranet: An extension of an organization's intranet, over the Internet, enabling communication between the institution and people with whom it deals.

Field: A unit of data within a record.

File: A collection of related data with a given structure.

Forecasting: Predicting the future by an analysis of data.

GUI (graphical user interface): A user interface to a computer based on graphics.

Hard copy: Printed computer output in the form of reports and documents.

Hardware: Physical computer equipment.

Information systems: Computer systems designed to store and manipulate information for communication and decision support.

Input/output (I/O): Transfer of data between an external source and internal storage.

Interface: Point at which independent systems or computers interact.

Internet: A worldwide network of computer networks that use the TCP/IP network protocols to facilitate data transmission and exchange.

Intranet: A privately maintained computer network that can be accessed only by authorized persons, especially members or employees of the organization that owns it.

Key: A field or fields within a record that makes that record unique with respect to other records in a file.

Kilobyte (KB): 1,024 bytes.

Local area network (LAN): Two or more computers connected for local resource sharing.

Mainframe computer: A powerful computer capable of being used and interacted with by hundreds of users, simultaneously.

Megabyte (MB): 1,024 kilobytes.

Microcomputer: A small computer built around a microprocessor.

Minicomputer: A midsize computer, smaller and less powerful than a mainframe but larger and more powerful than a microcomputer.

Modeling: Representation of a complex system used as a basis for simulation to allow for the prediction and understanding of the system's behavior.

Modem: Device that converts digital data from a computer to an analog signal that can be transmitted on a telecommunications line and that converts received analog transmissions to digital data.

Multimedia: Combination of different elements of media, such as text, graphics, audio, video, animation, and sound.

Multitasking: Mode of operation that provides for the concurrent execution of two or more tasks.

Online processing: System that provides for the immediate, interactive input and processing of data.

Operating system: Software designed to control the hardware of a specific computer system to allow users and application programs to use it.

Printer: Terminal or peripheral that produces hard copy or printed output.

Program: A set of computer instructions directing the computer to perform some operation.

Random access: A storage technique whereby a file can be addressed and accessed directly at its location on the media or a record can be addressed and accessed directly within a file.

Record: A group of related fields of data treated as a unit.

Robotics: Science or study of mechanical devices designed to perform tasks that might be otherwise done by humans.

Sequential access: Storage technique whereby a file can be addressed and accessed only after all those before it on the media have been or a record can be addressed and accessed only after all those before it in the file have been.

Simulation: Attempting to predict aspects of the behavior of some system by creating an approximate model of it.

Software: A program or set of programs written to tell the computer hardware how to do something.

Spreadsheet: Specialized type of software for manipulation of numbers.

Table: Collection of related records in a database management system.

Trend: Systematic pattern of change over time.

Ubiquitous computing: Human–computer interaction that involves sharing of computer technology with everyday activities and objects.

User friendly: Software considered easier to use for novices.

Virtual reality: Simulation of real environments.

Voice communication: Interaction with a computer by voice recognition.

Wide area network (WAN): A network of two or more groups of computers or computing devices that are remote from each other and connected by telecommunication equipment.

Word processor: Specialized type of software for the manipulation of words to produce printed material.

PART III

LEADING TO IMPROVE THE FUTURE QUALITY AND SAFETY OF HEALTHCARE DELIVERY

14

HEALTH POLICY, LAWS, AND REGULATORY ISSUES

Valorie Dearmon, RN, MSN, CNNAA, BC

LEARNING OBJECTIVES AND ACTIVITIES

- Describe policy and public policy and its relationship to healthcare issues.
- Outline a policy process.
- Describe the nurse's role in public policy.
- Describe the role and function of the U.S. Department of Health and Human Services.
- Review laws and regulations that impact health care.
- Differentiate between Medicare and Medicaid.
- Describe the licensure and credentialing processes.

CONCEPTS

Policy, public policy, agenda setting, nurse practice acts, licensure, certification, laws, regulations.

QUOTE

I find the great thing in this world is not so much where we stand, as in what direction we are moving—we must sail sometimes with the wind and sometimes against it—but we must sail, and not drift, nor lie at anchor.

—Oliver Wendell Holmes, Jr.,
Former U.S. Supreme Court Justice

NURSE MANAGER BEHAVIORS	NURSE EXECUTIVE BEHAVIORS
Complies with federal and state laws and regulations that affect the provision of patient care; participates in the legislative process through membership in professional organizations; identifies and eliminates sexual harassment, workplace violence, and verbal and physical abuse; complies with legal and regulatory guidelines for human resource management.	Possesses knowledge of health policy; articulates federal and state laws and regulations that affect the provision of patient care; participates in the legislative process concerning health care through membership in professional organizations and personal contact with public officials; educates patient care team members on the legislative and regulatory processes and methods for influencing both; interprets impact of state and federal legislation on nursing and healthcare organizations; identifies and eliminates sexual harassment, workplace violence, and verbal and physical abuse; interprets legal and regulatory guidelines for human resource management.

Introduction

All is not well on the home front. The United States, like other developed countries throughout the world, is struggling with how to best provide social services to its population, including the formidable challenge of providing health care. The difference, however, is that this country is spending more on health care than any other nation and still many outcomes fall below those of other countries.[1] Projections indicate that, without intervention, Medicare funds will be depleted within the next 10 years.[2] Furthermore, healthcare costs are estimated to rise to an unprecedented 20% of the gross domestic product by 2015.[3] Unlike most other developed countries, the United States does not have a national health system. Thus policy, or the lack of, implies that health care in America is a privilege and not a right for its citizens. Decentralization of policy leaves gaps and deficiencies in health care and allows for overlapping laws and regulations. Incongruent regulations pit providers against each other and providers against insurers and suppliers. Furthermore, regulation by multiple agencies burden providers with excessive requirements and costs. Policymakers are concerned about the increased number of uninsured and those requiring public assistance as well as the quality and cost of health care. However, consensus among stakeholders as to how to address these matters has yet to be achieved because of the complexity of issues, political agendas, and diversity in values.

Throughout the history of this country, laws and regulations governing the delivery of healthcare services have evolved. Needless to say, the end to healthcare woes is far from over and much work remains to be done. The knowledge and expertise of leaders is essential to tackle the multifaceted issues that face the nation. As the largest body of healthcare providers in this country, the voice of nursing must be heard. Participation in identifying and enacting workable solutions requires an understanding of health policy and the process used to establish governing regulations.

HEALTH POLICY

Health policy is an established plan of action usually made by governmental policymakers or healthcare organizations to achieve established outcomes pertaining to the healthcare system.[4] Figure 14-1 provides instances of health policy concerns within the United States for the federal, state, and local government and matters of concern for healthcare organizations and professional providers.[5] Many concerns overlap at different levels. Although there is much debate around the extent of healthcare regulation, most agree that regulation is required to protect the interest of the public. Health care in the United States is heavily regulated by federal, state, and local government as well as private accrediting and certifying organizations.[6]

Health policy can be described as an entity and a process. As an entity, policy serves to articulate the position or belief of the leaders or administration in power. The philosophy and mission held by the administration influences the direction of government policies. Policies can take the form of position statements, goals, programs, proposals, and laws. Development of public health policy occurs through a process. The economic climate and scarcity of resources have led countries throughout the world to

---

FIGURE 14-1 ILLUSTRATIVE HEALTH POLICY ISSUES FOR THE UNITED STATES

Federal level

- Adoption of a national healthcare plan
- What is the role of the federal government in managing malpractice suits and awards?
- Supply of healthcare professionals (How much is enough? Where should funding go?)
- Given that the Constitution does not recognize health care as a federal responsibility, what is the role of the federal government in supporting health care?
- What benefits should be offered by Medicare and state Medicaid programs?

State and local level

- Who should be eligible for Medicaid benefits? What benefits should be covered?
- Is it the state's responsibility to subsidize health care for the uninsured?
- How can the licensure process be improved to ensure quality, access, and proper competition?
- How should emergency planning measures be coordinated?

Health care organizations

- What proportion of charitable care (care not reimbursed) is appropriate beyond the mandated requirement?
- How can costs be controlled without jeopardizing access and quality?
- How can the organization balance the duty to provide services that meet the community needs within financial constraints?

Professional providers

- How should I influence local, state, and national professional organizations on health policy?
- How can I make the best decisions as to which managed care contract I should sign?
- Should I establish an independent practice or work for an established facility?

Source: Author.

reform healthcare policies. The World Health Organization describes the policy process as consisting of the following phases:

1. Problem identification and agenda setting
2. Formation
3. Legislative Process
4. Implementation
5. Evaluation

Problem Identification and Agenda Setting

During the problem identification phase of policy development, a societal problem within a community, state, or nation is identified. Establishing an accurate and appropriate definition of the problem is essential if resolution is to occur.[7]

Formation

Once an issue is defined, data are collected and the argument for policy development is introduced to government officials. During the formation phase, the policy statement is outlined, the purpose and results are well established, important political and socioeconomic aspects are considered, and anticipated resource consumption identified. During this phase, unspoken professional and personal values and beliefs of individuals participating in the policy process are likely to influence key decisions.[8] Sensitivity to these positions and assumptions are necessary to further policy development.

Adoption

Adoption is the process by which proposed policy becomes law, health programs are subsidized, and health policy is balanced in respect to other policies. Public agenda issues introduced as a bill must progress through the legislative process before enactment. During the legislative process, many factors influence the outcome of the proposed bill, including pressure from special interest groups, preference of voters, partisan views, and personal opinions. The voice of nursing cannot be overemphasized. Knowing legislators, writing letters, and supporting professional organizations can influence healthcare policy development.

Implementation

The implementation phase involves policy execution. This phase includes activities in which legislative mandates are carried out, often through programs. Legislators frequently look to experts to provide evidence-based information. "If government officials do not know qualified, appropriate experts, then decisions about program planning and design often are determined by legislators, bureaucrats, or staff who know little or nothing about the problem or the solutions."[9] Implementation of public policy frequently takes place through the regulatory process. Generally, a governmental agency is appointed to oversee the policy. The appointed agency is authorized to abide by a set of rules to operationalize the policy. A well-known example of legislation regulated by a government agency is a state nurse practice act. The nurse practice act is law that is administered through a board of nursing. Each board of nursing is authorized to establish rules and regulations for application of the law.

Evaluation

During the evaluation phase, the policy performance or program outcomes are appraised and policy is modified at times. Evaluation is a logical component of the policy process. "Evaluation research is a powerful tool for defending viable programs, and for providing rationale for program failure."[10] Evaluation should begin early on and continue throughout a program to avoid fatal flaws.[11] Milstead describes the Tuskegee experiment (1932–1972) in which a group of African-Americans was used as a control group and denied antibiotic treatment for syphilis even after treatment was validated as successful.[12] This example underscores the need for vigilant monitoring and evaluation to address moral and ethical concerns as part of the legislative and public policy process. Another example of sequential change to existing policy is seen in the Medicare program. Medicare originated in 1965 and was expanded in 1972 to include patients with end-stage renal disease. In 1973 Medicare was further expanded to include people of any age who meet the definition of Medicare established by Medicare. The latest revision to the program was the addition of the Medicare prescription program in 2006.

NURSES AND PUBLIC POLICY

Public health policy is adopted and shaped by the policy process. The process is highly impacted by the opinions and preferences of lawmakers, individuals, special interest groups, and organizations.[13] Professional nurses render more direct care than any other healthcare provider and thus are in a unique position to see firsthand the impact and needed changes of health policy, laws, and regulatory requirements. As the largest group of healthcare professionals in the country, the power base available to nurses established on numbers alone is enormous. According to the 2004 National Sample of Registered Nurses, there are 2.9 million registered nurses living in the United States.[14] Abood summarizes the sources of power for nurses and notes that the basis of power extends far beyond the numbers.[15] Figure 14-2 describes sources of power for nurses as expert, legitimate, referent, reward, and coercive. Legitimate power is afforded all nurses by virtue of licensure to practice nursing. Moreover, founding principles from the American Nurses Association's *Code of Ethics for Nurses With Interpretive Statements* (2001) and *Nursing's Social Policy Statement* (2003) as well as responsibilities established in American Nurses Association's *Scope and Standards for Nursing Administrators* (2004) and competencies from the American Organizations of Nurse Executives (2004) provide further evidence of legitimate power of the nurse. Nursing executives, by the nature of their positions, have the potential for all sources of power and, if used effectively, can influence both public and organizational policy. Importantly, successful leaders do not cling to personal power and recognize the power in each individual. Use of collective power magnifies influence and mobilizes resources to facilitate change.[16]

Today, health care is plagued with daunting challenges that continue to fuel public and political debate. Pressing issues confronting health care in the United States include, among others, access to care, quality and safety, cost, aging America, workforce shortage, and specialty population concerns. Nurses at all levels can affect change in health policy. Staying abreast of the issues is essential. Attending public

FIGURE 14-2   SOURCES OF POWER

Expert	Comes from having knowledge and skill needed by others
Legitimate	A result of the role of an individual
Referent	Obtained through admiration and respect
Reward	The power to give or withhold what others want
Coercive	The ability to punish

Source: Author.

meetings, reading the newspaper or journals, writing articles to influence opinion, contacting public officials, and participating in special interest organizations are numerous ways that nurses can become involved. Participation in professional organizations, especially those with political action committees, is one of the most effective means of influencing policy. Professional organizations with a political arm can be highly effective and influential in health policy development. These organizations study the issue, develop a stance, lobby, and provide financial contributions to candidates who support the legislative and regulatory agenda of the organization. The American Nurses Association Political Action Committee and the Political Action Committee of the American Organization of Nurse Executives in partnership with the American Hospital Association are two politically active nursing organizations striving to influence policy development. For years physicians have been considerably more successful than nurses in exercising sources of power to highly influence health policy. Imagine for just one moment the impact for nursing and patients if nurses collectively unified and actively engaged in policy development.

"As the largest group of healthcare professionals in the country, the power base of nurses established by numbers alone is enormous."

"The leader of today recognizes the power potential in each person."

"Pressing issues confronting health care in the United States include, among others, access to care, quality, safety, cost, aging America, and specialty population concerns."

DEPARTMENT OF HEALTH AND HUMAN SERVICES

The U.S. Department of Health and Human Services (DHHS) is the federal government's primary department for protecting the public's health and human services. Regulations pertaining to national health safety and well-being are administered by the DHHS. The budget for DHHS ($697 billion for fiscal year 2007) funds more than 300 programs and multiple agencies.[17] Some of the programs administered by DHHS are Social Security, Medicare, maternal and infant health, prevention of child abuse and domestic violence, services for older Americans, preventing disease and immunizations, and substance abuse and treatment. The Department's programs are administered by 11 divisions.[18]

FEDERAL AND STATE LAWS

Labor Laws

Federal and state labor laws regulate relationships between employers and employees. Healthcare organizations are not immune to these laws; thus, as with any other business, they are required to comply with established regulations. Laws cover such issues as working conditions, hours, compensation, union activity, workers' wages, occupational safety and health, and employment discrimination. Federal law is administered by the U.S. Department of Labor and is aimed at assisting every man and woman that needs or wants to work by guaranteeing safe working conditions, a minimum hourly wage, overtime pay, freedom from discrimination, unemployment insurance, and workers' compensation.[19] Special needs of those who desire to work such as the older American, minority groups, women, and handicapped, are addressed by federal law.

Title VII of the Civil Rights Act of 1964, a federal law enforced by the U.S and amended by the Equal Employment Opportunity Commission (EEOC), protects workers from discrimination because of race, color, religion, gender, national origin, disability, citizenship status, or age (if employee is at least 40 years old). The act prohibits harassment based on physical appearance or cultural practices (such as wearing a head scarf), religious affiliation, and association with other individuals or organization.[20] Title VII applies to businesses that employ a minimum of 15 full- or part-time employees. Under Title VII, employers are required to provide equal promotion opportunities to employees. If an employee who possesses certain characteristics protected by law is passed over for a promotion, the employer must be ready to demonstrate that the decision was based on sound criteria. On the other hand, if employee requirements for a position such as height or weight are imposed for valid reasons, the requirement is generally not interpreted as discriminatory, unless, however, it is imposed to prevent a candidate's selection for a position.

In *Buckley Nursing Home v. Massachusetts Commission against Discrimination,* a black applicant seeking a nurse's aide position sued the nursing home for discrimination after being interviewed but not hired for the position. Shortly after the interview, the nurse's aide was told that the position was filled. The position was subsequently advertised again and the nurse's aide reapplied for the position. When she called to inquire about the position she was told that she would be called as needed. During the trial, the court learned that other nurse's aides were hired after the aide's reapplication. Further testimony indicated that discussion had occurred by Buckley about the nurse's aide's color and that race was a determining factor for not hiring her. The nurse's aide was awarded money for lost wages and emotional distress.[21]

In 1980 the EEOC law expanded to include sexual harassment guidelines. These guidelines protect employees from unwelcome sexual advances or requests. Furthermore, the law prohibits verbal or physical conduct of a sexual nature when the behavior interferes with performance of work or creates intimidating, hostile, or offensive work situations.[22] To comply with the law, employers should have an anti-harassment policy in place describing the complaint procedure and must promptly act to prevent and correct harassment when a claim is made.

Managers should always take a complaint regarding alleged discrimination seriously and involve legal counsel. When the EEOC receives a complaint from an employee, an EEOC attorney is generally appointed to meet with the employee and review the complaint. After this interview, a meeting is held with the employer. Commonly, the EEOC attempts to negotiate a settlement between the employee and the employer. It is wise on the part of the employer to resolve the complaint through conciliation. If an agreement cannot be reached, the EEOC issues the employee a right to sue letter, giving permission to sue the institution. In the event that the EEOC finds the act of discrimination glaring, the EEOC may file a lawsuit on behalf of the employee. When the court finds the employer in violation of Title VII, the employer may have to "restore rightful economic status" of all those in the affected class. Even if the EEOC does not support the employee's claim of discrimination, the employee may still take legal action through the state for wrongful discharge, breach of contract, or discrimination under state law. Regardless of the outcome, it is illegal for an employer to retaliate against an employee who claims discrimination.

Figure 14-3 is a summary of other federal laws that further protect workers from unfair treatment or workplace discrimination.

State laws may further protect employees from discrimination, unfair treatment, or unsafe conditions in the workplace by expounding on factors such as testing positive for human immunodeficiency virus, marital status, obesity, sexual orientation, minimum wage, meal and break regulations, overtime, occupational safety and health practices, family and medical leave, drug and alcohol testing, employee arrest and conviction records, access to personnel records, and health insurance continuation.

The following discussion describes a few cases noted by Pozgar that involve labor relation litigation. The first case, *Theodore v. Department of Health and Human Services,* resulted in a finding of discrimination when a black nurse was improperly suspended after an altercation with a white nurse. Evidence indicated that the black nurse apologized after accidentally striking a white nurse while pushing a crib. The white nurse responded by striking the black nurse and blurting out inflammatory slurs. The court found no grounds for disciplinary action against the black nurse.[23] In *Schlitzer v. University of Iowa Hospital,* the State Supreme Court found that a nurse who had a weight-lifting limitation after an automobile accident did not meet the job requirements of a position. The court ruled that an employer

FIGURE 14-3   **FEDERAL LAWS, WORKER PROTECTION, AND CONSIDERATIONS**

Federal Law	Worker Protection	Considerations
Fair Labor Standards Act (FLSA)	Establishes minimum wage and overtime pay for nonexempt employees. Overtime occurs when worked hours <40 per week. All worked hours apply even if incidental, waiting, on-call, or if employee volunteers	Exempt employees are determined based on salary, duties, and responsibilities and do not qualify for overtime or minimum wage and are paid a salary and hours are not "clocked." Exempt employees are generally executives, administrative, and professional but titles alone do not determine status. (When state minimum wages are higher than federal standards, state standards apply.)
Child Labor Provisions of the FLSA	Establishes the minimum age of employment as 16 years	
Age Discrimination in Employment Act	Protects qualified individuals >40 years of age and <70 from discrimination; promotes employment based on ability	Private businesses with >20 employees
Immigration Reform and Control Act of 1986, 1990, & 1996	Protects lawfully admitted non-U.S. citizens from discrimination	The law requires employers to assess the legality of employees and imposes penalties for those who knowingly hire aliens.
The Rehabilitation Act of 1973	Protects handicapped employees from discrimination in the areas of recruitment, advertising, processing of applications, promotions, pay, benefits, and assignments.	Employers receiving federal monies must perform an assessment of compliance with the law.
Americans with Disability Act (ADA) of 1990	Protects people with a mental or physical disability from employment discrimination in hiring and promotion and requires that employer make "reasonable accommodations" for the employee to perform essential job requirements.	Employers with >15 employees for 20 or more weeks during a calendar year. Essential functions are usually defined in job descriptions.
Equal Pay Act of 1963	Equal pay for genders performing jobs within the same institution that require the same skill, effort, and responsibility	
Family and Medical Leave Act (FMLA) of 1993	Grants temporary medical leave for childbirth, adoptions, foster care placements, and employee's or family's serious health condition	Eligible employees have up to 12 work weeks of unpaid leave during any 12-month period. Following leave, the employee has a right to return to original position or an equivalent job with the same pay and benefits.
Pregnancy Discrimination Act	Prevents discrimination against pregnant women, childbirth, related medical conditions; must apply same employment policies to both pregnant and nonpregnant workers; women must be reinstated to work under same conditions of those after other disabilities	

continues

| | FIGURE 14-3 | FEDERAL LAWS, WORKER PROTECTION, AND CONSIDERATIONS (CONTINUED) |

Federal Law	Worker Protection	Considerations
Veteran's Readjustment Assistance Act	Provides reemployment rights for veterans to positions held before military duty	Reemployment rights are protected from 90 days post-discharge from training or service or 1 year from time of hospitalization
Occupational Safety and Health Act of 1970	Protects employees from workplace hazards such as hazardous chemicals, noise, fires, temperature and ventilation, blood and body fluid exposure; overseen by the Occupational Safety and Health Administration (OSHA)	Employers must enforce safety standards, provide employee training (right to know), supply protective apparel, post a federal or state notice of job safety and health protection, record all workplace injuries, and compensate employee for injury whether it is the employee's fault or not, and notify OSHA of job-related deaths. Inspections can occur at any time. Penalties apply including imprisonment if willful or repeated violations occur.
Consolidated Omnibus Budget Reconciliation Acts (COBRA)	Employees and their families must be offered by employers healthcare coverage for a specified period of time if employment has been terminated (except for gross misconduct), hours have been reduced, employees have become eligible for Medicare	Employers with >20 employees

Source: Author.

does not have a responsibility to modify the essential elements of a job to accommodate an individual's disability.[24] In *Odomes v. Nucare, Inc.*, the court ruled that pay discrimination occurred in a nursing facility when a female nurse's aide who performed similar work to male orderlies was paid less.[25]

Given that nurses comprise the greatest portion of the healthcare workforce, nurse managers and executives must be well informed about labor laws and regulations. Because a high volume of claims occur regarding discrimination, harassment, and wrongful discharge issues, nurses in management positions should work closely with the human resource department to ensure compliance with the laws.[26]

Federal and State Health Insurance

Medicare

Medicare, first established in 1965, is a federal health insurance plan covering citizens 65 years of age and older, people with certain disabilities, and individuals with end-stage renal disease. Medicare, administered by the Centers for Medicare and Medicaid Services, covers 40 million Americans and is the nation's largest health insurance program. Medicare consists of three provisions:

- Part A (Hospital Insurance) provides payment for inpatient care, including critical access hospitals and skilled nursing facilities. It does not cover custodial or long-term care. Part A also provides assistance for qualified individuals with expenses related to hospice care and home health.

Most individuals pay for this benefit during working years and therefore do not pay a premium to get these benefits.

- Part B (Medical Insurance) assists with payments for physician and outpatient care. It also pays for some of the expenses not covered by Part A such as physical and occupational and home health services as well as medically necessary supplies. A monthly premium is paid by most individuals receiving Part B benefits.
- Prescription Drug Coverage is an insurance that is provided to help lower prescription drug costs and protect against rising costs. The drug coverage became available in 2006. This is an optional benefit for a monthly premium.

Benefits of the Medicare program are provided to recipients regardless of means. Contribution from the workforce pay expenses related to hospital care. Major health policy debate is ongoing about the stability and viability of the Medicare program, particularly in light of the aging population.

Medicaid

Medicaid, also established in 1965, is a welfare program that provides public assistance for certain health expenses for low income children and their caregivers and adults with special needs such as age, disability, and pregnancy. The program is administered by the state, and thus each state sets its own guidelines. Matching funds are provided by the federal government based on the average income of resident's within the state. Participation in the Medicaid program is based on an individual's means; therefore income and resources are reviewed before eligibility for program.

REGULATORY ISSUES

Health care in America is one of the most highly regulated industries in our country. The government has a responsibility to protect the public and in doing so appraise and deem individuals and organizations safe to deliver health care. The keystone of health service regulation in the United States is regulation of licensure. The function of licensure is delegated by the federal government to the states. Therefore hospitals and other healthcare organizations along with clinical practitioners are licensed to provide services only after meeting criteria defined by the state in which they are located. American healthcare regulation inundates organizations from the federal, state, local, and even private sector. Of particular importance to nurses are the standards defined by The Joint Commission (TJC). A review of the agency's purpose and accreditation process follows.

The TJC is a private nonprofit organization established to define and apply standards of operation for healthcare entities. The TJC, consisting of healthcare members, hospitals, and organizations throughout the nation, provides a mechanism of self-governance known as accreditation. Board members consist of physicians, administrators, nurses, employers, a labor representative, health plan leaders, quality experts, ethicists, a consumer advocate, and educators representing a diverse background in healthcare policy and practice. Corporate members include the American College of Physicians, the American College of Surgeons, the American Dental Association, the American Hospital Association, and the American Medical Association. Of note, corporate membership does not include any nursing organizations.

Although participation in TJC is voluntary, Medicare, Medicaid, and most other insurance plans require providers to be accredited by either TJC or through state surveys to receive funds for services. Accreditation by TJC fulfills regulatory requirements in many states; thus most hospitals choose to participate in the accreditation process in spite of the costly fees associated with the review process and the rigorous standards.

TJC originated in 1910 when Dr. Ernest Codman proposed a system for hospitals to appraise patient results and to determine ineffective treatments.[27] In 1917 the American College of Surgeons established standards for hospitals that formed the basis of all subsequent review endeavors. In 1952 the

TJC was created to continue the work of the American College of Surgeons. In 1965, when the newly formed Medicare program was established, the TJC accrediting procedure was selected as the mechanism for determining qualifying hospitals for Medicare payment.

Accreditation is awarded for a maximum of 3 years. With the most recent changes, participating institutions are subject to unannounced visits from the TJC at any time during the 3-year cycle. Over the years the TJC has continued to expand the accreditation review process to other types of facilities. Today, TJC evaluates and accredits the following healthcare organizations:

- General, psychiatric, children's, and rehabilitation hospitals
- Critical access hospitals
- Medical equipment services, hospice services, and other home care organizations
- Nursing homes and other long-term care facilities
- Behavioral healthcare organizations, addiction services
- Rehabilitation centers, group practices, office-based surgeries, and other ambulatory care providers

Although participation by organizations in JCAHO is voluntary, Medicare, Medicaid, and most other insurance plans require providers to be accredited by either JCAHO or through survey by the state to receive funds for services.

TJC is widely known by healthcare professionals as an accrediting body for institutions. Nurse executives must be able to articulate patient care standards as published by TJC and Centers for Medicare and Medicaid Services and facilitate compliance within the organization.

Today, there is a wide range of compliance requirements from numerous accrediting and regulatory bodies that control health care, the breadth of which is beyond the scope of this text. Unfortunately, the networks of bureaucratic structures created by the regulations sometimes overlap, complement and contradict each other, making application difficult and costly for institutions.[28]

CREDENTIALING OF INDIVIDUAL PRACTITIONERS

Licensure is defined by the National Council of State Boards of Nursing (NCSBN) as "the process by which an agency of state government grants permission to an individual to engage in a given profession upon finding that the applicant has attained the essential degree of competency necessary to perform a unique scope of practice."[29] In the United States, surprisingly, licensure of healthcare practitioners did not begin until 1873 when Texas passed a law to regulate the practice of physicians. Until that time, physicians were plentiful; however, knowledge and quality was limited, to say the least.[30] Today, there are over 100 different health professions.[29] Healthcare practice, in most instances, is granted by a state in which services are delivered.[31]

Nursing Licensure/Credentialing

In 1899 nurse leaders in the United States decided that nursing had reached the stage of acknowledged indispensability as an occupation in the care of the ill and convalescent and furthermore that this occupation was so intimately bound up with the safety and health of the public that it required regulation and control in the education of those who desired to engage in it.[32] The leaders who inspired the struggle were keenly aware that, because all progress must have a beginning, some effective legislation was better than none at all; time would serve to improve the extent of control, to fill in the gaps, and to remedy the errors. The important thing was to get some law on the books. The first states to enact laws were North Carolina in 1902 and New Jersey, New York, Virginia, Maryland, Indiana, California, Connecticut, and Colorado in 1903.

Nurse Practice Acts in each state are laws designed first and foremost to protect the public and are the policing power of the state. The acts define nursing, mandate and set standards for licensure, mandate licensure examinations, regulate schools of nursing, set standards for curricula of schools of nursing, require continuing education for licensure renewal, mandate investigation of reports of violation of nursing practice, regulate the discipline of violators of nurse practice laws, and regulate advanced practice nurses.

"Nurse practice acts are designed, first and foremost, to protect the public and are the policing power of the state."

Each state has a nurse practice act that authorizes a board of nursing established to oversee the practice of nursing. The boards provide decisions as to which tasks may be delegated to licensed practical/vocational nurses and unlicensed personnel and that may become independent nurse functions.

To be eligible for licensure in any state, nurses must graduate from an approved school of nursing and successfully pass the National Council Licensure Examination for Registered Nurses (NCLEX-RN) or Practical Nurses (NCLEX-PN). Associate, diploma, and baccalaureate degrees sit for the same NCLEX examination. Though nurses are registered and granted licensure to practice in a given state, nurses may be allowed to practice in another state when reciprocity is granted by that state's board of nursing. There is a move toward the creation of legislative compacts between states to allow nurses the freedom to practice in nearby states without applying for reciprocity. In 2006, 20 states were members of the Nurse Licensure Compact, whereas 2 more were pending membership.[33]

"Nurses are ranked number one by the public on professional honesty and ethical standards."

Nursing is a profession built on ethical principles that has earned the trust of the public. According to the 2006 Gallup poll, nurses were ranked number one by the public on professional honesty and ethical standards.[34] Nurses have continued to hold this top position for all but 1 of the 8 years measured by the Gallup poll. However, in the event that nurses violate the tenets of their licensure, state boards of nursing are empowered to dis-

"Nurse executives, as leaders within an organization, are responsible to understand, articulate, and ensure compliance with the State Nurse Practice Act and the State Board of Nursing regulations."

cipline violators by probation, revocation of license, and referral to criminal courts. Nurse executives, as leaders within an organization, are responsible to understand, articulate, and ensure compliance with the State Nurse Practice Act and the State Board of Nursing regulations.

Advanced Practice Registered Nurses

The advanced practice nurse is a registered nurse prepared at the graduate level as a clinical nurse specialist, nurse practitioner, nurse mid-wife, or nurse anesthetist. Since the early 1990s the regulation of advanced practice registered nurses has been an issue of debate for the profession. Consensus exists for uniform regulation; however, the mechanism for ensuring competency and safe practice is yet to be clearly defined. In 1998 the American Association of Colleges of Nursing issued a position statement entitled, "Certification and Regulation of Advanced Practice Nurses," that called for uniformity in regulation of advanced practice registered nurses through certification rather than licensure. In 2000 the Delegate Assembly of the NCSBN adopted the following requirements to support uniformity in the licensure/authority process:

• Registered nurse licensure in good standing
• Graduation from a nationally accredited advanced practice program
• Advanced practice certification in the area of study by a national certification program
• Evidence of continued certification or competence

In 2002, a position paper was developed by the NCSBN on the regulation of advanced practice to provide guidance in state regulatory efforts. Additionally, the NCSBN board of directors, in an effort to further standardize regulation, approved criteria for both the certification programs and for the accrediting agencies. Still today, however, regulation varies greatly among state boards of nursing.[35]

Certification

Certification is another type of credential that recognizes a nurse's accomplishment after meeting specified requirements. Certification is awarded by a nongovernmental agency or association and therefore is not regulated by law. However, as mentioned above, many state boards of nursing use national certification programs as a requirement for granting authority for advanced practice nurses. Certification can be obtained from numerous professional nursing organizations recognizing various levels of practice for most specialty areas.

Evidence-Based Practice 14-1

Cliska, Hayward, Dobbins, Brunton, and Underwood designed a descriptive study to obtain an understanding of the needs of public policymakers as it related to decision making. Specifically addressed were research needs, perceptions of barriers to research utilization, and attitudes toward systematic reviews of decision makers in public health at the level of systems planning. In Ontario, public health consultants and managers were queried about barriers to research utilization and awareness of and attitudes toward systematic reviews as a method of translating research into policy practice. The public health consultants and managers were provided five completed reviews in summary, abstract, and full form and on diskette, hard copy, and Internet. Three-month surveys assessed use, relevance, application, and further dissemination of the reviews. Two-hundred forty-two individuals in public health policy and decision-making positions participated. Those responding described a significant, largely unmet, need for research evidence. Systematic reviews were reported as likely means to overcome the barriers to research use related to critical appraisal, time, timeliness, availability, cost, and credibility but not to barriers related to policy climate, authority, or implementation resources. Ninety-three percent said they would follow up, 91% remembered receiving it, 71% of these had read it, whereas 23% stated it played a part in program planning or decision making.[36]

SUMMARY

Health care in America is heavily regulated by federal, state, and local government as well as private accrediting and certifying organizations. Gaps and deficiencies in care for the public, overlapping laws, and excessive requirements for providers, insurers, and suppliers are the unintended consequence of decentralized health care. Health policy can occur in private or governmental organizations and is both an entity and a process. Nurses, as direct caregivers, are in a unique position to identify needed policy change. Given that nurses are the largest providers of health care, the numbers alone have the potential to highly influence policy development if nurses participate in the policy process.

The DHHS is responsible for overseeing the national health and human services policies. The DHHS administers many programs by various agencies. Laws and regulations that commonly impact nurses and patients include federal and state labor laws, federal and state health insurance, the TJC accreditation standards, and licensure laws. Nurse leaders need to be familiar with healthcare laws and regulations have an important duty to ensure compliance.

APPLICATION EXERCISES

Exercise 14-1

Select a healthcare policy currently in place in a healthcare organization (may be your work or field site). Using the policy process, outline how this policy was developed and implemented. What is the nurses' role in carrying out policy within the organization?

Exercise 14-2

Interview a nurse executive in a healthcare organization. Identify how the organization obtains and updates the licensure and certification of the professional nursing staff. What requirements are in place to ensure that the professional nursing staff remains competent? Is this a local, regional, and/or federal mandate?

Exercise 14-3

Interview the chief financial officer in a healthcare organization. What are the federal and state insurance plans in place in this system? What policy issues impact reimbursement in this setting?

Notes

1. McLaughlin, C., & McLaughlin, C. (2008). *Health policy: An interdisciplinary approach* (p. 4). Sudbury, MA: Jones and Bartlett.
2. Ibid., p. 23.
3. Borger, C., Smith, S., Truffer, C., Keehan, S., Sisko, A., & Smith, T. (2006). Health spending projections through 2015. *Health Affairs, 25*, 46–57.
4. Cherry, B., & Trotter, B. (2005). Health policy and politics: Get involved! In B. Cherry & S. Jacobs (Eds.), *Contemporary nursing: Issues, trends & management* (pp. 211–233). St. Louis, MO: Elsevier.
5. McLaughlin, C., & McLaughlin, C. (2008). *Health policy: An interdisciplinary approach* (pp. 4, 8, 10, 11). Sudbury, MA: Jones and Bartlett.
6. Field, R. (2007). *Health care regulation in America: Complexity, confrontation and compromise.* Oxford: Oxford University Press.
7. McLaughlin & McLaughlin, 2008, p. 180.
8. Ibid., p. 193.
9. Milstead, J. (2004). *Health policy and politics: A nurse's guide* (2nd ed., p. 27). Sudbury, MA: Jones and Bartlett Publishers.
10. Ibid., p. 22.
11. Longest, B. (2006). *Health policy making in the United States* (4th ed.). Chicago: Health Administration Press.
12. Milstead, 2004, p. 22.
13. Longest, 2006.
14. U.S. Department of Health and Human Services. (2004). *National sample of registered nurses.* Retrieved January 8, 2008, from ftp://ftp.hrsa.gov/bhpr/workforce/0306rnss.pdf
15. Abood, S. (2007). Influencing health care in the legislative arena. *Online Journal of Issues in Nursing, 12*, 3–5.
16. Porter-O'Grady, T., & Malloch, K. (2002). *Quantum leadership: A textbook of new leadership.* Gaithersburg, MD: Aspen.

17. U.S. Department of Health and Human Services. (2008). Department of Health & Human Services organizational chart. Retrieved January 17, 2008, from http://www.hhs.gov/about/orgchart.html

18. Ibid.

19. Pozgar, G. (2007). *Legal aspects of health care administration* (10th ed., p. 404). Sudbury, MA: Jones and Bartlett.

20. Ibid., p. 407.

21. Ibid., p. 417.

22. Ibid., p. 418.

23. Ibid., p. 417.

24. Ibid., p. 409.

25. Ibid., p. 416.

26. Warnick, M. (2001). Human resources issues. In R. Carroll (Ed.), *Risk management handbook for health care organizations* (3rd ed., p. 711). San Francisco: Jossey-Bass.

27. Field, 2007.

28. Ibid.

29. National Council of State Boards of Nursing. (2007). *Practice and discipline.* Retrieved January 10, 2008, from https://www.ncsbn.org/168.htm

30. Field, 2007, p. 20.

31. U.S. Department of Labor, Bureau of Labor Statistics. (2008). *Occupational outlook handbook* (2008–09 Edition). Retrieved January 9, 2008, from http://www.bls.gov/oco/home.htm

32. Lesnik, M., & Anderson, B. (1947). *Legal aspects of nursing* (pp. 25–26). Philadelphia: Lippincott.

33. U.S. Department of Labor, Bureau of Labor Statistics, 2008.

34. Saad, L. (2006). Nurses top list of most honest and ethical professions. Retrieved December 13, 2007, from http://www.gallup.com/poll/25888/Nurses-Top-List-Most-Honest-Ethical-Professions.aspx

35. National Council of State Boards of Nursing, 2007.

36. Cliska, D., Hayward, S., Dobbins, M., Brunton, G., & Underwood, J. (1999). Transferring public-health nursing research to health-system planning: assessing the relevance and accessibility of systematic reviews. *Canadian Journal of Nursing Research, 31,* 23–36.

15 RISK MANAGEMENT AND LEGAL ISSUES

Valorie Dearmon, RN, MSN, NEA, BC

LEARNING OBJECTIVES AND ACTIVITIES

- Describe laws impacting health care.
- Differentiate among the elements of a risk management program.
- Identify the risks professional nurses face regarding malpractice and other torts.
- Outline a plan for professional nurses to use to reduce the risks of legal actions.

CONCEPTS

Torts, civil and criminal law, negligence, malpractice, defamation, slander and libel, assault and battery, false imprisonment, standard of care, respondeat superior.

QUOTE

The only real mistake is the one from which we learn nothing.

—John Powell

Introduction

One could easily say that health care today is "risky business." In 1999 a seminal report was released from the Institute of Medicine indicating that medical errors contribute to the deaths of 44,000 to 98,000 hospitalized patients each year. It further indicated that more patients die each year from adverse events associated with health care than expire from automobile accidents (43,458), and that deaths resulting from medical errors surpass the number of deaths related to breast cancer, the eighth leading cause of death in the United States.[1] The report shook the public and healthcare community and generated a call for action. The Institute of Medicine report suggested that 90% of errors result from failures in the system and are not the blame of individuals.[2] Therefore a massive campaign was launched to increase patient safety through the transformation of complex systems within healthcare organizations. Despite enormous efforts by both private and governmental organizations to transform work environments and to improve patient safety, mistakes continue and the number of legal claims against healthcare providers continues to soar.[3] Inevitably, rendering patient care in imperfect work environments with broken systems and by humans (who are fallible) affords multiple opportunities for mishaps and misunderstandings. Given the complexities of health care today, managing risk poses major challenges for those in positions who lead. It is essential that nurse managers and executives possess a basic understanding of the law pertaining to health care and that every effort be made to institute safeguards for the protection of the public, employees, and organization.

> **❝Rendering patient care in imperfect work environments with broken systems and by humans (who are fallible) affords multiple opportunities for mishaps and misunderstandings.❞**

LAW IMPACTING HEALTH CARE

There are two distinct divisions of the law within the United States: criminal (public) and civil (private). In health care, both criminal and civil law apply, with the preponderance of litigation being civil in nature.

Civil Law

Civil law pertains to a wrongdoing between individuals or between an individual and the state, excluding criminal acts. In a civil case, defendants are found liable as opposed to guilty and are directed to pay monetary compensation for economic (financial loss) and or noneconomic damages (pain and suffering). Tort law, which addresses transgressions of one individual on the legal rights of another, is the foundation of civil law. There are two types of tort: unintentional and intentional.

Unintentional Torts

An unintentional tort or negligence may occur as a result of carelessness or accident and focuses on injury or harm. Unintentional torts are the basis of malpractice suits.

Negligence   Negligence is a part of tort or personal injury law and is defined as "a failure to use that degree of care that any reasonable and prudent person would use under the same or similar circumstances."[4] If a professional, such as a physician or nurse, is negligent while acting in his or her professional capacity, the term is coined medical negligence or malpractice. To recover damages when negligence is alleged, the burden of proof lies with the plaintiff to demonstrate each of the following four elements:

1. A legal duty to provide reasonable care
2. A breach of duty (an act or a failure to act)
3. Injury to another
4. Breach of duty must be the proximate (immediately related) cause of the injury

> **❝Being named in a lawsuit does not mean that wrongdoing has occurred, and injury does not necessarily indicate that someone was at fault.❞**

Generally speaking, anyone or any agency is susceptible to a suit for negligence for just about any act or omission. The essence of a negligence claim is that one's conduct fell below the expected care and the failure resulted in injury. Being named in a lawsuit does not mean that wrongdoing has occurred, and injury does not necessarily indicate that someone was at fault.

Medical Malpractice   Medical malpractice is "negligence on the part of a professional only while he or she is acting in the course of professional duties."[5] Malpractice contends that

1. One's conduct did not meet the expected professional standards or fell below the "standard of care," *and*
2. The failure caused harm to a patient.

Malpractice cases begin with an incident of alleged negligence and alleged injury. The injured party (plaintiff) retains an attorney and files a lawsuit against another (defendant). The plaintiff could be the patient, the patient's family, or a legal guardian. Depending on the allegations, there may be multiple defendants in the same lawsuit, including one or more hospitals, physicians, nurses, or others.

Medical malpractice is a serious concern for the healthcare industry. The Agency for Healthcare Research and Quality defines medical errors as "mistakes made in the process of care that result in or have the potential to do harm to patients."[6] Numerous reports indicate that medical errors are commonplace. Following a review of 30,000 medical records of patients discharged from 51 New York hospitals, a research team at Harvard University found that 3.7% of those hospitalized suffered adverse events, with 27.6% of the adverse events attributed to negligent care.[7] These findings are similar to other studies across the nation. Despite the high frequency of medical errors, only 1 of every 7.6 patients injured as a result of negligence file lawsuits, and even a smaller number receive compensation for injuries.[8] Furthermore, most individuals who file a malpractice suit have suffered a genuine injury or loss; thus a common belief that most lawsuits are fraudulent is unfounded.[9]

Malpractice lawsuits continue to escalate. The following cases represent a small sampling of medical malpractice events. In *Monk v. Doctor's Hospital*, the facility and physician were found negligent when a Bovie plate was inappropriately applied during surgery, resulting in a patient burn.[10] In an Alabama case, two nurses testified that they did not know a decubitus ulcer could be life threatening and a third nurse claimed ignorance in the need to call the doctor for symptoms of an infection. After their testimonies, the nursing facility employing these nurses was found negligent in providing training and supervision. The suit led to a judgment of 2 million dollars in damages for the plaintiff.[11] In *Lloyd Noland Hospital v. Durham*, the court ruled against the hospital when staff failed to administer a standing order of preoperative antibiotics to a patient.[12] Regrettably, the stories go on and on.

In many industries mistakes do not produce grave consequences, leaving organizations with more latitude to view errors as learning opportunities. However, in a business where one delivers quite personal and commonly invasive care to human beings, mistakes can have devastating and irreversible effects for those served. Healthcare leaders are in a difficult position of attempting to balance the multitude of good that occurs from the care and services provided to the majority with the potentially serious consequences of negligent incidents. The challenge to keep a "stiff upper lip" is tough when the reports of medical errors tarnish the reputation of the industry. Press releases and personal experiences continue to shake the confidence of healthcare consumers. In a recent national survey, findings revealed that 55% of participants were dissatisfied with the care they received and 34% reported that either they or a family member experienced a medical error.[13] These type of findings describe why today the public is more skeptical and leery of healthcare services and providers.

> **"The latest reports on malpractice claims indicate that the incidence of nurses personally named in lawsuits is greater today than ever before."**

The latest reports on malpractice claims indicate that the incidence of nurses personally named in lawsuits is greater now than ever before. According to the National Practitioner Data Bank, malpractice payments for nurses increased from 253 in 1998 to 5,567 in 2005.[14] These numbers do not reflect the incidence of nurses involved in lawsuits covered under the doctrine of corporate liability, which holds organizations responsible for the practice of all those within their walls.

In a review of more than 350 cases between 1995 and 2001, Croke identified six key areas for nursing negligence[15] summarized as the failure to

1. Follow standards of care
2. Use equipment in a responsible manner

| TABLE 15-1 | **NATIONAL PRACTITIONER DATA BANK, 2005 ANNUAL REPORT** |

Number of Medical Malpractice Payment Reports by Malpractice Reason—Nurses (Registered Nurses, Nurse Anesthetists, Nurse Midwives, Nurse Practitioners, and Advanced Practice Nurses/Clinical Nurse Specialists) National Practitioner Data Bank (September 1, 1990–December 31, 2005)

Malpractice Reason	RN (Professional) Nurse	Nurse Anesthetist	Nurse Midwife	Nurse Practitioner	Advanced Practice Nurse/ Clinical Nurse Specialist*	Total
Anesthesia related	128	915	1	8	1	1,053
Behavioral health related**	3	1	0	1	0	5
Diagnosis related	229	17	39	219	1	505
Equipment or product related	55	6	0	4	0	65
IV or blood products related	161	14	0	2	0	177
Medication related	555	29	3	62	1	650
Monitoring related	695	17	15	24	0	751
Obstetrics related	376	7	413	28	0	824
Surgery related	361	63	9	12	1	446
Treatment related	677	33	35	119	5	869
Miscellaneous	204	5	1	12	0	222
All reasons	**3,444**	**1,107**	**516**	**491**	**9**	**5,567**

Note: This table includes only disclosable reports in the NPDB as of the end of the current year. Voided reports have been excluded. Medical malpractice payment reports that are missing data necessary to determine the malpractice reason (8 reports for RNs) are excluded.
*Reporting using the "Advanced Nurse Practitioner" category began on March 5, 2002. The "Advanced Nurse Practitioner" category was changed to "Clinical Nurse Specialist" on September 9, 2002. Prior to March 5, 2002, these nurses were included in the "RN (Professional Nurse)" category.
**The "Behavioral Health" category was added on January 31, 2004. Reports involving behavioral health issues filed before January 31, 2004 used other reporting categories. Cumulative data in this category includes only reports filed after January 31, 2004.

3. Communicate
4. Document
5. Assess and monitor
6. Act as a patient advocate

Patient falls and medication errors continue to be leading incidents for nursing malpractice lawsuits. Identifying and implementing practices to improve patient safety is a priority in healthcare settings.

Standard of Care   The American Nurses Association describes a standard as an "authoritative statement defined and promoted by the profession by which the quality of practice, service or education can

TABLE 15-2	NATIONAL PRACTITIONER DATA BANK, 2005 ANNUAL REPORT

Mean and Median Medical Malpractice Payment Amounts by Malpractice Reason, 2005 and Cumulative through 2005—
Nurses (Registered Nurses, Nurse Anesthetists, Nurse Midwives, Nurse Practitioners, and Advanced Practice
Nurses/Clinical Nurse Specialists)
National Practitioner Data Bank (September 1, 1990–December 31, 2005)

| | 2005 Only | | | Cumulative through 2005 | | | | |
| | | | | | Actual | | Inflation-Adjusted | |
Malpractice reason	Number of Payments	Mean Payment	Median Payment	Number of Payments	Mean Payment	Median Payment	Mean Payment	Median Payment
Anesthesia related	68	$368,594	$110,938	1,053	$261,779	$100,000	$309,042	$123,867
Behavioral health related**	3	$236,667	$60,000	6	$126,851	$37,500	$127,062	$37,810
Diagnosis related	80	$263,207	$100,000	504	$290,458	$125,000	$335,067	$140,494
Equipment or product related	6	$64,002	$61,695	65	$155,682	$40,000	$193,125	$43,667
IV or blood products related	6	$102,500	$67,500	177	$222,399	$75,000	$264,523	$79,332
Medication related	62	$406,830	$87,500	650	$267,366	$62,500	$306,440	$70,087
Monitoring related	97	$267,559	$100,000	751	$297,705	$95,000	$345,137	$107,040
Obstetrics related	90	$675,032	$288,750	824	$533,086	$249,832	$598,187	$264,483
Surgery related	52	$124,505	$60,000	446	$148,716	$50,000	$173,544	$55,471
Treatment related	99	$192,159	$75,00	869	$168,650	$50,000	$191,070	$61,934
Miscellaneous	23	$95,952	$47,500	222	$237,216	$40,000	$268,997	$49,547
All reasons	**586**	**$319,905**	**$100,000**	**5,567**	**$282,821**	**$90,000**	**$324,929**	**$102,482**

Note: This table includes only disclosable reports in the NPDB as of the end of the current year. Voided reports have been excluded. Medical malpractice
payment reports that are missing data necessary to determine the malpractice reason (8 reports cumulatively) are excluded.
**The "Behavioral Health" category was added on January 31, 2004. Reports involving behavioral health issues filed before January 31, 2004 used other
reporting categories. Cumulative data in this category includes only reports filed after January 31, 2004.

be evaluated."[16] Nursing standards of care identify the skill level and knowledge of the professional and the expected level of care given a similar setting and under similar circumstances.[17] The standard of care or "customary practice" is the benchmark for measuring malpractice. The standard of care is commonly referenced in legal and nursing literature; however, if you ask most nurses to define the standard, the request tends to elicit a blank stare, at least momentarily. This is because the standard of care is not always easy to articulate. It is based on the circumstances surrounding the adverse event and the expected care of the "average" practitioner. If that were not complicated enough, add the uniqueness of individual patient needs and one can see why many times even experts have varying opinions about the standard. References such as standards and positions published by professional organizations, nurse practice acts, nursing texts, and other sources may be considered authoritative or "black lettered" reference materials and may be used to help clarify the standard. However, in a profession that holistically cares for the human elements of individuals, including the psychological, social, and physical components, these publications alone may not adequately define the standard of care. Furthermore, many traditional practices in nursing viewed as standard care have yet to undergo the rigor of scientific study and thus are not based on evidence. It is generally the culmination of many sources coupled with practice norms that establishes the standard.

Expert Nurse Witness   Because of the complexity of circumstances framing most alleged medical malpractice events, frequently an expert witness is called on to help the jurors interpret the applicable standard of care. Expert witnesses serve as agents in the legal process and are selected based on their experience in the specialty field and knowledge of the subject in question. Experts are asked to review the facts of the matter and to provide an opinion as to whether the care rendered by the defendant(s) met the ordinary or customary standard of practice. The expert is asked to testify regarding whether the care provided to the patient met the minimal requirement mandated by law, not the optimal level of care. Nurses are commonly asked to serve as expert witnesses by both defense or plaintiff attorneys. A nursing expert may be retained by an attorney to serve as a consultant or to give sworn testimony and generally receives payment for performing one or more of the following functions:

- Review records, charts, and depositions of other witnesses and give an opinion based on expert knowledge of standards related to the nursing care rendered to the patient at the center of the suit. Details of records and depositions are reviewed thoroughly to ensure understanding of the facts.
- Write a report of the review findings, sometimes referred to as a "downside review." When the expert is anticipated to testify, written critiques of the findings are discouraged because these may not be protected and thus admissible as evidence in the case.
- Perform a literature review for relevant information pertaining to the facts of the case.
- Testify under oath in deposition and at trial. In the event of testimony, the retaining attorney works closely with the expert in preparation for the deposition or trial. Giving sworn testimony can be stressful for the expert as the opposing attorney attempts to confuse the witness and diminish the expert's credibility. A nurse serving as an expert should take the responsibility of the role seriously and abide by an ethical code of conduct. Experts should rely on formal educational knowledge and experience to form opinions and should never adopt the opinion of others.

Nurses are qualified as an expert nurse based on formal education, licensure as a registered nurse, and experience. Nurses may become certified as legal nurse consultants through several accrediting organizations; however, certification is not a requirement to serve as an expert witness. Whether certified or not, preferred experts have published in peer-reviewed journals, possess the ability to speak convincingly and in language that a jury can understand, maintain good eye contact, have a record of accepting cases from both plaintiffs and defendants, and participate in professional organizations. The following case study describes a situation in which the testimony of an expert witness influenced the defense of the nursing care provided to an elderly patient.

Case Study

A Nurse Expert Witness Testified to the Nursing Standard   An elderly, blind, female patient in a hospital in Alabama fell and broke her hip. The family sued the hospital for negligence. The patient's chart indicated that the nursing personnel had planned her care with the patient and arranged the furniture in her room, including the position of her bed, so she could safely go to her chair and to the bathroom. It was the decision of the nursing personnel to leave the side rail at the foot of the bed nearest the bathroom down. The nursing personnel had documented that the patient was instructed to call for assistance, if needed. The patient complied with instructions and for several days safely ambulated to the bathroom without incident.

The plaintiff's lawyer argued that all four side rails should have been up on the bed and that the patient should have been instructed to call nursing personnel before getting up for any reason. The expert testified that nurses make ongoing judgments about the safety and well-being of patients and in this case assessed the patient to be safe to ambulate to the bathroom alone. Furthermore, the documentation and testimony of nurses indicated that the patient had been compliant with instructions and repeatedly demonstrated the ability to safely ambulate. Based on the expert's testimony, the jury ruled in favor of the hospital.

Medical Malpractice Tort Reform   Few issues in health care ignite as much emotion as the debates over medical malpractice. Over the last 30 years, states throughout the nation have experienced varying degrees of malpractice crisis. State legislators have intervened by enacting a number of laws known as tort reform to address issues such as the unavailability of insurance, rising premiums, and enormous pay outs. Since the mid-1970s the crises have calmed and resurged on numerous occasions. Once again, however, the frequency of claims and the size of pay outs are increasing. The latest tort crisis is characterized by both decreasing availability of medical malpractice insurance and rising premiums. Factors contributing to the crisis of today include increased public awareness of errors in health care, decreased confidence and trust among patients, advances in technology and increases in the intensity of medical services, higher expectations of the public, and less willingness of plaintiff lawyers to accept settlement offers.[18]

Patient Safety and the Tort System   Is the quest for patient safety and the current tort system compatible? Although evidence indicates that most errors are attributed to system error rather than the provider of care, society continues to punish practitioners for errors. The medical liability system appears to be in direct conflict with efforts of regulatory agencies, employers, and professional organizations attempting to change punitive cultures into cultures that discuss and analyze errors and redesign systems.[19] Although plaintiff lawyers argue that the threat of litigation improves patient safety, the "punitive, individualistic, adversarial approach of tort law is antithetical to the non-punitive, systems-oriented, and cooperative strategies promoted by leaders of the patient-safety movement."[20] Physicians are hesitant to disclose medical errors or to participate in activities to improve patient safety for fear of legal action.[21] Obviously, the tort system as we know it today is in need of restructuring to decrease reluctance of physicians and other healthcare professionals and organizations to fully disclose errors and to participate in patient safety initiatives without fear of retaliation.

> **Although plaintiff lawyers argue that the threat of litigation improves patient safety, the 'punitive, individualistic, adversarial approach of tort law is antithetical to the non-punitive, systems-oriented, and cooperative strategies promoted by leaders of the patient-safety movement.'**[22]

Intentional Torts

An intentional tort is a conscious decision to commit or omit an act and to either intend the result or to possess reasonable knowledge of the foreseeable consequences. Intentional torts that nurses may face include defamation, false imprisonment, and assault and battery, among others. Intentional torts possess all three of the following elements:[23]

1. An act that infringes on the rights of another with foreseeable consequences by the defendant
2. The individual carrying out the act or omission must deliberately intend the consequences
3. The consequences must be directly caused by the intended act or omission

Defamation Defamation is the issuance of a false statement about another person, which causes that individual to suffer harm. Libel involves the making of defamatory statements in a printed form, such as a magazine or newspaper. Slander, on the other hand, involves defamatory statements by oral representation. An example of slander is a malicious statement by a nurse that falsely accuses a patient or another individual of having an infectious disease or to be of immoral character. A person who defames the character of another and causes a loss of professional reputation must be able to prove the truth of the accusation. Truth is the absolute defense of an action in slander and libel. Claims of defamation are rare in health care.

> **A person who defames the character of another and causes a loss of professional reputation must be able to prove the truth of the accusation. Truth is the absolute defense of an action in slander and libel.**

False Imprisonment False imprisonment is the unlawful restraint of someone that affects the person's freedom of movement. False imprisonment could be alleged due to confinement by a locked door, physical restraint, chemical restraint, or even by the threat that force may be used. Recovery from a lawsuit based on false imprisonment includes damages for physical and psychological harm.

Years ago, it was common to see elderly people positioned in wheelchairs by vests or belt restraints to keep them from moving around independently. Today, it is possible that the application of restraints, unless used for medical reasons and in compliance with federal law or The Joint Commission (TJC) standards, may be interpreted as false imprisonment.[23] Strict guidelines exist in inpatient settings that define the appropriate use of restraints and seclusion along with required monitoring of those confined. Nurses should carefully adhere to these policies.

False imprisonment may also be alleged if an individual is prevented from leaving a facility by using restraint or coercion. There are legitimate reasons for detaining individuals that are legally justified. These include patients who are mentally incompetent or impaired and patients who are a threat to themselves or to others. In the event that there is question about the safety and well-being of a patient who desires to leave a facility against advice or when concern exists for another's welfare, legal advice should be sought immediately.[24]

Assault and Battery Assault is an intentional threat to inflict injury upon a person by another who has the ability to cause harm and thus puts the person in fear of an immediate danger. Battery is the intentional touching of or application of force to another person, in a harmful or offensive manner, and without consent. The most commonly alleged act of battery against nurses is the treatment without consent.

In the case of *Roberson v. Provident House*, a nurse inserted a catheter following a physician's as needed (PRN) Foley order.[25] The patient did not want to be catheterized and protested. The nurse was found to have committed assault and battery. Nurses must obtain permission from the patient before touching the patient. The consent procedure does not have to be formal and may be implied such as when the patient holds his arm out for the start of an intravenous line. Litigation regarding the requirement for informed consent has focused around the physician's failure to explain the risks, benefits, and alternatives to the procedure. However, hospitals and nurses may be held liable for lack of informed consent if they know or should have known there was not adequate disclosure or adequate consent.

> **A nurse who carries out any nursing intervention without the patient's consent, even if the intervention is beneficial, is potentially guilty of professional misconduct. The nurse may be disciplined by the state board of nursing and could be sued by the patient or face an allegation of assault and battery.**

How would you like to be in this circumstance? An older slightly confused patient is admitted to a medical-surgical unit for severe anemia of unknown etiology. The elderly man's appearance is unkempt. He has a scraggly beard consisting of long matted hair. A conscientious nurse, with good intention, decides to place the patient in the shower and thoroughly "scrub" the patient. After the bath, she trims his beard. When his son arrives, the son is irate about the beard being trimmed. The patient begins crying and accuses the nurse of restraining his hands while she cut his beard. He claims that despite his protests she continued to cut his beard. As innocent as the nurse may have been in this situation, claims of battery occurred. Fortunately, in this case, a letter of apology soothed this patient and son's ruffled feathers.

Criminal Law

Criminal law applies to an intentional wrongdoing against society as well as to an individual victim. A criminal offense is prosecuted by the state in which it occurs or by the U.S. Department of Justice. Crimes are defined as either misdemeanors or felonies. A misdemeanor is less serious than a felony, and guilt is generally punishable by fines or imprisonment for less than a year.[26] A felony such as rape or murder is punishable by confinement in a penitentiary for longer than 1 year.[27] Although less common than civil claims, healthcare providers have been accused of criminal negligence. Criminal negligence is an action that is considered to be "a reckless disregard for the safety of others."[28]

> *Although less common than civil claims, healthcare providers have been accused of criminal negligence. Criminal negligence is an action that is considered to be 'a reckless disregard for the safety of others.'*

One of the earliest and most famous cases of criminal negligence by a nurse is the Somera case, reported in *The International Review* (July 1, 1930, pp. 325–334). Lorenza Somera, as the head nurse, was directed by the operating surgeon to prepare 10% cocaine with adrenaline for administration to a patient for a tonsillectomy. Ms. Somera repeated and verified the order. A few moments after the injection was given, the patient showed symptoms of convulsions and died. The operating surgeon meant to say 10% procaine. Only Ms. Somera was found guilty of manslaughter due to negligence. The negligence consisted of following an order that the nurse should have known by reason of her training and experience was incorrect. Although the physician was negligent, the cause of death was the nurse's negligence.[29] According to the American Nurses Association's *Code of Ethics for Nurses with Interpretive Statements*, "Nurses are accountable for judgments made and actions taken in the course of nursing practice, irrespective of healthcare organizations' policies or providers' directives."[30]

> *Nurses are accountable for judgments made and actions taken in the course of nursing practice, irrespective of healthcare organizations' policies or providers' directives.*

In 1997, when a patient bled to death, a court in New Jersey charged five nurses with endangering the welfare of a patient. During the same year, in Colorado, three nurses were indicted for criminal negligence in the death of a newborn after an overdose of 10 times the prescribed amount of penicillin. In 2004, criminal charges were filed against an emergency room nurse who failed to report suspected child abuse for a 2-year-old boy. The child subsequently died at the hands of his stepfather. In Wisconsin, a nurse was charged with a felony after mistakenly administering an epidural anesthetic intravenously instead of the prescribed order of penicillin. The Wisconsin nurse failed to read the medication label carefully and neglected to follow the established bar code policy. These cases have raised serious concerns for nurses and other healthcare providers who are today exposed to both civil and criminal litigation for errors or misjudgments.

CORPORATE LIABILITY

Healthcare corporations are incorporated by the state and designated as either for-profit or not-for-profit. Not-for-profit organizations are exempt from federal taxes and, in most cases, state taxes. They also qualify for donations and charitable deductions.[31]

Board of Directors/Chief Operating Officers

Every institution is governed by a board of directors that has responsibility for the operation and viability of the institution. With the authority awarded a governing board, the board and its personal members have specific legal responsibilities and liabilities. The board and its members are accountable for the overall management of the institution. A chief operating officer is appointed by the board to carry out daily operations. The board reviews financial reports, approves strategic plans, and monitors internal operations. Furthermore, the governing body has the ultimate authority and responsibility to select medical staff. [32]

High ethical conduct is required of board members. Generally, strict rules of conduct are imposed on members to avoid conflicts of interest and self-gain. The members of the board are responsible for operating the organization in compliance with state, federal, and local laws. A case demonstrating how those in governing positions can face penalties when laws are not adhered to is that of *People v. Casa Blanca Convalescent Homes.* In this case the court found multiple violations of statutory regulations, including deficient staffing and inadequate care of residents. The operator of the facility was fined a significant amount for failure to comply with regulations.[33] Other instances of violations of the law have led to criminal prosecution.

Corporate Negligence

For years, hospitals and medical centers remained immune from liability for medical acts. With the erosion of charitable and governmental immunity, however, hospital risk for exposure increased. Under a doctrine of corporate law, hospitals are legally responsible for the safety and security of patients, employees, and visitors. The doctrine creates a duty of the hospital itself, directly to the patient. Thus hospitals cannot abdicate the responsibility to a third party. With a duty specific to the patient, hospitals are responsible to monitor the personnel involved in the processes within the organization, assess the overall operation of the facility, and make a conscious effort to identify potential risks. Corporate law in most states includes the following four duties:

1. The duty to use reasonable care in maintaining safe and adequate facilities and equipment
2. The duty to formulate adequate policies to ensure quality care for patients
3. The duty to oversee all persons who practice within its walls
4. The duty to select and retain competent physicians and staff

Respondeat Superior

The legal doctrine, *respondeat superior,* holds the employer responsible for torts committed by employees while on the job.[34] *Darling v. Charleston Community Hospital,* a landmark case, opened the door to corporate negligence liability of hospitals.[35] The case involved a young college football player who, after an injury, lost his leg after traction and cast application. Despite obvious signs of circulatory impairment and numerous attempts by the patient and family to seek assistance from staff, no remedial steps were taken. Although the patient was seen daily by a staff doctor, the court found the hospital negligent for not ensuring that the nurses reported important findings to physicians and notified supervisory personnel in the event that the doctor failed to act.[36]

As with physicians, hospitals are facing ever-increasing medical malpractice claims. The cost of hospital malpractice liability premiums are on the rise and can have a significant impact on operating funds. According to the Institute of Medicine, 54% of healthcare workers are nurses; therefore nurses have heightened opportunity for claims.[37] As indicated by the American Organization of Nurse Executives, an important skill for nurse managers is human resource leadership. Determining and providing for educational needs, assessing competency, appropriate evaluation, and having "crucial conversations" are key to enhancing patient safety and minimizing organizational liability.

Credentialing Liability

Corporate responsibility extends beyond the hospital's obligation to ensure sound management practices, safe operations, and appropriate behavior of employees and agents to liability for clinical competence and performance of all practitioners granted clinical privileges. As part of the credentialing process of any healthcare facility, organizations are responsible to appropriately investigate the qualifications and background of licensed independent practitioners applying to practice within the organization. Licensed independent practitioners are defined by the The Joint Commission (TJC) as "individuals permitted by law and by the organization to provide care and services without direction or supervision."[38] The TJC requires verification of licensure and credentials, work experience, and quality of care and encourages institutions to be thorough and deliberate when granting privileges.[39] Hospitals are mandated by law to query the National Practitioner Data Bank before granting physician privileges to practice within the facility and to recheck the file of healthcare practitioners every 2 years thereafter. The National Practitioner Data Bank, a nationwide tracking system, was established by federal law in1986 and formally inaugurated in 1990 to flag those who engage in unprofessional behavior and to restrict incompetent physicians and other healthcare practitioners from moving state to state without disclosure or discovery of previous medical malpractice payment and adverse action history.[40]

A landmark case in which a surgeon operated on a hip, injuring the femoral artery and nerve and causing permanent damage and paralysis, was the first legal case where a hospital was held liable for negligent credentialing.[41] A closer look at the physician revealed suspension from other hospitals and involvement in other cases of malpractice. The court held that hospitals have a duty to responsibly select medical staff.

Nurses who are victims of or who witness inappropriate behavior of a licensed independent practitioner are responsible to report such behavior. The same is true when a nurse observes competency issues. Nurse executives, as advocates for both the patient and staff, are expected to confront and address the matters utilizing processes defined within the organization to deal with behavioral or clinical performance matters.

OTHER AREAS OF LIABILITY FOR NURSES

Supervisor Liability

In 1994 the U.S. Supreme Court defined a nursing supervisor as a nurse who assigns, oversees, and provides direction to licensed or unlicensed personnel. This definition not only exposes nurses in formal supervisory positions to supervisory liability but expands the legal responsibility to staff nurses, particularly those who assume the responsibility of charge nurse. The "supervisor" may be found negligent if failing to assign or supervise appropriately. Furthermore, the corporation, under the doctrine of *respondeat superior*, is liable for the actions of both the nurse performing the assigned care and the nurse making the assignment.

Inadequate Staffing

Nursing facilities are responsible under federal law to provide adequate staffing.[42] Adequate staffing includes a sufficient number of competent staff to reasonably ensure safe care. An important nurse executive competency identified by the American Organization of Nurse Executives is the appropriate allocation of nursing resources based on patient acuity. This can be a major challenge for nurse administrators and other healthcare leaders of today, as organizations compete for dwindling numbers of healthcare providers.

Floating

Floating is common necessity in times of high acuity or short staffing. Floating has implications for both the nurse who is floating, the personnel reassigning the nurse, and the nurse delegating patient care to the floating nurse. The nurse who is being assigned to float has a professional duty to the organization and the patient to accept the assignment unless the nurse is lacking education and skill to perform the assigned duties. The nurse is obliged to provide for patients' safety. In extreme staffing circumstances, abandoning patients may potentially jeopardize patient care and safety. In these instances, "a nurse lacking in certain skills and experience is preferable to the patient lacking a nurse."[43] Thus fear or uncertainty is not a legitimate reason to refuse an assignment and used alone as a basis for refusing to float is considered unprofessional and may subject the nurse to the legal consequences of abandonment.

On the other hand, nurse managers and supervisors have a responsibility to appropriately staff the nursing units and when resources are limited must critically appraise the circumstances and carefully distribute personnel, striving to match the needs of the patients with the skills of the nurse. As indicated earlier, the supervisor, whether formally designated as such, or a staff nurse, who fails to assign and supervise appropriately, may be found negligent.

Following the Chain of Command

A nurse who fails to question an order of a patient when he or she believes that it is not in the best interest of the patient may be liable. Furthermore, nurses are responsible to contact a supervisor when a physician fails to take appropriate action or is unwilling to cooperate in a situation that threatens the well-being of a patient. Organizations should have a policy and procedure that clearly defines the chain of command. However, policy alone is not sufficient. Nurses need to be educated on their responsibility to notify an individual in authority to assist with unresolved or threatening situations. Commonly, by referring unusual or difficult situations to a higher level, action can be taken that can protect a patient's well-being. Therefore it is important to recognize that the nurse's duty to a patient extends beyond direct care and carries the responsibility of advocacy.

NURSES AND THE LITIGATION PROCESS

Nurses in an executive or manager role may be required to testify as a result of direct involvement in an alleged malpractice event, under the *respondeat superior* doctrine, or as the corporate representative. The designation of a corporate representative occurs following notice or subpoena of the organization to designate a person to testify on behalf of company policy. Staff nurses employed by the facility may be either personally named in a lawsuit or, more commonly, subjected to the litigation process as an agent of the facility. At any level, participation in the unfamiliar legal arena can be threatening and stressful. Figure 15-1 describes steps in the legal procedure. During the litigation process, communication between the attorney and client is considered privileged or protected by law and is inadmissible in court. However, if the client shares the discussion with others, the communication is no longer protected and may be entered as evidence in court. Unfortunately, the "code of silence" can magnify the anxiety of those involved in a lawsuit and can intensify feelings of shame, guilt, or isolation experienced by the defendants.[44] Education and emotional support of nurses going through the long and frightening litigation process is paramount.

FIGURE 15-1	STEPS IN A LEGAL PROCEDURE

1. A lawsuit begins when a complaint is filed by the plaintiff. Frequently, multiple parties are named in a lawsuit.

2. The insurance provider for the individual or entity is contacted and becomes involved in providing a legal team. When more than one party is named in the lawsuit, unfavorably for the defense, finger pointing between defendants may occur, especially if the parties are insured by different insurance carriers.

3. The discovery phase is the time whereby attorneys of opposing sides seek to identify the facts of the case in preparation for the legal battle. The discovery process can be quite lengthy as opposing attorneys exchange documents about the individuals, entities, policies, and medical records pertaining to the adverse event. Depositions of fact and expert witnesses on both sides are taken during the discovery phase.

4. As the case unfolds, commonly, there are attempts by the opposing attorneys to negotiate a settlement. It should be noted that settling a case does not confer guilt and may be the least risky and less costly resolution. The cost of the litigation process is high; thus settlement may be a reasonable compromise. However, some malpractice insurance providers may be reluctant to negotiate settlements for fear that bargaining encourages frivolous lawsuits.

5. If the parties cannot resolve the issue through settlement, a trial date is set by the court. Evidence and testimony is presented to a jury and a verdict is delivered.

6. Either side may appeal the decision of the court based on questions of law, not simple displeasure with the verdict. The cost associated with litigation must be weighed in the decision to appeal a verdict.

Source: Author.

RISK MANAGEMENT

Risk management in health care serves to provide a safe and effective environment for patients, visitors, and employees, thus averting or decreasing loss to the institution.[45] Identification, analysis, treatment, and evaluation of actual or potential hazards are the focus of risk management activities. Risk management has its beginnings in the transportation industry, particularly in investigations into aviation and traffic accidents. The primary reasons for these investigations were to determine patterns or causative factors in the accidents and then to eliminate, or at least control, as many factors as possible. Insurance carriers for institutions support risk management programs and commonly decrease the cost of premiums for providers who implement practices that reduce liability.[45]

Risk Management Responsibilities

Most healthcare institutions today have used the services of a risk manager. Because of the diversity in the size and organization of institutions, job descriptions of the risk manager vary considerably. Figure 15-2 defines competencies of a risk manager. Important areas of responsibilities include loss prevention and reduction, claims management, financial risk, and risk regulatory and accreditation compliance.[46]

Loss Prevention and Reduction

Loss prevention and reduction is the largest category of risk management and includes the following activities:

- Institution of a system to identify risk exposure such as incident or occurrence reporting, establishment of a communication system for referrals, and review of medical records, patient complaints,

---

| FIGURE 15-2 | RISK MANAGER COMPETENCIES |

1. Keep an up-to-date manual, including policies, lines of authority, safety roles, disaster plans, safety training, procedures, incident and claims reporting, procedures and schedule, and description of retention/insurance program.

2. Update programs with changes in properties, operations, or activities.

3. Review plans for new construction, alterations, and equipment installation.

4. Review contracts to avoid unnecessary assumptions of liability and transfer to others where possible.

5. Keep up-to-date property appraisal.

6. Maintain records of insurance policy renewal dates.

7. Review and monitor all premiums and other billings and approve payments.

8. Negotiate insurance coverage, premiums, and services.

9. Prepare specifications for competitive bids on property and liability insurance.

10. Review and make recommendations for coverage, services, and costs.

11. Maintain records and verify compliance for independent physicians, vendors, contractors, and subcontractors.

12. Maintain records of losses, claims, and all risk management expenses.

13. Supervise claim-reporting procedures.

14. Assist in adjusting losses.

15. Cooperate with the director of safety and the risk management committee to minimize all future losses involving employees, patients, visitors, other third parties, property, and earnings.

16. Keep risk management skills updated.

17. Assess the system for causes of errors and adverse events. Fix the system.

18. Use focus groups to identify unreported errors and adverse events. Eliminate punitive organizational culture.

19. Prepare annual report covering status, changes, new problems and solutions, summary of existing insurance and retention aspects of the program, summary of losses, costs, major claims, and future goals and objectives.

20. Prepare an annual budget.

Source: Author.

---

and performance improvement data. Developing early warning systems is crucial to the investigation of events. Early notification of events provides an opportunity to conduct timely interviews of involved parties and to secure medical records and malfunctioning equipment associated with the event.

- Development of policies and procedures that address key risk management areas, including confidentiality, informed consent, products recalls, and sentinel events

- Collaboration with quality management, nursing, medical staff, and infection control to promote loss reduction strategies. The TJC recommends the integration of risk management and quality assurance initiatives as a more efficient and cost-effective method for promoting quality and safety. Performance improvement data can identify potential risk areas and form the basis for action plans to reduce adverse occurrences. Quality and risk prevention go hand and hand. A thorough study of sentinel events using a root-cause analysis can provide valuable lessons for the organization. Aggregating and analyzing statistical data regarding quality and safety. These reports are presented to various committees and used by others, including the organization's board of directors, to determine the institution's risk for loss and to implement strategies to reduce exposure to liability.

- Coordination of education for staff on risk management issues
- Participation in the contract review process

Claims Management

All claims activities are generally handled by the risk management department. These functions include establishing files of potential or actual claims, coordinating claims activities, including negotiation of settlements, and serving as a liaison to administration as to the status of claims.[47] Claims management can be a time-consuming activity for a risk management department depending on the number and complexity of claims against an organization.

Financial Risk

A major concern of healthcare businesses is financial loss due to legal liability. Risk managers attempt to identify areas within the organization that may expose the institution to loss and estimate the potential and size of loss for exposure. When an adverse event occurs, effort is made to reduce the severity of loss through risk control strategies such as writing off hospital bills or personally meeting with the patient or family representative to resolve the grievance. The JCAHO mandates disclosure of sentinel events and other poor outcomes of care to patients and their families, when appropriate.[48] Unfortunately, many clinicians and institutions are reluctant to openly discuss bad outcomes for fear that discussion may be interpreted as an admission of guilt, even if not the case.[49] Furthermore, healthcare providers may incur legal obstacles with full disclosure.

In 2005, after the loss of a brother to a medical error, Doug Wojcieszak formed The Sorry Works! coalition. The coalition was formed based on this family's experience. The coalition advocates that in the event of medical error or negligence, the provider admits fault, provides the patient/family with an apology, explains plans to prevent the error from reoccurring, and offers fair compensation.[50] If medical error was not found to be the cause of the unexpected outcome, the coalition recommends that providers, accompanied by legal counsel, conduct a meeting with the patient/family and explain what happened and then apologize and offer empathy without acknowledging fault. Until safe systems are developed in health care that foster learning from mistakes while continuing to underscore individual accountability for wrongdoing, discomfort and debate about disclosure after an unexpected outcome will continue.

Compliance with Regulatory and Accreditation Agencies

Risk management includes the duty to comply with regulatory and accrediting bodies, such as the Occupational Safety and Health Administration, Emergency Medical Treatment and Active Labor Act, Health Insurance Portability and Accountability Act, and TJC, among many others. Additional regulatory activities may include mandatory reporting of deaths based on defined criteria to the coroner, compliance with safety codes, and requirements to report select incidents to state and federal agencies.[51]

Documentation

The medical record is an account of the patient's experience during a healthcare encounter. The primary purpose of the medical record is to accurately reflect in written form the medical and nursing care that a patient receives. It is important that nurses strive to document as accurately and timely as possible. Contradictions, inconsistencies, and unexplained gaps in the medical records are difficult to defend during litigation. It is recommended that documentation take place as soon after the occurrence as possible and that a minute-by-minute recording is done during an emergency. When time is of the essence, which is quite common in a busy clinical setting, brief notes with times, interventions, and other relevant information should be written on a piece of paper and transferred to the medical records as soon as time permits.

The old adage "if it wasn't documented, it wasn't done" is a good guideline to use in practice, but there is no legal basis for the premise. Every nurse knows that it is impractical for nurses to chart all nursing functions and patient care activities. To do so would leave many duties undone, possibly including patient care. However, when malpractice is alleged, the medical record is the primary source of information for determining whether the standard of care was met. Furthermore, failure to document appropriate information may be interpreted as a violation of the standard. In a New York case, *Gerner v. Long Island Jewish Hillside Medical Center*, an infant suffered brain damage after developing jaundice. Several events occurred that delayed diagnosis and treatment of the jaundiced condition, including the fact that the nurses failed to note the color of the baby's skin in the record until the third hospital day. Judgment was in favor of the plaintiff partially due to failure to document the patient's condition.[52]

Electronic documentation adds new dimensions of liability. Care must be taken to safeguard patient confidentiality and unauthorized access to information with computerized systems. Policies must be developed to protect computerized patient data and audits performed routinely to ensure that only those who have a "need to know" access records. Furthermore, nurses need to be fully educated to understand that when documenting electronically, the exact time that data are charted in the computer is captured automatically. Most nursing computerized documentation programs allow nurses to manually enter the time that an assessment or intervention occurs; however, when the time is different from the entry time, it may be difficult to explain the discrepancy in time. Therefore a procedure for late entries should be developed to guide staff on how to enter late entries. Finally, when implementing electronic documentation, it is essential that organizations minimize the need for duplicate documentation to prevent confusion; thus point-of-care documentation is preferable, whenever feasible.

The medical record is sacred ground and should never be altered after an entry is made. If it is found that a medical record has been modified, destroyed, or falsified in any fashion, the act may be construed as an attempt to conceal or manipulate facts and, under such instances, is considered a felony or criminal offense.[53] Moreover, manipulation of the record may be interpreted as malice in a medical negligence case and punitive damages may be awarded the plaintiff, even if the alteration of the record did not directly cause harm.[54] Figure 15-3 highlights a few tips for documentation.

Policies and Procedures

Policies and procedures are directives for the daily operations of an institution and are required for compliance with regulatory and accreditation agencies. Policy and procedure manuals are developed as a resource tool for employees to describe the general rules of conduct but are never intended to supersede the judgment of the employee. If a patient experiences an adverse outcome, the plaintiff's attorney ordinarily petitions the institution's policies and procedures to evaluate whether the practitioner's conduct was in compliance with the established internal practices.

Policies and procedures are expected to be followed unless there is a reasonable explanation as to why a deviation should occur. Plaintiff attorneys frequently argue that internal policies and procedures form the basis for the standard of care. However, "a policy and procedure manual is not necessarily the definitive source for standards of care."[55] Nevertheless, policies and procedures find their way into court rooms every day. For this reason, each version of a policy should be retained when revisions are

---

FIGURE 15-3	TIPS FOR DOCUMENTATION

- Never use the medical record as a forum to record complaints against another.

- Document instructions given to patients.

- Any corrections to the medical record should be done with a thin line drawn through the original entry, dated and initialed unless otherwise specified by hospital policy.

- Documented information should be factual and objective.

- Specific communication with physicians about the patient's condition should be recorded.

- Late entries should be recorded according to the facility's policy.

Source: Author.

made because often in lawsuits an organization is asked to produce the policy in effect at the time of the incident. Unfortunately, institutions may be remiss in ensuring that policies are updated timely and that the content reflects reasonable expectation rather than optimal practice. Organizations must be careful not to develop policies that specify conduct greater than recognized by authorities. This practice could result in the institution being held to a higher standard than the norm. Thus policies and procedures should be based on the best evidence and consistent with national standards.

This requires vigilance on the part of the organization to attend to details in the development, ongoing review, and revision of policies and procedures.[57] Finally, policies and procedures should be broad enough to allow for reasonable flexibility between departments and practitioners.

> 66 *The American Nurses Association defines evidence-based practice as "a process founded on the collection, interpretation, and integration of valid, important, and applicable patient-reported, clinician-observed, and research-derived evidence. The best available evidence, moderated by patient circumstances and preferences is applied to improve the quality of clinical judgments.* 99 [56]

Incident/Occurrence Reporting

An incident or occurrence report is an effective tool used to identify potential losses, opportunities, or potential claims. These reports are prepared for any unusual occurrence or near miss involving people or property, whether or not injury or damage occurs. Preferably, the report is generated at the time of the incident and by the individual(s) involved in the incident. However, if this is not possible, the incident report should be completed when it is first discovered.

Use of Incident Reports

Incident reports are used to collect and analyze future data for the purpose of determining risk-control strategies. Blake describes the use of a multiple causation model in incident report investigation. This theory suggests that causes, subcauses, and contributing factors weave together in particular sequences to cause incidents. An incident may have many concomitant causes; therefore seeking out as many causes as possible and rating them by their proximate or primary influence on the incident may be useful in reducing the chance of the incident recurring. Proximate causes are often referred to as parent and closest cause of the incident. Primary causes are procedural in nature, and such causes are discovered through back tracking from the proximate cause.[58]

Preparation of Incident Reports

Incident reports are commonly discovered during the legal process. Discoverability of incident reports depends on "state Quality Assurance and peer review statutes or statutes creating an attorney-client or insurer-insured privilege."[59]

Contents of incident reports may be either helpful in explaining facts of a case or incriminating. Commonly, defending attorneys argue against discovery, asserting that occurrence reports are part of the quality assurance process and must be protected to afford organizations the opportunity to assess and improve care without fear of legal exposure. In *Columbia/HCA Healthcare Corp. v. Eighth Judicial District Court*, the court ruled that because incident reports are part of the hospital's normal course of business, they remain open to discovery during the litigation process.[60] Incident reports should be objectively written, complete and factual. The incident report is corrected in the same manner as any other medical record and should not be altered or rewritten. It should contain no comments criticizing or blaming others. Figure 15-4 lists the dos and don'ts of incident reporting.

It may be institutional policy to send the incident report to the risk manager; however, if the event requires immediate attention, notification may need to be more prompt. The preparer can call the risk manager and nurse manager and give them verbal information on the need to investigate and evaluate events and to make needed corrections. To accomplish this, managers should establish a climate of trust that supports incident reporting by nurses. The TJC requires that incidents be reported.

FIGURE 15-4 **DOS AND DON'TS OF INCIDENT REPORTING**

Do

- Report any event involving patient mishap or serious expression of dissatisfaction with care.
- Report any event involving visitor mishap or property.
- Be complete.
- Follow established policy and procedure.
- Be prompt.
- Act to reduce fear in the nursing staff.
- Correct in the same manner as any medical record.
- Include names and identities of witnesses; record their statements on separate pages.
- Report equipment malfunctions, including control numbers. Remove equipment from service for testing.
- Keep the report confidential.
- Report to nurse manager.
- Confer with risk manager.
- Work to provide nursing care to meet established standards.
- Attend all staff development programs.
- Confirm all telephone orders in writing.

Don't

- Place blame on anyone.
- Place report on the patient's chart.
- Make entry about an incident report on the patient's chart.
- Alter or rewrite.
- Report hearsay or opinion.
- Be afraid to consult, ask questions, or complete incident reports. They can be part of your best defense and protection.
- Prescribe in the physician's domain.
- Be cold and impersonal to patients, families, or visitors.

Source: Author.

Risk Management and Nursing

Nursing leaders of today must challenge old practices and strive to build a culture of safety. Increasing demands for services and the rising cost of health care accompanied by diminishing reimbursement requires patients to move through the healthcare system quicker than ever before. The rapidity of patient turnover increases the chance of error and leaves potential gaps in communications. Further complicating the working conditions is the increase in patient acuity, high staff turnover, long work hours, increased interruptions and demands, and rapidly changing technology.[61] Moving from a culture of blame to one of safety begins with identifying the reason for errors rather than focusing on the individual making the error.[62] As the largest group of healthcare providers and those in closest contact to patients, nurses are in key positions to identify errors and to initiate measures to protect those they serve. However, studies indicate errors to be significantly underreported by nurses.[63] Improving systems that encourage reporting and ensure anonymity is necessary to identify and address safety issues. Safe working environments are built on open communication, properly prepared employees who are competent in performing required duties, adequate resources, and an infrastructure that allows staff to perform work successfully.[64] Lessons from other industries must be incorporated into health care. The aviation industry has created a culture of safety by closely monitoring the hours worked by pilots, redesigning systems, and promoting teamwork and communication to prevent errors.

Figure 15-5 lists innovative initiatives recently used to improve patient safety, and Figure 15-6 lists strategies to reduce malpractice claims. There is still much work to be done to ensure delivery systems

---

FIGURE 15-5 | **PATIENT SAFETY INITIATIVES**

- Development of rapid response teams (RRTs). As part of the Institute for Healthcare Improvement's campaign to save 5 million lives hospitals throughout the country have implemented RRTs to rescue medical-surgical patients from impending crisis. Studies have demonstrated a significant reduction in morbidity and mortality of hospitalized patients.[65]

- Implementation of communication models for reporting such as SBAR (situation, background, assessment, and recommendation)
  More than 60% of sentinel events reported to JCAHO identified communication as a root cause of the event.[66]

- Improvement of medication delivery systems including the use of bar coding. The Institute of Medicine reported that adverse drug events are the most common reason for medical errors and cost hospitals more than $20 billion per year.[67]

- Implementation of processes to improve the work environment such as transforming care at the bedside (TCAB). As many as 35% to 40% of unexpected hospital deaths occur in hospital medical-surgical units. TCAB projects sponsored by the Robert Wood Johnson and Institute of Healthcare Improvements aim to dramatically improve care on medical-surgical units by redesigning workspace, enhancing efficiency and reducing waste.[68]

- Development of teamwork. In the airline industry, "crew resource management" is a strategy to facilitate the team of flight attendants, pilots, and other crew.[69] Roles and responsibilities are clearly defined for numerous scenarios to ensure safety. This model is being used in some healthcare organizations such as obstetrical units where staffs "practice for emergencies."

- Development of clinical guidelines to promote standardization of care. A study of obstetrical patients indicated that when care failed to follow establish clinical guidelines, there was a sixfold increase in litigation cases.[70]

- Development of high-performing microsystems. High-performing microsystems yield better outcomes and effective care at lower cost and produce a more satisfying work environment.[71]

Source: Author.

FIGURE 15-6	STRATEGIES TO REDUCE MALPRACTICE CLAIMS

1. Ignorance of the law is not an excuse for wrongdoing. If a law exists but a person does not know it, that person will not be excused for breaking it.

2. Every person is responsible for his or her own actions. The nurse must know the cause and effect of all actions or will be subject to suit for malpractice when harm occurs to a patient.

3. A nurse will not carry out an illegal order of a physician or any other healthcare provider. The nurse must know that the order is a legal one before carrying it out.

4. New nurse graduates must not be assigned to duties beyond their competence.

5. An employer hiring a nurse is required to exercise ordinary, prudent policies and procedures.

6. By the "respondeat superior" or "master–servant" rule, injury by an employee because of negligence makes both employee and employer equally responsible to an injured party. The injured party may sue both employer and employee. Both may not necessarily be found guilty.

7. Professional nurses should carry malpractice insurance. Even when an employer insures an employee, the licensed employee is usually not covered outside the place of employment.

8. Malpractice litigation can be reduced by documenting telephone advice to patients, improving communication and listening skills, and effectively obtaining patients' informed consent.

9. Malpractice risks are increased when professional nurses supervise unlicensed employees.

10. Knowledge of state laws, such as mandatory reporting of abuse, is important for nurses.

11. Courts have interpreted ERISA (Employee Retirement Income Security Act) to limit physician autonomy and subordinate clinical decision making to cost-containment decisions made by managed care organizations.

12. Good provider–patient relationships contribute to preventing malpractice suits.

13. Iatrogenic injuries are a significant public health problem that must be addressed by professional nurses.

14. The costs of malpractice litigation can be reduced by managing risks rather than vindicating providers accused of malpractice. Successful risk management techniques include credentialing of professional staff, monitoring and tracking of complaints and incidents, and documenting in the patient's medical record.

15. The medical malpractice field appeared in the United States around 1840 and has been sustained by changing pressures on medicine, adoption of uniform standards, the advent of medical malpractice liability insurance, contingency fees, citizen juries, and the nature of tort pleading.

16. Human errors in clinical nursing practice are common and underreported.

17. With increased credentialing of advanced practice nurses in health maintenance organizations, there will be increased liability for their employers and increased need for personal malpractice insurance.

18. The nursing profession appears to hold its licensees to safer standards than does the medical profession; therefore nurses are disciplined more often and more harshly than are physicians.

19. Personal involvement with patients places the professional nurse in jeopardy of legal action by the state board of nursing.

20. Many charting practices can help decrease the liability risks for nurses.

Source: Author.

that are safe and effective and require commitment of the mass. Leaders must be willing to give power to others and trust in the skill and wisdom of the whole. The legendary management consultant Peter Drucker once said, "The leaders who work most effectively, it seems to me, never say 'I.' And that is not because they have trained themselves not to say 'I.' They don't think 'I.' They think 'we'; they think 'team.' They understand their job is to make the team function. They accept responsibility and don't sidestep it, but 'we' gets the credit. This is what creates trust, what enables you to get the job done."

Evidence-Based Practice 15-1

Sivell et al. reported on the significance of assessing risk as it relates to genetic screening. Per the researchers, as an individual perceives genetic risk such may influence risk management decisions, underscoring the need to understand the ways in which risk is constructed and interpreted. The authors systematically reviewed the literature, doing a narrative synthesis of 59 studies presenting data on the ways in which individuals perceive, construct, and interpret their risk and the subsequent effects. Although most studies assessed perceived risk from a quantitative perspective, the combined evidence noted that individuals find risk difficult to accurately quantify, with a tendency to overestimate. According to the researchers, rather than being a stand-alone concept, risk is something lived and experienced, and the process of constructing risk is complex and influenced by many factors. Although evidence of the effects of perceived risk is limited and inconsistent, there is some evidence that notes high risk estimations may adversely affect health and lead to inappropriate uptake of medical surveillance and preventative measures by some individuals. A more focused approach to research is needed with greater exploration of the ways in which risk is constructed, along with the development of stronger theoretical models, to facilitate effective and patient-centered counseling strategies.[72]

SUMMARY

There is an element of risk when practicing in the healthcare environment. Nurses and nurse leaders should be familiar with the potential liability associated with their chosen nursing role. Civil, criminal, and corporate laws apply to certain aspects of health care. Familiarity and compliance with laws is necessary to protect the nurse from liability. Medical malpractice claims continue to escalate as consumers of health care become more informed and expectations rise. Today, the public is less trusting of providers and less forgiving of mistakes. Good communication and rapport between providers and recipients of care accompanied by quality and safety measures are essential to decrease the incidence of malpractice claims. The litigation process is generally foreign territory for the nurses at any level of practice. Education and support is required to help the nurses through the lengthy and threatening experience of litigation. Risk management activities can identify potential risk for the organization and implement strategies to improve the safety and quality of care. Nurse leaders are responsible to ensure that risk management principles are practiced in the workplace.

APPLICATION EXERCISES

Exercise 15-1

Interview a risk manager. How do the risk manager's competencies compare with those outlined in Figure 15-2? What risk prevention strategies does the manager use? What has been the cost of losses caused by negligence during the past year?

Exercise 15-2

Examine the incident reporting program in a healthcare agency. What are the strengths? Weaknesses? How can it be improved?

Exercise 15-3

Interview a nurse executive. Using the patient safety initiatives outlined in Figure 15-5, review with the nurse executive patient safety concerns and strategies used in his or her healthcare organization.

Notes

1. Institute of Medicine. (2000). *To err is human: Building a safer health system.* Washington, DC: National Academies Press.
2. Institute of Medicine. (2004). *Keeping patients safe: Transforming the work environment of nurses.* Washington, DC: National Academies Press.
3. Studdert, D., Mello, M., & Brennan, T. (2004). Medical malpractice. *New England Journal of Medicine, 350,* 283.
4. Sharpe, C. (1999). *Nursing malpractice: Liability and risk management* (p. 5). Westport, CT: Reenwood Publishing Group.
5. Ibid., p. 17.
6. Agency for Healthcare Research and Quality. (2004). *AHRQ's patient safety initiative: Building foundations, reducing risk.* An Interim Report to the United States Committee on Appropriations (No. 4-RG005), p. 57.
7. Brennan, T., Leape, L., Laird, N., Hebert, L., Lawthers, A., & Newhouse, J. (1991). Incidence of adverse events and negligence in hospitalized patients: Results of the Harvard Medical Practice study. *New England Journal of Medicine, 324,* 370.
8. Localio, A., Lawthers, A., Brennan, T., Laird, N., Hebert, L., Peterson, L., et al. (1991). Relation between malpractice claims and adverse events due to negligence. Results of the Harvard Medical Practice study III. *New England Journal of Medicine, 325,* 245.
9. Dodge, A., & Fitzer, S. (2006). *When good doctors get sued* (2nd ed., p. 6). Olalla, CA: Dodge & Associates.
10. Pozgar, G. (2007). *Legal aspects of health care administration* (10th ed., p. 47). Sudbury, MA: Jones and Bartlett.
11. Ibid., p. 137.
12. Ibid., p. 204.
13. American Nurses Association. (2005). *The nurse's role in promoting a culture of patient safety* (p. 15). Silver Spring, MD: American Nurses Association.
14. Health Resources and Services Administration. (2007). National Practitioner's Data Bank. Retrieved January 3, 2008, from http://www.npdb-hipdb.hrsa.gov/npdb.html
15. Croke, E. M. (2003). Nurses, negligence, and malpractice: An analysis based on more than 250 cases against nurses. *American Journal of Nursing, 103,* 58.
16. American Nurses Association. (2004). *Nursing: Scope & standards of practice* (p. 49). Silver Spring, MD: American Nurses Association.
17. Sharpe, 1999, p. 33.
18. Studdert et al., 2004, p. 286.
19. Joint Commission on Accreditation of Healthcare Organizations. (2006a). *Health care at the crossroads: Strategies for improving the medical liability system and preventing patient injury* (p. 2). Washington, DC.
20. Studdert et al., 2004, p. 287.
21. Joint Commission on Accreditation of Healthcare Organizations, 2006a, p. 1.
22. Studdert et al., 2004, p. 287.
23. Sharpe, 1999, pp. 6–7.
24. Ibid., p. 10.
25. Pozgar, 2007, p. 39.
26. Ibid., p. 54.
27. Ibid., p. 54.
28. Ibid., p. 62.
29. Lesnik, M., & Anderson, B. (1947). *Legal aspects of nursing* (p. 258). Philadelphia: Lippincott.
30. American Nurses Association. (2001). *Code of ethics for nurses with interpretive statements* (p. 16). Silver Spring, MD: American Nurses Association.
31. Pozgar, 2007, p. 127.
32. Ibid., p. 161.
33. Ibid., p. 135.
34. Sharpe, 1999, p. 24.
35. West, J. (2001). Occupational and environmental risk exposures for health care facilities. In R. Carroll (Ed.), *Risk management handbook for health care organizations* (3rd ed., p. 327). San Francisco: Jossey-Bass.

36. Kearney, K., & McCord, E. (1992). A new era for hospital liability. *Risk Management, 39,* 31.

37. Institute of Medicine, 2004.

38. Joint Commission on Accreditation of Healthcare Organizations. (2006b). *Licensed independent practitioners.* Retrieved January 5, 2008, from http://www.jointcommission.org/AccreditationPrograms/Hospitals/Standards/FAQs/Surveillance+Prevention+and+Control+of+Infection/IC+Program/LIP_Health_Screening.htm

39. Joint Commission on Accreditation of Healthcare Organizations, 2006a, p. 2.

40. Health Resources and Services Administration, 2007.

41. Havlisch, R. (2001). Emerging liabilities in partnerships, joint ventures, and collaborative relationships. In R. Carroll (Ed.), *Risk management handbook for health care organizations* (3rd ed., pp. 327–328). San Francisco: Jossey-Bass.

42. Pozgar, 2007, p. 136.

43. Sharpe, 1999, p. 48.

44. Larson, K. (2006). The psychological impact of malpractice: The lived experience. *Nephrology Nursing Journal, 33,* 140.

45. Pozgar, 2007, p. 454.

46. Sewick, J., & Porto, G. G. (2001). The health care risk management professional. In R. Carroll (Ed.), *Risk management handbook for health care organizations* (3rd ed., pp. 3–4). San Francisco: Jossey-Bass.

47. Ibid., 5.

48. Joint Commission on Accreditation of Healthcare Organizations, 2006a, p. 9.

49. Sage, W. (2003). Medical liability and patient safety. *Health Affairs, 22,* 28.

50. Wojcieszak, D., Banja, J., & Houk, C. (2006). The sorry works! coalition: Making the case for full disclosure. *Journal on Quality and Patient Safety, 32,* 344–350.

51. Ibid., pp. 345–349.

52. Pozgar, 2007, p. 261.

53. Sharpe, 1999, p. 111.

54. Pozgar, 2007, p. 261.

55. Sharpe, 1999, p. 37.

56. American Nurses Association, 2004, p. 48.

57. Coben, M. (2001). Statutes, standards, and regulations. In R. Carroll (Ed.), *Risk management handbook for health care organizations* (3rd ed., p. 101). San Francisco: Jossey-Bass.

58. Blake, P. (1984). Incident investigation: A complete guide. *Nursing Management, 1,* 37–41.

59. Davis, K. S., & McConnel, J. C. (2001). Data management. In R. Carroll (Ed.), *Risk management handbook for health care organizations* (3rd ed., p. 126). San Francisco: Jossey-Bass.

60. Pozgar, 2007, p. 302.

61. Institute of Medicine, 2004.

62. American Nurses Association, 2005, p. 7.

63. Ibid.

64. Ibid., p. 15.

65. Institute for Healthcare Improvement. (2006). *Rapid response teams.* Retrieved January 5, 2008, from http://www.ihi.org/NR/rdonlyres/6541BE00-00BC-4AD8-A049-CD76EDE5F171/0/RRTHowtoGuide.doc

66. Joint Commission on Accreditation of Healthcare Organizations. (2006c). Sentinel events. Retrieved January 5, 2008, from http://www.jointcommission.org/SentinelEvents/Statistics/

67. Institute of Medicine, 2000.

68. Institute for Healthcare Improvement. (2003). *Transforming care at the bedside.* Retrieved November 19, 2007, from http://www.ihi.org/IHI/Programs/StrategicInitiatives/TransformingCareAtTheBedside.htm

69. Joint Commission on Accreditation of Healthcare Organizations, 2006, p. 4.

70. Ibid.

71. Ibid., p. 5.

72. Sivell, S., Elwyn, G., Gaff, C., Clarke, A., Iredale, R., Shaw, C., Dundon, J., Thornton, H., & Edwards, A. (2008). How risk is perceived, constructed and interpreted by clients in clinical genetics, and the effects on decision making: Systematic review. *Journal of Genetic Counseling, 17,* 30–63.

16 TOOLS FOR EVALUATING OPERATIONS AND CARE DELIVERY SYSTEMS

Amy Bearden, RN, MSN, NEA, BC

LEARNING OBJECTIVES AND ACTIVITIES

- Define the term *evaluating*.
- Describe the relationship of evaluating to the other major functions of management: planning, organizing, and directing (leading).
- Describe operations management.
- Describe transformation of organizational culture.
- Describe the use of controls as quality tools.
- Describe the use of controls as management tools.
- Describe the use of standards for controlling or evaluating.
- Demonstrate evaluating and controlling techniques.
- Use a set of standards in the evaluating function of a nursing agency or unit.
- Describe evidence-based management and its relevance to evaluation and control.

CONCEPTS

Controlling, evaluating, measuring, standards, transformation, Information Age, quantum leadership, microsystems, root cause analysis, Gantt chart, performance evaluation and review technique, benchmarking, evidence-based management, quality awards.

Defines goals within organizational departments in specific, measurable terms that include statements of performance related to standards; uses legal and accreditation standards to control, coordinate, and evaluate all activities of the organization; promotes implementation of processes that deliver data and information to empower staff in decision making; advocates for and supports a process of participative decision making; promotes the development of policies, procedures, and guidelines based on research findings and institutional measurement of quality outcomes.

Obtains input from representative nursing personnel to develop and implement a strategic master control plan incorporating legal and accreditation standards; supports information-handling processes and technologies to facilitate evaluation of effectiveness and efficiency of decisions, plans, and activities in relation to desired outcomes; ensures educational opportunities for staff based on evaluation findings, specific to the population served, professional practice, available technologies, or required skills, to enhance quality in healthcare delivery.

Introduction

Evaluating the effectiveness of healthcare operations and systems is critical to our continued improvement and success in providing healthcare services. Fayol defined evaluation or control as "verifying whether everything occurs in conformity with the plan adopted, the instructions issued, and principles established. It has for its object to point out weakness and error in order to rectify them and prevent recurrence."[1]

Additionally, Urwick defines controlling or evaluating as "seeing that everything is being carried out in accordance with the plan which has been adopted, the orders which have been given, and the principles which have been laid down."[2] Urwick refers to three principles of controlling:[3]

1. Uniformity ensures that controls are related to the organizational structure.
2. Comparison ensures that controls are stated in terms of the standards of performance required, including past performance. In this sense, controlling means setting a mark and examining and explaining the results in terms of the mark. This is often called benchmarking.
3. Exception provides summaries that identify exceptions to the standards.

❝The controlling process may be expressed as a formula:

$$Ss + Sa + F + C \rightarrow I$$

where Standards set + Standards applied + Feedback + Correction yield Improvement.❞

Figure 16-1 shows the control processes described by management authors.[4] According to Peters, vision, symbolic action, and recognition make up a control system in the truest sense of the word. Peters also states that "what gets measured gets done."[5]

EVALUATION AS A FUNCTION OF NURSING MANAGEMENT

Evaluation (control) is the management function in which performance is measured and corrective action is taken to ensure the accomplishment of organizational goals.[6] Control includes coordination of numerous activities, including decision making related to planning and organizing activities and information from directing and evaluating each worker's performance. Evaluation is also concerned with records, reports, organizational progress toward aims, and effective use of resources. Control uses evaluation and regulation; controlling is identical to evaluation.[7] Koontz and Weihrich defined controlling

---

FIGURE 16-1 CONTROL PROCESSES

Control Process

1. Establish standards to measure performance for all elements of management in terms of expected outcomes. Use specific operational terms to compare with organizational activities. These are the yardsticks by which achievement of objectives is measured.

2. Measure the actual performance. Apply the standards by collecting data and measuring the activities of nursing management, comparing standards with actual care.

3. Compare the performance with the established standards. Make any improvements deemed necessary from the feedback.

4. Take corrective actions. Keep the process continuous for all areas, including the following:
   a. Management of the nursing division and each subunit
   b. The performance of personnel

Nursing Example

a. Healthcare providers must use at least two patient identifiers when providing care, treatment or services.

a. Create and use a measurement tool to collect data by observing nurses in action and round on patients.
b. Obtain feedback from the patient about the identification process and what was used by the healthcare provider to make the identification.
c. Discuss and obtain recommendations from the nursing staff as to what identifiers would be the most efficient to use.

a. Identify how often the proper identification from the nurse did not happen and why.
b. Identify variations to the process or what other forms of identifying the patient may be occurring and why.

a. Make adjustments to the identification process and standardize the process with input from both healthcare providers and patients:
   i)   Ensure that the process is standardized and performed consistently within the division of nursing and each specialty unit.
   ii) Education about the patient identification standard and process should be provided to each nurse in orientation to the unit.
   iii) Continuously evaluate the individual staff nurse performance of the standard for patient identification through observation, peer evaluation and feedback from patient interviews.

Source: Author.

as "the measurement and correction of the performance in order to make sure that enterprise objectives and the plans devised to attain them are accomplished."[8]

Organizational control is the ongoing process of assigning, evaluating, and regulating resources to meet the goals of the organization. It involves managing people, equipment, technology, information, supplies, structure, and other resources. The act of controlling involves monitoring activities to ensure they are accomplished as planned and correcting any significant deviations or variations. An effective control system has standards, measuring tools, and a surveillance process culminating in corrective action. A quality control program for measuring patient care will have these same components.[9] Controlling is an important physical act of administration; another physical act is directing. It is often considered the final element of the administrative composite process, after directing, planning, and organizing. Functions of organizational management, such as planning, organizing, directing, and controlling, occur simultaneously.[10] These simultaneous actions are also called operations management.

> *Nurse managers use staffing reports, budget status reports, and other information to control the functioning system. These reports are both monitoring devices and feedback to the clinical nurses and care managers.*

OPERATIONS MANAGEMENT

Operations management is the central core function of every organization, including hospitals and other healthcare systems. The role of the operations manager within the organizational structure of a hospital or healthcare system is to transform and control an organization's inputs into the finished services of high quality.

Operational management is based on systems management theory and uses the four elements of inputs, transformation processes, outputs, and feedback.[11] Inputs that the nurse executive uses within the role of an operational manager include human resources, processes, materials, and supplies as well as technology and information. The nurse executive monitors the operations performance against a standard, goal, or plan by obtaining feedback or reactions from the working environment. Using the feedback obtained, the nurse executive makes adjustments or changes to the plan which transforms the operational processes to better meet the organizational goals. Controlling should be based on facts, because the ultimate purpose of control is to identify problems that in turn will assist nurse executives and managers to make informed decisions. Control as a function of operations management provides feedback as to whether the organization is effective (consistent high-quality results), efficient (lowest possible cost, productive), and has value-added processes.[12]

Organizational Transformation

Current literature identifies the adaptation of organizational structures to changes in our society. Technology and a focus on information continue to change our culture and the way we do business. In response to changes in the workplace, a horizontal versus a top-down or vertical hierarchy (Industrial Age) is necessary, focusing on creating new structures and processes. The transformation of the workplace is significant as the control hierarchy is one with multiple direction versus linear lines of control.[13] Porter O'Grady and Malloch describe organizations as existing internally in both worlds, that is, the top-down, linear, industrial control model and the ever-changing information technology–based multiple-direction world. Organizations are in the midst of major dramatic and dynamic transformational changes to adapt to increases in the portability of information. Porter O'Grady and Malloch identify the future as the "Quantum Age" and list the following quantum characteristics for organizational leaders[14]:

- Multifocal characteristics
- Nonlinear structures

- Focus on relatedness
- Multisystems scientific processes
- Center-out decision making
- Complexity-based models of design
- Value-driven action

Leaders in organizations are in constant flux as they transform from linear, top-down management structures to the creation of infrastructures, allowing individuals to own their work processes (autonomy) and participate in shared decision making. The multifocal characteristics of populations being cared for as well as those providing the care underscore the importance of using diversity in decision making to add value to care. Quantum theory considers these dimensions along with creating systems to support the ability to work through the interdependency of the workforce. An example of this adaptation is the development of shared governance councils within patient care areas. Leaders are managing a journey of transformation, chaos, and diversity.[15] Service is patient centered and care is relationship based with attention to quality, safety, and costs. We can no longer provide services that do not add value to the healthcare experience.

Organizations that deliver health care are complex and often cumbersome, making transformation difficult. Considering complexity science and chaos theory equips the nurse executives with additional knowledge and skills to reframe and rethink "business as usual." Conceptualizing the organization from a clinical microsystems perspective provides this option. Nelson and colleagues propose a clinical microsystem model for health care, an organizational structural design supporting small functional front-line units that provide patient care.[16] An intensive care nursery, a medical/surgical unit, and an adult neurointensive care unit are examples of clinical microsystems within a larger healthcare organization. Clinical microsystems are the front-line care structures built around patient care and supported by the larger mesosystem (programs and departments).[17] Each clinical microsystem takes its own personal journey toward excellence specific to the unit mission, which in turns contributes to the whole of the organization.

Following the complexity science model, small changes can make significant differences in outcomes. Clinical microsystems bear this concept out. The environment of clinical microsystems is promoted through the dynamics of a learning organization. A learning organization considers the concepts of systems thinking, mental models, personal master, building shared vision, and team learning.[18] A clinical microsystem is such a learning organization. Each microsystem analyzes its structure by identifying and working through the "5 Ps": Purpose, Patient, Professionals or caregivers, Processes, and Patterns. When the clinical microsystems has analyzed and evaluated the 5 Ps, intentional planned care and innovation can thrive. The clinical microsystems developmental journey has five stages that support transformation[19]:

1. Creating awareness of the clinical unit as an interdependent group of people with the capacity to make changes
2. Connecting routine daily work to the high purpose of benefiting patients as a system
3. Responding successfully to a strategic challenge
4. Measuring the performance of the microsystems as a system
5. Successfully juggling multiple improvements while taking excellent care of patients and continuing the development of an enhanced sense of the unit/department as system

Drilling down on the 5 Ps provides a systematic methodology in better understanding one's unit or department and evaluating outcomes. Without the attention to the interdisciplinary approach of the microsystem, valuable resources may be squandered from lack of understanding of how work really happens. Figure 16-2 provides the 5 Ps and points to consider when using this model to analyze and evaluate care.

FIGURE 16-2	THE 5 PS: MICROSYSTEMS THAT BENEFIT BY MASTERING THE 5 PS

1. Purpose: Know your purpose. Ask the following question: Our system exists to _____.

2. Patients: Know your patients. For whom are we caring?

3. Professionals: Know your professionals. Who provides patient care and what skills and talents do team members need to provide the right service and care at the right time?

4. Processes: Know your processes. How do we deliver care to meet our patients' need?

5. Patterns: Know your patterns. What are the regularly recurring work activities? What does it look like to work here?[20]

Source: Author.

SYSTEMS THINKING

In the role of evaluating processes within care delivery systems, nurse executives and mid-level managers need skills to become systems thinkers. Systems thinking is an individual discipline based on system dynamics; it is highly conceptual. Learning organizations integrate systems thinking where individuals enhance their capacity to create the results they truly desire by building teams and expanding and nurturing new patterns of thinking, which when done so collectively creates a shared vision. Learning organizations support flexibility and adaptive and productive ways of tapping the commitment of the workforce and their capacity to learn. Although all people have the capacity to learn, the structures in which they function are often not conducive to reflection and engagement. Furthermore, people may lack the tools and guiding ideas to make sense of the situations they face. Organizations that are continually expanding their capacity to create their future require a fundamental shift of mind among their members. Senge states in *The Fifth Discipline* (learning organizations)[21]

> The essence of the discipline of systems thinking lies in a shift of mind: Seeing interrelationships rather than linear cause and effect chains, and seeing processes of change rather than snapshots.

The practice of systems thinking starts with understanding a simple concept called "feedback" that shows how actions can reinforce or counteract (balance) each other. Eventually, systems thinking forms a rich language for describing a vast array of interrelationships and patterns of change. Ultimately, it simplifies life by helping us to see the deeper patterns lying behind the events and details.[21]

Nurse executives who have come up through the ranks may hold tight to ways of linear thinking and have difficulty putting into practice new insights and challenges of organizational systems and patient care delivery processes. Internal images about how patient care should be performed may be deeply held; thus visualizing a different "way of being" in the system is difficult at best. Using exercises to challenge one's mental models can provide insight and greater awareness of a viewpoint held. Additionally, evidence-based practice can also provide a methodology for securing evidence and information to support best practices. Without attention to our mental models and the possible need to shift our focus, evidence-based practice is provided in vain.

Operations management within health care requires a wide range of strategic and tactical decisions that control the outcomes of the organization. Strategic decisions are generally the primary focus of the role of the nurse executive; tactical decisions generally are attributed to nurse managers.[22]

Management Tools: Measurement Issues

For operations managers to be successful, standards, goals, and plans must be clearly communicated to all employees within the organization. All employees have to know the goals, mission, vision, and expected outcomes of the business for the service to achieve quality. Quality happens during human interaction moments at the bedside. It is a dynamic process because it is based on efficiency and effectiveness over a period of time. Leonard, Frankel, Simmonds, and Vega recommend frequent measurement and clear communication of results throughout the organization using newsletters, staff meetings, and data postings. They recommend the following basic types of measurement[23]:

- *Outcome measures:* Outcome measures chart progress toward the ultimate goal. Examples of outcome measures include mortality rates, length of stay, and frequency of ventilator-associated pneumonia.
- *Process measures:* Process measures show whether the change is resulting in improvement of the process. Examples include delays in admission and discharge and percentage of on-time administration of prophylactic antibiotic.
- *Balancing measures:* Balancing measures determine if the change is "robbing Peter to pay Paul." In other words, does the change improve one area but introduce problems in another? Examples include family satisfaction and readmission rates.

In the process of evaluation, policies and procedures are used as standards. Observations, questions, patient charts, patients, and healthcare team members also serve as sources of data. Corrective actions can be corroborative, disciplinary, or educational.[24] In the process of feedback, a positive experience stimulates motivation and contributes to the growth of employees.[25] A variety of tools can be useful in evaluating an organization's risks and its efficacy and efficiency.

Evaluation by Root Cause Analysis

Medical errors are an inherent problem for healthcare providers by virtue of the complexity of the systems encircling the care of patients. Although some medical errors are due to individual carelessness, most are not intentional; they are the result of the characteristics of the combination of routine and complex care.

Root cause analysis is an investigation looking at the multifaceted processes leading up to the event. A series of "what" and "why "questions are asked over and over again to get to the "root cause" of the event. The following questions are examples:

- What happened? What are the details leading up to the event?
- When did it happen?
- What area of service was impacted?
- Why did it happen? What were the steps in the process?
- What steps contributed to the event?
- What human factors, equipment factors, communication factors contributed?

An action plan with dates for implementation and measurement of effectiveness is then developed. Based on responses and feedback of such questions, strategies that impact the structure, process, and outcomes of an organization operational plan can be formulated, implemented, and evaluated (Figure 16-3). An organization may use a variety of computer-based tools that serve to facilitate a decision tree, which gives options to specific actions.

Management Tools: Performance Issues

Improvement of performance and high-value outcomes are the goals in health care. Among the controls are rules that let people know what is expected of them and how functions are to be coordinated.

| FIGURE 16-3 | ANSWER THE FOLLOWING QUESTIONS ABOUT THE HEALTHCARE SYSTEM WHERE YOU WORK |

Is there a confidential system to report errors?

Is it easy to report errors? (e.g., hotline, computerized form)

Is there a designated person who oversees error reporting?

Is there a mechanism for feedback to those who do report?

Following a sentinel event analysis, is there communication within the whole organization?

Source: Author.

Communication as information is essential to control. Self-control is essential to managerial control, because it is the highest form of control. Self-control is based on self-awareness, self-reflection, thoughtfulness, and intuitiveness. Self-control implies introspection and personal transformation.

Organizations rely on changes within individuals to transform the organization. As individuals change within an organization they create the collective intent (energy) that allows the organization to adapt (or not adapt) to internal and external factors.[26] The following are several tools leaders can access to increase introspection:

- Values clarification (writing down your internal values that motivate your decisions)
- Keirsey temperament sorter (http://www.keirsey.com)
- 360-degree evaluation
- Emotional intelligence (http://quiz.ivillage.co.uk/uk_work/tests/eqtest.htm)
- Strengths Finder 2.0 (http://sf2.strengthsfinder.com/research)
- Mentor–mentee relationship
- Performance evaluation

Self-control includes being up-to-date in knowledge, giving clear orders, being flexible, understanding reasons for behavior, helping others improve, increasing problem-solving skills, staying calm under pressure, and planning ahead. Employees should be told the facts in clear, deliberate language. Effective nursing managers hold employees accountable by establishing limits. Limits are developed by engaging staff input about acceptable behaviors and communicating the agreed on behaviors to their employees. Then, when a line is crossed, the appropriate disciplinary action can be taken. This is achieved by corrective action that is consistently applied after checking the facts.[27]

Controls can be separated into two elements: mechanical and sociological. There are three stages of control. The first two are mechanical elements and the third is sociological element[28]:

1. A predetermined definition of standards for a level of performance
2. Measurement of current performance against the standards
3. Corrective action when indicated

Nurse executives avoid the unintended consequence of control, that is, failure to adhere to standards. Because control can be perceived as a threat from unwanted power and authority, it can trigger defense mechanisms such as aggression and repression. Lemin advocated the following approaches to control: time, a high degree of mutual trust, a high degree of mutual support, open and authentic communications, clear understanding of objectives, respect for differences, use of member resources, and a supportive environment. These approaches lead to conflict resolution, changed beliefs and attitudes, genuine innovation, genuine commitment, strengthened management, and prevention of unintended consequences of control.[29]

In a good control system, controls should do the following[30]:

1. Reflect the nature of the activity and be fully integrated into the process.
2. Report errors promptly and accurately.
3. Be forward-looking in anticipation of further planning.
4. Point out exceptions at critical points where failure cannot be tolerated.
5. Be objective.
6. Be flexible, responsive to rapid change.
7. Reflect the organizational pattern.
8. Be economical comparing costs with the benefits.
9. Be easily understood and accepted by employees.
10. Indicate corrective action.

The best way to ensure the quality of nursing services provided in patient units is to establish the intended purpose of the unit, philosophy, standards of care, and objectives. At least two of these, philosophy and objectives, involve planning—further evidence that the major functions of management take place simultaneously.[31] Controlling mechanisms also include accreditation procedures, consultants, evaluation devices, rounds, reports, inspections, and nursing audits.[32]

Nurses activate the processes of control. This function involves the use of power and should be used by nurse executives to promote openness, honesty, trust, competence, and even confrontation. This function also involves value systems, ethical decision making, self-control, professional self-regulation, and control by an aggregate of professionals. Quality management programs excel in quality of care, including accessibility, beliefs, and attitudes of patients about health care; structure of health care; processes of care; professional competence; outcomes of care; and self-regulation. Audits and budgets are the major techniques of control.[33]

Control functions can be differentiated among levels of managers. For example, the nurse manager of a unit is concerned with short-term tactical operational activities, including daily and weekly schedules, assignments, and effective use of resources. This nurse manager also keeps records of absences and incidents and prepares personnel appraisals, which are control activities subject to quick changes. A variety of measurement methods can be useful in completing these tasks. Two measurement methods that can be used to assess achievement of nursing goals are task analysis and quality control. In task analysis, the nurse manager inspects the motions, actions, and procedures laid out in written guidelines, schedules, rules, records, and budgets. Task analysis is a study of the process of giving nursing care. It measures physical support only; a few tools have been developed to do task analysis in nursing. In quality control the nurse manager is concerned with measurement of the quality and effects of nursing care. The American Nurses Association (ANA), the The Joint Commission (TCJ), and other organizations have developed mechanisms or models for measuring nursing care. Many quality management techniques are referred to as audits.[34]

Nurse executives and managers generally work in organizations that provide their services in the presence of the customer; they are generally labor intensive and need short response times. Customers have direct contact and influence the outcome of the service provided.[35]

STANDARDS

Standardized organizational controls operationalized by the nurse executive can be structural, financial, budgetary, marketing, human resource management, and informational. Standards of care that impact nursing can be internal or external. Internal standards may include the job description, education and expertise, and the institution's policies and procedures. Performance standards should also be considered in the discussion of standardized organizational control measures.

Internal Standards

Internal standards are a prime element of the management of nursing services and can be used as a system for evaluation of the total effort, including evaluation of the management process, the practice of nursing, and all nursing care services. Evaluation requires standards that can be used to gauge the quality and quantity of services. The key source for these standards, which are available for both management and practice, is the ANA, whose publications include *Scope and Standards for Nurse Administrators* and *Standards of Clinical Nursing Practice*. Additional scope and standards for specialty practices are also available. These documents can be of assistance in developing the objectives of the division of nursing and of each unit and clinic. Objectives are developed into operational or management plans, and systematic and periodic review of accomplishment of these objectives are part of the evaluation system. A management evaluation system can be developed with a similar format. The nurse executive and nurse managers can effect further evaluation through development of criteria for nursing rounds.

External Standards

External standards consist of the following:

- Nurse practice acts
- Professional nursing organizations (e.g., American Organization of Nurse Executives, ANA)
- Nursing specialty practice organizations (e.g., Association of Operating Room Nurses, Emergency Nurses Association)
- Federal organizations and federal guidelines (e.g., TJC, Centers for Medicare and Medicaid [CMS])[36]

External standards continue to play an increasingly vital role in the evaluation of health care. The TJC's *National Patient Safety Goals Hospital Program, Core Measures,* and *Institutes of Hospital Improvements 5 Million Lives Campaign* are examples of external standards requiring the nurse administrator to evaluate a variety of performance measures of the healthcare organization.

External standards have played an increasingly vital role in the evaluation of health care. The TJC requires accredited hospitals to collect and submit performance data on acute myocardial infarction, heart failure, and pneumonia. This requirement was established to improve the safety and quality of care within hospitals. In July 2004 the CMS mandated public reporting of these measures. Public reporting implies that private health insurance companies, government agencies, and healthcare consumers have access to performance and the ability to make comparisons with other hospitals. This is a controlling measure called transparency. Transparency is essential because it increases the visibility of hospital performance, thereby making organizations accountable. Hospitals are financially motivated to participate with public reporting because CMS will withhold 4% of reimbursement if a hospital does not participate. Hospitals that do not meet minimum performance standards could end up suffering financially for providing suboptimal care and/or not being able to demonstrate appropriate care through documentation. Fact sheets detailing the quality measures are available at www.cms.hhs.gov/quality/hospital.

Performance Standards

Performance standards can be used for individual performance, and criteria can be developed for collective evaluation of patient care. The latter may include the standards for use during nursing rounds and the criteria for the quality management program. Standards are established criteria of performance, planning goals, strategic plans, physical or quantitative measurements of products, units of service, labor hours, speed, cost, capital, revenue, program, and intangible standards.[37] They have also been defined as "an acknowledged measure of comparison for quantitative or qualitative value, criterion, or norm . . . a standard rule or test on which a judgment or decision can be based." Nurse executives develop, in collaboration with clinical nurses, the "clinical nursing criteria against which to measure patient outcomes and the nursing process."[38] These standards are stated as patient outcomes, nursing care processes, incident reviews, and evidence-based practice.[39]

The following are eight categories of standards[40]:

1. Physical standards: Using patient acuity ratings to establish nursing hours per patient day
2. Cost standards: Cost per patient day for supplies
3. Capital standards: A new program of monetary investment, such as a patient teaching staff
4. Revenue standards: The revenue per hour of nursing care received by patients
5. Program standards: A program designed to develop a new nursing service for changing clients' behavior regarding exercise, eating, or other health activities
6. Intangible standards: Staff development costs in nursing
7. Goals: Intangible standards are frequently replaced by goals, including those for qualitative measurements.
8. Strategic plans, as control points for strategic control, are also used as standards.

The nurse executive's involvement in strategic planning necessitates knowledge of, abilities, and skills for strategic control.

MEASURING PRODUCTIVITY

Measuring productivity is a function of the controlling process. To perform this measure, management establishes a measurement of productivity as the standard for each department and unit. Inputs are reported to appropriate cost-center managers each month. Productivity measurement tools should be developed with input from the people being measured. This development may be done locally or through consultation. Nursing departments with computerized patient classification systems often have accurate productivity indices and reporting. A significant role for the nurse executive in regard to data collection is to ensure that documentation is complete, accurate, and consistent within the medical record to have accurate data for the reporting of performance measures.

Tools to evaluate productivity of independent nurse practitioners are available.[41] Figure 16-4 is an example of an evaluation or controlling plan for nursing services.

Preparing documentation for a Joint Commission visit, may include a system for maintaining ongoing documentation that is being adapted to changes in The Joint Commission (TJC) standards. Such a system ensures that standards are kept up-to-date and prevents last-minute crisis preparation for TJC visits. Self-study is also a method of meeting TJC safety requirements. Employees are held accountable for meeting the standard and are tested to verify competence.[41] Programs are written and distributed by education personnel, and records are maintained on education cards or by computer. Self-study methods can be used to meet other standards.

CONTROLLING TECHNIQUES

Specific controlling techniques include planned nursing rounds by nurse managers from all levels, checklists from the ANA *Scope and Standards of Nurse Administrators,* ANA *Standards of Clinical Nursing Practice,* TJC *Comprehensive Accreditation Manual for Hospitals,* and other published standards of third-party payers such as those put forth by the CMS.

Nursing Rounds

An effective controlling technique for nursing managers is planned nursing rounds, which can be placed on a schedule and can include all nursing personnel. Rounds cover issues such as patient care,

FIGURE 16-4 OPERATIONAL PLAN

Mission Statement to Which Objective Applies

The division of nursing has a stated philosophy and objectives. Personnel of each department or unit within the division will have their own philosophy and will set up their own objectives. The objectives will be continuously evaluated, and a written statement as to progress will be sent to the chair's office each August and February.

Philosophy Statement to Which Objective Applies

We believe that a continuous evaluation of the activities of the division of nursing is necessary to assess how effectively the needs of the patients are being met and to take action to improve nursing service when indicated. Research must be performed, and the results must be analyzed, adapted, and implemented to modify nursing procedures and practices for the attainment of more effective patient care.

Objective 6

The patient benefits from close nursing supervision of all nonprofessional personnel who give patient care, and the patient benefits from continuous evaluation of the nursing care given and of performances of all nursing service personnel based on professional standards.

Plans for Achieving Objective	Action and Accountability	Target Dates	Accomplishments
1. Plan and execute a system of continuous evaluation and appraisal of nursing services.	1. Make complete rounds throughout the hospital at least once a day from nursing office. Establish a system of formal nursing rounds by chair, assistants, and clinical nursing coordinators monthly.	Apr. 23, 20xx	Being done.
	2. Do a monthly nursing audit. Have committee chair brief the chair of the division of nursing afterward.	Dec. 1, 20xx	Criteria for major nursing diagnosis outcomes completed. Committee combined with other disciplines. Criteria applied to four nursing diagnosis outcomes with retrieval by medical records personnel and corrective actions taken.
	3. Develop standards for patient care. Use ANA *Standards of Clinical Nursing Practice* for evaluating patient care. Obtain copies for all head nurses.	Jan. 1, 20xx	Obtained. Being incorporated into system by committee of staff nurses. Will cross-check with job performance standards.
	4. Develop standards for personnel performance.	Dec. 31, 20xx	Completed for clinical nurses I, II, and III, charge nurse, in-service education coordinator, clinical coordinator, chair and assistants, operating room supervisor and staff nurses, public health nurse, and rehabilitation nurse.

(continues)

Plans for Achieving Objective	Action and Accountability	Target Dates	Accomplishments

	5. Set up a system whereby managers attend
	   a. Change-of-shift reports.
	   b. Unit conferences.
	   c. Unit in-service programs.
		July 1, 20xx	Receiving reports and need to plan for their use. Will discuss with managers.

	6. Review and use ANA *Scope and Standards for Nurse Administrators* to develop an evaluation and inspection checklist.	Dec. 1, 20xx	
2. Study organization.	1. Reorganize as needed. Have organization chart printed.	July 1, 20xx	Done as hospital policy.
	2. Write policy on unit policies and procedures.	July 1, 20xx	Done as nursing operating instruction 160-2-4.
3. Establish a counseling program for all nursing personnel.	1. Program counseling sessions for all head nurses. Have them do the same for those they supervise.	Jan. 1, 20xx	All done once by Jan. 1, 20xx.
	2. Use the job performance standards.		

Source: Author.

patient safety, nursing practice, and unit management. To be effective, the results should be discussed with appropriate nursing personnel in a follow-up conference. Part of the evaluation process takes place as a result of the communication occurring during the rounds. Figure 16-5 shows a protocol for planned monthly nursing rounds.

Nursing Operating Instructions

Nursing operating instructions or policies become standards for evaluation and controlling techniques (Figure 16-6). The ANA *Scope and Standards for Nurse Administrators* can be developed into a checklist for evaluating the management processes of nursing services. Figure 16-7 shows a format for converting these standards into a usable control tool. The ANA *Standards of Clinical Nursing Practice* can be implemented in several ways. One way is to convert the set of standards into a checklist, as in Figure 16-7. Written protocols should be developed to implement a program for the evaluation process. Another way these protocols may be implemented is by using them to develop the evaluation standards, as in Figure 16-8.

Gantt Charts

Early in the 20th century, Henry L. Gantt developed the Gantt chart as a means of controlling production. The chart, which is usually used for production activities, depicts a series of events essential to the completion of a project or program. Figure 16-9 shows a modified Gantt chart that could be applied to a major nursing administration program or project. The five major activities identified are segments of a total program or project. The chart could be applied to a project such as implementing a modality of primary nursing or implementing case management. The following are possible nursing activities for a project:

- Gather data.
- Analyze data.

FIGURE 16-5 — PROTOCOL FOR PLANNED MONTHLY NURSING ROUNDS

1. The chair, assistant chair, and other appropriate nursing personnel will make nursing rounds monthly.

2. Time is 10:00 to 11:00 A.M. unless otherwise indicated.

3. Schedule:

Unit	Day
1F	1st Tuesday
2A	1st Wednesday
2B	1st Thursday
2F	2nd Tuesday
ICU	2nd Wednesday
4A	2nd Thursday
3A	2nd Friday
3-OB	3rd Tuesday, 10:30 to 11:30 A.M.
3F	3rd Wednesday
4B	3rd Thursday, 11:00 A.M. to 12:00 noon
5A, CCU	4th Tuesday
5B	4th Wednesday

4. All unit nursing personnel are welcome to attend these rounds with their head nurse. Patient care needs come first. The following areas will be covered as rounds are made to each patient's bedside:
   a. Nursing histories
   b. Nursing care plans
   c. Nursing notes
   d. Nurses' signatures on necessary documents

5. Other management areas of note will be discussed after bedside rounds:
   a. Equipment and supplies
   b. Staffing and assignments
   c. Narcotic registers

Source: Author.

FIGURE 16-6 — OPERATING INSTRUCTIONS

1. Special care units will maintain policies and procedures relative to their mission. (These procedures will be reviewed, updated, and signed at least annually.)
   a. Intensive care unit
   b. Critical care unit
   c. Newborn/intensive care unit nursery
   d. Renal dialysis

2. Special care units will maintain a list of equipment needed to achieve their mission.

3. Supplies and equipment
   a. Blount resuscitator will have percent adaptor to increase oxygen concentration.
   b. Ambu resuscitator will have tail on to increase oxygen concentration.
   c. Humidification will not be used with oxygen with Ambu resuscitator.
   d. Trays from Central Sterile Supply will be returned as soon as used so that instruments will not be lost or misplaced.

Source: Author.

- Develop a plan.
- Implement the plan.
- Evaluate, give feedback, and modify the plan as needed.

Figure 16-9 is only an example. Application of this controlling process by nurse managers would be specific to the project or program, and the time elements for the various activities would vary. Using

---

FIGURE 16-7

FORMAT FOR CONVERTING THE ANA *SCOPE AND STANDARDS FOR NURSE ADMINISTRATORS* INTO A USABLE CONTROL TOOL

Standard No. _____ :

Measurement Criteria   Yes   No

(List)

Source: Author.

FIGURE 16-8

STANDARDS FOR EVALUATING THE CONTROLLING (EVALUATING) FUNCTION OF NURSING ADMINISTRATION OF A DIVISION, SERVICE, OR UNIT

1. An evaluation plan exists and is used for each nursing department, service, or unit.

2. Each evaluation plan is specific to the needs and activities of the individual department, service, or unit.

3. Evaluation findings are given in immediate feedback to subordinate nursing personnel.

4. Standards are accurate, suitable, and objective.

5. Standards are flexible and work when changes are made in plans and when unforeseen events and failures occur.

6. Standards mirror the organizational pattern of the nursing division, service, or unit.

7. Standards are economical to apply and do not produce unexpected results or effects.

8. Nursing personnel know and understand the standards.

9. Application of the standards results in correction of deficiencies.

Source: Author.

FIGURE 16-9

MODIFIED GRANT CHART

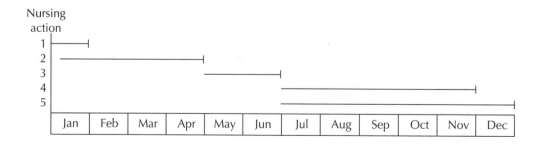

Source: Author.

Note: Five nursing actions are needed to complete a progam planned to start in January and end in December. In Figure 16-10, these five actions are translated into milestones and critical control points.

subcategories of activities with estimated completion times could also modify these five major activities. The nurse manager's goal is to complete each activity or phase on or before the projected date.

Critical Control Points and Milestones

Master evaluation plans should have critical control points: specific points in production of goods or services at which the nurse administrator judges whether the objectives are being met qualitatively and quantitatively. Critical control points tell whether the plan is progressing satisfactorily. They pinpoint successes and failures and their causes. Critical control points tell managers whether they are on target with regard to time, budget, and other resources. Milestones are segments or phases of specific activities of a project or program that are projected to occur within a time frame.

Figure 16-11 represents a modified Gantt chart with networks of milestones and critical control points. The critical path is

$$1 \rightarrow 2 \rightarrow 3 \rightarrow 4 \rightarrow 5 \rightarrow 6 \rightarrow 7 \rightarrow 8 \rightarrow 9 \rightarrow 17 \rightarrow 18$$

Line 5 in Figure 16-10 represents evaluation of all other nursing actions. This illustration is a simplified version of a control technique. Case management also uses critical paths with milestones and control points. Any major nursing program could have dozens or even hundreds of milestones and critical control points. This system also is known as the program evaluation and review technique (PERT).

Application of the milestone technique involves establishing a network of controllable pieces when planning a project or program. Each piece of the project or program is also allocated a prorated portion of the total budget. A nurse manager could use this technique to evaluate the actual expenditure amount versus the estimated budget at the end of each step of activity (or monthly) of the project or program. These are the critical control points, because each culminates in the achievement of a milestone. Each event may represent a budgeting allocation, a period of time or time span, or a continuum of several or all of these. Bar graphs are frequently used to depict milestone budgeting. Budgeting is a major controlling technique in any of its forms.[42]

Program Evaluation and Review Technique

PERT was developed by the Special Projects Office of the U.S. Navy and applied to the planning and control of the Polaris weapon system in 1958. The PERT system has been widely applied as a controlling process in business and industry.

PERT uses a network of activities, each of which is represented as a step on a chart. A time measurement and an estimated budget should be worked out that include the following[43]:

1. Finished product or service desired
2. Total time and budget needed to complete the project or program
3. Start and completion dates
4. Sequence of steps or activities required to accomplish the project or program
5. Estimated time and cost of each step or activity
6. Three paths for steps 4 and 5:
   a. Optimistic time
   b. Most likely time
   c. Pessimistic time
7. Calculation of the critical path, the sequence of the events that would take the longest time to complete the project or program by the planned completion date. This is the critical path because it will leave the least slack time.

FIGURE 16-10 · MODIFIED GRANT CHART

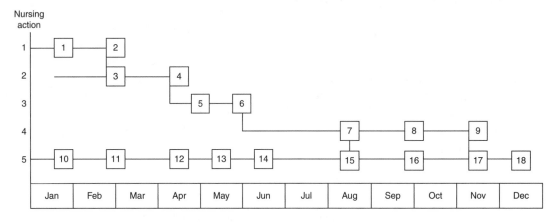

Modified Gantt chart
with milestones and critical control points
and network of milestones

Source: Author.

Why should nurse executives use the PERT system for controlling?

- It forces planning and shows how the pieces fit for all nursing line managers involved.
- It establishes a system for periodic evaluation and control at critical points in the program.
- It reveals problems and is forward looking.

The PERT system generally is used for complicated and extensive projects or programs, such as planning and implementing a system of nursing diagnoses, nursing interventions, and nursing outcomes.

❝ Multiple sites exist on the Internet as resources for information on controlling techniques, including Gantt and PERT charts. Many software programs are available for using these tools. ❞

Many records are used to control expenses and otherwise conserve the budget. These include personnel staffing reports, overtime reports, monthly financial reports, and expense and revenue reports. All these reports should be available to nurse managers to help them monitor, evaluate, and adjust the use of people and money as part of the controlling process.[44]

Benchmarking

Benchmarking, an offshoot of quality management, is a technique whereby an organization seeks out the best practices in its industry to improve its performance. Benchmarking is a standard, or point of reference, in measuring or judging factors such as quality, values, and costs. The following are examples of benchmarks that could apply to nursing[45]:

- Establishing a skill mix of nursing employees to obtain the highest quality of patient care at the lowest cost, which is called vertical leveraging. Horizontal leveraging uses cross-training to boost productivity. If the average for the industry was a ratio of 60% registered nurses to 40% other nursing personnel, the institution would make a decision to meet or exceed this ratio.

- An operating room utilization rate of 80% or higher if the industry rate is 75%.
- An average turnover time between cases of 15 minutes if the industry rate is 20 minutes.
- A reduction of 10% from the average-for-industry cost of supplies per patient day.
- A reduction of 50% from the average-for-industry rate of hospital-acquired infections.

Standards of care define the levels of care that a patient can expect to receive in a given situation or on a given nursing unit. They are clinical benchmarks and are the foundation for quality improvement programs.

Structure standards describe the environment in which care is delivered. Process standards describe a series of activities, changes, or functions that bring about result. Clinical standards, a subgroup of the process and outcome standards, are developed to include clinical issues specific to areas of practice. These include both standards of care and standards of professional practice. According to the ANA, standards of care are authoritative statements describing a competent level of practice. Standards of professional practice are authoritative statements describing a competent level of behavior in the professional role.[46] Outcome standards are the results to be achieved.

66 Standards of practice and standards of care are the benchmarks for nursing practice in all domains. 99

66 Benchmarking is enhanced when quality teams perform at the highest level of service by sharing their best practices and processes with similar committee teams in other institutions and organizations. 99

Standards of practice are used to structure the quality management program. They are linked to policy and procedure development and to job descriptions and performance appraisals. Implementation of standards is done through use of generic nursing care plans and the computer. Computers provide generic nursing care plans and nursing diagnoses, interventions, and outcomes.[47]

Quality management is a necessary element of benchmarking. The following are some benefits of benchmarking:

- Goals and objectives are set, and full team support to meet them is obtained.
- Performance regarding practices, processes, and outcomes is continually improved.
- Commitment and accountability for excellence exist.
- New approaches are sought out, learned, and adapted to.
- Organizational communication is improved.
- Clinical governance is improved.
- Patient satisfaction is improved.

The benchmarking program includes planning during team meetings, collection of specific data, data analysis to determine gaps, integration through keeping all team members informed, action, and follow-up and monitoring.[48]

MASTER CONTROL PLAN

To fulfill this important management function, nurse managers can use a master control or evaluation plan. It can be a general plan for all, with each manager adding specific items for his or her own management area. A sample master control plan is depicted in Figure 16-11.

EVIDENCE-BASED MANAGEMENT

"Evidence-based management means that managers, like their clinical practitioner counterparts, should search for, appraise, and apply empirical evidence from management research in their practice."[49] It is essential that managers document and systematically review their actions and decisions in such a way as to further add to the evidence base for effective management practices.[50]

FIGURE 16-11 **MASTER CONTROL PLAN**

Objective 1

Inspect for and identify the presence of written, current, and practical statements of mission, philosophy, vision, and objectives for the division of nursing and each of its component units. The statements should reflect the purposes of the healthcare organization and give direction to the nursing care program.

Actions

1. The written statements of mission, philosophy, and objectives were current (reviewed or revised within the past year).

2. They existed for the division of nursing and for each department, ward, unit, and clinic.

3. They were written by appropriate nursing personnel, representative of people who will accomplish them.

4. The philosophy reflected the meaning of clinical practice.

5. The philosophy was developed in collaboration with consumers, employees, and other healthcare workers.

6. The objectives were specified, written in behavioral terms, and achievable.

7. They guided the process of implementing the philosophy.

8. They were used for orientation of newly assigned personnel and were otherwise widely distributed and interpreted.

9. They supported the mission, philosophy, and objectives of the institution.

10. Nursing personnel knew the rights of individuals and served as advocates for these rights.

Objective 2

Inspect for and identify the presence of written operational or management plans for accomplishment of the objectives of the division of nursing and each of its component units.

Actions

1. The written operational or management plans were current (entries within past 30 days).

2. They existed for the division of nursing and for each department, ward, unit, and clinic.

3. They included specific actions to be taken to achieve objective, target dates, and names of personnel assigned responsibility for each action.

4. They were used to evaluate progress; accomplishments were listed.

Objective 3

Inspect for and identify the presence of an organizational plan for the division of nursing and each of its component units.

Actions

1. The organizational plan was current; it agreed with actual organization when checked.

2. It existed for the division of nursing and for each department, ward, unit, and clinic.

3. It showed the relationships among component parts, spelling out the major functions of each, and it showed relationships with other services.

4. The organizational plan supported the mission assigned to personnel.

5. All nursing functions were managed by the nurse administrator.

Objective 4

Inspect for and identify the presence of adequate policies and procedures for guidance of personnel of the division of nursing and each of its component units.

Actions

1. Policies and procedures of the division of nursing and of each department, ward, unit, and clinic were current (reviewed within past year).

2. Policies and procedures did not duplicate those of higher echelons.

3. Policies and procedures were not obsolete, restrictive, or inappropriate in context.

4. Content of location of policies and procedures was known by people who needed this information.

5. Policies and procedures for special care units included:
   a. Function and authority of unit director.
   b. Admission and discharge criteria.
   c. Criteria for performance of special procedures, including cardiopulmonary resuscitation, tracheostomy, ordering of medications, administration of parenteral fluids and other medication, and the obtaining of blood and other laboratory specimens.
   d. The use, location, and maintenance of equipment and supplies.
   e. Respiratory care.
   f. Infection control.
   g. Priorities for orders for laboratory tests.
   h. Standing orders, if any.
   i. Regulations for visitors and traffic control.

(continues)

6. The nursing annex to the disaster plan was current and included:
   a. Recall procedures.
   b. Assignment procedures.
   c. Training plan.

Objective 5

Inspect for and identify the presence of job descriptions and job standards for all personnel throughout the division of nursing.

Actions

1. Job descriptions and job standards existed and were current throughout the division of nursing (reviewed within past year).

2. Nursing personnel participated in formulating them.

3. Nursing personnel were classified according to competence, and salaries were commensurate with qualifications and positions of comparable responsibility within the agency and the community.

4. Job descriptions were used for purposes of counseling and helping employees to be productive.

5. They were used for orientation of newly assigned personnel.

6. They described the functions, qualifications, and authority of each position identified in the organizational plan.

7. They were readily available and known to each employee.

8. There was a designated nurse leader for the division of nursing who was a registered nurse with educational and experiential qualifications in nursing practice and the administration of nursing services.

Objective 6

Inspect for and identify the presence of a master staffing plan for the division of nursing and each of its component units.

Actions

1. A master staffing plan existed and was current for the division of nursing and each department, ward, unit, or clinic. It showed authorized versus assigned personnel and was reviewed at least monthly.

2. Adequate personnel policies existed to give guidance to nursing personnel in the planning of time schedules and to allow for mobility so that personnel could be matched to jobs.

3. Avenues of communication existed to give input from nursing personnel to the nurse administrator regarding staffing problems.

4. An active plan existed for sponsoring newly assigned personnel and for identifying their special training and experience and their desired assignments.

Objective 7

Inspect for and identify the presence of a planned counseling program for all personnel of the division of nursing.

Actions

1. The nurse executive had a planned program for counseling with managers, including charge nurses.

2. Counseling occurred at least every 6 months on a scheduled basis.

3. Charge nurses counseled with individual staff members on a scheduled basis at least once every 6 months.

4. The counseling process included discussion of progress toward personal objectives, and revisions resulted from the sessions. Job standards were reviewed, and special educational and experience goals were discussed and acted on.

5. Records of counseling sessions were available and were reviewed.

6. A career progression plan was operational.

Objective 8

Inspect for and identify the presence of a system of evaluation of nursing activities in the division of nursing and each of its component units.

Actions

1. A system for evaluation of the division of nursing and each of its departments, wards, units, and clinics was in operation.

2. Change-of-shift reports and ward conferences were being periodically evaluated (at least once every 6 months).

3. Management plans indicated current evaluation of accomplishment of objectives (within past 30 days).

4. Management personnel, including the nurse executive, made planned ward rounds at least monthly and checked all aspects of department, ward, unit, or clinic management, including the following:
   a. Narcotic registers
   b. Nursing histories
   c. Nursing care plans
   d. Nursing notes
   e. Drug levels and security
   f. Supplies and equipment
   g. Assignment procedures
   h. Patient records

5. The quality assurance program was in effect, and at least one problem per month had been evaluated since June 1.

(continues)

6. There was provision for inclusion of other healthcare disciplines and consumers in evaluating the nursing care programs.

7. Results of evaluation were used to assess planning for change.

Objective 9

Inspect for and identify the representation of division of nursing personnel on institution-wide and departmental boards, committees, and councils.

Actions

1. The division of nursing was represented on institutionwide boards, committees, and councils whose activities affected nursing personnel directly.
   a. Social actions
   b. Personnel boards such as awards and benefits

2. Nursing service committees had specific objectives.

3. Membership was current and representative of all appropriate segments of the nursing staff.

4. Minutes of meetings reflected progress toward objectives and followup of problems.

Objective 10

Inspect for and identify the existence of a working public relations program that serves as a means of communication between personnel of the division of nursing and the community they serve.

Actions

1. Evaluation programs existed to tell consumers of the nursing services available to them and to receive feedback from consumers on the types of services they needed.

2. There was a planned program to publicize nursing activities and recognize contributions and accomplishments of nursing personnel.

Objective 11

Inspect for and identify the existence of a planned program for training and continuing education for all divisions of nursing personnel.

Actions

1. Written statements of mission, philosophy, and objectives existed and were current (reviewed within past year).

2. An operational or management plan for the accomplishment of objectives was current (entries made within past 30 days).

3. The plan listed activities, set priorities and target dates, assigned responsibility, and provided for continuous evaluation.

4. The plan provided for identification of training and continuing education needs, including input from participants, translation of needs into objectives, and the accomplishment of objectives.

5. An orientation program existed and included philosophy and objectives of organization and nursing service, personnel policies, job descriptions, work environment, clinical practice policies and procedures, and operational policies and procedures.

6. Supplemental classes were taught to meet on-the-job training needs.

7. Training programs were documented.

8. The program supported career advancement.

Objective 12

Inspect for and identify the existence of procedures and policies for providing needed primary nursing care to patients.

Actions

1. Collection of data on each patient was sufficient to permit identification and assessment of the patient's needs and to institute an individual plan of care. Included were admission data and the patient's nursing history.

2. The nursing care plan included the nursing diagnosis, prescription for care, and patient's teaching needs.

3. The plan was used to provide care to the patient, and there was an ongoing reassessment of the patient's needs with appropriate changes made in the plan of care.

4. There was evidence that nursing actions required by physicians' orders, nursing care plans, and hospital policies were accomplished appropriately. Observations of patient's progress and response to actions were made and recorded.

5. There was evidence of interpretation and implementation of the *ANA Standards of Clinical Nursing Practice*.

6. Nursing administration had a plan for reviewing the requirements for giving credentials to individuals and healthcare organizations and for participating in their implementation.

7. Guidelines existed for assignment of personnel based on level of competence.

8. There were policies to use unit managers and ward clerks to perform clerical, managerial, and indirect service–roles.

9. Nursing administration provided resources to accomplish primary nursing care to patient: facilities, equipment, supplies, and personnel.

Source: Author.

Evidence-based management had been limited for a multitude of reasons: poorly indexed practical application, limited training in using evidence in making management decisions, and limited size and resources in some healthcare organizations to conduct and evaluate applied research.[51] The IOM identified five practices believed to provide an agenda for developing greater evidence-based management practices[52]:

1. Balancing the tension between efficiency and reliability
2. Creating and sustaining trust
3. Actively managing the process of change
4. Involving workers in work design and work flow decision making
5. Creating a learning organization

Evaluating critical management and operational functions and processes further underscores the need to provide evidence to improve patient and staff outcomes.

QUALITY AWARDS DEMONSTRATING ORGANIZATIONAL EXCELLENCE

The Malcolm Baldrige National Quality Award (www.baldrige.nist.gov) and the process for achieving this award were established in 1987, when Congress passed the Malcolm Baldrige National Quality Improvement Act. The award is designed to recognize organizations that demonstrate excellence in quality performance and establish best-practice standards in their industry. To compete for the award, organizations must choose one of three categories, manufacturing, service, or small business. If a hospital established a long-term goal of achieving this award, they would begin the process by submitting a lengthy application followed by an initial screening. If the hospital passed this screening, the next step would be to undergo a structured evaluation process conducted by certified Baldrige examiners. These examiners conduct site visits to examine processes and review hospital data based on seven categories. The requirements of the Criteria for Performance Excellence are embodied in seven categories as follows[50]:

- Leadership
- Strategic planning
- Customer and market focus
- Measurement, analysis, and knowledge management
- Workforce focus
- Process management
- Results

QUALITY AWARDS RECOGNIZING NURSING EXCELLENCE

The Magnet Recognition Program was developed by the American Nurses Credentialing Center, an affiliate of the ANA, to recognize healthcare organizations that provide nursing excellence. In 1983 The American Academy of Nursing's Task Force on Nursing Practice in Hospitals conducted a study of 163 hospitals to identify and describe variables that created an environment that attracted and retained well-qualified nurses who promoted quality patient/resident/client care. Fourteen of these hospitals had characteristics that seemed to attract and retain professional nurses within an organization. These became known as the "forces of magnetism."

In 1990 the America Nurses Credentialing Center was established as a separately incorporated non-profit organization, which currently offers the Magnet Recognition Program for individual healthcare organizations and for healthcare systems with multiple settings. A nurse executive who is considering application to obtain Magnet status must meet stringent criteria of personal leadership and nursing education, have the ANA's *Scope and Standards for Nurse Administrators* currently implemented throughout nursing within the organization, have policies and procedures that encourage nurses to confidentially express concerns about professional practice, and have enacted fair labor practices, regulatory compliance, and nurse-sensitive quality indicators. The certification includes self-assessment for preparation, site visit by a team of appraisers, submission of documentation, and annual monitoring of compliance to the criteria.

WHAT THE FUTURE HOLDS

Healthcare costs continue to escalate to meet the demands of the consumers. Despite advances in biomedical knowledge and technology, healthcare outcomes vary dramatically. It is in this context that the Robert Wood Johnson Foundation commissioned the IOM to evaluate how the nation uses scientific evidence in providing highly effective clinical services. In June 2006 the IOM appointed the Committee on Reviewing Evidence to Identify Highly Effective Clinical Services to respond to the foundation's request:

1. To recommend an approach to identifying highly effective clinical services across the full spectrum of healthcare services—from prevention, diagnosis, treatment, and rehabilitation, to end-of-life care and palliation.
2. To recommend a process to evaluate and report on evidence on clinical effectiveness.
3. To recommend an organizational framework for using evidence reports to develop recommendations on appropriate clinical applications for specified populations.

It was the committee's responsibility to make recommendation for a sustainable, replicable approach to identifying effective clinical services. Based on its work, the committee concluded that the nation must significantly expand its capacity to use scientific evidence to assess effective models in healthcare delivery systems. The report, *Knowing What Works in Healthcare,* proposes an organizational framework for a national clinical effectiveness assessment program, referred to throughout as "the Program." The Program's mission serves to maximize evidence to identify effective health services. Three functions are central to this mission: setting priorities for evidence assessment, assessing evidence (systematic review), and developing (or endorsing) standards for trusted clinical practice guidelines.[53] Evidence-based practice will continue to be at the forefront of health care service delivery, supporting the need to provide services that are safe, effective, patient-centered, timely, efficient, and equitable.[54]

Evidence-Based Practice 16-1

Duffy, Baldwin, and Mastorovich describe their work in an organization specifically centered on the benefits of adopting a professional practice model. The authors note that organizations of patient care in many acute care institutions lack a foundation in nursing theory. There has been support for organizing patient care according to a professional practice model. The researchers worked with an acute care setting and a school of nursing. A pilot implementation plan with formative and summative evaluation provided preliminary evidence used to expand the project. To evaluate the influence of the revised care delivery system, indicators were chosen that represented patient (satisfaction, pain, functional status) and nurse (vacancy rates, nurse satisfaction) outcomes indicators of interest. The researchers found that after 3 months, findings noted that patient satisfaction rose 2.71%, patient reported pain decreased 33% from a high of 3.5 to 1.1, and patient functional status remained unchanged. Nurse vacancy rates decreased 18.55% from 22.1% to 18%. Other findings indicated that overall nurse satisfaction rose 20% from 64% to 77%. Focus groups were also held with staff nurses from implementation units to gather feedback about the revised patient care delivery system. Responses from the focus groups indicated that purposeful interaction "makes patients feel special," the resource coordinator "allowed nurses more time to spend with patients and families," and the registered nurse staffing changes, although difficult, ensured that caring relationships were primary. Additional findings included the need for refining the revised roles and responsibilities of registered nurses and nursing assistants and open visitation.[55]

SUMMARY

Organizations are in the midst of operational change that is transforming every aspect of health care. The transformation is being driven by the increase in technology and the deepening need for communication leading to excellence in practice. Controlling/evaluating and coordinating are ongoing functions of nurse administrators that occur during planning, organizing, and directing activities. Through this process, standards are established and then applied, followed by feedback that leads to improvements. The process is continuous and systematic.

Each nurse manager should have a master control plan that incorporates all standards related to these actions. This plan can be applied to obtain immediate feedback and meet the objectives of control established for the unit, department, or division. The plan will verify results, provide instructions, and apply principles of uniformity, comparison, and exception.

Controls include policies, rules, procedures, self-control or self-regulation, discipline, rounds, reports, audits, evaluation devices, task analysis, quality control, and benchmarking. They should reflect the nature of the activity and be forward looking, objective, flexible, economical, and understandable. Controls should lead to continuous action.

Standards are the yardsticks for evaluation and include ANA's *Scope and Standards for Nurse Administrators* and *Standards of Clinical Nursing Practice*. Other standards include management plans, goals, programs, costs, revenues, and capital. Physical standards use Gantt charts, critical control points, milestones, and PERT. Each nurse manager should have a master evaluation plan, including a plan to further evaluate decisions with sound evidence.

APPLICATION EXERCISES

Exercise 16-1
With a group of your peers or colleagues, use Figures 16-9 and 16-11 to discuss developing a new evaluation plan for a nursing unit. Incorporate the standards from both exhibits. How can they be measured? Modify them as necessary. Use your final product to evaluate the nursing unit.

Exercise 16-2
Do an assessment of a healthcare organization's evaluation plan for quality improvement. Identify quality indicators, tools for measurement, and plans for improvement based on measurement results. How does this plan correspond to internal, external, performance, and productivity standards?

Exercise 16-3
From your assessment (Figure 16-2), consider one aspect of the quality improvement plan as it relates to evidence-based practice. How would you rate the evidence supporting this practice?

Notes

1. Fayol, H. (1949). *General and industrial management* (C. Storrs, Trans.) (p. 107). London: Sir Isaac Pitman & Sons.
2. Urwick, L. (1944). *The elements of administration* (p. 105). New York: Harper & Row.
3. Ibid., 107–110.
4. Koontz, H., & Weihrich, H. (1990). *Management* (5th ed., pp. 394–395). New York: McGraw-Hill; Hodgetts, R. M. (1990). *Management: Theory, process, and practice* (5th ed., pp. 226–229). Orlando, FL: Harcourt Brace; Fulmer, R. M., & Franklin, S. G. (1982). *Supervision: Principles of professional management* (2nd ed., pp. 214–216). New York: Macmillan; Rowland, H. S., & Rowland, B. L. (1997). *Nursing administration handbook* (4th ed., pp. 15–16, 35–44). Gaithersburg, MD: Aspen; Drucker, P. F. (1973). *Management: Tasks, responsibilities, practices* (pp. 495–505). New York: Harper & Row; Marriner-Tomey, A. (1996). *Guide to nursing management and leadership* (5th ed., p. 379). St. Louis, MO: Mosby; Mosley, D. C., Pietri, P. H., & Megginson, L. C. (1996). *Management: Leadership in action* (5th ed., pp. 492–512). New York: HarperCollins.
5. Peters, T. (1987). *Thriving on chaos* (pp. 587, 593). New York: Harper & Row.
6. Rowland & Rowland, 1997, p. 40.
7. Kron, T., & Gray, A. (1987). *The management of patient care: Putting leadership skills to work* (6th ed., p. 100). Philadelphia: W. B. Saunders.
8. Koontz & Weihrich, 1990, p. 393.
9. Barnum, B. S., & Kerfoot, M. (1995). *The nurse as executive* (4th ed., p. 229). Gaithersburg, MD: Aspen.
10. Arndt, C., & Huckebay, L. M. D. (1980). *Nursing administration: Theory for practice with a systems approach* (2nd ed., pp. 22–46). St. Louis, MO: Mosby.
11. Reed, D., & Sanders, N. (2005). *Operations management: An integrated approach* (2nd ed., p. 3). New Jersey: John Wiley & Sons.
12. Ibid., pp. 4–5.
13. Porter-O'Grady, T., & Malloch, K. (2007). *Quantum leadership: A resource for healthcare innovation* (2nd ed., pp. 5–6). Sudbury, MA: Jones and Bartlett Publishers.
14. Ibid., p. 20.
15. Ibid., p. 43.
16. Nelson, E., Batalden, P., & Godfrey, M. (2007). *Quality by design: A clinical microsystem approach* (1st ed., p. 35). New York: John Wiley & Sons.
17. Ibid., p. 75.
18. Ibid., pp. 131–135.
19. Ibid., p. 42.
20. Ibid.
21. Senge, P, (1990). *The fifth discipline.* New York: Doubleday.
22. Reed, D., & Sanders, N. (2005). *Operations management: An integrated approach* (2nd ed., p. 8). New York: John Wiley & Sons.
23. Leonard, M., Frankel, A., Simmonds, T., & Vega, K. (2004). *Achieving safe and reliable healthcare: Strategies and solutions* (p. 200). Chicago: Health Administration Press.
24. Franck, P., & Price, M. (1980). *Nursing management* (2nd ed., p. 135). New York: Springer Publishing.
25. Holle, M. L., & Blatchly, M. E. (1982). *Introduction to leadership and management in nursing* (pp. 178–185). Monterey, CA: Wadsworth Health Services Division.
26. Lloyd, R. (2004). *Quality healthcare: A guide to developing and using indicators* (1st ed., p. 297), Sudbury, MA: Jones and Bartlett Publishers.

27. Levenstein, A. (1981). *The nurse as manager* (M. J. F. Smith, Series Ed.) (pp. 17–33). Chicago: S-N Publications.
28. Lemin, B. (1977). *First line nursing management* (pp. 47–51). New York: Springer.
29. Ibid.
30. Fulmer & Franklin, 1982, pp. 216–217.
31. Ramey, G. (1976). Setting standards and evaluating care. In S. Stone & D. Elhart (Eds.), *Management for nurses* (p. 79). St. Louis, MO: Mosby.
32. Donovon, H. M. (1975). *Nursing service administration: Managing the enterprise* (pp. 160–169). St. Louis, MO: Mosby.
33. Beyers, M., & Phillips, C. (1979). *Nursing management for patient care* (2nd ed., pp. 109–141). Boston: Little, Brown.
34. Douglass, L. M. (1986). *The effective nurse: Leader and manager* (5th ed., pp. 245–278). St. Louis, MO: Mosby.
35. Koontz & Weihrich, 1990, pp. 394–395.
36. Reed, D., & Sanders, N. (2005). *Operations management: An integrated approach* (2nd ed., pp. 5–6). New York: John Wiley & Sons.
37. Berman, A., Snyder, S., Kozier, B., & Erb, G. (2008). *Kozier & Erbs, fundamentals of nursing, concept, processes and practice* (8th ed., pp. 57–58). New Jersey: Pearon Prentice Hall.
38. Ganong, J. M., & Ganong, W. L. (1980). *Nursing management* (2nd ed., p. 191). Gaithersburg, MD: Aspen.
39. Rosswurm, M. A., & Larrabee, J. H. (1999). A model for change to evidence-based practice. *Image: The Journal of Nursing Scholarship, 31,* 317–322; Matthews, P. (2000). Planning for successful outcomes in the new millennium. *Topics in Health Information Management,* 55–64; Silver, M. S. (1999). Incident review management: A systemic approach to performance improvements. *Journal of Healthcare Quality, 1,* 21–27.
40. Koontz & Weihrich, 1990, pp. 396–398; Harrington, C., Kovner, C., Mezey, M., Kayser-Jones, J., Burger, S., & Mohler, M. (2000). Experts recommend minimum nurse staffing standards for nursing facilities in the United States. *Gerontologist, 1,* 5–16.
41. Haggard, A. (1992). Using self-studies to meet JCAHO requirements. *Journal of Nursing Staff Development, 4,* 170–174.
42. Koontz & Weihrich, 1990, p. 424; Hodgetts, 1990, p. 243; Beyers & Phillips, 1979, pp. 134–135; Rowland & Rowland, 1997, p. 36; Fulmer & Franklin, 1982, pp. 221–227; http://www-mmd.eng.ac.uk/people 9/17/2004; http://gracie.santarosa.edu
43. Koontz & Weihrich, 1990, pp. 424–428; Hodgetts, 1990, pp. 240–242; http://www.criticaltools.com, 9/17/2004; http://www.infosystems.eku.edu
44. Ganong & Ganong, 1980, p. 257.
45. Patterson, (1993). Benchmarking study identifies hospitals' best practices. *OR Manager, 11,* 14–15.
46. American Nurses Association. (1991). *Standards of clinical nursing practice.* Washington, DC: Author.
47. McAllister, M. (1990). A nursing integration framework based on standards of practice. *Nursing Management, 4,* 28–31.
48. Murray, J. A., & Murray, M. H. (1992). Benchmarking: A tool for excellence in palliative care. *Journal of Palliative Care, 8,* 41–45; Woomer, N., Long, C. O., Anderson, C., & Greenberg, E. A. (1999). Benchmarking in home health care: A collaborative approach. *Caring,* 22–28; McGowan, S., Wynaden, D., Harding, N., Yassine, A., & Parker, J. (1999). Staff confidence in dealing with aggressive patients: A benchmarking exercise. *Australia New Zealand Journal of Mental Health Nursing,* 104–108; Voyles, C. R., & Boyd, K. B. (1999). Criteria and benchmarks for laparoscopic cholecystectomy in a free-standing ambulatory center. *JSLS,* 315–318; Gardner, D., & Winder, C. (1998). Using benchmarking to improve organizational communication. *Quality Assurance,* 201–211; Nurse staffing law may herald benchmarks. (1999). *Healthcare Benchmarks,* 137–138; Johnson, B. C., & Chambers, M. J. (2000). Foodservice benchmarking: Practices, attitudes, and beliefs of food-

service directors. *Journal of the American Dietetic Association,* 175–182; Bucknall, C. E., Ryland, I., Cooper, A., Coutts, I. I., Connolly, C. K., & Pearson, M. G. (2000). National benchmarking as a support system for clinical governance. *Journal of Royal College of Physicians London,* 52–56.

49. Axelsson, R. (1998). Towards an evidence-based health care management. *International Journal of Health Planning and Management, 13,* 307.

50. Walshe, K., & Rundall, T. (2001). Evidence-based management: From theory to practice in health care. *Milbank Quarterly, 79,* 429–458.

51. Page, A. (Ed.). (2004). *Keeping patients safe: Transforming the work environment of nurses.* Washington, DC: National Academies Press.

52. Ibid.

53. Eden, J., Wheatley, B., McNeil, B., & Sox, H. (Eds). (2008). *Knowing what works in health care: A roadmap for the nation.* Washington, DC: National Academies Press.

54. Institute of Medicine, Committee on Quality of Health Care in America. (2001). *Crossing the quality chasm.* Washington, DC: National Academies Press.

55. Duffy, J. R., Baldwin, J., & Mastorovich, M. J. (2007). Using the quality-caring model to organize patient care delivery. *Journal of Nursing Administration, 37,* 546–551.

References

American Nurses Association. (2004). *Scope and standards for nurse administrators.* Washington, DC: Author.

Balle, M. (1999). Making bureaucracy work. *Journal of Management in Medicine, 13,* 190–200.

Coombs, C. R., Doherty, N. F., & Loan-Clarke, J. (1999). Factors affecting the level of success of community information systems. *Journal of Management in Medicine, 13,* 142–153.

Dreachslin, J. L. (1999). Diversity leadership and organizational transformation: Performance indicators for health services organizations. *Journal of Healthcare Management, 8,* 427–439.

Eden, J., Wheatley, B., McNeil, B., & Sox, H. (Eds.). (2008). *Knowing what works in health care: A roadmap for the nation.* Washington, DC: National Academies Press.

Institute of Medicine, Committee on Quality of Health Care in America. (2001). *Crossing the quality chasm.* Washington, DC: National Academies Press.

Page, A. (Ed.). (2004). *Keeping patients safe: Transforming the work environment of nurses.* Washington, DC: National Academies Press.

17 QUALITY MANAGEMENT

Beverly Blain Wright, RN, MSN, CNA
Marylane Wade Koch, RN, MSN, CNA

LEARNING OBJECTIVES AND ACTIVITIES

- Differentiate between quality management and total quality management.
- Discuss Deming's 14 points of management theory.
- Discuss Deming's seven deadly management theory diseases.
- Identify nursing's external and internal customers.
- Identify and discuss seven components of a quality management program.
- Differentiate between quality management tools and describe when they should be used.

CONCEPTS

Quality management, total quality management, quality control, Shewhart cycle, internal customer, external customer, quality circles, structure, process, outcome.

NURSE MANAGER BEHAVIORS

Develops a quality management program demonstrating integration of standards. Selects elements of total quality management theory to increase customer satisfaction and improve staff productivity.

NURSE EXECUTIVE BEHAVIORS

Demonstrates theory of total quality management in development of quality management program that meets or exceeds accreditation requirements..

Introduction

One of the most challenging jobs of any nurse leader in the United States is to provide the best possible patient care at a reasonable cost. In this country $2 trillion each year is spent on health care with less than optimal results. Consumers, businesses, and politicians want quality care that matches the price paid, 50% more per capita than in other countries. The Institute of Medicine (IOM) reported that 90,000 or more patients die each year from preventable errors while in the hospital, estimating that 42% of Americans have received flawed medical care.

Nurses are in a unique position to enhance patient safety and minimize medical errors. They are in close proximity to the patient when they give care. In 2005, the Center for American Nurses published *The Nurse's Role in Promoting a Culture of Patient Safety*. This monograph was a step toward responding to IOM's report by improving patient safety through nurses.[2]

No longer can a nurse manager delegate the quality improvement function to a member of the staff or a department within the facility. The manager must be a knowledgeable leader, pursuing consumer and employee safety and demonstrating achievement of nursing care standards in every practice setting. Quality improvement, resource management, infection control, and risk management and safety are both manager and staff responsibility.

Effective quality management must be based on the philosophy that group behaviors can be transformed into a desirable culture. As costs, client expectations, and other aspects of health care become more demanding, it becomes more important that managers embrace and mentor total quality management (TQM) principles.

Evidence-Based Practice 17-1

The Kaiser Foundation study stated that hospital errors kill more patients than breast cancer. These figures demonstrate a loss of patient lives and personal function from medical errors that can be translated into lost income and escalating costs in disability and in corrective treatments. Some estimate the cost of medical errors may be as high as $29 billion each year.[1]

Quality can be defined as a state of mind or work ethic involving everyone in the healthcare agency. Decisions and commitment to improve care must be visible at all levels of the organization, seeking participation from front-line workers to reduce or eliminate errors.

Nursing quality assurance (QA) programs began in hospitals in the 1960s with the voluntary implementation of nursing audits. QA programs were designed to set standards for nursing care delivery and to establish criteria by which to evaluate these standards. However, professionals came to understand that quality cannot be ensured by audits. The Joint Commission (TJC) determined that to ensure quality, continuous improvement must be demonstrated. Synonyms for QM programs have emerged, such as quality improvement, continuous quality improvement, and performance improvement. Quality control, an aspect of QM, refers to sustaining conformance to standards.

Accreditation mandates that most aspects of health care must be incorporated into QM programs. Divisional or departmental programs must support an organization's mission. QM plans must incorporate customer satisfaction and patient rights. Leadership must step up and out to be sure quality is a continuous organizational goal.

Several groups besides TJC have stepped up to improve the quality of health care in this country. One of these is the IOM, who began focusing on assessment and improvement in 1996. In the IOM's 2001 quality chasm report, quality was defined as "the degree to which health services for individuals and populations increase the likelihood of desired health outcomes and are consistent with current professional knowledge." This report supports evaluation of quality based on Donabedian's quality theory based on structure, process, and outcome. Implementation of the IOM guidelines include establishing the mission and vision, creating a QM plan, providing the organizational framework that supports QM, using evidence-based clinical practice, and providing utilization management.[3] Other studies and reports from the IOM include *To Err is Human: Building a Safer Health System*; *Envisioning a National Healthcare Quality Report*; *Leadership by Example: Coordinating Government Roles in Improving Health Care Quality*; and *Priority Area for National Action: Transforming Health Care Quality*. All are available from the IOM website, http://www.iom.edu/CMS/8089.aspx

TOTAL QUALITY MANAGEMENT LEADERS

Health care looked outside the industry to leadership in achieving quality improvement. A number of leaders surfaced that offered promise and opportunity for achieving quality goals within the healthcare industry. Some of these leaders include Deming, Juran, Crosby, and Donabedian. Each model is worthy of study and understanding by the nurse manager, although not all principles will be applicable or adopted at the unit level. However, the nurse executive should note that in every model, management plays a key role in the agency's success.

W. Edwards Deming

Deming is considered by many as the pioneer in QM. An advocate for the principle of management for quality, he found that 80% to 85% of problems are with the system; only 15% to 20% are with workers. Workers should be told this and should be given the freedom to speak and contribute as thinking, creative human beings. Deming's theory of management includes 14 points (Figure 17-1). Deming also warned against the seven "deadly diseases" that decrease productivity and profitability because they destroy employee morale (Figure 17-2).

Application of Deming's Theory

General Douglas McArthur summoned W. Edwards Deming to set up quality circles for the Japanese in 1950.[4] When Deming presented the quality methods to 45 Japanese industrialists, they applied the methods. "Within six weeks, some of the industrialists were reporting gains of as much as 30% without purchasing any new equipment."[5]

FIGURE 17-1	DEMING'S 14 POINTS

1. Create constancy of purpose toward improvement of product and service. Everyone should have a clear goal every day, month after month. Satisfy the customer and reduce variation so all employees do not have to constantly shift their priorities.

2. Adopt a new philosophy by learning how to improve systems in the presence of variation, thus reducing variation in materials, people, processes, and products. End tampering and overreacting to variation.

3. Cease dependence on inspection to achieve quality by thoroughly understanding the sources of variation in processes and working to reduce variation.

4. End the practice of awarding business on the basis of price tag alone. Instead, minimize total cost by working with a single supplier.

5. Improve constantly and forever every process for planning, production, and service. Everyone uses PDCA (plan-do-check-act) cycle.

6. Institute training on the job. Know methods of performing tasks and standardize training. Accommodate variation in ways people learn.

7. Adopt and institute leadership. Work to help employees do their jobs better and with less effort. Learn which employees are within the system and which are not. Support company goals, focus on internal and external customers, coach, and nurture pride in workmanship.

8. Drive out fear, including fear of reprisal, fear of failure, fear of providing information, fear of not knowing, fear of giving up control, and fear of change. Fear makes accurate data nonexistent.

9. Break down barriers among staff areas, between departments. Promote cooperation. What is the constant, common goal?

10. Eliminate slogans, exhortations, and targets for the work force. Improvement requires changed methods and processes. Leaders change the system.

11. Eliminate numerical quotas for the work force and numerical goals for management. All people do not work at the same level of speed. There will be variation. Use realistic production standards. Eliminate management by objectives and use a system that rewards people's efforts toward improvement.

12. Remove barriers that rob people of pride of workmanship. Eliminate the annual rating or merit system.

13. Institute a vigorous program of education and self-improvement for everyone. This can be any education that improves self-esteem and potential to contribute to improvements in existing processes and advances in technology.

14. Put everyone in the company to work to accomplish the transformation.

Source: Reprinted from *Out of the Crisis* by W. Edwards Deming by permission of MIT and The W. Edwards Deming Institute. Published by MIT, Center for Advanced Engineering Study, Cambridge, MA 02139. Copyright 1986 by The W. Edwards Deming Institute. Dr. Deming rejected the concept of TQM, saying it was undefined.

| FIGURE 17-2 | DEMING'S SEVEN DEADLY DISEASES |

1. Lack of constancy of purpose.

2. Emphasis on short-term profits.

3. Evaluation of performance, merit rating, or annual review.

4. Management by use of only visible figures.

5. Mobility of management.

6. Excessive medical costs.

7. Excessive costs of liability.

Source: Author.

Using Deming's methods, managers and workers have a natural division of labor: The workers do the work of the system, and the managers improve the system. Thus the potential for improving the system never ends. Because workers know where the potential for improving the system lies, consultants are not needed. Managers know that the system is subject to a great variability and that problem events occur randomly. The common language for managers and workers is elementary statistics, which all workers learn.[6]

Variation Deming advocated the use of the language of statistics to identify which problems are caused by workers and which by the system. The most-used statistical tool is that of variation, which measures whether an activity is under control or, if it is not, to what degree it is out of control. Statistics enable workers to control variation by teaching them to work more intelligently. The common language of statistics may enhance discussion between participants of quality circles.[7] Variation is the concept that distinguishes normal routine changes in a process from unusual, abnormal changes that can be attributed to specific causes. Variations in performance are mostly attributable to the system. In some examples, Deming found 400% variation in performance attributable to the system.[8]

According to Deming, Shewhart, and others, there are chance (common) causes and special (assigned) causes of variation. Chance causes are common causes that are the fault of the system. They are system variations such as process input or conditions that are ever present and cause small, random shifts in daily output. They occur in 90% of cases and require fundamental system change by management. Chance causes are controlled causes. A system totally influenced by controlled variation or common causes is said to be in statistical control.

A special, or assigned, cause is specific to a particular group of workers, an area, or a machine. It is uncontrolled variation resulting from assignable causes or source. Special causes occur in less than 10% of cases. They require identification of the source and preventive action. Special causes require timely data to effect changes that will prevent bad causes and keep good causes happening (Figure 17-3).

Management by action uses the Deming (Shewhart) cycle. The cycle should be kept in constant motion and used at all levels of the organization. Reports should conform to the new system.[9]

Using control charts to determine whether the causes of accidents are common or special can lead to development of methods to prevent accidents. Employees can then set goals to reduce the special causes.[10]

Variation is a part of everything—of the supplies used by nurses, employee performance, and much more. Causes other than common and special causes exist. One such cause is tampering or making un-

FIGURE 17-3   **APPLICATION OF THE DEMING (SHEWHART) PDCA CYCLE TO TOTAL QUALITY MANAGEMENT**

PLAN
Common causes occur frequently (.90%) as a fault of the system and require a basic system change by management who will make the plan to fix them. Special causes occur infrequently (10%) and can be traced to a person or persons. The workers find the cause and plan preventive measures.

↓

DO
Plans are carried out by management and workers cooperatively.

Increased accidents and incidents may be due to common causes such as inadequate staffing (numbers and kinds) or special causes such as incompetent and inexperienced personnel.

↓

CHECK
The results are observed.

↓

ACT
The results are analyzed and lessons learned are noted and predictions made.

Source: Author.

necessary adjustments to compensate for common-cause variation. Another is structural variation caused by seasonal patterns and long-term trends.[11]

According to Deming, we should "measure the variations in a process in order to pinpoint the causes of poor quality." Quality improves as variability decreases.[12] Statistical charts are used to plot variations from the ideal in the production process and determine the right course to correct those variations.

Joseph Juran

Juran defined quality as fitness to serve, correct service the first time to meet customers' needs, and freedom from deficiencies. Quality necessitates employee involvement, with management leading the effort in planning, control, and improvement so that requirements are met. Quality requires identification of customers and their needs in a product-by-product and step-by-step process.[13]

Juran applies QM to all functions at all levels of the enterprise and incorporates the exercise of personal leadership and participation by top managers. In Juran's ideal workplace, all managers would be educated in QM techniques. The culture has a sense of unity, in which every employee knows the direction of the new course and is stimulated to go there. Resisting forces are multiple functions, levels in hierarchy, and product lines.[14] All these resisting forces are prominent in healthcare agencies.

Juran's philosophy of quality is based on three major premises: quality planning, quality control, and quality improvement. According to Juran, this quality trilogy can be grafted onto the strategic planning process (Figure 17-4).

Philip B. Crosby

Crosby earned his reputation as a quality leader at International Telephone and Telegraph. He defines quality by four absolutes,[15] as listed in Figure 17-5.

Culture and climate are important to achieving Crosby's absolutes. A climate of innovation is created because continuous innovation keeps customers coming back. The organizational culture often must experience change to raise every person's basic expectations. A small group of people may be used

---

FIGURE 17-4 | **JURAN'S QUALITY TRILOGY**

1. Quality planning creates a process for meeting goals under operating conditions.[17]
   - Identify customers, both internal and external
   - Determine customer needs
   - Develop product features that respond to customer needs
   - Set goals that meet needs of customers and suppliers
   - Develop process to produce the product features
   - Prove process meets quality goals during operations

2. Quality control, the second activity of the quality process, is performed by operations personnel who put the plan into effect by identifying deficiencies, correcting them, and monitoring the process. Quality control includes the following:[18]
   - Choose what to control
   - Choose units of measurement

   - Establish measurement
   - Establish standards of performance
   - Measure actual performance
   - Interpret the difference
   - Take action on the difference

3. The third and final premise of the Juran philosophy is quality improvement, which should be purposeful and in addition to quality control. Quality improvement includes the following:[19]
   - Prove the need for improvement
   - Identify projects for improvement
   - Organize to guide the projects
   - Diagnose to find the causes
   - Provide remedies
   - Prove remedies are effective under operating conditions
   - Provide for control to hold the gains

Source: Author.

FIGURE 17-5 | **PHILIP B. CROSBY'S FOUR ABSOLUTES**

1. Quality is "conformance to requirements." If the process is done right the first time, there is no need to redo it. Management sets the requirements and supplies the wherewithal to employees to do the job by encouraging and helping.

2. The system of quality is prevention rather than appraisal.

3. A performance standard of zero defects. A policy should be to deliver defect-free products on time.

4. The measurement of quality is the cost of nonconformance, because service companies spend half of their operating expenses on the cost of doing things wrong. Achieving these absolutes should be a constant priority. It requires the determination of management, the commitment of the entire organization, and the training and education of all employees. When they know and understand management's policy, employees will make TQM work. All levels of management are trained early.

Source: Author.

---

to uphold ethics and integrity. People will come to believe that quality is as important as financial management. An attitude that fosters change will be created. If managers think and operate in terms of quality, they will change the culture and create a climate of consideration for people, employees, customers, suppliers, and the community.

By policy, every department and unit has a quality strategy and a quality function. All managers participate in TQM; it becomes a part of how they think, feel, and act. Nurse managers may want to use Crosby's Quality Management Maturity Grid, shown in Figure 17-6, to measure quality improvement aspects of their department or unit and then expand use to other areas.

FIGURE 17-6	QUALITY MANAGEMENT MATURITY GRID

Measurement Categories	Stage One: Uncertainty	Stage Two: Awakening	Stage Three: Enlightenment	Stage Four: Wisdom	Stage Five: Certainty
Management understanding and attitude	No comprehension of quality as a management tool. Tend to blame quality department for "quality problems."	Recognize that quality management may be of value but not willing to provide money or time to make it all happen.	While going through quality improvement program, learn more about quality management; becoming supportive and helpful.	Participating. Understand absolutes of quality management. Recognize personal role in continuing emphasis.	Consider quality management an essential part of company system.
Quality organization status	Quality is hidden in manufacturing engineering departments. Inspection probably not part of organization. Emphasis on appraisal and sorting.	A stronger quality leader is appointed but main emphasis is still on appraisal and moving the product. Still part of manufacturing or other.	Quality department reports to top management, all appraisal is incorporated, and manager has role in management of company.	Quality manager is an officer of company; effective status reporting and preventive action. Involved with consumer affairs and special assignments.	Quality manager is on board of directors. Prevention is main concern. Quality is a thought leader.
Problem handling	Problems are fought as they occur; no resolution; inadequate definition; lots of yelling and accusation.	Teams are set up to attack major problems. Long-range solutions are not solicited.	Corrective action communication established. Problems are faced openly and resolved in an orderly way.	Problems are identified early in their development. All functions are open to suggestion and improvement.	Except in unusual cases, problems are prevented.
Cost of quality as percentage of sales	Reported: Unknown Actual: 20%	Reported: 3% Actual: 18%	Reported: 8% Actual: 12%	Reported: 6.5% Actual: 8%	Reported: 2.5% Actual: 2.5%
Quality improvement actions	No organized activities. No understanding of such activities.	Trying obvious "motivational" short-range efforts.	Implementation of the 14-step program with thorough understanding and establishment of each step.	Continuing the 14-step program and starting Make Certain.	Quality improvement is a normal and continued activity.
Summation of company quality posture	"We don't know why we have problems with quality."	"Is it absolutely necessary to always have problems with quality?"	"Through management commitment and quality improvement we are identifying and resolving our problems."	"Defect prevention is a routine part of our operation."	"We know why we do not have problems with quality."

Source: B. J. Deutsch. "A Conversation with Philip Crosby." Bank Marketing (April 1991), 25. Reprinted with permission from the Bank Marketing Association.

The Donabedian model is a classic way of assessing quality of care based on structure, process, and outcome where each part directly influences the next. This model is used by the IOM in performance measurement with their six aims of quality care that is safe, effective, patient centered, timely, efficient, and equitable.[16] Structure in this model refers to the healthcare setting and all available resources such as materials, staff, and setting structure. Process is defined as the action happening to the patient while receiving care given by the staff. Outcomes are the healthcare results that occur when the customer or patient has contact with the healthcare setting and staff.

Management should take the best of the theory of TQM and apply it assiduously. The best approach is to develop the philosophy that continuous improvement by all employees and managers is both desirable and possible.

CUSTOMERS

The customer is the focus of TQM philosophy. To provide quality services and products, the manager must first find out what the customer wants. The service that meets the customer's needs provides the income to the supplier, whether it is an educational institution or a healthcare agency. Quality is freedom from waste, trouble, and failure. The manager's goal is to meet and exceed customers' needs and expectations and then continue to improve.

Customers can be described as internal and external customers. In nursing management the external customers are patients, employers, and the community. Patients want quality care as evidenced by recovery from illness that allows them to return to their normal way of living. Patients facing death want a quality of care to keep their remaining time peaceful. The employer wants knowledgeable and skilled workers; the community wants productive citizens.

Internal customers are those who interact with each other within and among departments and disciplines, such as nursing, pharmacy, radiology, and medical laboratory. Clinical nurses are customers of nurse managers, admission services, and others. The customer should be satisfied quickly and economically if nurse managers are to stay in business. This core of customers includes those who generate a profit and inspire nurses to their best ideas and highest motivation.[17]

The focus of TQM is harmony, not competition or adversarial relations, and satisfying such customers, not confronting them. The continual quest for improvement would reduce variation, adversarial relationships within and among departments, and disharmony. This can be achieved by continuously using TQM, gathering and monitoring data, and using statistical tools to analyze the data.

QUALITY AS A PHILOSOPHY

QM is not a program but a philosophy and a way of life that must be adopted by each nursing manager to support optimal patient care. QM is customer-focused, decentralized, and empowering. Quality nurses aim for a world-class quality of care. This entails learning to deal with the most difficult patients and families. Nurse managers must educate and support clinical nurses as they deal with difficult customers.

Cross-functional teams and open, trusting, cooperative relationships are essential. Self-managed teams can perform multiple functions and schedule their own work, develop budgets, and deal directly with customers. They will be trained to develop needed relationships, do networking, deal with vendors, and manage projects.[18]

Successful customer relations require constant training and education programs. The need for staff development will increase as nursing staff address improved technology, greater product reliability, a customer-focused orientation, and flexibility in adapting to change. Nurse managers will continue to work with clinical staff to develop the best practice approaches and make decisions that affect all team members. An educated and well-trained work force is a nursing imperative. Every team member needs the skills of reading, understanding math, and conveying ideas to accomplish TQM.[19]

CULTURE AND CLIMATE

TQM requires a favorable environment in which values are shared as worthwhile or desirable and beliefs as truth. All employees in such an environment, including top management, believe in focusing on customers, both internal and external.

In this warm, friendly climate, employees feel positive about themselves, others, and their work. Employees trust managers who facilitate their work and treat them as equals. Managers drive out fear through leadership that promotes teamwork, respect, and trust.

Linkow suggests changing the culture through a total quality culture matrix tool (Figure 17-7) that follows these steps:

1. Describe the current culture through group brainstorming and interviewing.
2. Establish seven core total quality values and beliefs.
3. Correlate core values and beliefs with current culture.
4. Determine the strength of the current culture.
5. Identify targets for culture change. These will be core values and beliefs with negative or non-existent correlation or that are low in strength.
6. Use the group to change culture.
7. Use external threats to mobilize internal forces of change.[20]

FIGURE 17-7 TOTAL QUALITY CULTURE MATRIX

Cultural Media	Current Culture Examples	Customer Focus	Employee Focus	Teamwork	Safety	Candor	Total Involvement	Process Focus	Symbols
Heroes	Employee who got out of a hospital bed for important meeting with a client	●	△	△	△				
	Person who left his family on vacation to work with client	●	△	△					
	Understudy steps in at last minute for sick "star" and makes resoundingly successful presentation to tough clients	●		○					● = highly correlated
Myths and Artifacts	No titles on business cards		○	○			○		
	Stories of failures with clients are told with relish		○			●			○ = correlated
	Employees do whatever it takes to satisfy the client	●	△						
	Anyone may be interrupted at any time		△	○			○		△ = negatively correlated
Rites and Rituals	When a problem is identified a list of solutions is brainstormed by a group			●			○		
	CEO walks through headquarters many afternoons asking, "What are you working on?"		○	●			○		

Strength of Culture	Customer Focus	Employee Focus	Teamwork	Safety	Candor	Total Involvement	Process Focus	Symbols
Thickness	●	△	○	△	○	○	△	● = high
Extent of Sharing	●	○	●	△	●	○	△	○ = medium
Clarity of Ordering	●	○	●	△	○	○	△	△ = low

Source: Reprinted with permission of P. Linkow, Interaction Associates, Cambridge, Massachusetts.

QUALITY CIRCLES/QUALITY ACTION TEAMS

Quality circles are a participatory management technique that uses statistical analyses of activities to maintain quality products. The technique was initiated in Japan after World War II through Deming's teaching. The concept is to use statistical analysis to make quality improvements. Workers are taught the statistical concepts and use them through trained, organized, structured groups of 4 to 15 employees, called quality circles. Group members share common interests and problems and meet on a regular basis, usually an hour a week. They represent other employees from whom they gather information to bring to the meetings.[21]

Employees are trained to identify, analyze, and solve problems. Involved in the process, they make solutions work because they identify with ownership. As a result of being recognized, they develop good will toward their employers.

Quality circles are effective when facilitators, leaders, and members are trained in group dynamics and quality circle techniques. Leaders act as peers to generate ideas to improve operations and eliminate problems. In the process all quality circle members reach consensus before decisions are recommended or implemented. Training occurs during subsequent meetings.[22]

The objects of quality circles are participation, involvement, recognition, and self-actualization among clinical nurses caring for patients. Output from these objects of quality circles contributes to the knowledge base of human behavior and motivation, which is important to the development of nursing management theory. This theory will be learned and used by nurse managers concerned with developing job satisfaction of professional nurses in delivering quality nursing care.

Quality circles should meet successful group design guidelines, including the following[23]:

1. Participation groups process or have access to the necessary skills and knowledge to address problems systematically. All actors in the process receive training. Support people participate only as needed.

2. Formalized procedures enhance the effectiveness of the group. Systematic records are kept, and formal schedules of meetings adhered to.

3. To promote communication, participation groups are integrated horizontally and vertically with the rest of the organization. Accomplishments are publicized through award dinners and publicity in in-house newspapers. Organized higher level support groups hear the ideas of lower level groups. All are limited by usual formal and informal communication mechanisms and routes.

4. Groups are a regular part of the organization, not a special or extra activity. They are composed of members of natural work groups. Results are measured in terms of ongoing organizational objectives and goals.

5. Normal accountability processes operate using the same skills, habits, and expectations as general organizations.

6. Groups manage themselves and are assisted by leaders and facilitators who are peer group members.

7. Participation occurs in such areas as decisions about job enrichment; hiring; training in problem-solving skills, management skills, and business conditions; pay based on skill mastery; gain sharing; and union management relationships based on mutual interests.

Research indicates that productivity and morale improve when employees participate in decision making and planning for change. Participation includes goal setting, because participation leads to higher levels of acceptance and performance of these goals. Research also shows that highly nonparticipatory jobs cause psychological and physical harm.

Quality circles may use Pareto analysis, histograms, graphing techniques, control charts, stratification, scatter diagrams, brainstorming, cause-and-effect diagrams, run analysis, and conflict resolution.

Success factors of quality circles include management commitment and involvement, staff involvement, training, and patience. Tangible benefits include improved quality, increased productivity, and increased efficiency. Intangible benefits include improved work life quality, safety, morale, and job satisfaction.[24]

COMPONENTS OF A QUALITY MANAGEMENT PROGRAM

A quality management program is composed of the following components:

1. Clear and concise written statements of purpose, philosophy, values, and objectives.
2. Standards or indicators for measuring the quality of care.
3. Policies and procedures for using such standards for gathering data. These policies define the organizational structure for the program.
4. Analysis and reporting of the data gathered, with isolation of problems and variances.
5. Use of the results to prioritize, plan action, and correct problems and variances.
6. Monitoring of clinical and managerial performance and ongoing feedback to ensure that problems stay solved.
7. Evaluation of the QM system.

These components may be conceptualized in many different ways. One component builds on another. Batalden and Stoltz describe a framework for the continual improvement of health care (Figure 17-8) that incorporates underlying knowledge, policy for leadership, tools and methods, and daily work applications.[25] The mission, vision, guiding principles, and integration of values are critical to the policy for leadership. "For the continual improvement of health care, tools and methods are available that can accelerate building and using knowledge and communicating that understanding to others."[26] Tools and methods can be grouped into four major categories: process and system, group process and collaborative work, statistical thinking, and planning and analysis. Daily work applications include developing models for testing change and making adjustments as well as review of the improvements.

FIGURE 17-8	**THE FRAMEWORK FOR THE CONTINUAL IMPROVEMENT OF HEALTH CARE**

Underlying Knowledge

Professional knowledge:
- subject
- discipline
- values

Improvement knowledge:
- system
- variation
- psychology
- theory of knowledge

Policy for Leadership

Mission, vision, and quality definition
Guiding principles
Integration with values

Tools and Methods

Process, system
Group process and collaborative work
Statistical thinking
Planning and analysis

Daily Work Applications

Models for testing change and making improvement
Review of improvement

Source: P. B. Batalden and P. K. Stoltz. "A Framework for the Continual Improvement of Health Care: Building and Applying Professional and Improvement Knowledge to Test Changes in Daily Work." Joint Commission Journal on Quality Improvement (October 1993), 426. Oakbrook Terrace, IL: Joint Commission on Accreditation of Healthcare Organizations, 1993, p. 426. Reprinted with permission.

Conceptualizing quality management principles provides the nurse with tools for assisting the nursing department with the overall QM process.

Statements of Purpose, Philosophy, and Objectives

The initial planning of a QM program includes the development of clear and concise statements of purpose, philosophy, and objectives. The program's purpose and philosophy mirror the organizational purpose and philosophy and should be interwoven with the organization's values. The JCAHO gives specific guidelines designed to assess and improve quality of client care. Quality improvement theories—such as those of Deming, Crosby, and Juran—are recommended to healthcare organizations to better conceptualize the entire QM program.

An organization need not limit itself to one theory and may incorporate concepts from several to develop the best framework for the organization's purpose, philosophy, and objectives. Every QM program needs well-articulated objectives.

Standards for Measuring the Quality of Care

Standards define nursing care outcomes as well as nursing activities and the necessary structural resources. They are used to plan and evaluate nursing care. Outcomes include positive and negative indexes. Standards are directed at structure, process, and outcome issues and guide the review of systems function, staff performance, and client care. A number of healthcare organizations issue indexes. The Centers for Medicare and Medicaid Services annually disclose projected and actual hospital select indicator rates by diagnostic-related groups.

On January 1, 2004 TJC's National Patient Safety Goals (NPSGs) went into effect for all accreditation programs. The program-specific goals and objectives mandate implementation, measurement, and evidence of performance without negotiation. The purpose of the NPSGs is to promote specific improvement in patient safety. In June 2007 the TJC Board of Commissioners approved the 2008 NPSGs. For more information, go to http://www.jointcommission.org/PatientSafety/National PatientSafetyGoals. For hospitals, the TJC has issued accreditation performance measures involving the following functions:

1. Patient-focused functions: ethics, rights, and responsibilities; provision of care, treatment, and services; medication management; infection control
2. Organization functions: improving organizational performance; leadership; management of the environment of care, of human resources, and of information
3. Structures with functions: medical staff, nursing

TJC also requires measurement of core measures, one of the first steps in focusing on key treatment populations. An organization's results as well as national results for select core measures may be found on TJC's website: http://www.jointcommission.org/

TJC requires hospitals to proactively identify risks to patients, initiate actions to reduce risks (failure mode effect and analysis), and investigate unanticipated adverse "sentinel" events (root cause analysis). The failure mode effect analysis, initiated proactively, involves documenting the ways a process can fail (e.g., a flowchart), why this failure would occur (e.g., a cause and defect diagram), and how a redesign of the process may prevent failure (e.g., a flowchart). Hospitals are required to annually select one high-risk process based in part on TJC's published sentinel event alert. Hospital leaders are to provide education and resources to conduct proactive activities to reduce risk to patients.

Root Cause

Analysis is conducted to understand how and why an adverse sentinel event occurred and to prevent its reoccurrence. A sentinel event is an unexpected, unwanted occurrence involving death or serious physical injury. It is called "sentinel" because it signifies immediate attention. Root cause analysis includes assignment of a team to assess the event as soon as possible (within 72 hours). The team should include staff of all levels closest to the specific case, including those with decision-making authority. The process involves review of events, process failure, action plans, implementation of plans, and follow-up review.[27]

TJC is not the only group that collects quality data for measurement. Other organizations include the American Hospital Association, Voluntary Hospitals of America, National Committee for Quality Health Care, and the National Association of Health Data Organizations. These organizations gather, analyze, and publish data on quality of health care for consumers, employers, and the federal government. The standards include performance standards for providers. The objectives are to achieve improvement in the health status of clients, reduce unnecessary use of healthcare services, and meet specifications of clients and purchasers. These standards address improvement of healthcare quality, functions, and processes that must be carried out effectively to achieve good patient care outcomes, patient care, governance, and management. QM theory has been applied in the form of identifying common causes and special causes of performance variation.

Policies and Procedures

The third element of a QM program is the development of policies and procedures for using standards or indicators for gathering data to measure the quality of care. Batalden and Stoltz describe guiding principles that reflect the organization's assumptions about the responsibilities and desired actions of leaders that create a positive work environment. Integrating leadership policy with the values common to health professionals and underlying healthcare work is essential to contribute to shared ownership of the policy by everyone in the organization.[28] The policies and procedures define the organizational structure for the quality management program and prescribe the tools for gathering data.

DATA COLLECTION

Data collection tools may be in the form of questionnaires, rating scales, and interviews. Reliability and validity are important concepts in determining the worth of instruments used to measure variables in a study. Reliability is the extent to which an experiment, test, or measurement procedure yields the same results on repeated trials. Interrater reliability refers to the degree to which two raters, operating independently, assign the same ratings for an attribute being measured. Validity is the degree to which an instrument measures what it is intended to measure. Content (face) validity is the degree to which an instrument adequately represents the universe of content.[29]

The content of measure (standard, indicator, process step) could be written out with options to check "yes," "no," or "NA"—and to allow comments. Ideally, this could be done electronically (with a handheld device) and downloaded into a database if resources are available.

Nursing Audits

A basic form of quality data collection is the nursing audit. An audit is essentially an examination, verification, or accounting of predetermined indicators. There are three basic forms of nursing audits: structure audits, process audits, and outcome audits.

Structure Audits

Structure audits focus on the setting in which care takes place. They include physical facilities, equipment, caregivers, organization, policies, procedures, and medical records. A checklist that focuses on these categories measures standards or indicators. Structure can include such content as staff knowledge and expertise in addition to policies and procedures for nursing practice. Content related to specific nursing care to meet established standards are included in nursing process audits.

Process Audits

Process audits implement indicators for measuring nursing care to determine whether nursing standards are met. They are generally task oriented. Process audits were first used by Maria Phaneuf in 1964 and were based on the seven functions of nursing established by Lesnick and Anderson. The Phaneuf audit is retrospective, being applied to measure the quality of nursing care received by the client after a cycle of care has been completed and the client discharged. The Phaneuf audit has seven subsections[30]:

1. Application and execution of physicians' legal orders
2. Observations of symptoms and reactions
3. Supervision of the client
4. Supervision of those participating in care
5. Reporting and recording
6. Application and execution of nursing procedures and techniques
7. Promotion of physical and emotional health by direction and teaching

The Phaneuf model uses a Likert scoring system. It does not evaluate care recorded.

The Quality Patient-Care Scale is a process audit that measures the quality of nursing care concurrently with the cycle of care being given. It has six subsections:

1. Psychosocial–individual
2. Psychosocial–group
3. Physical
4. General
5. Communication
6. Professional implications

In this audit the nurse is evaluated by direct observation in a nurse–client interaction. A 15% sample of nurses on a unit is considered adequate. Both the Phaneuf and the Quality Patient-Care Scale process audits use the performance of the first-level staff nurse as a standard for safe, adequate, therapeutic, and supportive care.[31]

Other open-system audits include the Commission for Administrative Services in Hospital Scale and the Medicus Corporation Nurses' Audit. They also measure or monitor intervention, assessment, and clinical skills.

Outcome audits can be either concurrent or retrospective. They evaluate nursing performance in terms of establishing client outcome criteria. The National Center for Health Services developed an outcome audit based on Orem's description of nine categories of self-care requirements:

1. Air
2. Water and fluid intake
3. Food
4. Elimination
5. Rest, activity, and sleep
6. Social interaction and productive work
7. Protection from hazards
8. Normality
9. Health deviation

These categories are evaluated in terms of the following evidence[32]:

1. Evidence that the requirement is met
2. Evidence that the client has the necessary knowledge to meet the requirement

3. Evidence that the client has the necessary skill and performance abilities to meet the requirement

4. Evidence that the client has the necessary motivation to meet the requirement

Outcome criteria are set for populations. They can evaluate specific aspects of nursing care for particular groups, such as neonates, school-aged children, oncology, trauma, forensics, or long-term care. Client care goals should reflect an individual's optimal functioning given his or her current condition and resources for continued care. QA outcome indicators would capture if the goals, or outcome, were met or obtained.

The outcome variables as described by Evans and Ruff have face validity as outcomes of functional utility, and their value can be reliably assessed using descriptive statistics. These variables are considered important rehabilitation outcomes by clients, family members, and financial providers and have an impact on long-term functioning.[32]

Morbidity, disability, and mortality during and after provision of healthcare services are nationally recognized outcomes of health care. Nursing assessment and intervention may make a significant difference in the outcome variables, such as nosocomial infection rates in high-risk clients. McCormick illustrates the direction of outcomes that patients can take related to the assessment and treatments carried out.[33]

Another method of developing outcome criteria includes grouping of items for efficiency: diagnosis-related groups, specific protocols for treatment, life stages, and like standards. A determination is made as to whether the outcomes are met. If outcomes are not satisfactorily met, deficiencies are identified, corrected, and followed up.

QUALITY MANAGEMENT TOOLS

Statistical Techniques

Statistical techniques include measures of central tendency, measures of variability, tests of significance, and correlation. Central tendency refers to the middle value and general trend of the numbers. The three most common measures of central tendency are the mean, the median, and the mode. Measures of variability look at the dispersion of the measures. Three common measures of variability are the range, the standard deviation, and interpercentile measures.

The most common measure of interpercentile variability is the interquartile range, which is determined by ranking the order of the measures and then dividing the array into quarters. The range of scores comprising the middle 50% is the interquartile range. The t-test, regression analysis, and chi-square tests are tests of statistical significance.[34] Correlation refers to the extent to which two variables are related. The Pearson product–moment correlation coefficient of determination (r^2) is a method whereby cause and effect, or relationships, may be evaluated. This statistical analysis tool may be found in various computer software programs and is used with scatter diagrams. The coefficient of determination (r^2) is helpful in determining the percentage of variance on one variable that can be predicted by the variance on another variable.[35]

Data Analysis

Data analysis tools may be divided into three types: decision-making tools, data analysis charts, and relational charts. Brainstorming and multivoting are types of decision-making tools that involve groups or teams. With a degree of skill in the use of these tools and methods, workers can obtain and analyze data to validate their ideas about potential improvements and later test the results of changes implemented.

Brainstorming

Brainstorming is a free-flowing generation of ideas. This approach can generate excitement, equalize involvement, and result in original solutions to the problem. Ideas are not discussed as they are generated, but the team can build on the ideas of others. No judgments are made concerning an idea's worth or its feasibility. This discussion comes at a later point in the process. Brainstorming is useful when a list of possible ideas is needed. This technique works well to generate ideas for such tool: as the cause-and-effect diagram.

Multivoting

Multivoting is a method to determine the most popular or important items from a list, without a lot of discussion or difficulty. This method uses a series of votes to cut the list in half each time, thus reducing the number of items to be considered. This technique is used after a brainstorming session to identify the key items on which the group will focus.

Nominal Group Technique

This is a group decision-making process for generating a large number of ideas in which each member works by himself or herself. This technique is used when group members are new to each other or when they have different opinions and goals. This approach is more structured than that of brainstorming or multivoting.

Delphi Method

The Delphi method is a combination of the brainstorming, multivoting, and nominal group techniques. This tool is used when the group is not in one location, and it is frequently carried out through mail or e-mail. After each step in the process, the data are sent to one person, who compiles the data and sends out the next step to the participants for completion.

Prioritization Matrix

A prioritization matrix organizes (Figure 17-9) tasks, issues, or actions and prioritizes them by agreed on criteria. The tool combines the tree diagram and the L-shaped matrix diagram, displaying the best

---

FIGURE 17-9 **PRIORITIZATION MATRIX**

	Low Cost	High Strategic Priority	Meets Accreditation Standards	MD Concern	Staff Concern	Totals
Repair of roof	3	4	2	3	4	16
Purchase new X-ray machine	5	2	6	1	5	19
Develop Skilled Nursing Unit	4	1	6	2	2	15
Develop better communication with Home Health	2	3	1	4	3	13
Develop a staff newsletter	1	5	3	5	1	15

Key:
1 Strongly feel best choice
2 Feel best choice
3 Uncertain
4 Feel not good choice
5 Strongly feel not good choice
6 Not related at all
Least amount of points is the highest priority; highest amount of points is lowest priority.

Source: Author.

possible effect. The prioritization matrix is often used before more complex matrices are needed. The matrix applies options under discussion to priority considerations. This is used when issues are identified and options must be narrowed down, options have a strong relationship, or options all need to be done but prioritization or sequencing is needed.

Run Chart or Trend Chart

Run charts are graphic displays of data points over time. Run charts are control charts without the control limits. Their name comes from the fact that the user looks for trends in the data or a significant number of data points going in one direction or to one side of the average.

Trends generally indicate a statistically important event that needs further analysis. The tendency to see every variation in the data as significant should be resisted by waiting to interpret the results until at least 10 (or even better, 20) data points have been plotted. These charts are used to display variation, detect the presence or absence of special causes, or observe the effects of a process improvement (observe the effects of experiments on a process) (Figure 17-10).

Control Charts

Control charts are run charts to which control limits have been added above and below the mean. Generally, upper and lower control limits are statistically determined by adding and subtracting three standard deviations from the mean. Assuming a normal distribution and no special cause variation, a majority of the data points are expected to fall within the upper and lower control limits. Variance within the control limits results from aggregate common causes, and one should not tamper with the process performing as expected. As discussed earlier with regard to Deming's variance, special cause variance (data points outside the control limits) occurs in less than 10% of cases and requires evaluation. These charts are used to distinguish variation from common and special causes, assist with eliminating special cause variation, and observe effects of a process improvement (Figure 17-11).

FIGURE 17-10	**EXAMPLE OF A RUN CHART**

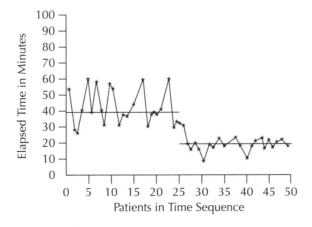

Source: P. B. Batalden, P. K. Stoltz. "A framework for the continual improvement of health care: building and applying professional and improvement knowledge to test change in daily work" Joint commission journal on quality Improvement (Oct 1993). 426. Oakbrook terrace, IL: Joint commission on Accreditation of healthcare organizations, 1993, p 426. Reprinted with permission.

FIGURE 17-11 STATISTICAL CONTROL CHART

Source: Author.

Process Flowchart

The process flowchart is a graphic display of a process as it is known to its authors or team. The flow-chart outlines the sequence and relationship of the pieces of the process. Through management of the data and information, the team comes to a common understanding and knowledge concerning the process. Information is discussed on the structure (who carries out the specific step in the identified process), what activity is occurring, and finally the outcome or the results.

Fishbone Cause-and-Effect Diagram

A cause-and-effect diagram is used to analyze and display the potential causes of a problem or the sources of variation. There are generally at least four categories in the diagram. Some of the common categories involve the "four Ms"—manpower, methods, machines, and materials—or the "five Ps"—patrons (users of the system), people (workers), provisions (supplies), places (work environment), and procedures (methods and rules). It is used to identify and organize possible causes of the problem or identify factors that will lead to success.

Histogram or Bar Chart

Before further analyzing a set of measured data, distribution of values is reviewed for each variable. The optimal tool for reviewing a distribution depends on how much data are available. A bar graph with a separate bar for each value may be used when data are sparse (fewer than 12 values), but as the data increase it becomes necessary to organize and summarize. A histogram, the most commonly used frequency distribution tool, does this by presenting the measurement scale of values along its *x*-axis (broken into equal intervals) and a frequency scale (as counts or percents) along the *y*-axis. Plotting the frequency of each interval reveals the pattern of the data showing its center and spread (including outliers) and whether there is symmetry or skew. This is important information because it may reveal signals of problems in the data and should influence the choice of measures of central tendency and spread. An important distinction must be made regarding bar charts and histograms. The *x*-axis consists of discreet categories, and each bar is a separate group. This chart is used to show the data's distribution or spread, whether the data are symmetric or skewed, or whether there are extreme data values (Figure 17-12).

Pareto Chart

A Pareto diagram displays a series of bars in which the priority can easily be seen by the varying height of the bars. The tallest bar is the most frequent. The bars are always arranged in descending height. The Pareto diagram is related to the Pareto principle (named after the 19th-century economist Vilfredo Pareto), which states that 80% of the problems or effects come from 20% of the causes. This chart is used to identify the most frequent or the most important factors contributing to costs, problems, and so on (Figure 17-13).

Quality Improvement Teams

One method of implementing a QM program is through a team or council. This team functions with a team leader, team members, and a facilitator. The team supports management in developing and implementing a QM program and may follow group dynamics. The American Nurses Association's *Guidelines for Review of Nursing Care at the Local Level* is pertinent in today's environment.

| FIGURE 17-12 | **A HISTOGRAM OF ERRORS** |

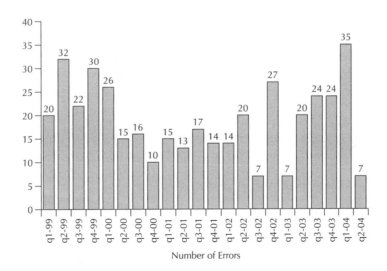

Source: Author.

FIGURE 17-13	**GENERALIZED PARETO DIAGRAM**

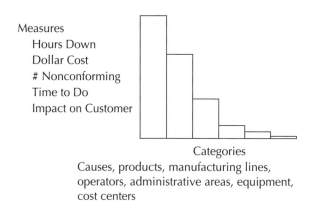

Measures
    Hours Down
    Dollar Cost
    # Nonconforming
    Time to Do
    Impact on Customer

Categories
Causes, products, manufacturing lines,
operators, administrative areas, equipment,
cost centers

Source: J. T. Burr, Center for Quality and applied statistics, Rochester Institute of Technology, one lomb Memorial Dr. P.O. Box 9887, Rochester, NY 14623-9887. Reprinted with permission.

PROBLEM IDENTIFICATION

Analysis and reporting of the data gathered from the evaluation process lead to problem identification and isolation. Evidence comes from primary sources, such as the client and nursing personnel, and from secondary sources, including the client's chart and family. Active client and family participation should be part of the process. QM addresses current problems. Nurses look for patterns or trends of deviation from normal. They also identify deficiencies relating to other departments that affect nursing care. If one takes a systems approach, problem identification is a team approach, with the client and family as major team players.

Problem Resolution

Once problems have been defined and isolated, plans are made to solve them on a priority basis. Critical problems are addressed first, and plans are immediately made and implemented to resolve them. Those involving the safety and welfare of the client take first priority. Other factors used in determining priority include severity, frequency, benefit, cost-effectiveness, elimination, reduction, association with professional liability, and impact on accreditation. The first consideration is always based on the impact on client care. Solutions and corrective action for problems are assigned to appropriate nursing departments, services, and units. The need is to resolve problems, not just evaluate them.

MONITORING AND FEEDBACK

The QM process is cyclic and requires monitoring of clinical and managerial performance and feedback to ensure that problems stay solved. Follow-up can be expensive and difficult. Problems of a multidisciplinary nature, such as those involving occupational therapy, physical therapy, speech pathology, and nursing, can be one consideration. The cyclic process will continue to set standards of care, take measurements according to those standards, evaluate care from multiple sources, recommend improvements, and, above all, ensure that improvements are carried out.

Involvement of Practicing Nurses

Practicing nurses can be motivated to embrace QM by a direct behavioral experience. Nurse managers should find out reasons nurses view QM unfavorably. Negative connotations may exist because of a lack of executive administrative support, views that the process is futile without changes in practice, and lack of physician involvement. Changing a negative viewpoint may be accomplished by the following strategies:

1. Ask clinical nurses to identify areas that need improvement.
2. Provide release time for clinical nurses to participate in QM activities, including attendance at committee meetings and time for QM audits.
3. Provide rewards, such as performance results achievement records, that can lead to pay raises, promotions, educational opportunities, or special assignments.
4. Target QM to patient care outcomes, the essence of nursing practice.
5. Involve clinical nurses in management through such techniques as quality circles, employee involvement programs, participatory management, decentralization, "adhocracy," and quality of work life.
6. Establish a peer review program involving nursing staff at all levels of patient care. Such a program can identify outcome criteria based on established standards for nursing practice. Peers determine if outcomes have been met based on ongoing and retrospective audits. Corrective action is determined by peers based on the outcome being adequately met.

Efficiency

Efficiency is concerned with the cost-to-benefit ratio. Can the appropriate standard be met with a cost acceptable to both consumer and provider? The computer is a labor-saving device for developing and conducting a QM program. Nurse managers will use it and teach other practicing nurses to use it. Standards will be kept up-to-date and accessible to all units in paper or electronic files. Standards should be cross-referenced.

Charts can be labeled for easy retrieval for nursing QM evaluation. In addition, the long-term care minimum data set can be an efficient QM tool for nursing homes. The minimum data set is a collection of baseline data (physical, social, and psychological factors) that can be used to assess, analyze, and plan care for residents in nursing homes. The 1987 Omnibus Budget Reconciliation Act mandated its specific elements.[36]

The following are some elements of efficiency and effectiveness:

1. Identification of the impact of nursing care on the health of the patient, that is, results or outcomes measured in terms of the patient's health status. Do the notes meet such a standard?
2. A program practical enough to be used in all clinical nursing settings
3. Random, unannounced samples
4. Nursing personnel who serve on committees long enough to be proficient
5. Grading by each person administering criteria
6. Higher patient acuity combined with shorter hospital stays
7. Interdisciplinary programs so nurses will not do the work of other disciplines. Nursing is ethically and operationally interdependent with other groups and organizations.
8. Planning for uncertain future by blueprinting scenarios for managing the future, changing the culture of nursing organizations, developing interpersonal skills, and making a creative response to risk taking[37]
9. Each nurse should be held responsible for self-improvement and for delivering a high standard of patient care.

Customer Satisfaction

Customer satisfaction is an integral part of QM. The satisfaction of not only the external client and family, but also the internal customers (an organization's staff and departments) should be assessed. Patient Rights and Human Resource standards specified by JCAHO and Centers for Medicare and Medicaid Services warrant measurement of these aspects.

Consumer satisfaction as an outcome of QM can be assessed through methods such as patient, family, and nurse interviews or surveys and observation checklists of nurse–patient interactions.

Quality in the healthcare marketplace is defined by employers, employee benefit consultants, physicians, and consumers—not by providers (even though physicians are providers, as are hospitals, nurses, and other caregivers). The reason physicians determine quality is that they have control over orders for diagnosis and treatment procedures. Only one-half of consumers, employers, and employee consultants ever differentiate between high- and low-quality hospitals.

Good employee relations and consumer relations programs are necessary for success in the healthcare marketplace, and their good quality must be communicated. Consumers want quality factors in this order[38]:

1. Warmth, caring, and concern
2. Expert medical staff that is concerned, thorough, and successful
3. Up-to-date technology and equipment
4. Specialization and scope of services available
5. Outcome

Training and Communication

Training and communication are important elements of a total quality program. Training includes interpersonal skills, stress management, and conflict management. Learning is a cyclic or continuous process. Nurse managers who play educator roles develop self-awareness by applying learning principles to their own behaviors. Patient education requires an interdisciplinary team approach.

Communication of QM findings, including problems, resolution of problems, and results, must be clear. Both physicians and nursing employees need to be kept up-to-date. Quality must be provided and communicated to be successful. This means that providers as well as consumers will know the status of the quality of care being rendered.

RESEARCH AND QUALITY MANAGEMENT

Nursing QM programs can be combined with research programs. Nursing research is being done in clinical settings to improve patient care outcomes. Research can provide prestige, advanced knowledge for nursing professionals, and a database for clinical nursing practice for the nurse manager.

Nursing research can be used to evaluate management issues such as staffing, cost management, and staff retention. It produces new knowledge of the relationship between process and outcome. Combining QM with research makes efficient use of personnel and other resources to link research with a mandatory process, to increase the probability that research will relate to patient care, and to increase sharing of successful quality management programs with others outside the institution.

SUMMARY

QM programs ensure that quality control standards are maintained and that care delivery continually evolves toward improvement. QM requires careful planning, development, data collection, resource allocation, and evaluation. Ideally, QM programs should be founded upon TQM, a proven theory for broad application. Leadership is paramount for successful integration of TQM into QM programs; leadership will change culture and climate to give workers the training they need to affect planning and productivity. Through effective use of QM tools, the efficiency of nursing interventions or actions can be demonstrated. QM programs may lend efficacy of results to research in support of establishing best practice for nursing.

APPLICATION EXERCISES

Exercise 17-1

Using a team that represents both nursing leaders within the organization and customers, construct a questionnaire for measuring external customer satisfaction. If such a questionnaire is currently available, review it and make changes only if changes are needed. Use the questionnaire to measure external customer satisfaction with nursing. Analyze the results using appropriate QM tools, and plan for changes to improve external customer satisfaction.

Exercise 17-2

Using a team representing nursing leaders within the organization, discuss abolishing the current performance appraisal system. Use brainstorming to generate ideas for pros and cons, then use multivoting to select the first choices from the list.

Exercise 17-3

Using a team representing nursing leaders within the organization, identify a major problem. Decide on the data to be measured. Proceed to gather and analyze data and solve the problem using Deming (Shewhart) cycle or other QM methodology.

Exercise 17-4

Using a team representing nursing leaders within the organization, describe the culture of the organization. Discuss how QM may be incorporated into research. How could best practice be identified and set standards?

Exercise 17-5

Make a plan for a quality circle using the guidelines described in this chapter.

Exercise 17-6

Examine the QM program of a healthcare agency. How does it support the overall mission, vision, and values of the organization?

Notes

1. Pellet, J. (2007). A prescription for health care: What can be done to improve the cost and quality of medical care. *Chief Executive, 52,* 230.
2. Friesen, M., Farquhar, M., & Hughes, R. (2005). *The nurses's role in promoting a culture of patient safety* (p. 905). Silver Spring, MD: Center for American Nurses.
3. Staskon, F. C., Kopera, A., & Wilson, R. C. (2007). Taking the IOM quality challenge: Providers can do a lot to meet the Institute of Medicine's call for improving the quality of healthcare (Institute of Medicine's quality control measures to improve the performance of healthcare services). *Behavioral Healthcare, 24,* 27–35.
4. Piczak, M. W. (1988). Quality circles come home. *Quality Progress, 1,* 37–39.
5. Tritus, M. (1988). Deming's way. *Mechanical Engineering, 28,* 38–45.
6. Ibid., pp. 26–30.
7. Ibid.
8. Duncan, W. J., & Van Matre, J. G. (1990). The gospel according to Deming: Is it really new? *Business Horizons, 32,* 3–9.

9. Francis, A. E., & Germels, J. M. (1989). Building a better budget. *Quality Progress, 21,* 70–75.

10. Smith, T. A. (1989). Why you should put your safety system under statistical control. *Professional Safety,* 31–36.

11. Joiner, B. L., & Gaudard, M. A. (1990). Variation, management, and W. Edwards Deming. *Quality Progress, 1,* 29–39.

12. Heinzlmeir, L. A. (1991). Under the spell of the quality gurus. *Canadian Manager, 22.*

13. Heinzlmeir, T. R. (1991). Quality can't be delegated. *Supervision,* 6–7.

14. Juran, J. M. (1989). Universal approach to managing for quality. *Executive Excellence,* 15–17.

15. Vasilash, G. S. (1981). Crosby says get fit for quality. *Production,* 51–52, 54; Heinzlmeir, T. R., 1991; Oberle, J., & Deutsch, B. J. (1991). A conversation with Philip Crosby. *Bank Marketing,* 22–27; Crosby, P. B. (1984). *Quality without tears: The art of hassle-free management.* New York: McGraw-Hill.

16. Institute of Medicine. (2006). *Performance measurement: Accelerating improvement—pathways to quality health care* (p. 171).

17. Schaaf, D. (1991). Beating the drum for quality. *Quality,* 5–6, 8, 11–12.

18. Peters, T. (1991, November 12). Family gives "teams" plenty of experience. *San Antonio Light,* p. E3.

19. Konstam, P. (1992, January 1). Making productivity grow takes work. *San Antonio Light,* p. 1E.

20. Linkow, P. (1989). Is your culture ready for total quality? *Quality Progress,* 69–71.

21. The theory of quality circles was actually developed by Frederick Herzberg and W. Edwards Deming of the United States approximately 50 years ago. Johnson, S. (1985). Quality control circles: Negotiating an efficient work environment. *Nursing Management,* 34A–34B, 34D–34G; Goldberg, A. M., & Pegels, C. C. (1984). *Quality circles in health-care facilities.* Gaithersburg, MD: Aspen.

22. Ibid.

23. Morhman, S. A., & Ledford, G. E., Jr. (1985). The design and use of effective employee participation groups: Implication for human resource management. *Human Resource Management,* 413–428.

24. Piczak, 1988.

25. Batalden, P. B., & Stoltz, P. K. (1993). A framework for the continual improvement of health care: Building and applying professional and improvement knowledge to test changes in daily work. *Joint Commission Journal on Quality Improvement,* 424–450.

26. Ibid.

27. Ibid.

28. Ibid., p. 434.

29. Sweitzer, S. C., & Silver, M. P. (1997). Measurement tools for analysis. In *NAHQ guide to quality management* (7th ed., pp. 81–105). Glenview, IL: NAHQ.

30. Curtis, B. J., & Simpson, L. J. (1985). Auditing: A method for evaluating quality of care. *Journal of Nursing Administration,* 14–21.

31. Ibid.

32. Evans, R. W., & Ruff, R. M. (1992). Outcome and value: A perspective on rehabilitation outcomes achieved in acquired brain injury. *Journal of Head Trauma,* 24–36.

33. McCormick, K. A. (1991). Future data needs for quality care monitoring, DRG considerations, reimbursement and outcome measurements. *Image: Journal of Nursing Scholarship,* 29–32.

34. Sweitzer, S. C., & Silver, M. P. (1997). Measurement tools for analysis. In *NAHQ guide to quality management* (7th ed., pp. 81–105). Glenview, IL: NAHQ.

35. Pyrczak, F. (2003). *Making sense of statistics: A conceptual overview* (3rd ed., pp. 44–66). Los Angeles: Pyrczak Publishers.

36. Spuck, J. (1999). Using the long-term care minimum data set as a tool for CQI in nursing homes. In J. Dieneman (Ed.), *Nursing administration: Managing patient care* (2nd ed., pp. 95–105). Stamford, CT: Appleton & Lange.

37. Allio, R. (1986). Forecasting: The myth of control [Interview with Donald Michal]. *Planning Review, 1,* 6–11.

38. Coddington, D. C., & Moore, K. D. (1987). Quality of care as a business strategy. *Healthcare Forum Journal, 1,* 29–34.

18 PERFORMANCE APPRAISAL

Amy Bearden, RN, MSN, NEA, BC

LEARNING OBJECTIVES AND ACTIVITIES

- Outline the need to do performance appraisals.
- Define performance appraisal.
- Describe the purposes of performance appraisal.
- Differentiate among the standards for performance appraisal.
- Describe training approaches for performance.
- Distinguish among performance appraisal methodologies.
- Describe performance appraisal problem areas.
- Distinguish among the major types of pay for performance.
- Identify the criteria used in a pay-for-performance plan.
- Discuss the design of a pay-for-performance plan.

CONCEPTS

Performance appraisal, performance standards, job analysis, job description, job evaluation, feedback, work redesign, peer ratings, self-ratings, pay for performance, merit pay, gain sharing

QUOTE

The test of a first-rate intelligence is the ability to hold two opposing ideas in mind at the same time and still retain the ability to function. One should, for example, be able to see that things are hopeless yet be determined to make them otherwise.

—F. Scott Fitzgerald

Maintains a system of introductory and annual performance appraisals based on job descriptions as standards, bases all pay increases on a merit pay system, seeks constructive feedback regarding his or her own practice, takes action to achieve plans for improvement, and participates in peer review as appropriate. Coaches and acts as a mentor for career development of others.

Develops a system of performance appraisal that uses a combination of supervisor, peer, and self-ratings. Feedback is provided based on input from the nursing staff. Human resource personnel use job analysis, job evaluation, and work redesign techniques to improve employee productivity. Employs a variety of pay-for-performance compensation plans as a part of the annual budget. Identifies industry trends and competencies in nursing administration and nursing practice. Engages in self-assessment of role accountabilities on a regular basis, identifying areas of strength as well as areas for professional and practice development. Evaluates accomplishment of the strategic plan and the vision for professional nursing.

Introduction

Employees make or break service-driven healthcare organizations; they deliver the patient care that the organization exists to provide. As feedback is obtained about the service from customers such as patients, physicians, regulatory agencies, and financial data, the organization providing the service responds by making changes in goals and direction. The organization depends on each individual employee to make changes in their performance in alignment with the goals of the larger system to be successful. Performance appraisal is a control process in which employees' performances are evaluated against standards important to the operations of an organization. It is a form of communication and consists of a disciplined interaction between a manager and an employee. The process consists of the job description, performance standard, performance appraisal and performance ratings, and/or pay for performance or rewards. Pay for performance incorporates the principles of performance appraisal. The literature on performance appraisal is voluminous, indicating its value to management.

Considerable research has been done on various aspects of the performance appraisal process. In the guidebook, *What You Accept Is What You Teach*, Michael Henry Cohen sets standards for employee accountability. He states, "the three most important decisions you will ever make as a manager are whom you hire, whom you promote, and whom you allow to remain on your team."[1] He further identifies the expectations the nurse executive has the right to require from employees[2]:

- *Competence:* Every employee should strive to be excellent at what they do. As a nurse administrator, there is an expectation that nurses know their scope and standards of practice as defined in the American Nurses Association (ANA) *Nursing Scope and Standards of Practice,* have membership in their clinical professional organization, hold professional certification in their field, and have knowledge of specific disease processes, effective pharmaceuticals, and evidence-based practice. There is the expectation of being accountable for one's professional development.
- *Excellent customer service:* Every employee should know and exceed customer expectations. Staff members are expected to know their patients, to include demographics and the most frequent disease process, and to have excellent communication skills of listening, teaching, and validating understanding. They should have the integrity to do what is right even when no one is looking.
- *Teamwork:* Staff members should exhibit behavior that is collaborative and respectful of others. There is an expectation that employees will come to work on time; avoid bickering, back biting, or complaining; and be perceived as approachable by peers and other professionals. They should participate in decision making as part of the solution as patient care problems arise. Teamwork is the number one indicator for improving quality.
- *Fiscal responsibility:* All resources should be used prudently. It is expected that employees will take care of medical equipment, identifying items that need repair, remain productive, keep the work environment clean by putting away supplies, and not abuse meal or break times.

In turn, the nurse executive and manager must

- *Communicate expectations:* There should be a structured systematic process to communicate clear expectations and feedback of performance to the employee.
- *Document communication:* Written accounts of praise for performance should be provided, as well as counseling for improvement.
- *Have reasonable expectations:* Expectations must be in line with professional standards of practice.
- *Have safe, legal and ethical expectations:* Human resource policies and procedures, the organizations grievance procedure, and legal and regulatory requirements must be known and communicated.
- *Have nondiscriminatory expectations:* Laws that provide employee protection should be known; these are described in Chapter 8.

PERFORMANCE APPRAISAL AS AN UNCOMFORTABLE TASK

Employees and managers can be uncomfortable with the performance appraisal process because it involves changing behaviors in individuals. Some employees view performance appraisal as being more valued by top management than by themselves and their supervisors. Some managers do not like to do performance appraisal because it makes them feel guilty: "Did I do justice by the employee?" As writers of performance appraisals, nurse managers are concerned that they may "cast something in stone" that is inaccurate, be criticized on written grammar and spelling, say something illegal about the ratee, or be unable to substantiate their comments.[1] Other managers are afraid of employees' reactions to ratings. Performance appraisal requires careful planning, information gathering, and an extensive formal interview, all of which is time consuming. Managers perform activities of short duration, attend ad-hoc meetings, perform nonroutine duties, and focus on current information, all of which are short-term activities compared with the ongoing performance appraisal process.[2] The process is usually not interactive, moves slowly, is passive, is isolated, and is not people oriented.[3]

Measurement of performance is imprecise. Often, the focus is on the format, not the people. In some organizations, the human resource department sends the rating forms to the departments shortly before the end of the fiscal year. The forms must be completed immediately and are done with little or no training or preparation of the rater or ratee. The result is distrust by employees and dread by managers.

Evidence-Based Practice 18-1

A survey of Fortune 1300 companies (1,000 industrial and 300 nonindustrial) indicated that 29% of hourly workers are not evaluated by a formal appraisal system; 39% of respondents indicated that where used, performance appraisal systems are "extremely effective" or "very effective." Performance appraisal systems are underappreciated.[4]

Performance appraisal systems require top management commitment. They can be tied to the planning cycle by being related to personnel budgets or included as a management plan. Performance appraisal systems are most helpful when managers commit to using them for purposes beneficial both to employees and to the organization.

Research in performance appraisal domains has little effect on the process or the outcome. Some suggest that research and practice focus on fair and accurate performance appraisal as a process before attempting to use it to improve performance.[5]

Performance appraisal literature indicates the following results[6]:

- U.S. industry has used performance appraisal systems for an average of 11 years. Performance appraisal systems had little input from line managers, employees, and customers.
- Most formats use management by objectives for executives, managers, and professional employees. Trait-based rating scales are the norm for nonexempt employees. Behavioral-anchored rating scales (BARS), forced-choice scales, or mixed standard scales are seldom used. Executives and hourly employees are least likely to be evaluated.
- Supervisor ratings are most common. Self, peer, and subordinate ratings are seldom used.
- Very few organizations allow decisions about performance appraisal policies or practice to be made at the level at which they are executed.
- Some raters receive rater training; however, employee training has seldom been welcomed.
- Only 25% of raters are held accountable for managing the appraisal process.
- Few employee opinions about the appraisal process are solicited.
- Managers are concerned with fairness, justice, and future performance.
- Of an organizational workforce, 60% to 70% is rated in the top two performance levels.
- A more comprehensive theory of the performance appraisal process is needed.

"Research indicates that high levels of organizational politics relate to the conscientious job performance of workers."[7]

PURPOSES OF PERFORMANCE APPRAISAL

Performance appraisal may be a nurse manager's most valuable tool in controlling human resources and productivity. The performance appraisal process can be used effectively to govern employee behavior to produce goods and services in high volume and of high quality. Nurse executives can also use the performance appraisal process to govern corporate direction in selecting, training, career planning with personnel, and rewarding personnel. The Fortune 1300 survey indicated that 80% used appraisal systems to justify merit increases, provide feedback, and identify candidates for promotion, all of which are considered short-term goals. These goals were linked to long-term goals of performance potential for succession planning and career planning but could be much more useful in strategic planning. Of these companies, 58% used performance appraisal to identify strengths and weaknesses, whereas 39%

used performance appraisal for career planning; 89% used performance appraisal for general guidelines for salary increases, whereas only 1% used performance appraisal for forced distribution of bonuses. Forced distribution sets a limit on the number of high-level ratings.[8]

In addition to being used for succession planning, promotions, counseling, training and development, staff planning, retention, termination, selections, and compensations, performance monitoring has been found to make employees effective. It is a managerial tool that can facilitate performance levels that achieve the company's mission and objectives.[9]

Appraisal systems are needed to meet legal requirements, including those for standardized forms and procedures, clear and relevant job analysis, and trained raters. When they do not meet such requirements, disciplinary actions, including termination, do not stand up in court.[10]

Motivation

> **It is the nature of man to rise to greatness if greatness is expected of him.**
>
> —John Steinbeck

A goal of performance appraisal is to stimulate motivation of the employee to perform the tasks and accomplish the mission of the organization. Promotions, assignments, selections for education, and increased pay are some goals that stimulate this motivation.

Salary Problems

Performance evaluation is used to determine and provide equitable salary treatment. Jobs within groups of professionals, such as engineers, physicians, chemists, physicists, and nurses, have the same basic characteristics. Differences exist in the complexity of jobs. One could say that the job of a nurse assigned to a special care unit is more complex than is that of a nurse assigned to an intermediate care unit. Contrast this with the complexity of managing the care of an active intermediate care unit of 20 to 45 patients. The complexity of providing nursing care to many patients who have differing problems and are being treated by many physicians, in addition to directing many medical care plans and many nonprofessional workers, appears to be equivalent to the complexity of intensive nursing care. In fact, some nurses want to be assigned to special care units not because of the dynamics of the situation but because their sphere of operations is limited. Is a nurse in one of these units entitled to a higher salary than a nurse in the other? The job analysts say yes, if special training is required, complicated specialized equipment is being used, and the nurse is required to make more independent and critical judgments.

The jobs of all professionals can be evaluated using conventional performance appraisal techniques. However, arguments abound regarding the relationship of performance appraisals to salaries and promotion. Some writers recommend not performing performance appraisals in times of salary increases and promotions.[11] According to a survey of 875 companies, 32% experimented with some form of performance-based pay.[12] Kirkpatrick recommends separating appraisals for merit salary increases from appraisals for performance improvement. Appraisals used for merit salary increases look backward at past performance, look at total performance, compare one individual with others doing the same job, are subjective, and are done in an emotional climate. Appraisals used to improve performance look ahead; are concerned with detailed performance; are compared with what is expected regarding standards, goals, and objectives; and are conducted in a calm climate.[13]

For performance reviews related to salary administration, nurse managers should explain to associates the basis of decisions. The reviews should be fair and should be completely understood by the managers, who should allow employees to react even to the point of discussing the reviews with higher management. When a high salary increase results, the nurse manager communicates the good news to the employee. Three months should elapse between appraisals for salary administration and those for improved performance.[14]

Expectancy theory states that "the greater a person's expectancy (i.e., subjective probability) that effort expenditure will lead to various rewards, the greater the person's motivation to work hard."[15] Rewards of high value should be obtainable and related to job performance. Employees repeat rewarded behavior and will be retained, thus maintaining productivity. Research indicates that productivity increased from 29% to 63% with output-based pay plans versus time-based pay plans. Individual incentive plans are better than group incentive plans.[16]

Adequate pay is the most powerful motivator of performance, and people will not work without it. Other financial incentives, such as shift differentials, education pay, and certification pay, are positive motivators. Research reveals that productivity actually drops with time-based rewards and hourly wages. Good employees leave rather than work with poorly performing ones. Rewards should be related to job performance. The results can be seen by correlating rewards across individual performances. There should be substantial differences in the rewards.[16]

Kopelman suggests a mixed-consequence system: rewards for good performance and deductions for poor performance. The latter requires coaching, training, counseling, reassigning, or terminating. Important job responsibilities and behaviors deserving of high rewards can be determined from job analysis and should be related to difficult performance standards or goals.[17]

The Xerox Experience

Before 1983 Xerox had a traditional appraisal system, tying merit pay increases to performance rating. Employees were dissatisfied with the lack of an equitable rating distribution. Of employees, 95% were at the level three or four in a four-level rating system. Forced distribution was used to control the numbers of employees above or below a specific level. There were no planned objectives, and the focus was on the summary rating. A task force was used to develop a performance feedback and development process with the following characteristics[18]:

1. Objectives were set between manager and employee.
2. The evaluation was documented and approved by a second-level manager.
3. An appraisal review was held at the end of 6 months, with review and discussion of objectives and progress. Both manager and employee signed the written report.
4. A final review was held at 1 year.
5. The process emphasized performance feedback and improvements.
6. A merit increase discussion was held 1 to 2 months later.
7. There was agreement on personal goals related to communications, planning, time management, human relations, and professional goals (specialty and job).
8. There were financial and human resource management objectives.
9. Managers were trained in the process.

Regular surveys of the Xerox system indicated that 81% of employees understood their work group objectives better, 84% considered the appraisals to be fair, 72% understood how merit pay was determined, 70% met personal and professional objectives, and 77% favored the system.

Other Purposes

An effective appraisal generates understanding and commitment, leading to productivity. Career development and succession planning and performance appraisal support each other if they share objectives, recognition, concern, and communication. Usually, nurse managers take charge of performance appraisal and nurses take charge of career development. They can come together for mutual benefits.

Talent development can be a mutual goal and benefit of the two programs. Performance input supports future options and paths for growth and development of employees.[19] Accreditation and professional standards may require or suggest the use of performance evaluation.

Performance appraisals can also be used to confirm hiring decisions, particularly when new employees have an introductory period before becoming permanent. This period is crucial because employees can be terminated without the extended termination process. The premise is that a new employee is performing at their best in essential qualities of attitude and work ethic in this introductory period. Effective nurse managers use this period to counsel and coach the employee to perform effectively or terminate the relationship if performance is unsatisfactory. The performance appraisal documents the process.

Performance appraisal has multiple purposes. Management should determine purposes that fit organizational needs.[20] Perhaps the ultimate purpose of performance appraisal is to measure accountability and improve practice standards. Performance appraisal systems can promote professionalism and a professional practice model. In nursing, the delivery of care is a major area to be evaluated. Evaluation addresses strengths and weaknesses, new or altered policies, and the need for more knowledge. Feedback increases self-awareness and professionalism.[21]

DEVELOPING AND USING STANDARDS

Performance Standards

Performance standards are derived from job analysis, job descriptions, job evaluation, and other documents detailing the qualitative and quantitative aspects of jobs. Performance standards are established by authority, which may be the agency in which they are used or a professional association, such as the American Nurses Association (ANA). They are measuring sticks for qualitative and quantitative evaluation of the individual's performance. These standards should be based on appropriate knowledge, and they should be practical enough to be attained. Like other documents, they must be kept up-to-date.

Job or performance standards for the nurse executives and nurse manager may be developed using the ANA *Scope and Standards for Nurse Administrators*. Performance standards for a job are written and used to measure the performance of the individual filling the job. Employees should know these standards are being used and know what they are. They may be asked to bring copies of the standards to their supervisor for scheduled counseling. Employees also may be asked to list their accomplishments in relation to the standards. Doing so makes performance counseling less of a threat and allows employees to recognize and discuss their accomplishments. Employees may be guided to recognize areas in which their performance falls short and may be encouraged to voice goals for improvement in these areas. This method of using performance standards has been found to be effective.

The ANA Congress for Nursing Practice developed and published standards of practice in several specialty areas. The ANA *Standards of Clinical Nursing Practice* can be used in the development of performance standards. Figure 18-1 is an example of performance standards for a clinical nurse. The nurse manager evaluates nursing productivity with standards that measure nursing performance. Standards are based on history or past experience and "gut-level appraisal by the person in charge."[22] They include establishment of criteria, planning goals, and physical or quantitative measurements of products, units of service, labor hours, speed, and the like.[23]

A standard is "a unit of measurement that can serve as a reference point for evaluating results."[24] In collaboration with clinical nurses, nurse managers develop the units of measurement as both process (intervention) and outcome criteria. Accuracy and fairness of performance appraisal come from having an objective, standards-oriented performance appraisal plan. The plan should have objectively defined task standards that can be measured in terms of output and observable behavioral change. These performance standards should relate to both quantity and quality—that is, the who, how, when, where, and what of the work. They include production standards.[25]

Performance evaluation includes standards for experience, complexities of the job, level of trust, and understanding of work and mission. Friedman recommends developing job standards based on

FIGURE 18-1 PERFORMANCE STANDARDS—CLINICAL NURSE

Performance Standards

1. Type of work: Nursing care of patients
   Major duty: Performs the primary functions of a professional nurse (50% of working hours).
   a. Obtains nursing histories on all newly admitted patients.
   b. Reviews nursing histories of all transfer patients.
   c. Uses nursing histories to make nursing diagnoses determining patients' needs and problems. Using this information:
      i. Initiates a nursing care plan for each patient.
      ii. Lists goal(s) for each nursing need or problem.
      iii. Writes nursing prescription or orders for each patient to meet each need or problem and goal.
      iv. Applies the plan of care, giving evidence of knowledge of scientific and legal principles.
      v. Executes physicians' orders.

2. Type of work: Management of nursing personnel
   Major duty: Plans nursing care of patients on a daily basis (14% of working hours).
   a. Rates each patient according to number and complexity of needs and goals.
   b. Knows abilities of each team member.
   c. Makes a daily assignment for each team member.
   d. Discusses assignment with each team member at the beginning of each shift.
      i. Listens to taped report with team members.
      ii. Sees that team members review physicians' orders and nursing care plans.
      iii. Answers questions arising from these activities.
   e. Confers with charge nurse and ward clerk periodically to ascertain whether there are any new orders.
   f. Plans for a team conference at a specific time and place and tells team members.
   g. Incorporates division and unit philosophy and objectives into team activities.
   h. Assists with assignment of LPN and RN students, including them as active team members according to their backgrounds and learning needs.

3. Type of work: Management of nursing personnel
   Major duty: Supervises team activities (10% of working hours).
   a. Makes frequent rounds to assist team members with care of patients. At the same time, talks to and observes patients to determine:
      i. New needs or problems.
      ii. Progress. Confirms these observations with patient if possible.
   b. Conducts 15- to 20-minute team conference using a specific agenda that has been made known to team members at previous day's conference.
      i. Involves all team members.
      ii. Solicits comments on new problems or special problems of patients and updates selected nursing care plans as needed.
      iii. Assigns roles for next day's team conference.
   c. Writes nursing progress notes and updates remaining nursing care plans.
      i. Assists technicians with writing notes as needed for training. Otherwise reads and countersigns their notes. Writes own notes.
      ii. Updates those nursing care plans not done at team conference. Recognizes this is a professional nurse's responsibility.
      iii. Reads notes of LPNs and RNs.
   d. Communicates nursing service and hospital policies to team members on a daily basis through referral to information such as daily bulletins, minutes of meetings, and changes in regulations.

4. Type of work: Management of equipment and supplies
   Major duty: Identifies needs; plans and submits requests for new and replacement equipment and supplies to charge nurse (1% of working hours).
   a. While working with team members, identifies malfunctioning equipment and supply shortages and reports same to charge nurse and ward clerk on a daily basis.
   b. Submits requests for new equipment and supplies to charge nurse on a quarterly basis.

5. Type of work: Training
   Major duty: Identifies training needs of team members and plans activities to meet needs (5% of working hours).

(continues)

a. Identifies specific training needs of individual team members through daily observation of their performance and interviews.
b. Evaluates performance through use of performance standards. Makes these standards known to each team member, and holds each responsible for meeting standards.
c. Plans counseling and guidance of each team member on an individual basis and at least quarterly.
d. Plans and conducts unit in-service education programs at least monthly. Involves team members.
e. Recommends team members for seminars, short courses, college programs, and correspondence courses.
f. Thoroughly orients all new team members. Conducts skill inventory during initial interview and plans on-the-job training for those needed skills in which team member is not proficient.
g. Annually submits budget requests for training materials and programs to charge nurse.
h. Makes reading assignments and allows time for team members to use library resources.

6. Type of work: Planning patient care
   Major duty: Coordinates nursing resources essential to meeting each patient's total needs and goals (5% of working hours).
   a. Consults with patients' physicians daily.
   b. Requests consultations of clinical nurse specialists. This may include clinical nurse specialists in pediatrics, mental health, medical/surgical, radiology, public health, and rehabilitation.
   c. Consults with other personnel as needed, including chaplain, social worker, recreation worker, occupational therapist, physical therapist, pharmacist, and inhalation therapist. Coordinates with physicians and charge nurse as needed.
   d. Supports philosophy of having ward clerks assume nonnursing activities by assisting with their training as needed on a daily basis to help them become proficient in their duties.
   e. Aggressively pursues having ward clerks do administrative tasks and nursing team members perform the primary functions of nursing. The latter most commonly occurs at patients' bedsides.

7. Type of work: Teaching patients
   Major duty: Teaches patients to care for themselves after discharge from the hospital (5% of working hours).
   a. Plans teaching as a major rehabilitation goal for each newly admitted patient. Includes it as part of nursing assessment and enters it on the nursing care plan.
   b. Reviews and updates teaching plans daily.
   c. Involves resource people in teaching program.
   d. Refers cases to visiting nurse for followup.
   e. Makes followup appointments for assessment of progress toward nursing goals with a clinical nurse.
   f. Involves families in teaching as indicated.

8. Type of work: Evaluation of care process
   Major duty: Conducts audits of nursing care (3% of working hours).
   a. Audits nursing records on a daily basis.
   b. Performs bedside audit on a weekly basis.
   c. Audits closed charts of discharged patients monthly.
   d. Reviews patient questionnaires.
   e. Discusses results of all audits with team members as a group and on an individual basis.

9. Type of work: Personnel administration
   Major duty: Rates performances of team members (2% of working hours).
   a. Writes performance reports.
   b. Discusses reports with individuals to learn their personal goals.

10. Type of work: Self-development
    Major duty: Pursues a program of continuing education activities (5% of working hours).
    a. Sets own goals for self-development, including a reading program and a set of educational goals for short courses, conventions, workshops, college courses, and management courses.
    b. Participates in division and departmental in-service education programs.
    c. Participates in nursing service committee activities.
    d. Participates in research projects.
    e. Participates as a citizen in the community through involvement in professional organizations and service projects.
    f. Assumes responsibility for knowledge of, progress in, and utilization of community resources such as:
       i. Health groups
       ii. Civic groups
       iii. General education groups
       iv. Nursing recruitment
       v. Others

Source: Author.

four to eight core responsibilities. For nurse managers, these core responsibilities could be in the major management functions of planning, organizing, directing (leading), and controlling (evaluating). They could also be related to the roles of clinician, teacher, administrator, consultant, and researcher. Finally, these core responsibilities could be related to self-development. Desired behaviors, outputs, or results under each core responsibility are then developed as performance objectives. Objectives are related to or combined with behaviors as standards for performance evaluation.[26] Job analysis, job descriptions, and job evaluations are important sources of standards for performance evaluation.

66 Standards include the dimensions of evidence-based nursing practice, measurable outcomes, and accountability. 99 27

JOB ANALYSIS

Edwards and Sproull list objective performance dimensions developed by management and employees as a necessity for effective performance appraisal. These performance dimensions are developed from job analysis. "Performance criteria should be: (1) measurable through observation of behaviors of the job, (2) clearly defined, and (3) job-related." Nurse managers and nursing employees should agree on the meaning and priority of each measurement. These standards do not need to be quantifiable but must be keyed to observable behavior[28]:

Observable behavior → Job analysis → Job standards

Basing performance appraisal on job analysis makes it more relevant and establishes content validity.[29] Job analysis systematically gathers information about a particular job. It "identifies, specifies, organizes, and displays the duties, tasks, and responsibilities actually performed by the incumbent in a given job."[30] Job analysis begins with identification of the domain of content to be measured. The domain of content may be stated in terms of the tasks to be performed, the knowledge base required, the skills or abilities needed for the work, or personal characteristics deemed necessary.[31]

Job analysis reveals overlap among jobs so they can be modified. It can be used to improve efficiency and proficiency by identifying skills certification, altering staffing levels, reassigning staff, selecting new employees, altering management, establishing training objectives and standards, developing career ladders, and improving job satisfaction.[32] A procedure for doing job analysis is as follows[33]:

1. Name the job specifically, for example, nurse manager–oncology.
2. Go to the workplace, identify the target nurses working in the job family, and talk to them. Ask these questions:
   a. What are the characteristics of a good nurse manager?
   b. What are the characteristics of a poor nurse manager?
   c. How does a good nurse manager differ from a poor nurse manager?
   d. How does a good nurse manager perform tasks better than others?
   e. What are examples of effective performance by a nurse manager?
   f. Why is this nurse manager effective?
   g. What are examples of ineffective performance by a nurse manager?
   h. Why is this nurse manager ineffective?
   i. Describe a nurse manager who performs the job better than anyone else. Why?
   j. Which job skills would you look for if you had to hire someone to be a nurse manager? Why?
   k. Describe the prior training or experience needed to effectively perform as a nurse manager. Why is this so?

3. Have the job incumbents list all duties, tasks, and responsibilities, or DTRs, that they perform. Cover a specific time period.

4. List on index cards all DTRs that the job incumbents perform. Do this by observation for a specific time period that coincides with the period covered in item 3 above. DTRs can be listed one to each index card.

5. Compare the two lists, and aim for a consensus between job incumbents' lists and yours.

6. State the duties, tasks, and responsibilities in specific, clear, behavioral terms.

7. Determine the four to eight categories of job tasks to be used, such as managerial, direct care, maintenance, and interpersonal.

8. Classify each DTR into the four to eight core job categories.

9. List the DTRs by priority, and use consensus to improve efficiency.

10. Evaluate DTRs for specificity, indicating how and when they will be performed.

11. Review DTRs with the team, eliminating those with low priority. Rewrite items as needed, making each a unique job skill stated in understandable language.

12. Set standards of performance, including the percentage of time each is to be done.

13. List constraints: educational, experiential, physical, and emotional.

14. Write a summary of the unique facets of the job.

15. Prepare a job analysis questionnaire and administer it to all personnel with the same job title.

Research on job analysis information has shown no significant differences between effective and ineffective retail store managers. Research also has shown no significant differences among police officers between high-job-performers' perceptions of the demands of their jobs compared with low-job-performers' perceptions. Because these research studies are few and inconclusive in relation to the literature on the subject, nursing researchers should do research in these areas. The described method of developing a master inventory of knowledge, skills, and abilities could be used to develop job analysis for other jobs.[34]

Recent downsizing and demassing of organizations have caused managers to plan and restructure the work of remaining employees. This includes eliminating, simplifying, and combining steps, tasks, or jobs to make work easier and more enjoyable. One goal is to reduce stress by eliminating unneeded rules, procedures, reviews, reports, and approvals. Another goal is to redesign physical work by analyzing jobs using the overall process described by Denton observe and understand the current decision-making process; use a flow chart to document decisions; evaluate each decision-making step, both current and proposed; implement the change; and evaluate the results after a reasonable time has passed. Money is saved by eliminating ineffective bureaucracy.

> *Oryx, a Dallas-based oil and gas company, used teams to eliminate 25% of internal reports and reduced signatures for capital expenditures from 20 to 4. It reduced the annual budget time from 7 months to 6 weeks and saved $70 million in operating costs in 1 year.*

Sometimes money is saved by adding employees and slowing the production process to improve quality.[35]

Motorola uses these six steps to achieve statistical process control[36]:

1. What do I do?
2. For whom do I work?
3. What do I need to do my work better?

> *Job analysis is used to establish board certification in nursing specialties, ergonomic criteria for shift workers, licensure examination for registered nurses (NCLEX-RN), job descriptions for nurse editors, compensation systems, redesigns for effective and efficient systems of care, and interviewing techniques for hiring the right applicants.[37]*

4. How can I specifically design my work?

5. How can I do my work better?

6. Do benchmarking: Measure, analyze, and control the improvement process.

Job analysis leads to a job description of the work expected by the institution, which can be used for performance appraisal.

JOB DESCRIPTION

Job Description as a Contract

A job description is a contract that should include the job's functions and obligations and specify the person to whom the employee is responsible. It is a written report outlining duties, responsibilities, and conditions of the work assignment.[38] It is a description of a job, not of a person who happens to hold that job. Most formats for job descriptions include a job title and statements of basic functions (one sentence), scope, duties, responsibilities (areas in which achievements are measured), organizational relationships (for communication), limits of authority, and criteria for performance evaluation. Job descriptions should be one to two pages long.[39]

Use of Job Descriptions

Job descriptions are used for many purposes, including the following:

- Establishing a rational basis for the salary structure
- Clarifying relationships among jobs
- Helping analyze employees' duties
- Defining the organizational structure and support
- Reassigning and fixing functions and responsibilities in the entire agency
- Evaluating job performance
- Orienting new employees
- Assisting with hiring and placement
- Establishing lines of promotion
- Identifying potential training needs
- Critically reviewing the existing work practices within the agency
- Maintaining continuity of all operations
- Improving the work flow
- Providing data about proper channels of communication
- Developing job specifications
- Serving as a basis for planning staffing levels

Many changes in the dynamic environment of a healthcare agency (such as changes in personnel, departmental or agency objectives, budget, and technology) create the need for periodic review and revision of job descriptions. Time should not be wasted preparing job descriptions that will not be put to use. Job descriptions should be available to all personnel so they know the dimensions of their jobs, which in the agency can help them in their work, how their performances will be evaluated, and the opportunities for advancement. To make the data more useful, numerical values may be assigned to the important elements of the specific duties, as in Figure 18-1.

> **❝**Role development of nurse specialists is defined in evolving job descriptions of practice from novice to expert. This role development is being shaped by healthcare policy, particularly that related to managed care; available resources; increased job complexity; and relationships between job satisfaction and organizational climate. The new career models are founded on self-responsibility, entrepreneurial aptitude, vision, and personal empowerment. The case manager nurse of the 21st century is forward thinking, flexible, and solution oriented.**❞**[40]

To avoid bias, data for job descriptions should be gathered from several sources. Data may be collected by interviewing the job incumbent, having an incumbent keep a log of duties performed during a specific time period, observing the person, and having the person fill out a questionnaire (job analysis).

The person preparing the job descriptions should determine how they will be used so the needed information is included. It is probably best to introduce job descriptions during a time of favorable economic outlook, when this action is less threatening to employees. Job descriptions should be introduced to the staff registered nurses first. Managers may fear increased work loads and grievances. It is important to consult with all employees and allow them to discuss, comment on, and recommend changes in the job descriptions for positions. Doing so makes development of job descriptions a cooperative venture, leading to consensus, effective management, and effective performance appraisal. Language used in the job descriptions should be simple and understandable.

> *Because job descriptions are guides, rigid application of them can result in negative behavior.*

Job descriptions should define minimum standards for effective job performance and employment and should not be too detailed. The catch-all phrase "performs other duties as directed" is evasive and should not be put in a job description. A format is needed for quality and thoroughness of job descriptions. Kennedy recommends the following 11 elements[41]:

1. Header: job title, name and location of incumbent, immediate superiors
2. Principal purpose or summary; overall contribution of incumbent
3. Principal responsibilities, including percentage of time spent on each
4. Job skills: knowledge, skills, and education
5. Dimension or scope: quantifies areas such as the budget, size of reporting organizations, and impact on the bottom line
6. Organizational chart
7. Problem-solving examples
8. Environment
9. Key contacts
10. References guiding the incumbent's actions
11. Supervision given and received

Job descriptions can be written to comply with some legal, regulatory, and accrediting requirements and used to[42]:

- Meet the licensing laws of the state, rules of accrediting agencies, and Medicare and Medicaid regulations
- Determine job ratings and classifications
- Determine whether jobs are exempt or nonexempt
- Recruit, select, evaluate, and retain employees

Figure 18-2 presents a job description for a bedside nurse in a U.S. hospital around 1887. Figure 18-3 is a current job description for a generalized clinical nurse.

PERFORMANCE APPRAISAL AND JOB DESCRIPTIONS

Peters in *Thriving on Chaos* has a low opinion of job descriptions.[43] "Performance appraisal should be ongoing, based on a simple, written 'contract' between the person being appraised and his or her boss. Limit objectives to no more than three per period (quarter, year). Eliminate job descriptions."

Performance appraisal, the setting of objectives, and job descriptions are control devices. As such, Peters claims, they are increasingly bureaucratic, run by "experts," and out of touch with the world of

---

FIGURE 18-2 **1887 JOB DESCRIPTION**

In its publication, *Bright Corridor*, Cleveland's Lutheran Hospital published this job description for a bedside nurse in a U.S. hospital in 1887.

In addition to caring for your fifty patients, each bedside nurse will follow these regulations:

1. Daily sweep and mop the floors of your ward; dust the patient's furniture and window sills.

2. Maintain an even temperature in your ward by bringing in a scuttle of coal for the day's business.

3. Light is important to observe the patient's condition. Therefore, each day fill kerosene lamps, clean chimneys, and trim wicks. Wash the windows once a week.

4. The nurse's notes are important in aiding the physician's work. Make your pens carefully; you may whittle nibs to your individual tastes.

5. Each nurse on day duty will report every day at 7:00 A.M. and leave at 8:00 P.M., except on the Sabbath, on which day you will be off from 12:00 noon to 2:00 P.M.

6. Graduate nurses in good standing with the director of nursing will be given an evening off each week for courting purposes, or two a week if you go regularly to church.

7. Each nurse should lay aside from each payday a goodly sum of [her] earnings for her benefits during her declining years, so that she will not become a burden. For example, if you earn $30 a month you should set aside $15.

8. Any nurse who smokes, uses liquor in any form, gets her hair done at a beauty shop, or frequents dance halls will give the director of nurses good reason to suspect her worth, intentions, and integrity.

9. The nurse who performs her labors, serves her patients and doctors faithfully and without fault for a period of 5 years will be given an increase by the hospital administration of $.05 a day, providing there are no hospital debts that are outstanding.

Source: Author.

---

human relations, because they promote stability at the expense of flexibility. Most job descriptions are not read or followed by successful workers. The alternative is coaching and teaching values.[44] Using performance appraisal as ways to enhance the work experience rather than "boxing" it in can facilitate productivity and joy in the workplace. Knowing the standards can provide a degree of comfort and security and thus be a useful tool rather than a control mechanism.

Job Evaluation

Job evaluation is a process used to measure exact amounts of base elements found in a job. Laws require men and women to be paid equally for equal work requiring equal skill, knowledge, effort, and responsibility under similar working conditions. This factor is important in the fight to achieve pay equity for women and hence for nurses.[45]

Job evaluation rates jobs within a given agency. Although several job evaluation systems exist, The Hay Job Evaluation System is the best known. It was developed in 1951 by the Hay Group, a Philadelphia-based consulting firm, to approve managerial, technical, and professional positions.[46] The Hay System attempts to measure exact amounts of base elements found in all jobs, including know-how, problem solving, and accountability. Know-how includes practical procedures, specialized techniques, scientific disciplines, managerial knowledge, and human relations skills. Problem solving includes the thinking challenge created by the environment. Accountability includes freedom to act, input of the job on the corporation, and the magnitude of the job. Observations of use of the Hay

FIGURE 18-3 POSITION DESCRIPTION

Title: Generalized Clinical Nurse (GCN)

General Description. The GCN is a professional nurse with academic preparation at the BSN level or above who provides expert nursing care based on scientific principles; delivers direct patient care and serves as a consultant or technical advisor in the area of health professions; and serves as a role model in the leadership, management, and delivery of quality nursing care by integrating the role components of clinician, administrator, teacher, consultant, and researcher.

Qualifications

1. Educational
   a. Graduation from an accredited school of nursing.
   b. Bachelor of Science in Nursing degree required.
2. Personal and professional
   a. Current state professional nursing license.
   b. Knowledge of and experience in preventive care (screening and teaching).
   c. Demonstrated knowledge and competence in nursing, communication, and leadership skills.
   d. Ability to analyze situations, recognize problems, search for pertinent facts, and make appropriate decisions.
   e. Ability to coordinate orientation and continuing education of clinic staff utilizing appropriate teaching strategies.
   f. Ability to apply principles of change, organizational theory, and decision making.
   g. Membership and participation in professional organizations desirable.
   h. Recognition of civic responsibilities of nursing.
   i. Ability to communicate effectively both in writing and verbally.
   j. Evidence of professional manner and conduct.
   k. Optimum physical and emotional health.

Organizational Relationships. The GCN is administratively responsible and accountable to the nurse administrator. He or she is responsible for assessing, teaching, coordinating, providing appropriate care, and making referrals when necessary.

Activities

1. Clinician
   a. Give direct patient care in selected patient situations and serve as a behavioral model for excellence in practice.
   b. Assist the nursing personnel in assessing individual patient needs and formulation of a plan of nursing care; write nursing orders, when appropriate, for implementation of nursing plan; assist the nursing personnel in documenting the effectiveness of the individualized care.
   c. Set, evaluate, and reevaluate standards of nursing practice; communicate these standards to the nursing personnel; change standards as necessary.
   d. Evaluate nursing care given to patients within the clinical area (assessing and teaching); when appropriate, make recommendations for improvement of that care.
   e. Function as a change agent; identify the barriers to more comprehensive healthcare delivery, modify behavior, and introduce new approaches to patient care.
   f. Collaborate with other healthcare providers and make appropriate referrals when necessary.

2. Teacher
   a. Provide an atmosphere conducive to learning.
   b. Teach appropriate preventive measures to clients.
   c. Direct the orientation of new staff and student nurses to ease their role transition and improve their skills, attitudes, and practices.
   d. Consider the needs of the adult learners (nursing personnel) as well as the clinicians' knowledge and expertise when planning continuing education to the clinical practice.
   e. Initiate or assist with the planning, presenting, and evaluating continuing education programs for clinic staff.
   f. Guide and assist staff and nursing students as they assume the responsibility of patient teaching.

3. Administrator
   a. Function as a change agent and appraise leadership, communication, and change processes in the organization and assist with direct strategies for change as necessary.

    b. Work collaboratively with hospital personnel and other healthcare providers in planning care and making referrals.

    c. Make recommendations relative to improving patient care and staff and student requirements to the appropriate administrative personnel.

    d. Support and interpret the clinical policies and procedures.

4. Self-Development
    a. Assume responsibility for identifying own educational needs and upgrade deficit areas through independent study, seminar attendance, or requesting staff development programs.
    b. Evaluate own nursing practice and instruction of others and the effect these have on the quality of patient care.

5. Consultant
    a. Conduct informal conferences with nursing personnel concerning patient care of specific health problems, the problem patient, or other pertinent problems related to nursing as suggested by the staff.
    b. Assist personnel to develop awareness of community agencies/resources available in planning patient care.
    c. Serve as a resource person to patients and their families.

6. Researcher
    a. Determine research problems related to preventive care, nursing clinics, and so on.
    b. Conduct research studies to upgrade independent nursing practice.
    c. Demonstrate knowledge of the current research applicable to the clinical area, and apply this knowledge in nursing care when appropriate.
    d. Research clinical nursing problems through the development and testing of relevant theories, evaluation, and implementation of research findings for nursing practice.
    e. Promote interest in reading and reviewing of current publications dealing with the delivery of preventive care to ambulatory patients.

Source: Author.

System indicate that the percentage of specialized know-how decreases with high-level positions, making problem solving and accountability the real payoff factors.[47]

Work Classification

Helton reports a system for work classification to improve white-collar work. The system includes four categories: specialist, professional, support, and clerical. Professional and specialist jobs involve a significant amount of cognitive effort, are not routine, and are challenging. Criteria used to classify white-collar work are work range, work structure, control, and cognitive effort. Applied to nursing, the nurse with a master's degree is a specialist; the nurse with a baccalaureate degree a professional; the nurse with a diploma, an associate degree, or a licensed practical nurse a support person; and aides and clerks equivalent to clerical workers. It would be economical to develop or integrate aides and clerks into one job classification.[48]

> *Some people believe that autonomy and bureaucracy are incompatible; however, bureaucratic activities that support professional nurses' autonomy are desirable.*

Job redesign uses job enlargement and job enrichment. Job enlargement uses horizontal loading to add tasks of equal difficulty and responsibility to jobs. Job enrichment uses vertical loading to add tasks that increase the difficulty and responsibility of jobs. Job enlargement and job enrichment have beneficial results, including increased productivity. In 32 experiments involving job redesign, 30 indicated impact; the median increase in productivity was 6.4%. Employee satisfaction increased in 20 cases and was tied to more pay for increased work, less supervision, and more worker autonomy.

To make job redesign effective, nurse managers need to make accurate diagnosis and real job changes. They need to address technological and personnel system constraints, support autonomy, have a bureaucratic climate, have union cooperation and top management and supervising management support, have individuals ready to fill the jobs, and have contextual satisfaction with pay, supervision, promotion opportunities, and coworkers.[49]

Work Redesign

Work redesign needs to encompass the entire nursing care system. Work redesign should incorporate cultural issues, management structure, practice patterns, task and operating system alignment, and commitment to continuous quality improvement. Work redesign is serious work.[50] A hostile internal culture fostering competition depresses performance because players tend to attempt to beat rivals rather than perform tasks well. The weaker party may give up, whereas the stronger one feels dangerously invincible. Friendly competition is replaced by mistrust, suspicion, and scorn. Change this type of environment to one of cooperation and higher performance. Outside competition can stimulate employees.[51]

Other suggestions for work redesign include the following[52]:

- Define the existing culture; identify the desired culture. Identify gaps, and plan to close them in a manner consistent with the vision and strategies of the healthcare system.
- Change structures to those that facilitate autonomy, multidisciplinary teams, new work designs, and participation in reward and risk.
- Change unwanted patient outcomes by identifying and changing practices and processes that create them.
- Because treatment design drives work redesign, gather and analyze data about treatment types and number.
- Redesign operating policies, systems, and jobs. Assess all of them using teams of practitioners who decide which to eliminate, modify, or add. Assess everything.
- Create a customer–supplier model of quality improvement to provide quality and quantity of products and services that customers want. Consider all these as management work.

Training

Nurse managers should be educated to do effective performance appraisals that maintain employee productivity. Training entails coverage of subjects such as motivational environment, appropriate job assignment, proper supervision, establishing job expectancies, appropriate job training, interpersonal relationships, providing feedback, interviewing, coaching, counseling, and performance appraisal methods. Performance-based appraisal systems consider how the employee actually performs in his or her role, taking into account the degree of interdependency and collaboration in the role.

Training raters make performance appraisal work. The goal of such training is improved productivity. A training program can give nurse managers a conceptual understanding of performance appraisal as a management system for transmitting, reinforcing, and rewarding the behaviors desired by the organization. Raters need to know how performance appraisals will be used. Research indicates that raters have been found to vary ratings depending on their use. Refresher training is recommended after 1 year. Performance appraisal training can be conducted with other management development programs.[53]

An effective appraisal system has an objective, reliable method to evaluate whether raters are qualified. Training of raters should focus on specific evaluating errors. Research indicates that rater training decreases accuracy because the raters become more sensitive to typical rating error and change their responses, thus creating new errors. Training programs should be designed to increase awareness of this fact and correct for it. Raters are trained to capture all components of an individual's contribution to the organization, including qualitative behavior. All behavior does not reduce to quantitatively measurable performance.[54]

Training based on feedback is specific. Train the raters in behavior observation, documentation of critical performance incidents that support the consensus of a team evaluation, sensitivity to employees in legally protected categories, and performance criteria.[55]

Feedback

An analysis of 69 articles reporting 126 experiments in which feedback was applied indicated that feedback with goal setting, behavioral consequences, or both was much more consistently effective than was feedback alone. Daily and weekly feedback produced more consistent effects than did monthly feedback. Also, feedback accompanied by money or benefits of food and gasoline produced improvements in behavior more often than did praise. Graphs were used to illustrate feedback results, demonstrating the highest proportion of consistent effects. The conclusion is that feedback graphically presented at least weekly along with tangible rewards yields effective work performance.[56]

Training includes providing specific feedback to raters on timeliness, completeness, rating errors, and quality and consistency of ratings. Training methods include case studies, role plays, behavioral modeling, discussion, and writing exercises that evaluate actual appraisals, relating them to job descriptions.[57]

Feedback closes the loops by tying together the appraisal process. Feedback informs the ratee of achievements compared with expectations. It must be timely, constructive, and objective, and it must ensure that the ratee knows and can respond. The goal is to have good results continue by eliminating frustrations, which lead to lowering of goals and performance.[58]

Rater feedback from team evaluation consensus (TEC) addresses systematic inconsistencies, including unlawful bias. Correction by feedback creates improved accuracy of the system, improved morale, increased worth, and increased productivity. TEC identifies inaccurate raters for directed training or elimination as raters.[59] Feedback can be provided through coaching, counseling, and interviewing.

Coaching

The appraisal rater is a leader and a coach. Coaching for job performance is similar to coaching for athletic performance. As a coach, the rater does continuous reinforcement of tasks done well and helps with other tasks. In addition, the rater uses knowledge of adult education to train the employees to accomplish assigned work, does two-way communication, and has the necessary resources to do the job.

Coaching can include observing and listening for examples of work, good or bad. The rater coach praises the good and helps improve the bad with a joint action plan. Coaching makes performance evaluation useful.[60] Coaching is a yearlong evaluation and discussion of performance, which eliminates surprises. Progress discussions can be brief, regular, frank, open, and factual and can include the employee's viewpoint. The rater does not try to achieve truth but tries to discuss perceptions. The coach also removes obstacles to satisfactory performance. If the consequences are not working to improve unsatisfactory performance, the coach changes them. The ultimate step is to transfer or terminate the employee.[61]

Progressive discipline protects the employer from unwarranted liability resulting from discrimination charges and lawsuits, but it fails to bring about behavioral change in employees to make them fully functioning, committed team members. Employees already perceive performance appraisal to be evaluative and judgmental, not developmental. Progressive discipline combined with performance evaluation results in compliant employees. Effective leaders are coaches who gain commitment from employees. Today's employees will put forth effort if stimulated, challenged, and recognized for their efforts. They do not want to be managed; therefore managers must manage, lead, and coach.

Coaching can reduce discipline. The nurse manager as coach is available to observe behavior, provide feedback, and encourage employees to do their best. Coaching is done on a regular basis and is nonjudgmental. Employees believe the coach manager is supporting them to do better, to be successful, and to excel.

The following are some actions of an effective coach manager[62]:

- Listens
- Views the employee as a person
- Cares about the employee and helps with personal problems
- Sets a good example
- Stretches the employee
- Encourages the employee
- Helps get the work done
- Keeps the employee informed
- Praises the employee for a job well done, and provides criticism in a forthright manner

An employee who can do the job effectively may not need coaching. Coaching is personal. It is a process that involves time, interviews, observation, feedback, and help to make employees successful. The process may be repeated as necessary. A written coaching plan is helpful. It should be positive and upbeat. The manager writes the suggestions to be used for employee improvement. These suggestions should not be overstated but should describe behaviors, not characteristics. Appropriate alternative behaviors should be included in all coaching plans and sessions. The rater observes and gives feedback to correct wrong behavior or reinforce improvements by praise, factoring him- or herself into the problem as a possible contributor to it. Coaching should be done frequently and feedback given immediately with incremental changes so that employees are not stretched to the breaking point. The goal is to build a relationship that helps an employee do a good job or move on.[63]

Counseling

Counseling can be the most productive function of supervision. Counseling interviews are for the purpose of advising and assisting an individual to grow and develop self-direction, self-discipline, and individual responsibility. The counseling interview is a helping relationship involving direct interaction between the counselor (rater) and the counselee (ratee). In a counseling interview, a personal face-to-face relationship takes place. One person helps another recognize, accept, examine, and solve a certain problem.

Nurse managers can use the counseling interview to offer support and to

- Help workers develop realistic pictures of themselves, their abilities, their potential, and their deficiencies
- Explore courses of action
- Explore sources of assistance
- Accept incontestable limitations and learn to live with them, whether physical, emotional, or intellectual
- Make choices and improve capabilities

Unless they have had special training, most nurse managers are not qualified for in-depth, extensive counseling in areas involving personality structure or analysis of psychological or emotional conditions. Nurse managers must be wary of tampering with the psyche of the worker. In such cases, nurse managers should know and be able to recommend sources of help. Referring the employee to the organization's employee assistance program is appropriate when counseling begins to cross the line regarding serving as a means of assisting the employee to improve performance versus dealing with personality or behavioral issues.

Although counseling interviews are conducted to promote desirable behavior, the term *counseling* should not be used synonymously with the term *reprimand*. Reprimands belong more properly in the progress and informational type of interview.

Three approaches can be used for the counseling interview: directive, nondirective, and elective. When using the directive approach, the interviewer knows in advance what will be discussed. In this approach the interviewer gives advice, makes suggestions, helps the individual make meaningful decisions, and may even take action on some of the decisions made. This approach can be quite successful in career counseling.

66One often hears supervisors say, 'I have counseled him on what will happen if he does not improve.' This is not counseling; this is informing a worker of the consequences of certain types of behavior or performance. 99

The nondirective approach starts with the individual being counseled on strengths and weaknesses, potential, and problems. The individual takes responsibility for solving the problems; the counselor aids by listening. This approach is ideal for personal counseling but requires skill. The person being counseled says what he or she wants and freely expresses feelings; the interviewer must hide personal feelings and not express personal ideas. The counselor is a mirror only, reflecting the thoughts, ideas, and emotions of the counselee. This technique gives the individual an opportunity to think through problems out loud. Usually, the employee will come up with some kind of answer or course of action. In using the nondirective approach, it is most important that there be no interruptions or advice on a course of action.

With the exception of the preemployment interview, it is advisable to keep notes during the interview and write a summary afterward. The summary should indicate any decisions made during the interview and any follow-up action required. A comment should be made in terms of how well the interview accomplished its purpose. No notes should be taken during the preemployment interview, although a summary of the interview and the decision reached should be written up immediately afterward. Taking notes during the interview discourages the applicant and makes it difficult to obtain the information needed.

Career progression depends on present and past duty performance, personal initiative, motivation, professional development, and growth potential. Performance counseling of subordinates is vitally important so they know where they stand, how well they are doing, and where they can improve. The goal of this counseling is to improve present and future performance, not to make a critical examination of the past. Informal, day-to-day performance counseling dealing with current activities and immediate performance is important and must be continuous; however, it is not enough. Planned, careful performance counseling, scheduled at regular intervals, is needed to encourage self-improvement and to further development. During the counseling interview, the supervisor and subordinate work together to set targets in response to the job description requirements and targets for future job progression. The targets are put into writing, and progress is reviewed at the next session.

Performance counseling results from observation and evaluation of performance based on job standards. Anecdotal records may be kept and yield facts to support written ratings or reports. When counseling employees on performance problems, the rater uses a problem-solving approach. Such an approach includes reaching agreement that a problem exists, discussing alternative solutions, agreeing on a solution, and following up on progress.[64]

Interviewing

Interviewing is covered more fully in Chapter 8. For appraisal interviews, the problem-solving approach is also more effective than are the tell-and-see and tell-and-listen methods. High ratee participation produces high rater satisfaction. The problem-solving rater has a helpful and constructive attitude, does mutual goal setting with the ratee, and focuses on solutions to problems. The rater also acts with the knowledge that being very critical does not improve behaviors.[65]

Good performance appraisal interviews follow these basic guidelines[66]:

- They are based on detailed, specific notes that address accomplishments and shortcomings.
- They produce no surprises from the coach.

- The drafted appraisal is discussed with the ratee and then finalized.
- Work is started and ended with positive accomplishments.
- Needed changes are specified.
- Criticism is respectful.
- Written responses are allowed.
- Staff members are invited to assess the manager's performance.

Topics for performance appraisal review include the following[67]:

- Regular job duties (based on job description)
- Special assignments and miscellaneous projects
- Service and professional development
- Working relations
- Communication skills

PEER RATINGS

Research has shown that an individual's peers, that is, those people the individual works with from day to day, are a more reliable source for identifying the capacity for leadership than are the person's superiors. The armed services have found that peer nominations for leadership are significant predictors of future performance, a finding that could be tested in the nursing population. Democratic procedures, that is, having peers select the person to be promoted, would probably be threatening to many nurse managers. It has been found that peer selection differs little from selections by superiors. Occasionally, peers see a member of their group as a leader when superiors do not. Peer rating is valid when the group members have sufficient interaction and when group membership is reasonably stable over time. Peer rating is also valid if the position is important within the organization. Peer rating does help to identify potential leaders who go unnoticed by superiors. When several individuals are equally qualified for a position, peer ratings may single out the one with the highest informal leadership status.[68]

Peer evaluation may begin in high school with the Peer and Self-Evaluation System.[69] Peer rating is the professional model of appraisal used by physicians and is gaining interest and use among professional nurses. Peer rating is advocated as part of a system to make performance appraisals more objective, the theory being that multiple ratings give a more objective appraisal. Ratings can be obtained from multiple managers, project leaders, peers, and even patients.[70] Peer review is a performance appraisal process among persons with similar competencies who are in active practice. These persons critically review the practice of others using established standards of performance.[71] Peer review is self-regulation and supports the principle of autonomy.[72] It consists of colleagues examining the goal-directed care of colleagues with standards that are specific, critical indicators of care written by colleagues.[73]

The purposes of peer review are to measure accountability, evaluate and improve delivery of care, identify strengths and weaknesses, develop new or altered policies, identify a worker's need for more knowledge (competence), increase workers' self-awareness from feedback (critical reflection), and increase professionalism.[74]

Implementation of a peer review rating or evaluation system includes the following[75]:

- Planning by management and clinical nurses. It may be a steering committee representing these categories of nurses plus those from the domains of research and education.
- Having a shared governance type of environment
- Defining the peer review process and who is a peer
- Setting goals
- Outlining the process through consultation with management, human resources personnel, and a labor attorney. A decision is made as to who gathers the data. It can be the employee, with a clin-

ical nurse specialist as coordinator. Decisions are also made as to when and how often the interview will be done and how the outcome will be handled.

- Developing a tool using the job description
- Obtaining multiple inputs: peer reports, self-reports, and coach reports. The manager acts as coach and counselor.

The peer review process may be developed using three distinct phases of establishing a peer review program: familiarization, utilization, and internalization.[76] Phase 1, familiarization, is characterized by the development of trust, talking through the process, and establishing that the performance, not human worth, is being evaluated. Phase 2, utilization, is defined as trial-and-error responses in which objectives are refined; the peer review process takes a sharper focus. Phase 3, internalization, occurs when there is complete actualization of the entire peer review process; on-site, hands-on evaluations are conducted and findings are acted upon.

A new performance evaluation system is needed for flattened organizations with only one manager for 30 to 100 employees. Peer evaluation meets this need and, when done within a team, should be anonymous. Peers are more knowledgeable about each other's performance than is the manager. Peer review can improve teamwork. Rigg recommends using one rating category of overall capability, with a bell-shaped curve ranking criteria. Written comments are made for only those results falling outside the range.[77]

> *A survey of advanced practice nurses indicated peers evaluated only 17.5% of their job performance, with the most frequent evaluation parameters being appropriateness of care, patient satisfaction, patient outcomes, and patient volumes. Patient outcomes fell into four categories: clinical end points, complications, compliance, and functional status.* [79]

Peer review can be taught using videotapes developed locally. Studies of peer review indicate that professional nurses view it favorably, although some consider it a threat to friendship, time consuming, and artificially inflated. It does not always change the level of staff satisfaction with performance appraisals. Because nurses are more often directly accountable to their employers than to their customers, peer review requires strong management support.[78]

SELF-RATING

Self-rating is another method of performance appraisal that is seldom used. In the Fortune 1300 study, immediate supervisors did 96% of appraisals.[80] Problems with self-raters are the same as with supervisor raters, indicating the need for training of both.[81]

Employee-developed performance appraisals have been found to be tougher than those of supervisors. Employees are the subject-matter experts and do wider coverage of their jobs. Proactive, they establish expectations beforehand. Appraisal interviews are done after self-evaluation, with a common agenda and without surprises; therefore conversations are more productive. Objectives are under the employee's control. Because they come from employees and supervisors, the job elements and performance indicators are legally defensible and broad in perspective, and they elicit employee commitment.[82]

Self-evaluation can be developed by using small groups. Having a good job description facilitates development of good behavioral expectation appraisal forms that become customized for each position. The human resources department can provide a facilitator and other support. The following questions facilitate performance indicators[83]:

- Think of who has been most effective at this element or task. What behaviors and results can you cite to support your choice?
- Think of the behaviors or results that made you say to yourself, "It would be good if everyone did that." What are they?

- What are the tricks of the trade related to this task or element?
- Think about times when you perform this task well and other times when you are not as successful. What causes the difference?
- How is the average performer different from the excellent one?
- If you were training someone, what would you emphasize?

Self-rating has been found to be threatening because the employee must place him- or herself in view of others. Self-rating is a participatory management approach supported by research. Employees who view the organization as being open are more favorable to participating in performance appraisals.[84] Employees can be trained to research their own performance and the work environment. They can do self-assessments of and then analyze goals and expectations. Employees can also be trained to influence management communication skills to obtain information and advice, express their needs, and learn the style of influence to use on the manager. Thus employees become protégés of proactive performers.[85]

Although self-appraisals increase employee understanding of performance feedback and provide unique information, they are not used often. To be effective, self-evaluation should measure similar attitudes as do evaluations by supervisors. To be effective, self-appraisals should measure actual performance, relate to same time period as the criterion, be done by individuals who are experienced in self-evaluation, and be tied to a criterion group (coworkers).

Somers and Birnbaum studied a sample of 198 staff nurses in a large urban hospital. They found "no evidence of leniency error or restriction of range in self-appraisal job performance." Convergence between self- and supervisory ratings was also evident and was interpreted as an effect of halo error, that is, a tendency to rate all employees as outstanding. Self-rating requires that employees be trained in its use and focus on core job skills to make it work.[86]

A two-part format for self- and peer evaluation can be used in a peer-review evaluation process. The objective of an emergency medical services unit that used this format was to determine competence. Qualification for peer evaluation included the amount of time peers worked together. Results indicated the following[87]:

- Peers rated partners higher than partners rated themselves in intubation, electrocardiogram recognition, advanced cardiac life support, skills as an emergency medical technician–paramedic, and skills as an emergency medical technician–ambulance.
- Self-ratings were higher than were peer ratings in communication, scene management, trauma, patient assessment, and report-rating skills, which are more subjective areas.
- Both peer and self-ratings indicated that patients who were system abusers received the lowest quality of care and that the higher the socioeconomic group, the better the care received.

Research indicates that employee ratings do not differ by age; however, supervisors may view the capabilities of younger employees more positively than those of older employees.[88]

Peer and supervisor ratings have been found to be relatively highly correlated; self–supervisor and self–peer ratings are only moderately correlated. In an assessment center study, peer evaluations were better predictors of subsequent job advancement than were other ratings, including self-ratings. Peer and self-ratings predicted management potential. Behavioral information was important to peer and self-evaluation.[89]

OTHER RATING METHODOLOGIES

Other rating methodologies are less common than are supervisor, peer, and self-ratings. They include Team Evaluation Consensus (TEC), Behavior-Anchored Rating Scaler (BARS), and Task-Oriented Performance Evaluation System (TOPES). These methodologies measure job-related behaviors.

Team Evaluation Consensus

TEC uses multiple raters, a method claimed to minimize rater bias and inaccuracies. TEC uses peers, managers, and immediate supervisors for a total of two to eight raters. Direct comparisons are made with other employees or with performance benchmarks of "outstanding" or "consistently exceeds."[90]

Behavior-Anchored Rating Scales

BARS list specific descriptors of good, average, and poor performance for each of several to many job aspects. Extensive analysis is required to develop these descriptions, making them time consuming and difficult to develop. Returns are small.[91]

Descriptions of particular jobs are used to identify key job elements. Key job elements are used to develop descriptive statements of good and bad behavior. An individual's behavior is rated by closeness to behavior descriptions for key job elements (performance dimensions). Job elements, in turn, lead to behavior descriptions for each category of excellent, good, average, poor, and unacceptable, and finally lead to rating of an individual's behavior.

Raters and ratees develop the description list. Personnel time makes BARS expensive to develop. There is no composite performance score. The system is defensible in court. There have been favorable employee response and performance improvement. The results of BARS are more realistic because this system is less threatening than are most performance appraisal systems.[92]

Task-Oriented Performance Evaluation System

TOPES concentrates on job tasks rather than behavior, although it is behaviorally based because it measures task accomplishments. TOPES is also legally defensible because it relates directly to the job. Job tasks are weighted for a composite performance score. Employees can be compared across jobs. TOPES is more objective than are other methodologies because it can be used to measure quantifiable performance. Task elements are evaluated by statements that support an excellent, good, average, weak, or unacceptable rating. The score on each task is multiplied by its weight, and scores are added for a composite score.[93]

PROBLEM AREAS IN PERFORMANCE EVALUATION

It is largely assumed that merit rating systems of performance evaluation help to develop subordinates and attest to their readiness for pay increases, promotions, selected assignments, or penalties. When such systems have been scrutinized, three main problem areas have been found[94]:

1. Associates have not been motivated to want to change.
2. Even when people recognize a need for change, they are unable to make that change.
3. Associates become resentful and anxious when the merit system is conscientiously implemented.

Effectiveness

Contrast two situations in which the same job standards are applied. In the first situation, the associate is handed a completed rating form and is told to read and sign it. He or she does so but immediately appeals to the next highest level of management. The associate says that this rating is the lowest received in his or her 15-year career and that he or she has never been told the quality of his or her performance was slipping. Although the situation is resolved in favor of the associate, he or she is no longer satisfied with working for the manager and must be transferred.

In the second situation, the job standards are discussed with the associate before they are used. The associate is asked to identify those performance factors and responsibilities that are really important to the success of the unit. He or she is also asked to write out the goals of his or her job as they are seen. The goals are fully discussed by the manager and associate. Progress is discussed at the request of the associate and at stated intervals. As a result, the associate is assisted in planning educational activities that will be accomplished in preparation for the career desired.

Which of the two situations meets the criteria of an effective performance appraisal?

Weaknesses

Many pitfalls and deficiencies exist in the performance appraisal process. Many managers defend performance appraisal as a system for improving performance. As used, it probably has negative influences because most people know their shortcomings better than does their manager. Criticisms by people who have not been adequately trained to manage an appraisal system cause employees to be anxious and frustrated, to see themselves as failures, and, in some cases, to withdraw.

The rater is influenced by the most recent period of performance, an influence that may be positive or negative. Without objective measurements and records, raters tend to focus on the few outstanding activities that are vivid in their minds. Personal feelings can influence raters, causing positive "halo" or negative "horns" effects. In many instances, the performance is appraised without clear job definitions, job descriptions, and job standards. The employee seldom knows the yardsticks by which performance is being measured. Raters are either lenient or tough, causing a great variance in value judgments. Attitudes about whether the employee deserves a pay increase influence the rater. Some managers believe that all employees are average, and they project their beliefs by rating everyone the same.[95]

Other rating errors include the following:

- *Leniency/stringency error:* The rater tends to assign extreme ratings of either poor or excellent.
- *Similar-to-me error:* The rater rates according to how he or she views him or herself.
- *Central tendency error:* All ratings are at the middle of the scale.
- *First impression error:* The rater views early behavior that may be good or bad and rates all subsequent behaviors similarly.

Other problems of performance appraisal include racial bias, focus on longevity, and complacency of managers. In their usual form, performance appraisals are intrinsically confrontational, emotional, judgmental, and complex. A survey of 360 managers in 190 corporations on the performance appraisal process indicated the following[96]:

- 69% viewed objectives as unclear.
- 40% saw some payoff.
- 29% saw minimal benefits.
- 45% were only partially involved in setting objectives for their own performance.
- 81% said regular progress reviews were not conducted.
- 52% said guidelines for collecting performance data were haphazard or nonexistent.
- Only 19% viewed performance appraisal as properly planned.
- Only 37% viewed meetings as highly productive.
- 30% saw no worthwhile results.

Performance appraisals are extrinsically affected when format is improper because of lack of manager preparation, confusion about objectives, once-a-year activity, and over-reliance on forms. There are also the extrinsic areas of inappropriate values and attitudes: avoidance of conflict to avoid unpleasantness, lack of respect by failing to take the appraisal seriously, and misuse of power, causing the ratee to be beaten down, resentful, and uncommitted.[97]

FUTURE OF PERFORMANCE APPRAISAL

Deming advocated the abolition of performance appraisals. Performance appraisal is the deadliest of Deming's "deadly diseases" that stand in the way of quality management. According to Deming, performance appraisals embody a win–lose philosophy that destroys people psychologically and poisons healthy relationships. A win–win philosophy emphasizes cooperation, participation, and leadership, directed at continuous improvement of quality.[98]

Deming's system provides for three ratings for performance appraisal using process data. Using the statistic of variation, ratings fall within the system, outside the system on the high side, or outside the system on the low side. If the rating is within the system, pay corresponds to seniority; if outside the system on the high side, pay should be based on merit; and if outside the system on the low side, the employee should be coached or replaced.[99]

Effective Management of Performance Appraisals

How do we overcome these pitfalls or deficiencies? First, we must be aware of them. Second, we can learn the management-by-objectives approach and treat people as people. As a result, employees know by which yardsticks they are measured. The performance appraisal will be a joint project. It will be a helpful situation for rater and ratee. If the situation is working correctly, ratees usually push themselves.

A complex and lengthy evaluation form has not proved effective in rating personnel. Many managers have reduced their rating system to a limited checklist and a write-up that asks for strengths and weaknesses, with specific examples to justify each. Many managers agree to the following principles for a rating system:

1. The system should be simple, effective, efficient, and administratively feasible.
2. The procedures and uses of the system should be understood and agreed on by line management and the employees being rated.
3. Factors to be rated should be measurable and agreed on by managers and subordinates.
4. Raters should understand the purpose and nature of the performance review. They should be taught to use the system, observe, and write notes, including a critical incident file; organize notes and write evaluations that include examples of evidence; edit their reports; and conduct effective review interviews.
5. Raters should understand the meanings of the dimensions rated, including the dimensions' relative weights. Managers are reported to be able to distinguish among only three levels of performance: poor, satisfactory, and outstanding.
6. Criticism should promote warmth and the building of self-esteem for both ratee and rater.
7. The process should be organized and used to manage employees on a daily basis according to their needs to be coached.
8. Praise or suggestions for improvement should be done at the time of the event.
9. Standards of performance should be set and modified at the time of the event.
10. Performance standards should be valid, reliable, and fair.
11. Managers should be rewarded for good performance evaluation skills.
12. Professionally accepted procedures should be used for job analysis, development of job-related observable performance criteria, and job classifications. Fairness is ensured when processes are applied systematically and uniformly throughout the organization.
13. A fair employment posture committed to equal opportunity should be used. A conscientious and equitable appraisal system reduces lawsuits and ensures fairness and confidence. Such a system should be congruent with administrative and legal guidelines.

14. Work output, not habits and traits such as loyalty, should be measured unless the habits or traits are described by specific examples of observed behavior.

15. Quality, constant innovation, and functional barrier distraction should be emphasized.

16. Appraisal should be less time consuming through time management: daily feedback, preparation time for annual or semiannual evaluation, execution time that is spread out, and group time for consultation and coordination of appraisal criteria with peers. The last provides for fairness and equity throughout the organization.

17. The number of performance categories should be small, and no forced ranking should be used. Raters should keep it simple: 10% to 20% of the total, superior (bonus $\times$ 2); 70% to 85%, satisfactory (bonus); and 5% to 10%, questionable or unsatisfactory (no bonus).

18. The form and process should be kept simple: a one- to two-page written contract drafted with the subordinate and containing one to two specific annual or semiannual objectives; one to two personal, group, or team growth or career-enhancement objectives; one to two objectives to improve skills; and one objective related to the team's strategic theme (such as quality improvement). The manager should use open-ended prose as the format, do formal reviews bimonthly or more often, and be able to recall the content of each contract.

19. Performance goals should be straightforward, emphasizing the manager's desired results and considering what is important to the continuing success of the business.

20. Pay decisions should be made public. No one will be embarrassed if there is equity.

21. Formal appraisal should be made a small part of overall recognition that includes listening, recognition, pay, and involvement.

22. Multiple ratings, including those of ratees' subordinates, should be used.[100]

23. To get employees to buy into performance improvement, managers should create a relationship to individual and organizational performance improvement and in turn—to add value to the success of each individual—the department and the organization, identify a measurement for each critical point in the process, and present reports and celebrate monthly at staff meetings.[101]

Evaluating performance can be challenging with the differing conceptual models offered as well as tools to be used to document tasks and roles. Paying for performance is a method that has been successful and rewards value-added behaviors and activities in the workplace.

PAY FOR PERFORMANCE

Pay for performance is based on equity theory, expectancy theory, the law of effect, and psychological fulfillment. Equity theory indicates that people want to be treated equally and fairly by employers. Expectancy theory says that people believe they can achieve certain levels of performance and, if they do, they expect to be rewarded. The law of effect states that behavior will be rewarded when repeated. Equity theory, expectancy theory, and the law of effect, individually or combined, apply when the employee says, "I believe that when I increase my efforts or inputs to produce sustained greater outputs, my employer will increase my rewards." Increased pay that is linked as a reward to increased employee inputs and outputs is pay for performance. When used effectively, the compensation system rewards superior, excellent, and satisfactory performance. People perceive an imbalance in this theory when they put forth greater effort than others but receive the same rewards. They perceive compensation to be inequitable, and pay becomes a dissatisfier.[102] Pay for performance is an incentive program that links pay to employee or corporate performance.[103]

Performance, not longevity, is fast becoming the basis for pay increases in institutions of all sizes. This may apply only to the managerial staff, or it can apply down to the lowest-paid employees in an organization.[104] Pay for performance falls in line with healthcare organizations need for accountability of health care outcomes. Without positive outcomes, reimbursement is affected.

Since the recession of 1982, pay for performance has become the mode for pay increases in business and industry. Of 1,080 Canadian companies surveyed, 64% indicated they would use a merit-only pay increase; 32% would use a general-plus-merit system for pay in-creases.[105] A survey of 250 manufacturers indicated that 76% had incentive-based programs.[106] A 1993 survey of 2,000 U.S. companies indicated that 6% used pay for performance.[107]

> **Results of longitudinal research conducted by the Italian National Health Service indicate that performance-related pay for health service professionals requires a careful implementation process to be a powerful tool at management's disposal to increase employees' performance and commitment.** [108]

Expected Outcomes

Expectancy theory postulates that individuals will choose among alternatives in a rational manner to maximize expected rewards. A study designed to test subjects' choice of a pay plan from among piece rate, fixed rate, and bonus concluded the following[109]:

- Pay choice has a strong impact on subjects' behavior.
- High-ability individuals choose a piece-rate plan or a bonus plan over a fixed-rate plan.
- Individuals tend to choose a pay plan that maximizes their expected rewards.
- Pay choice results in higher pay satisfaction.

Studies of managers and administrators show a positive relationship between pay-for-performance perception and pay satisfaction. A pay rate higher than that of the outside market also results in greater employee satisfaction. Pay system fairness is a function of factors that pertain to organizational justice, such as participation in pay system development, perceived fairness of allocation procedures, and greater understanding of the pay system.[110]

A company's ability to compete and its company–employee relations are improved by creatively managed compensation systems. Performance-based pay affects profitability, with profits increasing when high or good performance is rewarded with pay incentives. Variable pay affects profitability more than does base pay.[111]

There may be a limit to the ratio of pay for performance. A study of 75 college students that related performance to 0%, 10%, 30%, 60%, or 100% of base pay as incentive indicated that whereas 0% pro-duced no significant incentive, "the productivity of subjects in the 10%, 30%, 60% and 100% incentive groups did not differ. They all produced significant incentive."[112]

Compensation is a part of business strategy. A direct link exists between compensation and achieve-ment of established goals. Increased compensation is an incentive for employees to do well. An em-ployee will work to achieve predetermined goals if there are predetermined rewards.[113]

The following are some reasons for basing pay on performance[114]:

1. Increases job satisfaction. Associates who are involved in developing a work plan feel ownership of the process; as a result, they work harder to make their plan successful.
2. Reduces absenteeism
3. Increases productivity. Workers will perform clearly identified behaviors that are rewarded. (Mediocrity should not be rewarded.)
4. Decreases voluntary turnover, which says, "I believe I am worth more. Other employers will pay me more."
5. Improves the quality of the employee mix. This system attracts and keeps higher-level performers.

Zenger reported on a study of 984 engineering employees of two large U.S. high tech companies. The study found that offering pay incentive awards confirmed that "extremely high and moderately low per-formers are likely to remain in firms offering these contracts while moderately high and extremely low per-formers are likely to depart." The contracts with these companies aggressively rewarded extreme performance and largely ignored moderate performance limits. To correct this, the employer can design a system to retain above-average performers and reduce turnover for only the extremely low performers.[115]

Pay for performance rewards what is valued by the employer, which may be time-in-grade and longevity. In a competitive business environment, however, employers are more apt to value new job skills and new knowledge by paying more for performance that demonstrates their use than for longevity.[116]

TYPES OF COMPENSATION PROGRAMS

Figure 18-4 lists the major types of compensation programs.[117]

Pay-for-Performance Process

The following are elements of a pay-for-performance process:[118]

1. Compensation should be part of the strategic planning process. When done with employees or their representatives as part of a task force, the compensation plan is more apt to be perceived as fair and to elicit employees' trust. Company mission, philosophy, objectives, vision, values, and business plans can be guides to developing a compensation plan. Decisions are made on how to link compensation to employee or company performance and hence to individuals ver-

---

FIGURE 18-4 | **MAJOR TYPES OF PAY-FOR-PERFORMANCE (COMPENSATION) PROGRAMS**

Type	Characteristics
Merit Pay	Probably most common. Usually a percentage of base pay. Sometimes part of a pay raise—a percentage for merit and a percentage for longevity. Pay raises are established for each job or group of jobs. Progression at fixed intervals is based on observation of performance. Standards of employees' success are not established a priori. When given as a merit bonus, it is not added to base pay. An individual incentive plan.
Gain Sharing	A profit-sharing plan, usually a group incentive plan. A specific share of the organization's profits is distributed to a group of employees based on production measures, financial performance, and quality of service.
Cash or Lump Sum Bonuses	Usually a share of the profits. Also a group incentive. May be a uniform bonus paid to all or most employees organization-wide.
Pay for Knowledge	Pay is linked to learning new skills and being able to work at a higher level or at more than one specialty.
Employee Stock	Profit-sharing plan. Some pay cash from interest and dividends. Most are deferred plans.
Ownership Plans	Risky link (ESOPs) between pay and performance for these plans. The direct pay contingency is typically quite small and linked to company performance.
Individual Incentive	Compensation is paid for individual performance.
Small Group Incentive	Each member of a group is compensated for achieving predetermined objectives.
Instant Incentive	Individual compensation for noteworthy achievements.
Recognition Programs	Performance awards to individuals or groups. May be money, educational programs, vacation/travel, certificates, or other symbolic award.

Source: Author.

sus groups. It is best to use more than one kind of incentive. The plan should be customized to the organizational culture and core values of a pay system. An obvious link exists between effort and performance and the need for rewards. The organization should consider the need for change and the level(s) of organizational participation. The current compensation system should be assessed for gaps, holes, and overfunding. Potential plan types should then be assigned to close the gaps.

2. Goals should be carefully set. They should be achievable to avoid system errors. When goals are set with employees, they assume ownership of the goals. Organizational performance goals may relate to improving employee motivation, engendering a culture of employees who genuinely care about organizational effectiveness, and tying labor costs to the organization's ability to pay specific amounts. Goals should be made job specific. Consideration of costs of the plan, consistency with plant and division objectives, and fitting the culture of the organization is taken when developing the plan.

3. Standards for measurement should be precise because they are the benchmarks against which performance is met. Participants should be able to influence standards. Standards may include the following:

- Quality standards related to total quality management or continuous quality improvement for eliminating defects or errors
- Safety standards related to all customers, internal and external
- Attendance standards such as pay for unused sick time or paid days off
- Productivity standards related to volume of inputs versus outputs
- A pay-for-performance matrix
- Job descriptions that include specific objectives of each position and measure the accomplishments of those objectives.
- Job descriptions can be developed with input from incumbents. When job descriptions are related to pay for knowledge, new technology may require help from experts and outside vendors. Results of these job descriptions include items such as "trained and motivated crew" and "safety." Each result has one to three or four measures of accomplishment, such as "responsiveness to customer's needs" and "number of machine breakdowns." Preparation to meet pay for knowledge includes massive training efforts that may be done in cooperation with vendors, consultants, and educational institutions. An extensive set of training modules can be developed so that training is directly related to the job description.
- Organizational performance: profitability and financial performance
- Management by objectives
- Critical incidents: innovation, new products and services, market penetration, and targets
- Economic value-added (EVA)
- Some companies are awarding bonuses and stock options to managers on the basis of EVA, which is a way of increasing a company's real profitability. EVA equals the operating profits minus taxes minus the total annual cost of capital. The cost of capital includes interest paid on borrowed capital (less the deductible tax) plus equity capital, the money provided by the shareholders. Equity includes investment in human capital. A positive EVA means wealth is being created, whereas a negative EVA means that capital is being destroyed. EVA can be used for service businesses. EVA can be raised by using less capital and giving shareholders higher dividends. Stock prices go up.
- Cooperation among individuals or groups
- Specific competencies, such as communication, customer focus, adaptability, interpersonal skills, team relationships, and leadership
- Cultural diversity

4. An objective performance appraisal system needs to be established that measures the achievement of the standards as employee outputs. The following are some examples:
   - Completion of specific education and training programs
   - Absence or reduction (including prevention) of accidents, injuries, and illnesses, and measurably reduced pollution
   - Specific problems solved
   - Reduced supply inventories and supply use
   - Reduced patient stays
   - Increased responsibility
   - Reduced costs
   - Demonstrated mastery of knowledge, skills, and abilities

Supervisors should be trained to use the (performance appraisal) system effectively. The performance appraisal system must be objective. Some companies separate performance appraisals from salary reviews. During performance appraisals career development—improvement, job skills, and career growth—is the focus. During the salary review, the focus is on worth—objectives and potential to learn new skills.

Performance standards should not be confused with results or accomplishments. If cultural diversity is a standard that is measured and rewarded, it will be accomplished.

5. A plan needs to be chosen (see Figure 18-4). The structure should be tailored to the performance dimensions of the job.
6. Necessary policies and procedures for implementing the plan must be written and communicated to the participants. All employees need to understand the system, that is, what it is and how it works.
7. The plan is then implemented and monitored.
8. The effectiveness of the plan is evaluated.

GROUP VERSUS INDIVIDUAL PLANS

Group Plans

Group incentive plans include small groups or work units to which rewards are allocated for group performance exceeding predefined standards, productivity improvement plans, and profit-sharing plans. These plans are designed to encourage teamwork and cooperation with shared profits, information, responsibility, accountability, and participation in decision making.

Group variable pay is used for meeting goals based on collaborative performance and teamwork and thus encourages communication. Quality can become a team sport and a win–win situation. Group variable pay is flexible and can respond to multiple goals and measures and to change. Group variable pay should be funded independently of other pay plans.[119]

Most compensation plans tend to be indecisive. People expect to be rewarded when they increase their output because of work redesign. Managers act as their coaches and facilitators in the process.[120] Teams, not individuals, increasingly are being rewarded for good work that results in innovation, increased cost control, and higher morale. Team leaders or managers set up worthwhile goals that are easy to measure. Everyone from plant manager on down receives the same annual raise for achieving or exceeding goals. The percentage of pay is set by goals that may be divided between those of the unit and organization. Employees are involved in designing team-based incentive programs. A trusting work relationship is needed. Some companies have teams of 25 to 50 employees who supervise themselves; they have no time clock and no foreperson. After a 3-month probation period, teams take over evaluation. When employee performance is substandard, the team recommends improvement programs, probation, or termination. The team helps hire new employees. Team members identify free riders and layabouts.[120]

Individual Plans

Individual merit pay can create internal competition for pay raises and the withholding of information from each other by competing employees. It encourages individuals to try to improve the system on their own, a difficult job to accomplish. Individual merit pay also uses individual quality outcome measures, which are difficult to develop meaningfully. It encourages a microfocus, decreases flexibility, and produces anxiety.

Competency Model

Individual accomplishments are temporary and variable, whereas competencies and salaries are additive over time. Competency reflects individual performance; accomplishments can result from individual or group efforts. A value-added pay system combines base salary to employee competency and rewards individual or team accomplishment with one-time lump-sum awards. Employees are paid and rewarded for actual accomplishments, and fixed payroll costs are reduced. As employees move through competency levels, the salaries are planned to reflect this. Thus employees are paid what they are worth to the organization. Employees who exceed goals add value to their positions. The value-added compensation approach is motivational and controls costs.[120]

Benner's research, using the Dreyfuss Model of Skills Acquisition, could be used as the competency model for a pay-for-performance system. Base pay would mirror the five levels of proficiency: novice, advanced beginner, competent, proficient, and expert. A nurse who bettered the time line for achieving a higher level of proficiency could be paid a lump-sum bonus for the accomplishment.[121]

PAY DESIGNS

Many employees are willing to risk fat bonuses for superb results. The risk is that bonuses go down with recession. Bonuses hold down fixed costs; merit raises increase costs, driving up retirement benefits.

A study by Schwab and Olson produced a number of findings. These findings included that the implementation of a conventional merit system achieved a considerably better link between pay and performance than did a bonus system. A bonus system without periodic adjustments in base wages also performed less well than a conventional merit system, because merit systems benefit from the consistency of true performance over time. One surprising finding was that even a very substantial error in the measurement of performance had only a modest effect on the pay–performance correlation.[122]

Rewards should be consistent, fair, timely, and related to work. They should also be ample. In a pay-for-performance system, the outcomes include increased productivity from "overpaid" performers and rewards for underpaid performers.

> *Money to fund programs sometimes comes from senior managers who give up their bonuses. Companies also use money from attrition.*

The Quaker Oats pet food plant at Lawrence, Kansas paid employees 5% to 10% above market to attract and retain above-average employees and remain nonunion.[123] To achieve maximal effect on employees, base pay must be kept at a level at or above the industry average. Also, labor costs must be reduced by using incentives not added into base pay.

HOW TO DO A MERIT PAY INCREASE

Merit is a term that is becoming increasingly associated with performance and pay increases for nurses. Merit may be based on the current market value within the geographical region for the position. Currently, nurses are valuable because of the nursing shortage, so market value is high. If the nurse shortage resolves and nurses become plentiful, then merit pay may adjust downward in response. Merit means that employees receive what they deserve. Pay and rewards are based on the degree of competence employees demonstrate in performing their jobs. Merit systems can include both rewards and punishments. The general goal of a merit performance and pay system is to reward people on an incremental scale so that the top achievers or performers are paid the highest salaries. A merit pay system must have four components:

1. Individual performance standards
2. Measurement scales
3. A budget
4. An award procedure

Merit pay increases are an employee incentive program. Employees who have their competencies developed, encouraged, and recognized have better attitudes about their work and their employers. These employees work to achieve organizational objectives that support their personal objectives. Merit rewards or punishments are extrinsic. The reward or punishment can be in the form of promotion, praise, recognition, criticism, social acceptance or rejection, or benefits.[124]

Many of these rewards or punishments are activated with a total merit pay system. Extrinsic rewards need to be associated with the intrinsic rewards that come from employees' participation in making decisions about their work and the conditions under which they perform their work. Professional nurses want control of their nursing practice. They want to participate in management decisions about how they accomplish this. As a result, they receive intrinsic rewards from having made the organization successful, because they have contributed to that success.

Performance Standards

Individual performance standards are written criteria developed by the supervisor in conference with the individual to be evaluated. They evolve from an established, more generalized set of job performance criteria, the job description. These performance standards are tailored to the individual's abilities and goals and to the common expectations of the individual and that person's supervisor. These standards should be measurable, and they should be objectively applied. The supervisor and employee can both observe or know that the standards have been met. These standards can be written in the format of a performance results contract related to the job description. Figure 18-5 represents a division of nursing policy. The procedure for implementing this policy involves use of a job description and a performance results contract (Figure 18-6).

Measurement Scales

The weights assigned to each key results area can be in terms of units or percentages. It is more practical to assign up to 1.0 unit to each key results area and determine the percentage of achievement at the annual or final conference. Doing so allows objectives to be added, modified, or deleted without readjusting the percentage weight. In Figure 18-7, the weights are the numbers assigned to each key results area. The total of these is 100. If the employee achieves 90, then the percentage of achievement for merit pay purposes is 90%. This percentage is used to allocate budgeted wage and salary increases.

Budget

Personnel pay increases are usually projected in the operational budget represented by the excerpt in Figure 18-7. They can be related to increases in the consumer price index, to the marketplace, or to the financial status of the institution. The financial status must be a major consideration. The human re-

| **FIGURE 18-5** | **POLICY AND EVALUATION OF EMPLOYEE PERFORMANCE** |

All nursing service employees will have a criteria-based performance evaluation as follows:

1. Initiated on nursing service employee orientation.

2. At the end of the probationary period (3 months).

3. Annually (to be initiated during the following evaluation period for all employees). The annual performance evaluation will be cosigned by the head nurse or supervisor and employee, and filed in the employee's personnel file.

4. When an employee terminates employment or transfers, there will be an evaluation conference. A completed performance results contract will be cosigned by the employee and head nurse/supervisor, then placed in the personnel file.

Conferences and renegotiations concerning the criteria-based performance evaluation may occur as often as the employee/supervisor deems necessary.

Source: Author.

| **FIGURE 18-6** | **SAMPLE PERFORMANCE RESULTS CONTRACT** |

1. Scope of Responsibility

As clinical nurse consultant, assumes responsibility to improve the quality of health care received by the patient in the defined clinical area of expertise through role modeling, teaching, consultation, and research. The consultant assists nursing personnel to achieve their full potential and satisfaction in providing effective, efficient, and individualized care to patients and their families. The clinical nurse consultant is self-directed, determining the priorities of the role through inter- and intradisciplinary collaboration. Evaluates own practice based on the attainment of individual objectives. Responsible to the director of nursing for staff development.

2. Key Results Areas

Performance Results	**Individual's Performance**
a. Schedule monthly meetings with head nurse of each unit to discuss needs and to plan for utilization of clinical consultant in meeting those needs.	I would like to see more assertive behavior in this area. Meetings were often put off and not enough consistent followup—head nurses to set a time. 8%
b. Present in-service for each area as contracted with head nurses.	Observations and needs should be made by both parties in setting up classes. This area has improved since January in some units. 7%
c. Work with department members to evaluate and revise nursing orientation program.	Done. New schedule completed. Meeting held—head nurses of 5th, 6th, 7th, and 8th floors. 10%
d. Orient new staff to orientation program.	Worked with [Name]. 10%
e. Coordinate nursing orientation program with Staff Development, Personnel Relations, and Nursing Service.	Continuous need for smooth coordination and double-checking on dates. 9%
f. Review and revise medication exam as necessary.	Recommendation made to [Name]. 10%
g. Assist in teaching CPR as directed.	Class taught as scheduled. 10%
h. Continue to coordinate and present Drug Update.	Aminoglycoside (antihypertensive agents, penicillin—March). Series started in September—was delayed in starting. Need for assertion in meeting this objective. 9%

(continues)

Performance Results	Individual's Performance
i. Present classes based on needs survey.	Equipment Fair done. Coordinated with [Name]. 10%
j. Participate in critical care course—present emergency reinsertion of tracheostomy tube.	Content approved by Alabama Board of Nursing. Very poor evaluations from second class, with many negative comments written and verbalized. 7%

Complete for Terminal Evaluation Only

	Excellent	Good	Fair	Poor
Attendance				
Initiative				
Quantity of work				
Cooperation				

Eligible for rehire ____Yes ____No

3. Authority Codes
   A. Does without reporting
   B. Does and reports
   C. Gets approval before doing
   D. Participates in
   E. Recommends to supervisor
   F. Assists supervisor under direction

Summary

[Name] has been flexible in coming in for in-service programs on 7–3 and 11–7 shifts. Has completed most of the areas on the performance contract satisfactorily. Is generally well received by new employees and helpful in their orientation to Metropolitan Medical Center.

I would like for [Name] to take more initiative and to be more assertive in identifying needs with the head nurses of the clinical units and in addressing those needs promptly and consistently. [Name] has been active in emergency admission unit and I would like to see more activity on 7th and 8th floors and the NITU.

I would also ask [Name] to address concerns and questions to me directly.

Director Staff Development	May 8, 20xx

Source: Courtesy of the University of South Alabama Medical Center, Mobile, AL.

sources department usually prepares a cost analysis by position (Figure 18-8). This cost analysis is the bridge for merit pay increases for the total nursing division.

Award Procedure

Nurse administrators take all performance results contracts for each category of nursing personnel and add up the percent totals for all persons (for the nurse in Figure 18-7, this was 90%.). The total for registered teaching nurse II (RTN II) was 1.911%. This number is divided into the total budgeted dollars for RTN II, which was $19,263 (the sum of the amounts for filled and vacant positions labeled "Cost" in Figure 18-8). For each percent, each person in this category will be allocated $10.08. A person who receives a 90% merit pay increase will receive 90 × $10.08 = $907.20 (Figure 18-9). This amount is transferred to a personnel action memorandum and processed through payroll. Each employee is told by the supervisor how much merit pay he or she will receive.

FIGURE 18-7   CALCULATING MONETARY–MERIT INCREASE FOR RTN II POSITIONS

Percent	Amount	Percent	Amount
100	$1,008	71	$716
99	998	70	706
98	988	69	696
97	978	68	685
96	968	67	675
95	958	66	665
94	948	65	655
93	937	64	645
92	927	63	635
91	917	62	625
90	907	61	615
89	897	60	605
88	887	50	504
87	877	40	403
86	867	30	302
85	857	20	202

Source: Author.

The Process

- Step 1. Employee and supervisor have a conference at an appointed time to establish the key results (objectives) that the employee will accomplish over an agreed-on period of time. These results include organizational objectives from the supervisor and personal objectives of the employee. Each will come to the conference table prepared to present the objectives in an atmosphere of mutual trust and cooperation. At this conference the wording of the key results areas will be negotiated, weights will be assigned to each, time frames will be established, controls or reporting authority will be established, and the approximate date will be set for the next evaluation conference.
- Step 2. A definitive date is established, and the next conference is held. At this conference the supervisor and employee discuss progress in accomplishment of key results areas. The supervisor and employee modify objectives by negotiation, discard those they agree are no longer relevant, add new ones as needed, and discuss and record progress in the accomplishment of each objective. This conference and all succeeding ones can be scheduled at earlier dates on supervisor or employee request.
- Step 3. Conferences are scheduled at 1- to 3-month intervals until the probationary period is completed, the annual rating is required, or the employee transfers or terminates. At these times the contract is summarized, signed by employee and supervisor, and filed in the employee's personnel folder. The weights assigned by negotiated discussion are totaled, and a number is assigned. This number is used in allocating the merit pay increase.

FIGURE 18-8 **BUDGET FOR 4% MERIT PAY INCREASE**

Nursing Positions		FTE	Total Current		FTE	Total Current
Position Classification	Filled	Salaries	Cost	Vacant	Salaries	Cost
Licensed practical nurse	84.50	$1,108,339	$44,334	9.00	$110,021	$4,401
RTN I—clinical level I	249.00	4,607,379	184,295	18.00	312,794	$12,512
RTN I—clinical level II	14.00	292,921	11,717	1.00	20,255	810
RTN I—clinical level IIII	1.00	22,755	910	0.00	0	0
RTN I (working supervisor)	45.00	893,820	35,753	0.00	0	0
Registered teaching nurse II	20.00	443,126	17,725	2.00	38,438	1,538
Nursing service supervisor I	11.50	266,910	10,676	2.00	40,228	1,609
	425.00	$7,635,250	$305,410	32.00	$521,736	$20,869
Total cost: Annual			$305,410			$20,869
Monthly			$25,451			$1,739

Source: Author.

FIGURE 18-9 **STANDARDS FOR EVALUATION OF PAY-FOR-PERFORMANCE PROGRAMS**

1. There are pay-for-performance programs.
2. They were developed with input from employees.
3. They are based on company philosophy, goals, objectives, and vision.
4. They have policies and procedures.
5. The goals are job-specific.
6. There are standards for measurement.
7. They are linked to an objective performance appraisal system.
8. Rewards are linked to effort and performance.
9. Employees are informed about the programs.
10. Employees trust the programs.
11. Managers are well trained and skilled in administering the programs.
12. The programs are funded or budgeted.
13. An evaluation program is in place to monitor the programs.
14. Productivity and performance outcomes are being measured.
15. The plans are accomplishing the stated objectives.

Source: Author.

Merit pay is a difficult procedure to accomplish because employees may not agree with the outcome. Also, supervisors are hesitant to make decisions that give employees variable pay increases. Some experts suggest that merit performance appraisal for pay be separated from performance appraisal done for other purposes. We found that the two can work together when planned, communicated, and fairly applied.

SUMMARY

Performance appraisal is a major component of the evaluating or controlling function of nursing management. Organizations are successful when employees are held accountable for performance. If used appropriately and conscientiously, the performance appraisal process governs employee behavior to produce goods and services in high volume and of high quality. Pay for performance integrates concepts from performance appraisal to enhance further this evaluation process.

Performance appraisal is a part of the science of behavioral technology and should be viewed as part of that body of knowledge. Nurse managers need this knowledge to manage the clinical nurse effectively and efficiently as a human resource.

When used for merit pay increases, a retrospective use, performance appraisal should be separated from appraisal that looks to the future. Output-based pay plans are more effective than are time-based pay plans.

Performance appraisal should be done as a system with

1. Clearly defined performance standards developed by rater and ratee
2. Objective application of the performance standards, with both rater and ratee measuring the ratee's performance against the standards
3. Planned interval feedback with agreed-on improvements when indicated
4. A continuous cycle (Raters and ratees should trust each other.)

Job analysis and job description are essential instruments of behavior technology used in performance appraisal that provide objectivity and discriminate among jobs. Coaching, counseling, and interviewing are skills of an effective performance appraisal system. In addition to supervisor ratings, performance appraisal can include peer ratings, self-ratings, TEC, BARS, and TOPES.

"Teams are effective in implementing pay-for-performance plans."

The purposes or uses of performance appraisal are multiple. In nursing, performance appraisal is used to motivate employees to produce high-quality patient care. The results of performance appraisal are often used for promotion, selection, and termination and to improve performance. Incentive programs are very common in organizations. The trend is to link pay to employee or corporate performance. Doing so motivates employees to increase productivity, especially when tied to operational measures such as attendance, quality, and safety. The most common individual performance-based pay plans are merit, awards, piece rates, and commissions.

A pay-for-performance plan should be communicated well, have measures that can be influenced by participants, be consistent and fair, provide ample and timely rewards, and be trustworthy.

Participants in a pay-for-performance plan often risk the choice of earning less for the chance to earn more later through higher retirement benefits. Pay for performance starts with reduced wages and salaries, although the base should equal or slightly exceed the industry standard.

Equity theory, expectancy theory, and the law of effect are the basis for pay for performance. People expect equal pay for equal work and increased rewards for increased output.

Problems with performance appraisal systems (as well as pay-for-performance plans) include poor preparation of raters and ratees, problems of recency, halo and horns effects, lack of use of standards, leniency/stringency errors, similar-to-me errors, central tendency errors, and first impression errors.

A simple, well-planned performance appraisal system can be devised. It will be successful when understood by employees and will require considerable supervisory effort using nursing management theory.

APPLICATION EXERCISES

Exercise 18-1

If a pay-for-performance program does not exist in your organization, prepare a proposal for one. Present it to your supervisor and the director of human resources. You may want to do this as a group exercise.

Results of longitudinal research conducted by the Italian National Health Service indicate that performance-related pay for health service professionals requires a careful implementation process to be a powerful tool at management's disposal to increase employees' performance and commitment.

Exercise 18-2

Use Figure 18-9 to evaluate the pay-for-performance programs in a healthcare organization. These may be individual awards, such as merit awards, piece rate, or individual commissions, or they may be group awards, such as gain sharing, profit sharing, stock options, or bonuses.

How can the programs be improved? Make a management plan for improving them and present it to your supervisor and the director of human resources.

Exercise 18-3

Determine the extent to which a nurse manager exhibits coaching behaviors. Apply these coaching behaviors to yourself or have a group of peers apply it to themselves, and use the results for discussion.

Exercise 18-4

With a group of peers, discuss whether the performance appraisal system is too complicated. If it is, how can it be simplified and still meet accreditation and legal requirements? Are these requirements keeping the system too complicated? If so, how?

Exercise 18-5

With a group of peers, discuss how the job descriptions can be modified in a manner that is consistent with the vision of the organization. The goal is to make them objective and usable.

Notes

1. Cohen, M. (2007). *What you accept is what you teach, setting standards for employee accountability.* Minnesota: Creative Health Care Management, Inc.
2. Ibid., pp. 14–21.
3. Krantz, S. (1983). Five steps to making performance appraisal writing. *Supervisory Management, 1,* 7–10.
4. Zemke, R. (1985). Is performance appraisal a paper tiger? *Training, 1,* 24–32.
5. Krantz, 1983.
6. Fombrun, C. J., & Land, R. L. (1983). Strategic issues in performance appraisal: Theory and practice. *Personnel, 1,* 23–31.
7. Moroney, B. P., & Buckley, M. R. (1992). Does research in performance appraisal influence the practice of performance appraisal? Regretfully not! *Public Personnel Management, 4,* 185–195.
8. Bretz, R. D., Milkovich, G. T., & Read, W. (1992). The current state of performance appraisal research and practice: Concerns, directions and implications. *Journal of Management, 8,* 321–352.
9. Hochwarter, W. A., Witt, L. A., & Kacmar, K. M. (2000). Perceptions of organizational politics as a moderator of the relationship between conscientiousness and job performance. *Journal of Applied Psychology, 9,* 472–478.

10. Fombrun & Land, 1983.

11. Schneier, C. E., Geis, A., & Wert, J. A. (1987). Performance appraisals: No appointment needed. *Personnel Journal, 1,* 80–87.

12. Zemke, 1985.

13. Levenstein, A. (1984). Feedback improves performance. *Nursing Management, 1,* 65–66.

14. Zemke, 1985.

15. Kirkpatrick, D. L. (1986). Performance appraisal: When two jobs are too many. *Training, 65,* 67–69.

16. Ibid.

17. Kopelman, R. E. (1983). Linking pay to performance is a proven management tool. *Personnel Administrator, 9,* 60–68.

18. Ibid.

19. Ibid.

20. Deets, N. R., & Tyler, D. T. (1986). How Xerox improved its performance appraisals. *Personnel Journal,* 50–52.

21. Jacobson, B., & Kaye, B. L. (1986). Career development and performance appraisal: It takes two to tango. *Personnel Magazine,* 26–32.

22. Kelly, K. J. (1990). Administrator's forum. *Journal of Nursing Staff Development,* 255–257.

23. Jambunathan, J. (1992). Planning a peer review program. *Journal of Nursing Staff Development,* 235–239.

24. Fulmer, R. M., & Franklin, S. G. (1982). *Supervision: Principles of professional management* (2nd ed., pp. 214–215). New York: Macmillan.

25. Koontz, H., & Weihrich, H. (1988). *Management* (9th ed., pp. 490–494). New York: McGraw-Hill.

26. Ganong, J. M., & Ganong, W. L. (1980). *Nursing management* (2nd ed., p. 191). Gaithersburg, MD: Aspen.

27. Blai, B. (1983). An appraisal system that yields results. *Supervisory Management,* 39–42.

28. Friedman, M. G. (1986). 10 steps to objective appraisals. *Personnel Journal,* 66–71.

29. Rambur, B. (1999). Fostering evidence-based practice in nursing education. *Journal of Professional Nursing,* 270–274; Aliotta, S. L. (2000). Focus on case management: Linking outcomes and accountability. *Topics in Health Information Management,* 11–16; Frankel, A. J., & Heft-LaPorte, H. (1998). Tracking case management accountability: A systems approach. *Journal of Case Management,* 105–111.

30. Edwards, M. R., & Sproull, J. R. (1985). Safeguarding your employee rating system. *Business,* 17–27.

31. Price, S., & Graber, J. (1986). Employee-made appraisals. *Management World,* 34–36.

32. Ignatavicius, D., & Griffith, J. (1982). Job analysis: The basis for effective appraisal. *Journal of Nursing Administration,* 37–41.

33. Dienemann, J., & Shaffer, C. (1992). Faculty performance appraisal systems: Procedures and criteria. *Journal of Professional Nursing,* 148–154.

34. Markowitz, J. (1987). Managing the job analysis process. *Training and Development Journal,* 64–66.

35. Ignatavicius & Griffith, 1982; Markowitz, 1987; Prien, E. P., Goldstein, I. L., & Macey, W. H. (1987). Multidomain job analysis: Procedures and applications. *Training and Development Journal,* 68–72.

36. Coaly, P. R., & Sackett, P. R. (1987). Effects of using high- versus low-performing job incumbents as sources of job analysis information. *Journal of Applied Psychology,* 434–437.

37. Denton, D. K. (1992). Redesigning a job by simplifying every task and responsibility. *Industrial Engineering,* 46–48.

38. Ibid.

39. Wolfe, M. N., & Coggins, S. (1997). The value of job analysis, job description and performance. *Medical Group Management Journal,* 42–44, 46–48, 50–52; Conn, V. S., Davis, N. K., & Occena, L. G. (1996). Analyzing jobs for redesign decisions. *Nursing Economics,* 145–150.

40. Berenson, C., & Ruhnke, H. O. (1966). Job descriptions: Guidelines for personnel management. *Personnel Journal,* 14–19.

41. Webb, P. R., & Cantone, R. J. (1993). Performance evaluation: Triumph or torture? *Journal of Home Health Care Practice,* 14–19.

42. Kleinpell, R. M. (1999). Evolving role descriptions of the acute care nurse practitioner. *Critical Care Nursing Quarterly,* 9–15; Quaal, S. J. (1999). Clinical nurse specialist: Role restructuring to advanced practice registered nurse. *Critical Care Nursing Quarterly,* 37–49; Nemeth, L. (1999). Leadership for coordinated care: Role of a project manager. *Critical Care Nursing Quarterly,* 50–58.

43. Kennedy, W. R. (1987). Train managers to write winning job descriptions. *Training and Development Journal,* 62–64.

44. Rowland, H. S., & Rowland, B. L. (Eds.). (1987). *Hospital legal forms, checklists, and guidelines* (pp. 23–28). Gaithersburg, MD: Aspen.

45. Peters, T. (1987). *Thriving on chaos* (pp. 596–597). New York: Harper & Row.

46. Ibid.

47. Waintroob, A. (1985). Comparable worth issue: The employers side. *The Hospital Manager,* 6–7.

48. TNA's Professional Services Committee. (1985). Nurses and the comparable worth concept. *Texas Nursing,* 12–16.

49. How to establish the comparable worth of a job: Or one way to compare apples and oranges. (1982). *California Nurse,* 10–11; TNA's Professional Services Committee, 1985.

50. Helton, B. R. (1987). Will the real knowledge worker please stand up? *Industrial Management,* 26–29.

51. Kopelman, R. G. (1985). Job redesign and productivity: A review of the evidence. *National Productivity Review,* 237–255.

52. Bolster, C. J. (1991). Work redesign: More than rearranging furniture on the Titanic. *Aspen's Advisor for Nurse Executives,* 4–7.

53. Kanter, R. M. (1990). *When giants learn to dance* (pp. 75–82). New York: Simon & Schuster.

54. Bolster, 1991.

55. Martin, D. C., & Bardol, K. M. (1986). Training the raters: A key to effective performance appraisal. *Public Personnel Management,* 101–109.

56. Edwards & Sproull, 1985.

57. Ibid.

58. Balcazar, F., Hopkin, B. L., & Suarez, Y. (1985). A critical, objective review of performance feedback. *Journal of Organizational Behavior Management, 1,* 65–89.

59. Martin & Bardol, 1986; Friedman, 1986.

60. Ratcliffe, T. A., & Logsdon, D. J. (1980). The business planning process: A behavioral perspective. *Managerial Planning,* 32–38.

61. Edward & Sproull, 1985.

62. Schneier, Geis, & Wert, 1987.

63. Lachman, V. D. (1984). Increasing productivity through performance evaluation. *Journal of Nursing Administration, 1,* 7–14.

64. Frankel, L. P., & Ofuzo, K. L. (1992). Employee coaching: The way to gain compliance. *Employment Relations Today, 5,* 311–320.

65. Ibid.

66. Lachman, 1984.

67. Martin & Bardol, 1986.

68. Wilbers, S. (1993, May 23). Performance reviews can be easier. *San Antonio Express-News,* p. 3G.

69. Ibid.

70. Booker, G. S., & Miller, R. W. (1966). A closer look at peer ratings. *Personnel, 1,* 42–47.

71. Strom, P. S., Strom, R. D., & Moore, E. G. (1999). Peer and self-evaluation of teamwork skills. *Journal of Adolescence, 9,* 539–553.

72. Friedman, 1986.

73. Jambunathan, 1992.

74. Jurf, J. B., Ecoff, L., Haley, W., Keegan, P. L., & Williams, P. A. (1992). First steps toward peer review. *Journal of Nursing Staff Development,* 184–186.

75. Jacobs, M. E., & Vail, J. D. (1986). Quality assurance: A unit-based plan. *Journal of the Association of Nurse Anesthetists,* 265–271.

76. Ibid.; Jambunathan, 1992.

77. Jacobs & Vail, 1986; Jurf et al., 1992; Jambunathan, 1992.

78. Ibid.

79. Rigg, M. (1992). Reasons for removing employee evaluations from management control. *Industrial Engineering,* 17.

80. Jambunathan, 1992; Jurf et al., 1992.

81. Gregg, A. C., & Bloom, K. C. (1999). Performance evaluation and patient outcomes monitored by nurse practitioners and certified nurse–midwives in Florida. *Clinical Excellence in Nursing Practice,* 279–285.
82. Fombrun & Land, 1983.
83. Zemke, 1985.
84. Price, S., & Graber, J. (1986). Employee-made appraisals. *Management World,* 34–36; Andrusyszyn, M. A. (1990). Faculty evaluation: A closer look at peer review. *Nurse Education Today,* 410–414.
85. Ibid.
86. Lovrich, M. P. (1985). The dangers of participative management: A test of unexamined assumptions concerning employee involvement. *Review of Public Personnel Administration,* 9–25.
87. Jacobson & Kaye, 1986.
88. Somers, M. J., & Birnbaum, D. (1991). Assessing self-appraisal of job performance as an evaluation device: Are the poor results a function of method or methodology? *Human Relations,* 1081–1091.
89. Ballinger, J., & Ferko, J., III. (1989). Peer evaluations. *Emergency,* 28–31.
90. Van der Heijden, B. I. (2000). Professional expertise of higher level employees: Age stereotyping in self-assessments and supervisor ratings. *Tijdschrift voor Gerontologie en Geriatrie,* 62–69.
91. Shore, I. H., Shole, L. H., & Thornton, G. C., III. (1992). Construct validity of self- and peer evaluation of performance dimensions in an assessment center. *Journal of Applied Psychology,* 42–54.
92. Edwards & Sproull, 1985.
93. Zemke, 1985; Edwards & Sproull, 1985.
94. Bushardt, S. C., & Fowler, A. R., Jr. (1988). Performance evaluation alternatives. *Journal of Nursing Administration,* 40–44.
95. Ibid.
96. Fox, W. M. (1969). Evaluating and developing subordinates. *Notes and Quotes,* 4.
97. Coyant, J. C. (1973). The performance appraisal: A critique and an alternative. *Business Horizons,* 73–78.
98. Lofton, R. E. (1985). Performance appraisal: Why they go wrong and how to do them right. *National Productivity Review,* 54–63.
99. Ibid.
100. Moen, J. T. (2004). Performance appraisal systems. *Public Personnel Management, 5,* 243–248.
101. Mainstone, L. E., & Levi, A. S. (1987). Fundamentals of statistical process control. *Journal of Organizational Behavior Management, 9,* 5–21.
102. Krantz, 1983; Martin & Bardol, 1986; Logan, C. (1985). Praise: The powerhouse of self-esteem. *Nursing Management, 36,* 38; Friedman, 1986; Schneier et al., 1987; Edwards & Sproull, 1985; Breeze, E. Y. (1968). The performance review. *Manage,* 6–11; Dienemann & Shaffer, 1992; Peters, 1987.
103. MacFalda, P. A. (1998). Performance improvement: How to get employee buy-in. *Radiology Management,* 35–44.
104. Appelbaum, S. H., & Shapiro, B. T. (1992). Pay for performance: Implementation of individual and group plans. *Management Decision: Quarterly Review of Management Technology,* 86–91.
105. Grossmann, J. (1992). Pay, performance and productivity. *Small Business Reports,* 50–59.
106. Browdy, J. D. (1989). Performance appraisal and pay for performance start at the top. *Health Care Supervisor,* 31–41.
107. Appelbaum & Shapiro, 1992.
108. Grossmann, 1992.
109. Tully, S. (1993, November 1). Your paycheck gets exciting. *Fortune,* 83–84, 88, 95, 98.
110. Adinolfi, P. (1998). Performance-related pay for health service professionals: The Italian experience. *Health Service Management Research,* 211–220.
111. Farh, J.-L., Griffith, R. W., & Balkin, D. B. (1991). Effects of choice of pay plans on satisfaction, goal setting, and performance. *Journal of Organizational Behavior, 12,* 55–62.
112. Miceli, M. P., Jung, I., Near, J. P., & Greenberger, D. B. (1991). Predictions and outcomes of reactions to pay-for-performance plans. *Journal of Applied Psychology,* 508–521.
113. Milkovich, G., & Milkovich, C. (1992). Strengthening the pay–performance relationship: The research. *Compensation & Benefits Review,* 53–62.
114. Frisch, C. J., & Dickinson, M. A. (1990). Work productivity as a function of the percentage of monetary incentives to base pay. *Journal of Organizational Behavior Management, 11,* 13–33.

115. Berger, S., & Moyer, J. (1991, August 19). Launching a performance-based pay plan. *Modern Healthcare,* 64.

116. Parnell, J. A. Performance appraisals and paying for excellence. *Journal of Organizational Behavior, 10,* 48–52.

117. Zenger, T. R. (1992). Why do employers only reward extreme performance? Examining the relationships among performance, pay, and turnover. *Administrative Science Quarterly,* 198–219.

118. Williamson, R. M. (1992). Reward what you value and reach new maintenance performance levels. *Plant Engineering,* 113–114.

119. Appelbaum & Shapiro, 1992; Grossman, 1992; Conte, M. A., & Kruse, D. (1991). ESOPs and profit-sharing plans: Do they link employee pay to company performance? *Financial Management,* 91–100; Schwab, D. P., & Olson, C. A. (1990). Merit-pay practice implications for pay–performance relationships. *Industrial and Labor Relations Review,* 237S–255S; Jones, D. W., & Hanser, M. C. (1991). Putting teeth into pay-for-performance programs. *Healthcare Financial Management, 32,* 34–35, 40, 42.

120. Grossmann, 1992; Appelbaum & Shapiro, 1992; Guthrie, J. P., & Cunningham, E. P. (1992). Pay for performance for hourly workers: The Quaker Oats alternative. *Compensation & Benefits Review,* 18–23; Meng, G. J. (1992). Using job descriptions, performance and pay innovations to support quality: A paper company's experience. *National Productivity Review,* 247–255; Performance reviews key in pay for performance and pay. (1993, May 10). *Wall Street Journal,* p. B1; Milkovich & Milkovich, 1992; Berger & Moyer, 1991; Tully, S. (1993, September 20). The real key to creating wealth. *Fortune,* 38–39, 44–45, 48, 50; MacLean, B. P. (1990). Value-added pay beats traditional merit programs. *Personnel Journal,* 46, 48–50, 52; Greenwald, J. (1991, April 15). Workers: Risks and rewards. *Time,* 42–43; Thornburg, L. (1992a). Pay for performance: What you should know. *HR Magazine,* 58–61; Thornburg, L. (1992b). How do you cut the cake? *HR Magazine,* 66–68, 70, 72; McNally, K. A. (1992). Compensation as a strategic tool. *HR Magazine,* 38–40; Browdy, 1989.

121. Benner, P. (1984). From novice to expert: Excellence and power in clinical nursing practice. Menlo Park, CA: Addison-Wesley.
122. Schwab, D. P., & Olson, C. A. Merit pay practices: Implications of pay-performance relationships, *Industrial Labor Relations Review, 43*, Special Issues, 237.
123. Guthrie, J. P., & Cunningham, E. P. (1992). Pay for performance for hourly workers: The Quaker Oats Alternative, *Compensation Benefits Review, 24*, 18–23.
124. Sturman, M. C. (2006). Using your pay system to improve employees' performance: How you pay makes a difference. *Cornell Hospitality Reports 6*, 13, October, 8–14.

References

Falcone, P. (2007). *Productive performance appraisals.* AMAC, American Management Association. Washington, DC.

Fallon, L. F., & McConnell, C. R. (2007). *Human resource management in health care: Principles and practice.* Sudbury, MA: Jones and Bartlett Publishers.

Marqulus, L. S., & Melin, J. A. (2005). *Performance appraisals made easy.* Corwin Press.

Niespodziani, C. A. (2007). The CMS-JCAHO crosswalk: A side-by-side analysis of the CMS conditions. HC Pro, Inc.

Shi, L. (2007). *Managing human resources in health care organizations.* Sudbury, MA: Jones and Bartlett Publishers.

19 THE PROFESSIONAL NURSING STAFF EDUCATOR

Debbie Faulk, PhD, RN
Arlene Morris, EdD, RN

LEARNING OBJECTIVES AND ACTIVITIES

- Describe the staff development process.
- Synthesize the impact of the American Organization of Nurse Executives' guiding principles on the role of the staff development educator.
- Describe the roles of staff development educators and factors that impact roles and responsibilities.
- Distinguish the characteristics of adult learners.
- Integrate adult learning principles into program design.
- Apply strategies to promote critical thinking.
- Describe current trends impacting the healthcare delivery system and the impact on professional nurse staff development educators.
- Examine future issues related to the staff development educator role.

CONCEPTS

Staff development, adult learning, critical thinking, quality and safety, evidence-based practice.

> ### QUOTE
>
> *The important thing to realize is that without necessarily being creative, a leader plays an indispensable role in the process of creation. As a crucial member of the field, a gatekeeper to the domain, the individual in a leadership position holds the keys for turning wild ideas into practical reality.*
>
> —Mihaly Csikszentmihalyi

NURSE MANAGER BEHAVIORS	NURSE EXECUTIVE BEHAVIORS
Utilizes the staff development process to coordinate learning experiences for nursing staff.	Meets legal and accreditation standards for personnel competency through professional staff development; provides financial and human resources; establishes policies for staff development; provides release time for staff to attend continuing education offerings; motivates employees to assume personal responsibility for professional development; provides mechanisms to identify staff growth needs; evaluates the effects of staff participation in continuing education offerings on quality of client care.

Introduction

After two decades of dramatic, rapid changes to the healthcare delivery system, nurses employed in clinical practice settings continue to adjust to multiple roles while striving to maintain a value of "client first." Economic constraints brought on by policy changes for reimbursement, rapid changes in technologies, and restructuring/corporate mergers continue to drive changes in healthcare delivery systems across settings. Staff development departments have been changed by these events, resulting in doubts and concerns related to how quality and client outcomes are impacted by educational endeavors. Marquis and Huston, however, believe that staff development can actually be a "cost-effective method of increasing productivity."[1] Staff development is vital to clarify the role expectations of multiple nursing education levels of preparation and to promote quality, safe, client-centered care. As staff and client needs change, staff development becomes the lifeblood of a professional nurse, allowing application of new research and methods in practice, which then translates to improved client outcomes.

In 2003 the American Organization of Nurse Executives (AONE) identified guiding principles for future patient care delivery.[2] AONE described knowledge as critical to the future of client care and stated that this knowledge must be access based and synthesized to ensure coordinated care across multiple levels, disciplines, and settings. This vision for future delivery of client care will influence the staff development educator's ability to fulfill roles and responsibilities. Given the sociopolitical and economic changes impacting today's complex healthcare delivery systems, professional staff development educators have a greater challenge to develop and provide consistent high-quality, evidence-based education to adult learners.

STAFF DEVELOPMENT EDUCATOR ROLES

As mentioned previously, staff development departments have undergone numerous structure and process changes over several decades. As a result of changes to staff development organization, the role of the staff development educator has evolved and expanded; in many situations the nurse manager assumes the role of professional staff development educator. Changes to the role also included title changes such as staff development instructor, clinical educator, staff development specialist, or professional development specialists.[3]

The National Nursing Staff Development Organization defines staff development as the "systematic process of assessment, planning, development, and evaluation that enhances the performance or professional development of healthcare providers and their continuing competence."[4] Staff development activities include orientation, in-service education, staff development, continuing education, and academic education.[5] Although these activities can overlap somewhat, the desired learning outcomes are the important factors.

Grasmick describes six roles of the professional staff development educator: educator, facilitator, change agent, consultant, researcher, and leader.[6] Responsibilities within each of the roles vary according to the institution and the needs of learners. In the educator role, the staff development process is used to provide educational programs for nursing personnel as well as non-nursing staff. These programs address nursing skills and knowledge and evaluation of outcomes related to increased professional development and competency levels and may be provided through staff orientations, in-services, and evidence-based practice updates. To address role changes of the staff, in-service education is needed to refine and develop new skills and knowledge related to job performance. These learning experiences usually are brief and narrow in scope because they are aimed at only one competency or knowledge area. Technological advances now allow for in-service education programs to be delivered in a variety of formats, such as computer-assisted instruction, simulations, on-line programs, or use of intranets to deliver mandatory programs unique to the healthcare setting or those programs necessary to meet regulatory standards.

Continuing education responsibilities include planning and organizing learning experiences in a variety of settings intended to build on the previous education and experience of staff nurses. Also, state board–approved continuing education offerings provide nurses with new approaches to healthcare delivery and enhance practice, education, administration, research, and theory development for state license renewal.[7] Examples include workshops, conferences, self-learning modules, seminars, and on-line programs.

In the role of facilitator, the staff development educator assists learners to identify individual needs, the resources appropriate for meeting these needs, and how to access the appropriate resources. In the past this may have included organization of expert presenters in a classroom. Today, however, widely accepted changes in delivery methods such as web-based learning allow innovative teaching strategies. The staff development educator must be aware of and use evidenced-based teaching–learning strategies related to new technology mediums.

Evidence-Based Practice 19-1

Findings from a pilot study indicated that interactive videoconferencing is an "effective, accepted format for educational opportunities" and does not "compromise student learning or assessment by external assessors."[8]

As a change agent, the staff educator participates in evaluating client outcomes and staff needs to identify areas in which change is needed and acts to facilitate the change process within the healthcare environment. The staff educator also serves as a change advocate by serving on institutional committees and by being a member of professional nursing organizations to ensure that client and practice issues are addressed.

In the consultant role, the staff educator serves as a resource in the problem-solving process throughout the healthcare delivery system. Administration, units of care, and intraprofessional staff need the expertise of the professional staff educator in collaborating to identify the root cause of issues related to quality client outcomes, then to plan strategies for educating those involved. Additionally, staff educators consult with schools of nursing to provide optimal student clinical experiences through a preceptorship while maintaining a safe, effective care environment for the client. School of nursing faculty, the preceptor, and staff development educators collaborate to identify learning needs of nursing students based on clinical learning objectives. Professional staff development educators create a positive climate and join with nurse managers to prepare the preceptor for the role. Staff development educators and nurse managers, along with nursing faculty, can facilitate the preceptor role by offering educational programs. Furthermore, staff educators in the consultant role provide feedback to nursing education programs regarding the quality of graduates and collaborate to develop methods that enhance quality.

As a researcher, the staff educator utilizes and facilitates the research process. This includes assisting staff in the recognition and development of research questions related to clinical nursing interventions as well as administrative procedures. The staff development educator also develops questions that inform the educator role. Evidence generated from research is disseminated for utilization through presentations and scholarly writings. The staff development educator must promote development of writing and presentations skills.

AONE recognizes that "excellent leadership is essential to ensure excellent patient care."[9] As a leader, the professional staff development educator must model lifelong learning because this is crucial in nursing. Additionally, the role of leader involves awareness of the group process and interpersonal skills such as coaching, mentoring, relationship building, dissemination of information, and determination of resources. A critical and often less recognized leadership activity is job-related counseling. This responsibility is extremely important given today's complex healthcare delivery system. Job-related counseling involves promoting the professional growth of employees by assisting them to deliver high-quality care within current standards. Counseling also includes evaluating promotion possibilities and assistance in obtaining formal training. In the leader role, today's nursing professional staff educator is in a unique position to advocate for nursing as a profession. Expanded roles may require the staff educator to embody the organization within the community, including representing the institution to non–healthcare consumers, serving on community or professional organization boards or advisory councils, and providing information to official policy decision makers in areas of expertise.

Within each of the staff development educator roles there are overlapping responsibilities. It is difficult to determine which role or responsibility is of the greatest importance. However, at any given time, the staff development educator may find that one or two responsibilities take precedence. As staff needs, resources, and abilities change, the staff development educator must be flexible and embrace the changes to provide quality staff education.

EDUCATOR COMPETENCIES

To function effectively and efficiently within the demanding multifaceted roles, staff development educators must possess skills in education, leading and managing, interpersonal and advanced communication skills, clinical expertise, and political acumen. Wolff categorized critical staff educator competencies within the cognitive, psychomotor, and affective learning domains.[10] Figure 19-1 lists the suggested competencies within these three domains.

FIGURE 19-1	STAFF DEVELOPMENT EDUCATOR COMPETENCIES

Cognitive Domain	Affective Domain	Psychomotor Domain
• Nursing, organization, and education philosophies and theories	• Awareness of personal values and philosophy	• Learner skills
• Adult educational principles and strategies	• Emotional intelligence	• Teaching skills
• Clinical nursing knowledge	• Valuing of individuals	• Communication skills
• Diversity awareness	• Valuing of lifelong learning	• Clinical nursing skills
• Effective communication strategies	• Valuing political acumen	• Technology skills

Source: Author.

Clinical nurses often transition to staff development roles and may not have had formal education in the roles and competencies. Staff development educators model lifelong learning by progressing from self-learning to development of teaching skills, eventually leading to confidence in the ability to integrate competencies by shifting the focus to the learner.

ORGANIZATIONAL FACTORS

Each organization needs a statement of beliefs, or philosophy, about how and why it will accomplish staff development. Important to the development of a philosophy is the recognition that the primary goal of professional development is to provide quality care with the result being positive client outcomes. Flowing from the mission and philosophy of the organization of which it is a part, the staff development philosophy should be written by a representative group, rather than an individual, and be accepted by staff and administrators. In writing a philosophy for staff development for healthcare professionals, the group needs to address the following areas:

- Commitment to quality and safety
- Importance or valuing of staff development
- Costs and benefits of staff development
- How learning occurs, including theoretical bases
- Teaching–learning strategies
- Employees' responsibility for learning
- Organizational responsibility for providing staff development

Organization

A staff development department can be organized in a number of ways, depending on the philosophy, mission, and goals of the organization. A centralized model includes one agency-wide staff development department, with nurse and/or non-nurse educators. In this model, all departments collaborate to determine and plan for the needs of staff. In the decentralized model, the nursing department has its own organized in-service or staff development program. The nursing staff development department may then adopt a central unit-based model.

Changes in the healthcare delivery system have led to new models or paradigms in staff development. Instead of focusing on organizational-wide models such as centralized or decentralized, Cooper and Bulmer consider staff development department structure in light of the type of customers that are served.[11] For example, staff development educators may provide programs for (a) all nursing personnel, (b) all providers of care for the client, (c) all employees of an organization, or (d) all employees of a multisite corporation.

Personnel

The number of staff development personnel depends on the size of the agency and the organizational structure. In small agencies the coordinator may be the only staff member. The management or governance of the staff development program also depends on the size and structure of the organization. However, in all types of agencies, the nursing leadership is essential to enabling effective nursing education programs.

Advisory Groups

An advisory group represents the customers receiving the education and is important regardless of the size of the agency, type of governance, or staff development structure. This group may be composed of persons from within the organization, those outside the organization, or a combination of both and is useful for identifying needs and creative strategies and resources for planning programs. The advisory group members may increase participation by communicating the purpose of staff development programs directly to the people represented.

Budgets

In the era of cost containment, cost and benefit data must be collected and analyzed. The manager of staff development may be responsible for developing and implementing the budget. The amount of monies allocated for staff development may vary according to staff size, the number of anticipated new employees, and existing resources. The organization must demonstrate a commitment to staff development through allocation of necessary resources.

STAFF DEVELOPMENT PROCESS

Staff development is based on a philosophy of adult education that uses teaching and learning principles and concepts that apply to people with a combination of responsibilities, including family and financial obligations, employment commitment(s), and identified areas of interest or specialization. Consideration of employees' learning style, as well as level of motivation, should be a factor in planning staff development programs. While working within the philosophy of the organization, the staff development educator seeks ways to incorporate the individual learner's goals, aspirations, and personal philosophy of nursing.

Staff development educators motivate adult learners to consider that learning is a continuing process throughout a professional career. Lifelong learning involves self-direction in identifying needs and areas for growth, which in turn promotes motivation for involvement and selection of methods for learning. Lifelong learning is essential in nursing because of rapid changes in healthcare delivery systems and changing roles within that system to keep current. Nursing is influenced by public policy, technology, and societal and economic changes. Technology, which continually increases in complexity and scope, and innovations in health care are major forces motivating nurses to pursue lifelong learning. Nurses must adjust quickly to the demands associated with high-tech skills in many areas. Effective staff development programs respond to the needs of nurses practicing under such increased demands.

Characteristics of Adult Learners

Galbraith[12] suggests that adult learners individually fall at various points between the maxim "you can't teach an old dog new tricks" and the super learner idea proposed by Knowles.[13] Adult learner variability occurs from diverse previous experiences, the wide span of age cohorts, and unique individual learner needs. "Adult learners have never been more diverse and we as teachers must be attuned to the influence of diversity and culture on motivation and hence on learning."[14] Staff development educators need to recognize that adult learners may share similar characteristics, as listed in Figure 19-2.

Motivation may be defined as the energy that causes adults to strive toward competence in matters believed to be important. A common culture is created when the staff development educator values and engages the needs of adults. Staff educator acumen in determining what adult learner characteristics prevail in various teaching–learning situations is a skill that influences learning and transfer of information. Strategies must be developed in planning for specific learners, anticipated outcomes of the learning, and types of evaluation to be done.

Principles and Strategies of Adult Learning

There are various well-known principles of adult learning that can guide the staff development educator. Greater learner motivation and self-initiation can be encouraged by identifying learner needs before the teaching session. This can occur by simply asking the learner what knowledge is desired from the session or the anticipated use of the information. The information may be viewed as more pertinent and interesting if it can be related to an immediate need or problem. New material should build on past experiences, and teaching should be designed with a review of related material or experiences to provide scaffolding for transition to the new material. Videos, computer-based programs, education modules, or group work may enable learners to control the rate and/or repetition of the presentation. Group work, collaboration, and teams may promote the social aspects of learning, and variety in learning activities can help maintain interest. The teacher assumes the role of facilitator, with mutual respect for learners who actively contribute and partner in the learning situations. An environment of respect, comfort, and free of distractions promotes learning, and any perception of threats or fear of failure should be avoided.

FIGURE 19-2 | **ADULT LEARNER CHARACTERISTICS**

1. Prior knowledge impacts readiness to learn.

2. Life experiences and knowledge is not necessarily organized sequentially.

3. Individuals vary in preferred style of learning.

4. The role of the learner is active rather than passive and may involve conflicts in maintaining performance of multiple roles.

5. Active participation with feedback and repetition of information may be important for retention of knowledge.

6. Variations in sensory and physical abilities may impact learner motivation and/or ability to participate in various teaching strategies.

Source: Author.

Evidence-Based Practice 19-2

East and Jacoby used a quasi-experimental design to determine the effectiveness of an educational module on staff compliance with central line policy. Findings indicated that educational modules were an effective teaching strategy.[15]

Critical Thinking

Critical thinking is near and dear to the heart of adult educators because of its connection to the democratic principle of allowing all to question concepts and rationales. Critical thinking may provide the template for adult education practices.[16] Critical thinking is a process of logical reasoning that involves the recognition of assumptions underlying beliefs and behaviors as well as justification for ideas and actions. Information should be analyzed to make sense of experiences. Critical thinking requires comprehension and analysis of variables that impact situations, including use of inductive and deductive reasoning.

The staff development educator can model critical thinking by the manner in which content is presented. The teaching strategy of lecture may lead to a passive approach to learning. However, interactive strategies can encourage sharing the thinking and experiences of various learners. For example, Socratic questioning may be used as a strategy to explore underlying premises, help recognize assumptions, evaluate various points of view, consider rationales, and prompt consideration of implications and consequences. Encouraging discussion can promote learners' evaluation of previous ways of thinking and assumptions, including critical reflection of conflicts in values and behaviors. Other examples of interactive techniques, such as case-based learning (Figure 19-3), scenario or vignette analyses, and simulations, can allow learners to problem solve, to identify assumptions, and to seek additional information that increases both engagement in the learning and retention for future application. In evaluating the use of simulation specifically to measure competencies, the staff development educator must be aware of the need for further research related to this teaching–learning method (Figure 19-4). Development of effective simulation scenarios is challenging and may require additional education for the staff development professional.

Personal teacher/learner attitudes that foster critical thinking include intellectual humility, confidence and independence in thinking, courage to challenge the status quo, examination of personal bias, being fair-minded, integrity, perseverance, and curiosity.[20] The activities suggested in Figure 19-5 encourage development of critical thinking.

FIGURE 19-3   **CASE-BASED LEARNING STRATEGY**

Case-based learning defined as "a teaching method which requires students to actively participate in real or hypothetical problem situations, reflecting the kind of experiences naturally encountered in the discipline under study,"[17] is a proven teaching and learning method to motivate learners and to fill the gap between theory and practice. Benefits of this teaching method include knowledge acquisition, problem-solving skills, and positive attitudes.[18] Additionally, improved understanding, retention, and recall of information is an advantage of this learning method.[19]

Source: Author.

FIGURE 19-4	SIMULATION IN STAFF DEVELOPMENT

Simulation-based assessments "have the potential to evaluate clinical competencies . . . and is an essential component both for the research to establish the assessment and criterion setting methodologies, and also to provide equivalent cases to different personnel and teams for testing competency."[21]

Dillon, Boulet, Hawkins, and Swanson suggest the need for more simulation research to determine what can or can not be measured with simulation, what content and skills are essential in a summative discipline-specific evaluation, and whether performance in simulated experiences can be translated into effective practice behaviors in clinical settings.[22]

Source: Author.

FIGURE 19-5	ACTIVITIES TO STIMULATE CRITICAL-THINKING SKILLS

1. Allow time for identifying personal assumptions.

2. Include alternative perspectives (may have debate).

3. Use critical incident questionnaires.

4. Include demonstrations or scenarios.

5. Use case stories or case studies.

6. Deliberately end each teaching session with unanswered questions.

Source: Author.

Evidence-Based Practice 19-3

In a systematic review, O'Brien et al. found that passive, didactic sessions are less likely to result in a change in professional practice, whereas interactive workshops result in moderate changes in professional behaviors.[23]

EVALUATION OF STAFF DEVELOPMENT

Staff development evaluation is multifaceted and involves learner and program evaluation. Learner evaluation includes measurement of learner outcomes in comparison with predetermined objectives and judgments related to effectiveness of teaching strategies. Program evaluation includes the determination of whether specific programs should be continued. Each course, seminar, class, or workshop is evaluated when it is completed to determine whether the program met the needs for which it was designed. Wilson, Crockett, and Curtis suggest a five-level framework for evaluation of staff development[24]:

- *Level 1:* Evaluation of participant satisfaction related to the educational offering (e.g., questionnaires)
- *Level 2:* Assessment of the degree of learning (e.g., pre- and posttest comparison, rubrics, or percentage of participants scoring a predetermined level). Bloom's levels of taxonomy can provide

structure from simple to complex learning. For example, performance of a psychomotor skill may initially be at the imitation level, or the evaluation standard may be set at the level of application of performing the skill for a different type of client population or setting; a level of learning in the cognitive domain may be initially set at recall of facts that have been presented, progressing to analysis of a client situation.[25]

- *Level 3:* Evaluation of behavior changes or transfer of learning to the actual work environment (e.g., principles of client care learned in an educational program are applied on the unit to impact client outcomes)
- *Level 4:* Evaluation of the educational offering on the institution as an organization (e.g., education regarding prevention of nosocomial acquired urinary tract infections decrease in the month following in-services regarding meatal care for those having indwelling catheters)
- *Level 5:* Assessment of cost-to-benefit of the educational offering in which the total program costs are divided into the potential or actual benefits (e.g., the total costs for a program to prevent nosocomial acquired urinary tract infections is $6,000, but the outcome of the program is 90% reduction in urinary tract infections in clients with indwelling catheters on the unit where the in-service was presented). Challenges related to cost-to-benefit analysis include the difficulty in quantifying some types of data and attributing the client care activities directly to the effects of the educational offering.

Wilson et al. acknowledge that all five evaluation levels may not be necessary in every educational situation. However, the highest level that is applicable should also include evaluation of the lower supportive levels.[24]

Organizations must provide a supportive environment in which changes in behavior can lead to increased quality of care and thereby increase client health outcomes. Translation of evaluation data into reports or executive summaries can then allow evaluation of the effectiveness of each staff development offering. This in turn can foster awareness of the potential impact of staff education to help develop an organizational culture of quality improvement.

TRENDS AND ISSUES IN STAFF DEVELOPMENT

Legal and Ethical Issues

A number of ethical and legal issues are related to staff development. Ethical issues such as promotion of products made by sponsors of educational programs and integrity in dating mandatory staff competency requirements must be addressed.[26] Confidentiality regarding personal information of staff and clients is another ethical consideration for the staff development educator. Staff educators must have knowledge and adhere to legal limitations related to releasing confidential information. For example, use of patient's names and other identifying information during classes must be avoided as well as use of this private information on hard copies of materials.[26] Other laws that have an impact on staff development include the Americans with Disability Act, copyrights, and scope of practice.

Workforce Diversity

The healthcare workforce of the 21st century is composed of diverse ethnicities, genders, and generations, leading to a number of challenges for the professional staff development educator. Among these challenges are diverse learning styles, cultural backgrounds, language barriers, levels of experience, and generational expectations. Knowledge and skills related to diversity is important throughout the staff development process. Helping staff assess personal assumptions, biases, and prejudices may be the first step to overcoming problems related to ethnic, gender, and generational diversities. According to Haase-Herrick "the ability of all nurses to work well with a culturally diverse staff is essential."[27] The realization that each staff member is an individual, with strengths and needs, can form a foundation that fosters communication. Planning staff teaching–learning activities that incorporate strategies to identify personal stereotypical assumptions may include role play, movies, simulations, case studies, and process recordings.

Quality and Safety

In 1996 the Institute of Medicine (IOM) began a coordinated approach focused on assessing and improving the quality of health care within the United States. The IOM's definition of quality is "the degree to which health services for individuals and populations increase the likelihood of desired health outcomes and are consistent with current professional knowledge."[28] Interdisciplinary healthcare providers are purported to lack adequate preparation to provide high-quality and safe health care and require an ongoing assessment of competency. Staff development educators should provide programs that address the five identified core areas for developing and maintaining competency:

1. Delivering patient-centered care
2. Working as part of an interdisciplinary team
3. Practicing evidence-based health care
4. Focusing on quality improvement
5. Using information technology[29]

The IOM made further recommendations regarding client safety in its report on transforming the work environment for nurses. This report suggests actions for healthcare organizations specifically related to management practices, competency of the healthcare providers, design of healthcare provision, and a total organizational commitment to focus on client safety.[30]

Finkelman and Kenner believe the IOM reports are central to changes in the healthcare delivery system and the movement toward interprofessional collaboration and should be the primary focus of nursing education.[31] Healthcare team members should be skilled in root cause analysis to begin effective problem-solving strategies with the goal of increasing safety and thereby positive client outcomes. Figure 19-6 shows examples of specific teaching–learning activities using IOM recommendations.

EVIDENCE-BASED PRACTICE

Evidence-based practice differs from research utilization in that client preferences and values and the expertise of the healthcare provider are necessary to determine which evidence is most applicable and appropriate in a given situation.[32] Motivating interprofessional staff to use research findings and evidence-based practice guidelines may be a challenge for the staff development educator. However, use of current best practice standards is essential for improving quality client outcomes. Motivation can be increased by including teaching about the linkage between an area in which client outcomes need improvement, how client care interventions are related to client satisfaction and outcomes, and how changing practice may lead to improved outcomes. Knowing where to find quality, consistent, and replicated accurate information can also increase motivation for using research findings.

The staff development educator must incorporate teaching that systematic reviews and evidence-based guidelines can be obtained from focused database searches, including the Cochrane database, the Johanna Brigg's Institute, the Cumulative Index to Nursing & Allied Health Literature (CINAHL), ProQuest, and others. Methods for grading evidence must also be included in teaching healthcare providers. Recognition of barriers for information access such as lack of staff time, lack of available resources (e.g., Cochrane database), and lack of knowledge regarding database searches is important in planning learning activities. Teaching may include skills for determining levels of evidence from on-line resources and systematic reviews. Critical appraisal of the evidence is an important skill in evidence-

FIGURE 19-6	TEACHING–LEARNING ACTIVITIES TO PROMOTE IOM COMPETENCIES

IOM Core Competencies	Learning Activity	Expected Learner Outcomes
Patient-centered care	• Experiential learning activities in which learners participate as the client • Case scenarios • Videotaped simulations • Role play situations of intercultural client/health care provider interactions	• Identify breakdown in communication or fragmentation of care • Accurate use of interpreters or identify alternative communication strategies
Working in interdisciplinary teams	• Simulated experiences • Chart review • Videotaped scenarios • Case study	• Learning the roles of the interdisciplinary team members in high-stress or high-risk situations
Evidence-based practice	• Develop clinical question(s) for review of current research • Develop question(s) regarding increasing quality of client outcomes • Develop question(s) regarding effective organizational environments of care	• Skills in writing questions for research • Development of database search skills
Applying quality improvement	• Use root-cause analysis in a prepared scenario	• Determine areas of needed improvement as teams work toward the goal of meeting the client's needs
Using informatics	• Annual offerings relating to HIPAA requirements, computer systems, access to client information at the point of care	• To reduce errors in client care and documentation

Source: HIPAA, Healthcare Insurance Portability and Accountability Act.

based practice. The staff development educator, along with biomedical librarians and statisticians, can facilitate this learning process. Staff development educators can use a simple tool designed by Oermann, Floyd, Galvin, and Roop to teach nurses in clinical settings how to evaluate systematic reviews.[33]

Awareness of healthcare trends and issues provide a foundation for planning staff development programs. The staff development educator may play a huge role in deciding which evidence-based practice model is adopted by the organization. Interaction with organizational structure is a necessary first step, including incorporating (or possibly revising) the philosophy, mission, and administrative support to ensure a focus on quality and safety in health care. Commitment of all stakeholders is necessary to transform to a culture of quality.

FUTURE PLANNING FOR STAFF DEVELOPMENT

Staff development educators must be proactive in planning strategies for meeting the future educational needs of interprofessional staff in light of current and potential challenges. The staff development process must be used to ensure competencies in the following areas:

- Emergency preparedness
- Bioterrorism

- Pandemics
- Effective interpersonal communication and emotional competencies
- Aging population
- End-of-life concerns
- Integration of leadership and management into team building for socialization and resocialization of staff
- Leadership and management skills, specifically conflict management and delegation

These topics are not all inclusive but are the prevailing issues facing nursing and healthcare delivery as a whole. A number of considerations are intertwined within each of these topics and are critical to staff development. Two such concepts are coherence and trust. Ponte, Kruger, DeMarco, Hanley, and Conlin define coherence as "a pervasive, enduring, and dynamic feeling of confidence that one's internal and external environments are predictable, and that there is a high probability that things will work out as well as can reasonably be expected."[34] Coherence, as proposed by these authors, is important in creating a work environment where high-quality care is valued and where professional development is encouraged. Ponte et al. suggested a framework for reshaping nursing practice environments where competency in practice development, leadership development, and quality and safety are major themes.[34] Effective staff development requires addressing each of these areas. Information obtained from nurses in focus groups revealed a desire for ongoing support, development and maintenance of skill in new technologies, increased development of nursing practice skills, and more education regarding professionalism.[34] Perception that professional development and nursing care are valued by the organization's leaders is crucial to developing coherence. An environment of coherence promotes a "more satisfied work force, a safer work environment, and improved patient care."[34]

Further considerations for future teaching–learning endeavors include focusing on the staff's feelings and development of emotional competencies. "Evidence suggests that emotionally intelligent leadership is key to creating a working climate that nurtures its employees and encourages them to do their best with enthusiasm, in turn this pays off in improved business performance."[35] A nurse's intelligence is important but must include critical emotional competencies. Emotional competencies are defined by Goleman as "a learning capability based on emotional intelligence that results in outstanding performance at work."[36] These competencies occur in clusters and include self-awareness, self-management, social awareness, and relationship management.

Issues of cost containment, nurse staffing patterns, and access to care must also be considered in light of any future healthcare educational initiatives. For example, nurses are ever more aware of containing costs in all practice settings and adhering to new reimbursement regulations. The nursing shortage has impacted nurse staffing, challenging staff development educators to plan offerings for a variety of staff educated at different levels (i.e., LPN/VPN, ADN, diploma, BSN, CNL, CNS, APRN, DNP, etc.). Various nurse-to-client ratios and staffing mix patterns will be developed and evaluated for effectiveness in attaining desired client outcomes, which will then lead to public or institutional policy development.

Other changes influencing professional development include use of various technologies (such as telemedicine) to assess and monitor clients with acute or chronic conditions in areas with limited healthcare services. Nurse-managed services may increase in response to a need for health promotion and disease prevention as well as to manage chronic conditions of an aging population.

Strategies to address the issues discussed above require evaluation of techniques that have shown previous effectiveness and the development of new paradigms. The professional nurse will need the ability to access and use evolving knowledge for practice. This knowledge requires the nurse to expand critical-thinking skills to include critical synthesis of the information to allow coordinated care across multiple levels, disciplines, and practice settings. Strategies are needed to support relationship building with clients, families, populations, and other professionals, including the span of generations, diversity, and interdependency. The synergy of these relationships is greater than what would be enabled by any of the individual parts.

According to Pacini, using the eight nurse characteristics (i.e., clinical judgment, clinical inquiry, caring practices, response to diversity, advocacy/moral agency, facilitation of learning, collaboration, systems thinking), one can conceptualize and construct an educational program that integrates knowledge development that can only be acquired by being in the presence of patients and families and that which can be enhanced or facilitated using didactic methods.[37]

Finally, any future plans for staff development must revolve around a focus on communication for safe, quality care. Specific techniques such as SBAR (situation, background, assessment, and recommendation) may be incorporated into teaching–learning strategies such as case studies, role plays, or evaluated in simulation activities.

SUMMARY

Professional nursing staff development educators are challenged by multiple demands and evolving issues in health care. Issues of cost containment, nurse staffing patterns and access to care must also be considered in light of any future healthcare educational initiatives. Competency in teaching diverse staff can have a tremendous impact on the quality of health care.

Nurses in all practice environments have struggled through the "re era" (redesigning, restructuring, and reengineering). These struggles have resulted in a frustrated, stressed, and angry workforce.[38] Professional staff development educators must be aware of these feelings and how the feelings may impact the healthcare delivery system as whole and individual providers' competencies. According to Huber, "Staff development has been identified in the literature as an important factor in job satisfaction. It provides employees with an opportunity to improve their practice, level of competency, or other areas of self-interest."[39]

To create a successful future for health care, skills such as creative thinking, access to information, synthesis of knowledge, reflection to evaluate varying paradigms, and an emphasis on valuing improved client outcomes are needed across disciplines. Staff development educators must continue to use adult education principles and strategies in the development, implementation, and evaluation of multidisciplinary programs that focus on the delivery of quality, safe, cost-effective, client-centered care. Additionally, using evidence regarding the link between quality nursing care and improved client outcomes can help leaders, staff, employers, and educators develop an appreciation of the importance of the nursing discipline.

APPLICATION EXERCISES

Exercise 19-1 Critical Thinking

Staff educators orienting nurses to a new unit may use a chart in which identifying client information has been removed. From the chart, the orientee identifies the following:

- Appropriate and inappropriate documentation
- Teaching (or lack of) related to the client and family's identified needs
- Evaluation (or lack of) regarding effectiveness of medications
- Any iatrogenic complications that could have been prevented
- Use of evidence-base for nursing interventions
- Other pertinent data for the unit

In a group setting, the staff development educator uses Socratic questioning to elicit responses regarding how improvements could be made for each area.

Exercise 19-2 Diversity

Staff educators responsible for educating intraprofessional staff may use a DVD that includes persons from multiple cultures and generations. With the audio muted, the learners identify meanings from the nonverbal cues of the actors. This can be used as a prompt for discussion regarding potential assumptions that can be made based on nonverbal behaviors or incongruence between anticipated nonverbal cues and verbal communication. Each learner can be asked to keep a journal of occurrences of interactions in which incongruence was perceived and attempts to clarify meaning perspectives while avoiding assumptions or stereotypes.

Exercise 19-3 Accessing Information

The staff development educator poses a clinical question. Participants are required to search CINAHL, ProQuest, and Cochrane database to find various levels of evidence related to the clinical question. Key search words, limits for the search (age, gender, client population, dates of research, etc.), and Boolean connectors are identified. Participants then determine if any of the findings can be applied to the clinical question.

Exercise 19-4 Quality

Participants in a staff education program are asked to define criteria for quality nursing care, including specific behaviors, and how these can impact client outcomes. Participants are then asked if quality nursing care can be measured and in what way(s).

Notes

1. Marquis, B. L., & Huston, C. J. (2009). *Leadership Roles and Management Functions in Nursing: Theory and Application* (6th ed.). Philadelphia, PA: Wolters Kluwer Health/Lippincott, Williams & Wilkins.
2. American Organization of Nurse Executives. Guiding principles for future care delivery. Retrieved February 7, 2008, from http://www.aone.org/aone/resource/guidingprinciples.html
3. American Nurses Association. (2000). *Scope and standards of practice for nursing professional development.* Washington, DC: The Association.
4. National Nursing Staff Development Organization. (1999). *Strategic plan 2000.* Pensacola, FL.
5. Lockhart, J. S. (2004). *Unit-based staff development for clinical nurses.* Pittsburgh, PA: Oncology Nursing Society.
6. Grasmick, L. L. (2002). Roles of the staff development educator. In K. L. O'Shea (Ed.), *Staff development nursing secrets* (pp. 7–15). Philadelphia: Hanley & Belfus.
7. Furze, G., & Pearcey, P. (1999). Continuing education in nursing: A review of the literature. *Journal of Advanced Nursing, 29,* 355–363.
8. Daria, M., Zerr, K., & Pulcher, L. (2008). Using interactive video technology in nursing education: A pilot study. *Journal of Nursing Education, 47,* 87–92.
9. American Organization of Nurse Executives. Nurse executive competencies. Retrieved January 23, 2008, from http://www.aone.org/aone/pdf/February%20Nurse%20Leader—final%20draft—for%20web.pdf
10. Wolff, A. C. (2002). Educator competencies. In K. L. O'Shea (Ed.), *Staff development nursing secrets* (pp. 27–37). Philadelphia: Hanley & Belfus.
11. Cooper, D. C., & Bulmer, J. M. (2002). Staff development department management. K. L. O'Shea (Ed.), *Staff development nursing secrets* (pp. 47–58). Philadelphia: Hanley & Belfus.
12. Galbraith, M. W. (2004). *Adult learning methods: A guide for effective instruction* (3rd ed.). Malabar, FL: Krieger.
13. Knowles, M. (1984). *Andragogy in action.* San Francisco: Jossey-Bass.
14. Wlodkowski, R. J. (1999). *Enhancing adult motivation to learn* (rev. ed.). San Francisco: Jossey-Bass.

15. East, D., & Jacoby, K. (2005). The effect of a nursing staff education program on compliance with central line care policy in the cardiac intensive care unit. *Pediatric Nursing, 31,* 182–184.

16. Brookfield, S. D. (2004). Critical thinking techniques. In M. Galbraith (Ed.), *Adult learning methods: A guide for effective instruction* (3rd ed., pp. 341–360). Malabar, FL: Krieger.

17. Ertmer, P. A., & Russell, J. D. (1995). Using case studies to enhance instructional design education. *Educational Technology, 55,* 23–31.

18. Cliff, W. H., & Wright, A. W. (1996). Directed case study method for teaching human anatomy and physiology. *Advanced Physiology Education, 15,* S19–S28.

19. Specht, L. B., & Sandlin, P. K. (1991). The differential effects of experiential learning activities and traditional lecture classes in accounting. *Simulation and Gaming, 22,* 196–210.

20. Paul, R., & Elder, L. (2005). *A guide for educators to critical thinking competency standards.* Dillon Beach, CA: Foundation for Critical Thinking.

21. Gaba, D. M. (2004). The future vision of simulation in health care. *Quality and Safety in Health Care, 131*(Suppl. 1), i2–i10.

22. Dillon, G. F., Boulet, J. R., Hawkins, R. E., & Swanson, D. B. (2004). Simulations in the United States Medical Licensing Examination. *Quality & Safety in Health Care, 1*(Suppl. 1), i41–i45.

23. O'Brien, M. A., Freemantle, N., Oxman, A. D., Wolf, F., Davis, D. A., & Herrin, J. (2001). Continuing education meetings and workshops: Effects on professional practice and healthcare outcomes [Cochrane Review]. *The Cochrane Library,* Issue 1.

24. Wilson, R., Crockett, C., & Curtis, B. (2002). Evaluation. In K. L. O'Shea (Ed.), *Staff development nursing secrets* (pp. 149–160). Philadelphia: Hanley & Belfus.

25. Bloom, B. S., Engelhart, M. D., Furst, E. J., Hill, W. H., & Krathwohl, D. R. (1956). *Taxonomy of educational objectives: Handbook I: Cognitive domain.* New York: David McKay.

26. O'Shea, L., & Robinson, C. B. (2002). Legal and ethical issues in education. In K. L. O'Shea (Ed.), *Staff development nursing secrets* (pp. 47–58). Philadelphia: Hanley & Belfus.

27. Haase-Herrick, K. (2008). Socializing and educating staff for team building. In B. L. Marquis & C. J. Huston (Eds.), *Leadership roles and management functions in nursing* (6th ed.). Philadelphia: Lippincott, Williams & Wilkins.

28. Institute of Medicine. *Crossing the quality chasm: The IOM health care quality initiative.* Retrieved January 23, 2008, from http://www.iom.edu/CMS/8089.aspx?

29. Institute of Medicine. *Health professions education: A bridge to quality.* Retrieved January 23, 2008, from http://www.iom.edu/report.asp?.id=5914

30. Institute of Medicine. *Keeping patients safe: Transforming the work environment for nurses.* Retrieved January 23, 2008, from http://www.iom.edu/report.asp?id=16173

31. Finkelman, A., & Kenner, C. (2007). *Teaching IOM: Implications of the Institute of Medicine reports for nursing education.* Silver Springs, MD: ANA Nursebooks.

32. LoBiondo-Wood, G., & Haber, J. (2006). *Nursing research: Methods and critical appraisal for evidence-based practice* (6th ed.). St. Louis, MO: Mosby/Elsevier.

33. Oermann, M. H., Floyd, J. A., Galvin, E. A., & Roop, J. C. Brief reports for disseminating systematic reviews to nurses. Retrieved February 7, 2008, from http://www.nursingcenter.com/library/journalarticleprint.asp?Article_ID=667360

34. Ponte, P. R., Kruger, N., DeMarco, R., Hanley, D., & Conlin, G. (2004). Reshaping the practice environment: The importance of coherence. *JONA, 34,* 173–179.

35. Goleman, D. (2001). An EI theory of performance. In C. Cherniss & D. Goleman (Eds.), *The emotionally intelligent workplace* (pp. 27–44). San Francisco: Jossey-Bass.

36. Goleman, D. (1998). *Working with emotional intelligence.* New York: Bantam Books.

37. Pacini, C. M. (2007). The synergy model: A framework for professional development and transformation. In M. A. Q. Curley (Ed.), *Synergy: The unique relationship between nurse and patients* (pp. 26–32). Indianapolis, IN: Sigma Theta Tau International.

38. Thomas, S. P. (2004). *Transforming nurses' stress and anger* (2nd ed.). New York: Springer.

39. Huber, D. L. (2006). *Leadership and nursing care management* (3rd ed.). St. Louis, MO: Saunders/Elsevier.

20 BUILDING A PORTFOLIO FOR ACADEMIC AND CLINICAL PARTNERSHIP

James L. Harris, DSN, APRN-BC, MBA, CNL
Sandra E. Walters, MSN, RN

LEARNING OBJECTIVES AND ACTIVITIES

- Identify benefits of an academic and clinical partnership.
- Define portfolio and provide examples of evidence.
- Outline the role of an academic partner.
- Outline the role of a clinical partner.
- Discuss the significance of the clinical nurse leader in academic partnerships.
- Describe the role of an academic partner in relation to the development of a portfolio.
- Identify the components of an academic and clinical portfolio and the development process.
- Identify elements and frameworks to consider when designing markers of success.
- Describe techniques used to manage academic and clinical partnerships.

CONCEPTS

Partnerships, communication, data collection and analysis, directing (leading), coaching, portfolio development, delegation, evidence-based practice, synergy, accountability.

NURSE MANAGER BEHAVIORS	NURSE EXECUTIVE BEHAVIORS
Applies communication techniques and frameworks when developing an academic and clinical portfolio and maintains effective partnerships.	Designs systems and processes that result in successful academic and clinical partnerships to ensure consultant resources are available to staff; uses frameworks to develop successful portfolios; disseminates information to stakeholders.

Introduction

Diversity helps to sustain complex adaptive systems and contributes to information and novelty within organizations. One strategy for increasing the level of diversity in an organization is the development of relationships and linkages with other organizations, as occurs with the formation of academic and clinical partnerships.[1] In addition to increasing the capacity of the healthcare system to bring additional information to the decision-making table, multiple benefits can be derived from these partnerships:

- Improved education of nursing students as the needs of the healthcare system drive curriculum changes in academic institutions[2]
- Increased availability of faculty to teach nursing students through support of adjunct faculty appointments
- Increased availability of clinical sites for the education of nursing students
- Enhanced opportunity for clinical nurses to participate in an academic milieu that can offer resources, mentoring, and consideration for pursuit of doctoral education
- Decreased orientation costs for clinical sites related to new graduates
- Enhanced ability of clinical sites to identify and attract future registered nurse employees[3]
- Maximized use of limited equipment and other resources and avoidance of duplication in nursing programs[4]
- Increased competence and training availability for nursing staff[5]
- Improved community relations as outreach programs result in the perception of the organization as being a positive corporate citizen[6]

As partnerships are formed, the evaluation of program outcomes presents a challenge to nursing leaders at all levels of an organization. Tools developed to aid in the evaluation process must be robust enough to encompass a range of clinical and academic settings while allowing the collection of information regarding specific performance elements. The process of building a portfolio for clinical and academic partnership requires the establishment of strategic directions and governance arrangements for each organization.[7] Building a relationship between academic and clinical entities may mean breaking fresh ground inside one or both organizations as a means of capitalizing on individual assets. It is important that each member of an academic and clinical partnership be cognizant of the fact that not all activities that serve to strengthen a partnership must have a basis in business practices. Oftentimes, sharing fun can be as important as collaborating on work initiatives.

THE PORTFOLIO

The portfolio has gained acceptance in nursing as a tool for the demonstration of professional competence and as a means for reflecting learning in the educational process. The portfolio has been defined as a collection of evidence of both the products and processes of learning such that past experiences form the basis for continued development and new experiences.[8] Many view the central concept of the portfolio as that of personal and professional reflection[9] or a determination of how well activities and programs have met their stated goals. Whatever the specific definition used, the portfolio must have a clearly stated purpose such as the evaluation of outcomes of a clinical and academic partnership. The responsibility on the part of nurse managers to develop, nurture, and support their profession, coupled with the need to provide accountability for the equitable distribution of resources, makes the portfolio a practical mechanism for documentation of program goals and outcomes.[10] The portfolio can be used to

1. Explore specific learning outcomes or competencies to be developed such as those related to the quality of academic/clinical presentation expected of the portfolio for individual participants
2. Develop a standardized performance/learning contract that includes program aims, each with an action plan of activities and indicators that will be used as evidence of success
3. Assemble evidence of contract completion and complete summary reflection for each item in the learning contract. This often consists of a synoptic statement of what evidence is present to demonstrate desired outcomes together with a critical evaluation of the quality of the evidence.

ROLE OF THE ACADEMIC PARTNER

Academic institutions do not operate in a vacuum or silo. They respond to numerous private, government, and community interests and requests and create visionary opportunities for successful outcomes. Otherwise, the academic institution is not contacted to form partnerships or engage in collaborative projects. Those academic institutions that are visionary and welcome partnerships form rich collaborative relationships that become the foundations for successful enterprises. Strong partnerships create dynamic portfolios beneficial to societal needs and benchmarks for others who transform knowledge, skills, and best practices into innovative models and deliverables. Unparalleled opportunity and the capability to address critical issues in health care are an example of the ardent call for academia and healthcare agencies to form partnerships.

Partnerships and portfolios do not magically emerge. The academic partner must be in a ready state to address needs and open to change when contacted by an agency. Change may require shifting from the traditional approaches to ones that meet diverse and cultural needs, while addressing numerous learning needs and high technological skill sets of individuals. Recognizing what does not work is as critical to success as what does work. Extracting these lessons is not always smooth, so listing them can promote engagement in all sorts of initiatives. A personal belief that partnerships are essential can be a powerful tenet and is useful when agendas and goals are in conflict. Void the belief, and a natural blaming culture persists and the partnership is doomed to failure or to diminished outcomes and deliverables.

Evidence-Based Practice 20-1

Open dialogue during planning and delivery of the requested product or project is beneficial to create a diversity of opportunities and creative use of academic and agency intellectual properties. Recognizing that as a partner in a collaborative endeavor, a teacher and learner perspective is assumed and requisite for success.[11]

Coleman suggests that using emotional intelligence (link between social and emotional abilities) is vital to working with and leading others.[12] It allows one to listen carefully and authentically express oneself as others are motivated and use their talents to the fullest. An engaged partner must demonstrate the skill sets and commitment to team building, communication, promoting change, motivating colleagues, and respecting and understanding workplace culture.[13]

Visibility by the partner beyond the academic setting creates the stage for buy-in from others. If a change in standard operating procedures or approaches is desired, sustained visibility and contact can limit the obstacles that often manifest themselves during the phases of planned change. Adopting a mutually acceptable framework can guide activities and engage multiple individuals and departments toward accomplishment of a goal. The framework should include a common purpose, identified values and beliefs, a plan to engage and educate staff, use improvement techniques, build contingencies, and adopt a style of encouragement and engagement.[14] If changes in roles are required, skill set education should follow to strengthen staff competencies, especially those of communication, delegation, assessment, data analysis, and evidence-based methods. If systems change is required, pilots can offer opportunities for evaluation, role clarity, system efficiency, communication flow, and satisfaction.

What can start serendipitously at one institution or agency can become reality when an academic partner is open to change and sustained partnerships. The benefits of a partnership are numerous and may include enhanced relationships and communications, cost efficiency, responsiveness to identified needs, improved access to development opportunities, and potential for additional developments through the partnership.

ROLE OF THE CLINICAL PARTNER

The clinical partner must begin the partnership process by conducting an assessment of its resources, strengths, and weaknesses. Figures 20-1, 20-2, and 20-3 provide examples of the type of information that should be collected in preparation for discussions with partner.

Once the initial assessment has been completed, a determination of additional points for discussion with academic partners should be developed. This should include assignment of an individual to function as a liaison, establishment of goals, data to be collected for evaluation of outcomes, frequency of meetings, communication strategies, and specific legal or contractual requirements for implementation of the partnership.

ROLE OF THE LIAISONS AND PARTNERSHIP COMMITTEES

It should be understood that the academic and clinical partnership is created with the thought that it will require modification in response to changes in either the academic or clinical setting. Because of

FIGURE 20-1 **HOSPITAL-SPECIFIC STAFFING DATA**

Nursing Unit	Unit Type	Number of Beds	Total RN staff	BSN Degrees	MSN Degrees
2 Alpha	Medical	40	30	16	2
2 Beta	Surgical	40	32	17	3
3 Zeus	Oncology	15	12	8	2
MICU	Intensive Care	15	40	25	5
Total		110	114	66	12

Source: Author.

FIGURE 20-2 **HOSPITAL-SPECIFIC RESOURCES AVAILABLE**

Resource Available	Capacity	Availability	Considerations
Library	8 students per visit	Monday through Friday 8 A.M. to 6 P.M.	Requires facility identification, unlimited copies, no materials can be removed.
Conference room	16	Monday, Wednesday, Fridays 1–3 P.M.	Can be reserved in advance up to 3 months. Other times available on a week to week basis.
Education classroom	10	Monday through Friday 8–10 A.M.	Contains CPR mannequins and other teaching equipment for skills lab. Must be reserved in advance.
Computer instruction room	15	Wednesday and Fridays 1–3 P.M.	Requires 2 weeks advanced scheduling for informatics support staff that must be present.

Source: Author.

the dynamic nature of the healthcare industry, changes brought by external regulatory agencies, stakeholder demands, and healthcare innovations, there needs to be a mechanism available by which the partnership can be modified to the degree possible in response to emerging needs. Needs are met and stakeholder expectations are realized through alignment of resources.

PARTNERSHIP PERFORMANCE ISSUES

Successful academic and clinical partnerships must be underpinned by performance-based outcomes if markers of success are realized and communicated. At the inception of the partnership, agreement to use an existing portfolio format or create one is essential. However basic, many partnerships often scramble to document outcomes at the completion of a partnership project because a portfolio format was not adopted, losing a wealth of rich data that could have been captured throughout the process and as certain milestones were reached.

FIGURE 20-3 HOSPITAL-SPECIFIC EDUCATIONAL RESOURCES AVAILABLE

Need	Frequency	Considerations
Patient education forum presenters	Monthly on either first or second Wednesday 1–2 P.M.	Topics target high-risk groups: diabetes, obesity, heart disease, etc.
Continuing education presenters	Monthly on Thursday mornings 10–11 A.M.	Topics of broad interest to registered nurses: Infection control, infusion therapy, research utilization, etc. CEUs* given.
Critical care core curriculum	Course taught quarterly	Lecture topics from core curriculum. 30-minute to 1-hour lectures for most topics. CEUs given.
Basic cardiac life support instruction	Weekly course Wednesdays 2–3 P.M. or any evening 4–8 P.M.	Certified American Heart Association instructor required.
Nurse manager development	As available	Leadership development topics for current or aspiring managers. CEUs available.

Source: Author.
*Continuing Education Units (CEUs)

What is a portfolio as it relates to an academic and clinical partnership? The portfolio is a roadmap of outcomes-based indicators and subsequent documentation that tracks the successes throughout the partnership and can support future endeavors. Emphasis is on higher order skills such as application, analysis, synthesis and evaluation, problem solving, and real work situations.[15–18] Integral to the portfolio process is showcasing and celebrating successes as the partnership matures. Sustained successes (quantitative and qualitative) create opportunities for the creation and development of additional measures, partnerships, and research proposals that can substantiate evidence-based practice.

The clinical nurse leader project initiated by the American Association of Colleges of Nursing (AACN) outlined guidelines for a partnership model.[19] What started as a pilot project by engaging clinical agencies and academic institutions to form a partnership has transcended into a project with sustained outcomes. Avenues have been created whereby staff can meet the daily challenges in health care and educators can successfully prepare students for practice. Inherent in the AACN guidelines is the use of information and outcomes as a fundamental component when assembling an outcomes portfolio. The portfolio becomes a key element useful for managers to document the merits to sustain a role and supports organizational stewardship whereby resources are effectively utilized. Portfolios can be a tool useful to faculty in assessing the progression by a student and by practitioners who document clinical markers of their successes. Data gleaned from the portfolios can be used by the partnership to market outcomes.

Kaplan and Norton support the development of a portfolio using a strategy map as the framework.[20] The framework links assets to behaviors that support values creation using four interrelated perspectives: financial, customer, internal processes, and learning and growth. The financial perspective captures the tangible outcomes such as profits, revenue, and product costs. The customer perceptive focuses on how an organization or partnership intends to generate sales, outcomes, and loyalty from valued customers or stakeholders. The internal processes perspective details operations management, customer management, and innovation. The learning and growth perspective concentrates on human, information, and organization capital within the organization or partnership. As portfolios are built, one can align outcomes when developing future strategy and measurement tools.

DESIGNING MARKERS OF SUCCESS

The portfolio is a tool used to track and communicate individual and partnership successes. However, if markers of success are not identified early in the partnership and periodically reviewed, successes may not be realized and the potential for individual and organizational growth are often obstructed. When designing markers of success, partnerships should question assumptions, beliefs, and values and consider multiple points of view while attempting to verify reasoning.[21] Boundaries are another critical consideration. They must be explicitly identified, and challenges to meeting target outcomes must be considered. Goldsmith identified three key considerations that should be addressed as markers of success are crafted[22]:

1. Control results, not processes.
2. Be flexible while remaining accountable.
3. Design markers that are purposeful and meaningful to the partnership.

Such efforts may or may not morph into a predictable and standardized process early on, but as the partnership evolves, success is realized, innovation is introduced, and outcomes are demonstrated. Rogers described "by which an innovation is communicated . . . among the members of the . . . system" for the purpose of providing exposure to the innovation.[23] To achieve success, the partnership must continuously engage in and monitor activities that support the innovation. Creativity must be fostered by both the academic and clinical participants. Feedback from key informants cannot be overlooked as outcomes data are tracked, trended, and presented. Often, infrastructures are created without seeking input or considering needs of stakeholders. An example is the creation of clinical services that satisfies a small group while ignoring population-based needs.

In 2004 the AACN introduced the clinical nurse leader role. Successful markers followed as academic and clinical sites formed partnerships and developed a new nursing role, the first in over 35 years. Clinical outcomes have followed that include reduced fragmentation in care, increased staff and patient satisfaction, and a number of anecdotal reports of nurses remaining at the bedside as opposed to seeking other career opportunities. Successful organizations and individuals have mapped outcomes that illustrate how clinical indicators are met and sustained. The marker of the success lies in how they have brokered opportunities using clinical activities that can be measured and disseminated widely. Without developing markers of success, a roadmap is not created and organizations and individuals take for granted their successes and valued outcomes.

MANAGING ACADEMIC AND CLINICAL PARTNERS

Opportunities for academic and clinical partners to improve performance, quality of services, and educate individuals to provide care require commitment and dedication. Pivotal to achieving such is how the academic and clinical partners are managed. Identifying a lead individual or champion is an initial step. Selection can require delicate facilitation, influence, and persuasion. Otherwise, conflicts manifest and paralysis occurs, leading to unmet goals and frustrated partners. The selected leader or champion must be knowledgeable of both the academic and clinical setting or a steep learning curve follows and many opportunities for success may be lost. The designated leader or champion must engage all partners to build systems and processes that will support the identified goal. Communication at all levels is central to success. Without open communication, roles become blurred and individuals may start operating in different directions void of the identified goal. Plsek wrote that "islands of improvement" cannot be sustained in an organization or partnership without a permanent champion.[24] As one manages academic and clinical partners, synergy is created and innovation and diffusion follow.[25] Webster defines synergy as the interaction of agencies, agents, or conditions such that the total effect is greater than the sum of the individual effects.[26]

The synergy model can be used as a template when managing academic and clinical partners.[27] It pairs the needs of both organizations with the talents of faculty and staff. Senge described "mental models" as a determinant of how we make sense of the world and how we take action.[28] As such, the partner leader or champion takes the shared vision and communicates it with others while continuously creating and mapping outcomes. Organizational and personal incentives can be matched, forming the capability for sustained successes. For example, what started as an idea by an academic and clinical partner was developed into clinical guidelines that led to evidence-based inquiry and a joint publication. A return on investment helps individuals focus on projects with sustainable pay back over time. Future growth and development is fostered, and people are inspired to commit to more activities. Competencies and new skill sets can be built by partner participation that stretch people to effectively use talents and engage others in outcomes management.

SUMMARY

Academic and clinical partnerships are not new. The clinical nurse leader role has propelled the need and importance for education and practice to forge new avenues to improve patient outcomes. Academic and clinical partners improve collaboration by increased availability of faculty to teach nursing students through support of adjunct faculty appointments, thereby increasing availability of clinical sites for the education of nursing students. These partnerships, built on a portfolio model, can increase competency and training availability for nursing staff and improve community relations as outreach programs result in the perception of the organization as being a positive corporate citizen.

APPLICATION EXERCISES

Exercise 20-1
Develop a list of rights, norms, rules, agreements, and enforcement mechanisms that academic and clinical partners could share. One example would be development of a common dress code for nurses.

Exercise 20-2
Discuss communication and interaction protocols found in various organizations. Formulate a plan for how communication could be enhanced by adoption of common protocols and/or bylaws for the conduct of business meetings.

Exercise 20-3
An understanding of organizational goals is important for each member of a partnership. Develop a list of goals for a clinical site and identify specific strategies an academic partner might use to participate in their attainment. Develop a list of goals for an academic partner and identify specific strategies a clinical partner might use to participate in their attainment.

Exercise 20-4
Identify external stakeholders in clinical and academic settings. List specific activities to benefit external stakeholders that would allow participation by the clinical and academic partners.

Notes

1. McDaniel, R. R., & Driebe, D. J. (2001). Complexity science and healthcare management. *Advances in Health Care Management, 2,* 11–36.
2. Steefel, L. (2005). Partnerships pilot CNL programs. Retrieved December 2, 2007, from http://www.nurse-week.com/news/Features/05-05/CNLPrograms.asp
3. Murray, T. (2007). Expanding educational capacity through an innovative practice-education partnership. *Journal of Nursing Education, 46,* 330–333.
4. Tennessee Center for Nursing. (2005). *Curing the crisis in nursing education: A master plan for Tennessee.* Retrieved December 2, 2007, from http://www.centerfornursing.org/Nursing_News_and_reports/CuringtheCrisisinNursingEducation.pdf
5. Bartels, J. E., & Bednash, G. (2005). Answering the call for quality nursing care and patient safety: A new model for nursing education. *Nursing Administration Quarterly, 29,* 5–13.
6. American Nurses Credentialing Center. (2005). *ANCC Magnet Recognition Program application manual* (pp. 42–44). Washington, DC.
7. Thompson, H. (2007). Portfolio development. *Nursing Management, 14,* 14–15.
8. McMullan, M., Endacott, R., Gray, M. A., Jasper, M., Miller, C. M. & Scholes, J., (2003) Portfolios and assessment of competence: A review of the literature. *Journal of Advanced Nursing, 41,* 283–294.
9. McEwan, A., & Taylor, D. (2007). Assessing practice through portfolio learning. *Journal of Community Nursing, 21,* 4–6.
10. Curtin, L., & Arnold, L. (2005). A framework for analysis, Part II. *Nursing Administration Quarterly, 29,* 288–291.
11. Ward-Smith, P., Hunt, C., Smith, J. B., Teasley, S. L., Carroll, C. A., & Sexton, K. (2007). Issues and opportunities for retaining experienced nurses at the bedside. *Journal of Nursing Administration, 37,* 485–487.
12. Coleman, D. (1995). *Emotional intelligence: Why it matters more than IQ.* New York: Bantam Books.
13. Conley, S. B., Branowicki, P., & Hanley, D. (2007). A competency and preceptor model to facilitate new leader success. *Journal of Nursing Administration, 37,* 491–498.
14. Reinertsen, J. L., Gosfield, A. G., Rupp, W., & Whittington, J. W. (2007). *Engaging physicians in a shared quality agenda* (pp. 1–48). Innovative Series 2007. Institute for Healthcare Improvement, Washington, DC.
15. Farr, R. C., & Tone, B. (1994). *Portfolio and performance assessment: Helping students evaluate their progress as readers and writers in growing to meet your needs.* New York: Harcourt Brace College.
16. Stiggins, R. J. (1997). *Students-Centered classroom assessment* (2nd ed.). Upper Saddle River, NJ: Prentice-Hall.
17. Spandel, V., & Cullham, R. (1995). *Writing from the inside out: Revising for quality.* Portland, OR: Northwest Regional Educational Laboratory. Distributed through IOX Assessment Associates, Los Angeles.
18. McMillian, J. H. (1997). *Classroom assessment: What teachers need to know* (2nd ed.). Boston: Allyn and Bacon.
19. American Association of Colleges of Nursing. (2007). White paper of the education and role of the clinical nurse leader. *AACN,* 1–40. Washington, DC.

20. Kaplan, R. S., & Norton, D. P. (2004). Measuring the strategic readiness of intangible assets. *Harvard Business Review, 2,* 52–63.
21. Boyd, R. D., & Myers, J. G. (1988). Transformative education. *International Journal of Lifelong Education, 7,* 261–284.
22. Goldsmith, S. (2006). Crisis breeds innovation. Harvard University Government Innovators Network [serial online]. Retrieved January 3, 2008, from www.ksg.harvard.edu/innovations/Management/index.html?p=./Goldsmith
23. Rogers, E. M. (1983). *Diffusion of innovations.* New York: Free Press.
24. Plsek, P. (2000). *Spreading good ideas for better health care: A practical toolkit, tools, perspectives, and information for health care providers.* Irving, TX: HDC/Tools/Organization/Docs.
25. Tachibana, C., & Nelson-Peterson, D. L. (2007). Implementing the clinical nurse leader role using the Virginia Mason production system. *Journal of Nursing Administration, 37,* 477–483.
26. *Merriam-Webster's collegiate dictionary* (10th ed.). (1997). Springfield, MA: Merriam-Webster.
27. Curley, M. A. Q. (2004). Synergy: From theory to practice. *Excellent Nursing Knowledge, 1* [serial online]. Retrieved January 3, 2008, from www.nursingknowledge.org/enk
28. Senge, P. M. (1994). *The fifth discipline: The art and practice of the learning organization.* New York: Currency Doubleday.

References

American Nurses Credentialing Committee announces market of Critical Portfolio. (2006, March). *South Dakota Nurse,* Retrieved December 23, 2007, from CINAHL Plus with Full Text database.

Billings, D., & Kowalski, K. (2005, July). Teaching tips. Learning portfolios. *Journal of Continuing Education in Nursing, 36,* 149–150. Retrieved December 23, 2007, from CINAHL Plus with Full Text database.

Cole, G. (2005, November). The definition of "portfolio." *Medical Education, 39,* 1141. Retrieved December 23, 2007, from CINAHL Plus with Full Text database.

Kear, M., & Bear, M. (2007, March). Using portfolio evaluation for program outcome assessment. *Journal of Nursing Education, 46,* 109–114. Retrieved December 23, 2007, from CINAHL Plus with Full Text database.

Mullen, P. (2007, March 28). The good portfolio. *Nursing Standard, 21,* 62–63. Retrieved December 23, 2007, from CINAHL Plus with Full Text database.

Rees, C. (2005, November). "Portfolio" definitions: Do we need a wider debate? *Medical Education, 39,* 1142. Retrieved December 23, 2007, from CINAHL Plus with Full Text database.

Williams, M., & Jordan, K. (2007, May). The nursing professional portfolio: A pathway to career development. *Journal for Nurses in Staff Development, 23,* 125–131. Retrieved December 23, 2007, from CINAHL Plus with Full Text database.

21 TRANSFORMATIONAL LEADERSHIP AND EVIDENCE-BASED MANAGEMENT IN A CHANGING WORLD

Linda Roussel, RN, DSN, NEA, BC

LEARNING OBJECTIVES AND ACTIVITIES

- Describe transformational leadership and evidence-based management.
- Define leadership.
- Explain trait theories of leadership.
- Match examples to Gardner's nine tasks to be performed by leaders.
- Match examples to individual leadership behavioral theorists.
- Match examples to the theory of transformational leadership.
- Discuss similarities between leadership and management.
- Match examples to interpersonal bases of power.
- Describe quantum leadership in a new age of health care.

CONCEPTS

Transformational leadership, evidence-based management, trait theories of leadership, behavioral theories of leadership, leadership styles, gender issues of leadership, buffering, quantum leadership.

QUOTE

I must follow the people. Am I not their leader?

—Benjamin Disraeli, British Statesman

NURSE MANAGER BEHAVIORS	NURSE EXECUTIVE BEHAVIORS
Facilitates involvement of registered nurses, other staff members, and patients/clients/residents in interdisciplinary identification of desired outcomes; emphasizes problem solving, results, analysis of failure, tasks, control, and decision making; collaborates with appropriate departments in promoting integrated systems to support nursing service delivery and decision analysis.	Facilitates the establishment and continuous improvement of clinical guidelines related to outcomes that provide direction for continuity of care and that are attainable with available resources; focuses on creating spirit and commitment, seeking advice and feedback, empowering constituents, and modeling appropriate behavior as symbols of values and norms.

Introduction

Transformational leadership is needed for change required in health care and critical to successful organizational outcomes. Leadership is central to safety in a variety of industries as well as to an organization's competitive cost position after a change initiative.[1–3] Transformational leadership has been specifically identified by the Institute of Medicine in its work on medical error and patient safety.[4] Changes in nursing leadership have been underscored in creating safe environments for patients and staff, particularly as the weakening of clinical leadership has been cited as a cause of organizational concerns and issues.[5] The Institute of Medicine described factors of problematic leadership[6]:

- Increased emphasis on production efficiency (bottom-line management)
- Weakened trust (reengineering initiatives, poor communication patterns)
- Poor change management (inadequate communication, insufficient worker training, lack of measurement and feedback, short-lived attention, limited worker involvement in developing change initiatives)
- Limited involvement in decision making pertaining to work design and work flow (hierarchical structures, limited voice on councils, committees)
- Limited knowledge management (process failures, limited second-order attention)

To address these challenges, the following recommendations were made by the Institute of Medicine for healthcare organizations, particularly related to acquiring nurse leaders for all levels of management (e.g., at the organization-wide and patient care unit levels). Nurse leaders should do the following[7]:

- Participate in executive decisions within the healthcare organizations.
- Represent nursing staff to organization management and facilitate their mutual trust.
- Achieve effective communication between nursing and other clinical leadership.
- Facilitate input of direct-care nursing staff into operational decision making and design of work processes and work flow.
- Be provided with organizational resources to support the acquisition, management, and dissemination to nursing staff of the knowledge needed to support their clinical decision making and actions.

Although no one particular organizational structure for locating nursing leadership across all healthcare organizations was identified, the focus of the recommendations was on well-prepared clinical nurse leaders at the most senior level of management. Magnet hospitals have found some positive outcomes related to staff and patient satisfaction that correlated with participatory and transformational leadership. Clearly, transformational leadership is called for to address these challenges, to improve quality outcomes for patients and staff, and to heighten overall organizational effectiveness.[8]

HISTORY

Florence Nightingale, after leaving the Crimea, exercised extraordinary leadership in health care for decades with no organization under her command.[9] She was also one of the purest examples of the leader as agenda setter. Her public image is that of the lady of mercy, but under her gentle, soft-spoken manner she was a rugged spirit, a fighter, and a tough-minded system changer. In mid-19th century England, a woman had no place in public life, least of all in the fiercely masculine world of the military establishment. Nightingale took on the establishment and revolutionized health care in the British military services. Yet she never made public appearances or speeches and, except for her 2 years in the Crimea, held no public position. She was a formidable authority on the evils to be remedied, she knew exactly what to do about them, and she used public opinion to goad top officials into adopting her agenda. Florence Nightingale was both leader and manager.[10]

LEADERSHIP DEFINED

Researchers have studied leadership for decades, but experts still do not agree on exactly what it is. Many persons use the term *leadership* as if it were a magic quality, something one is born with or for which one simply has a talent. However, like talent for music and art, talent for leadership involves much knowledge and disciplined practice. Many definitions of leadership have been written, including that of Stogdill, who defines it as "the process of influencing the activities of an organized group in its efforts toward goal setting and goal achievement."[11] A difference in responsibilities exists among group members, and each member influences the group's activities. A leader is one others follow willingly and voluntarily.[12]

Stogdill's definition of leadership can be applied to nursing. In nursing practice, goals of patient care are set. Each patient has a nursing care plan that lists the problems that interfere with achieving physical, emotional, and social needs. For each problem, a goal is set and an approach or nursing prescription is written. An interdisciplinary team may identify problems, set goals, and write prescriptions. The team is influenced by the most highly skilled nurse available, the registered nurse who coordinates the care. Each interdisciplinary team member assumes different responsibilities in performing the total team functions.

The same principles may be applied to the entire division of nursing. Usually, the title of the head of the division is assistant administrator, vice president, chair, or director of nursing services. The division head is responsible for influencing all nursing employees toward achieving the stated purpose and objectives of the division of nursing. The nurse administrator is influenced by a stated philosophy or statement of beliefs about the kinds of services to be rendered by the personnel of the division of nursing. The total staff includes personnel in different job categories, including nurse managers, nursing case managers of shifts, and clinical nursing personnel, each with different responsibilities.

Gardner defines leadership as "the process of persuasion and example by which an individual (or leadership team) induces a group to take action that is in accord with the leader's purposes or the shared purposes of all."[13] Numerous other definitions of leadership exist. These definitions include the terms leader, follower or constituent, group, process, and goals. One can conclude that leadership is a process in which a person inspires a group of constituents to work together using appropriate means to achieve a common mission and common goals. Constituents are influenced to work together willingly and cooperatively with zeal and confidence and to their greatest potential.[14]

Leadership is a social transaction in which one person influences others. People in authority do not necessarily exert leadership. Rather, effective people in authoritative positions combine authority and leadership to assist an organization to achieve its goals. Effective leadership satisfies four primary conditions[15]:

1. A person receiving a communication understands it.
2. This person has the resources to do what is being asked of him or her.
3. The person believes the behavior being asked of him or her is consistent with personal interests and values.
4. The person believes the request is consistent with the purposes and values of the organization.

According to McGregor,[16] there are at least four major variables now known to be involved in leadership:

1. Characteristics of the leader
2. Attitudes, needs, and other personal characteristics of the followers
3. Characteristics of the organization, such as its purpose, its structure, the nature of the task to be performed
4. Social, economic, and political milieu.

Leadership is a highly complex relationship that changes with the times. Such changes are brought about by management, unions, or outside forces. In nursing, changes in leadership are wrought by nursing management, nursing educators, nursing organizations, unions, and the expectations of the clientele (patients and their families).

Talbott said, "Leadership is the vital ingredient that transforms a crowd into a functioning, useful organization."[17] The theme in these definitions seems always to be the same: "Leadership is the process of sustaining an initiated action. It is certainly not a matter of pointing in a direction and just letting things happen. Leadership is the conception of a goal and a method of achieving it; the mobilization of the means necessary for attainment; and the adjustment of values and environmental factors in the light of the desired end."[18]

In all definitions, leadership is viewed as a dynamic, interactive process that involves three dimensions: the leader, the follower(s), and the situation. Each dimension influences the others. For instance, the accomplishment of goals depends not only on the personal attributes of the leader but also on the follower's needs and the type of situation.[19]

Leadership Theories

Trait Theory

Much of the early work on leadership focused on the leader. This research was directed toward identifying intellectual, emotional, physical, and other personal traits of effective leaders. The underlying assumption was that leaders are born, not made.

After many years of research, no particular set of traits has been found that predicts leadership potential. There are several possible reasons for this failure. According to McGregor, "Research findings to date suggest that it is more fruitful to consider leadership as a relationship between the leader and the situation than as a universal pattern of characteristics possessed by certain people."[20] This statement implies that leadership is a human relations function and that different situations may require quite different characteristics from a leader. It is generally accepted in nursing that authoritarian power is effective in times of crisis but that otherwise it promotes instability.

Despite the shortcomings of the trait theory, some traits have been identified that are common to all good leaders. Such traits as honesty, trustworthiness, integrity, fair, skilled communicator, goal-oriented, dedicated, committed, and hard working continue to surface in the literature.

Gardner's Leadership Studies

Two major treatises of Gardner's writings that relate to the traits of leadership are the tasks of leadership and leader–constituent interaction.[21] Gardner identifies nine tasks to be performed by leaders[22]:

1. *Envisioning goals:* These include envisioning the best a group can be, solving problems, and unifying constituencies. Goals may involve extensive research. They may be shared, and they come from many sources. Long-term goals lend greater stability than do short-term goals.

2. *Affirming values:* Communities have "shared assumptions, beliefs, customs, ideas that give meaning, ideas that motivate." These include norms or values. Values embody religious beliefs and secular philosophy. Society celebrates its values in art, song, ritual, historic documents, and textbooks. People will strive to meet standards that affirm their values and motivate them. Values must be continually rebuilt or regenerated, with leaders assisting to rediscover and adapt traditions to the present. Leaders reaffirm values through words, policy decisions, and conduct.

3. *Motivating:* Leaders stimulate people to serve society and solve its problems. They balance positive attitudes and acts with reality. They look toward the future with confidence, hope, and energy. Loss of confidence breeds rigidity, fatalism, and passivity. Poverty negatively affects morale, learning, and performance. Leaders correct the circumstances of negative attitudes and defeat. Involving employees in decisions gives them a sense of power and ownership. Leaders resolve failure, frustration, and doubt and use intuition and empathy to solve problems.

4. *Managing:* Leadership and management overlap. Leaders set goals, plan, fix priorities, choose means, and formulate policy. They also build organizations and institutions that outlast them. Leaders keep the system functioning by setting agendas and making decisions. Leaders mold public opinion and exercise political judgments.

5. *Achieving workable unity:* Leaders function in a pluralistic society in which conflict is necessary if there are grievances to be settled. Conflict is also necessary in competing commercially, settling civil suits, and bringing justice to the oppressed. Conflict must be resolved to achieve cohesion and mutual tolerance, internally and externally. Society is fragmented and must not be polarized. Conflict resolution requires political skills: brokering, forming coalitions, mediating conflicting views, de-escalating rhetoric and posturing, saving face, and seeking common ground. People must trust each other most of the time to prevent or resolve conflict. Leaders raise the level of trust.

6. *Explaining:* Leaders must communicate effectively. They teach.

7. *Serving as a symbol:* Leaders speak for others. They represent unity, collective identity, and continuity.

8. *Representing the group:* All human systems are interdependent. Leaders take a broad view of events.

9. *Renewing:* Leaders blend continuity with change. They are innovators who awaken the potential

of others. They visit the front lines and keep in touch. Leaders sustain diversity and dissent, and they change the social order.

Leader–Constituent Interaction

Charismatic Leaders   Gardner defines charisma as the quality that sets one person apart from others: supernatural, superhuman, endowed with exceptional qualities or powers. Charismatic leadership can be good or evil. Charismatic leaders emerge in troubled times and in relation to the state of mind of constituents. They eventually run out of miracles and "white horses," even though the leaders are magnetic, persuasive, and spellbinding.

Masses of people often follow the charismatic leader. Such masses have historically been labeled unstable. Worry about mob rule and instability still exists. Social disorder is embodied in the Constitution of the United States.

Influence of Constituents on Leaders   Constituents and leaders have an equal influence on each other. Constituents confer the leadership role. Good constituents select good leaders and make them better. In politics, constituents may follow any leader unless they are bureaucratic constituents (such as government employees) who feel constrained to mute their support. Loyal constituents support leaders who help them meet their needs and solve problems.

Influence of Leaders on Constituents   Leaders choose to be leaders. They must adapt their leadership style to the situation and their constituents. In doing so, they weigh the following considerations: the degree of structure they want in relationships with constituents; the degree or hierarchy of authority, formality, discipline, constraint, and control; and the degree of focus on task versus that on people.

Leaders influence their superiors and their subordinates and have the courage to defy their constituents. Sam Houston was a leader of this type. He opposed the secession of Texas from the United States, going against his constituents. A leader may show different faces to pluralistic groups of constituents, including special interest groups.

Transforming Leaders

Transforming leaders respond to people's basic needs, wants, hopes, and expectations. They may transcend the political system or even attempt to construct it in order to operate within it. Transforming leadership is innovative, and it evolves.

The best leadership may be that which focuses on self-development and self-actualization. Leaders should develop the strengths of constituents and make them independent.[23]

Behavioral Theories

Behavioral theories include Douglas McGregor's Theory X and Theory Y, Rensis Likert's Michigan studies, Blake and Mouton's Managerial Grid, and Kurt Lewin's studies. Each of these is described here in more detail.

McGregor's Theory X and Theory Y   McGregor related his theories to the motivation theories of Maslow. McGregor states that each person is a whole individual living and interacting within a world of other individuals. What happens to this person happens as a result of the behavior of other people. The attitudes and emotions of others affect this person. The constituent is dependent on the leader and desires to be treated fairly. A successful relationship is desired by both and depends on the action taken by the leader.

Security is a condition of leadership. Constituents need security and will fight to protect themselves against real or imagined threats to these needs in the work situation. Leaders must act to give constituents this security through avenues such as fair pay and fringe benefits. Unions act to solidify job security.

An effective leader creates an atmosphere of approval for constituents. Such an atmosphere is created through the leader's manner and attitude. Given the genuine approval of their leader, constituents will be secure. Otherwise, they will feel threatened, fearful, and insecure.

Knowledge is another condition of effective leadership espoused by McGregor. Employees have security when they know what is expected of them, including the following[24]:

- Knowledge of overall company policy and management philosophy
- Knowledge of procedures, rules, and regulations
- Knowledge of the requirements of the subordinate's job duties, responsibilities, and place in the organization
- Knowledge of the personal peculiarities of the constituent's immediate leader
- Knowledge by the constituent of the leader's opinion of his or her performance
- Advance knowledge of changes that may affect the constituent

Consistent discipline is another condition for effective leadership. People are met with approval when they do their jobs according to expectations. They should know what to expect in terms of disapproval when they do not meet expectations. Leaders should be consistent in setting standards and expecting constituents to meet them. Even discipline must occur in an atmosphere of approval.

Security encourages independence, another condition for effective leadership. Insecurity causes a reactive fight for freedom. Security that stimulates independence is desired. Constituents need to become actively independent by being involved in contributing ideas and suggestions concerning activities that affect them. When workers are secure and encouraged to participate in solving the problems of work, they provide new approaches to solutions. They work to achieve the goals of the organization and feel they are a part of it.

With security and independence, constituents develop a desire to accept responsibility. The level of responsibility can be increased at a pace commensurate with preservation of constituents' security. Having security gives constituents pleasure and pride. Leaders need security before they can delegate responsibility to constituents.

All constituents need a provision for appeal, that is, an adequate grievance procedure by which they can take their differences with their superiors to a higher level in the organization. Leaders who do the jobs expected of them and who treat constituents in ways that meet their needs and give them security achieve self-realization and self-development.[25]

Likert's Michigan Studies Likert and his associates at the Institute for Social Research at the University of Michigan conducted extensive leadership research. They identified four basic styles or systems of leadership: system I, exploitative-authoritative; system II, benevolent-authoritative; system III, consultative-democratic; and system IV, participative-democratic.

A measuring instrument for evaluating an organization's leadership style was developed by Likert's group. It contains 51 items and encompasses variables of the concepts of "leadership, motivation, communication, interaction-influence, decision making, goal setting, control, and performance goals."[26]

It is generally conceded that leadership behavior improves in effectiveness as it approaches system IV.

Blake and Mouton's Managerial Grid The managerial grid is a two-dimensional leadership model. Dimensions of this model are tasks or production and the employee or people orientations of managers.[27]

Two key dimensions of managerial thinking are depicted on the grid: concern for production on the horizontal axis, and concern for people on the vertical axis. They are shown as 9-point scales: 1 represents low concern, 5 represents an average amount of concern, and 9 is high concern.

These two concerns are interdependent; that is, although concern for one or the other may be high or low, they are integrated in the manager's thinking. Thus both concerns are present to some degree in any management style. Study of the grid enables one to sort out various possibilities and the attitudes, values, beliefs, and assumptions that underlie each approach. When one is able to objectively see one's own behavior compared with the soundest approach, it provides motivation to change to more closely approximate the soundest management. When group members come to share 9, 9 values, beliefs, attitudes, and assumptions, they develop personal commitment to achieving group goals as well as their individual goals. In doing so they develop standards of mutual trust and respect that cause them to elevate cooperation and communication.

Blake and Mouton contend that the 9, 9 style is the one most likely to achieve highest quality results over an extended period of time. The 9, 9 style, unlike the others, is based on the assumption that there is no inherent conflict between the needs of the organization for performance and the needs of people for job satisfaction.

Finally, as an orienting framework, the grid serves as a map to more effective ways of working with and through others. When group members have this common frame of reference for what constitutes effective and ineffective approaches to issues of mutual concern, they are able to take corrective action based on common understanding and agreement about the soundest approach and an objectivity when actions taken are less than fully sound.

Kurt Lewin's Studies   Lewin's leadership studies were done in the 1930s. Lewin examined three leadership styles related to forces within the leader, within the group members, and within the situation. From Lewin's studies, the leadership styles emerging were autocratic, democratic, and laissez-faire. The autocratic leader makes decisions alone and tends to be more concerned with task accomplishment than with concern for people. In contrast, the democratic leader involves followers in the decision-making process and is people-oriented, focusing on human relations and teamwork. The laissez-faire leader is permissive and generally abstains from leading the staff, which often results in low productivity and employee frustration.

Other behavioral studies include the Ohio State studies, which use a quadrant structure that relates leadership effectiveness to initiating structure (with emphasis on the task or production) and consideration (with emphasis on the employee). These studies identified four primary leadership styles relating to those leaders with high initiating structure to low initiating structure and those with low consideration to high consideration.

The Ohio State Researchers used the Leader Behavior Description Questionnaire. Items related to initiating structure and to consideration describe how leaders carry out their activities. Both factors are considered simultaneously rather than on a continuum. As to which combination works best, the situation determines the style.[28]

Problems with Leadership Questionnaires   According to Phillips and Lord, the accuracy of leadership questionnaires is debatable. Yet they are often the only feasible way to measure leadership in real-world settings. Some researchers consider reliable questionnaires accurate. However, these authors contend that any systematic sources of variance, such as leniency error, halo, or implicit theories, can produce high internal consistency. Factor structures produced solely on the basis of implicit leadership theories do not tell users of these questionnaires anything about accuracy.

The Leader Behavior Description Questionnaire was flawed because its subjects form an overall leadership impression before completing it. Questionnaires can be improved by requiring "observers to distinguish between the presence and absence of specific, conceptually equivalent behaviors in video-taped stimulus materials."[29]

Most questionnaire-based leadership research has been conducted in laboratory settings. The results are biased by the fact that some conditions do not exist in typical field settings. Research participants

do not know or have contact with the target leader; thus the behavioral-level accuracy of their responses is limited. Phillips and Lord make the following suggestions to improve research techniques of
existing behavioral description questionnaires[30]:

1. Assess whether the level of accuracy required for the purpose is classification or behavioral.
2. Assess whether the level of accuracy produced by the chosen measurement technique is classification or behavioral.
3. Evaluate the research setting for potential biases "such as rote knowledge of performance, leniency in describing superiors, or other relevant rater characteristics."
4. If biases exist, judge whether they are likely to be confounded with substantive variables of interest to the user.
5. Collect global measures of leadership and leniency during the measurement process.

Leadership Style

Other studies of leadership focus on style, including contingency-situational leadership models that
focus on a combination of factors, such as the people, the task, the situation, the organization, and environmental factors. These models combine theories of Fred F. Fiedler; Paul Hersey, Kenneth H.
Blanchard, and D. E. Johnson; and William J. Reddin.

Fiedler's Contingency Model of Leadership Effectiveness

There must be a group before there can be a leader. Fiedler describes three classifications that measure the kind of power and influence the group gives its leader. The first and most important of these
is the relationship between the leader and the group members. Personality is a factor, but its influence depends on the group's perception of the leader. Second is the task structure, the degree to
which details of the group's assignment are programmed. If the assignment is highly structured, the
leader will have less power. If the assignment requires planning and thinking, the leader will be in a
position to exert greater power. Third is the positional power of the leader: Great power does not always yield better group performance. The best leader has been found to be one who has a task-
oriented leadership style. This style works best when the leader has great influence and power
over group members. When the leader has moderate influence over group members, a relationship-
oriented style works best.

The organization shares responsibility for a leader's success or failure. Leaders can be trained to
learn in which situations they do well and in which they fail. The job can be fitted to the leader. The appointee can be given a higher rank or can be assigned constituents who are nearly equal in rank and
status. Most appointees can be given sole authority or can be required to consult with the group. The
appointee can be given detailed instructions or independence. A highly successful and effective leader
avoids situations in which failure is likely. That leader seeks out situations that fit his or her leadership
style. Knowledge of strengths and weaknesses helps in choosing this style.[31]

Fiedler's theory is one of situations: leadership style will be effective or ineffective depending on
the situation.

Life Cycle Theory of Hersey, Blanchard, and Johnson

Hersey, Blanchard, and Johnson follow a situational approach to leadership. A person's leadership style
focuses on a combination of task behaviors and relationship behaviors. Focus on task behaviors is
"characterized by endeavoring to establish well-defined patterns of organization, channels of communication, and ways of getting jobs accomplished." Focus on relationship behavior relates to "opening up
channels of communication, providing socio-emotional support, actively listening, 'psychological
strokes,' and facilitating behaviors."[32]

Reddin's Three-Dimensional Theory of Management

Reddin combined Blake and Mouton's managerial grid with Fiedler's contingency leadership model. The outcome was a three-dimensional theory of management; the dimensions are adapted from managerial grid theory, contingency leadership style theory, and effectiveness theory. These possible combinations result in four basic leadership styles:

1. Separated, in which both task orientation and relationship orientation are minimal.
2. Dedicated, in which task orientation is high and relationship orientation is low. Dedicated leaders are dedicated only to the job.
3. Related, in which relationship orientation is high and task orientation is low. Related leaders relate primarily to their constituents.
4. Integrated, in which both task orientation and relationship orientations are high. Integrated leaders focus on managerial behavior, combining task orientation and relationship orientation.

These management styles are identified below:

- Executive leaders are integrated and more effective than are compromiser leaders, who are less effective integrated leaders.
- Developer leaders are related and more effective than missionary leaders, who are less effective related leaders.
- Bureaucrat leaders are separated and more effective than deserter leaders, who are less effective separated leaders.
- Benevolent autocrat leaders are dedicated and more effective than autocrat leaders, who are less effective dedicated leaders.

The range of effectiveness is a continuum. As in other theories of leadership, the effective behavior of the leader is relative to the situation. Effective leaders apply leadership styles after assessing situations.[33]

Transformational Leadership

The healthcare system is experiencing tremendous change and chaos, and the problems of organizations are increasingly complex. Healthcare organizations are restructuring and redesigning the way patient care is delivered to meet the challenges of these changes. In addition, health care is prohibitively expensive for many Americans. Hospitals and emergency rooms are financially burdened by the uninsured who suffer from violence, drug overdose, and HIV infection. Many people, especially in rural areas and inner cities, do not have access to health care because hospitals are downsizing and a shortage of healthcare personnel exists. Leaders must find ways to keep staff motivated in this chaotic, unstable environment. Therefore effective leaders in this atmosphere of rapid change will acknowledge uncertainty, be flexible, and consider the values and needs of constituents.[34]

Bennis and Nanus describe a theory of leadership called transformational leadership. They define a transformational leader as one who "commits people to action, who converts followers into leaders, and who may convert leaders into agents of change."[35] These authors believe that the nucleus of leadership is power, which they define as the "basic energy to initiate and sustain action translating intention into reality."[36] Transformational leaders do not use power to control and repress constituents. These leaders instead empower constituents to have a vision about the organization and trust the leaders so they work for goals that benefit the organization and themselves.

Leadership is thus not so much the exercise of power itself as it is the empowerment of others. This does not mean that leaders must relinquish power, but rather that reciprocity, an exchange between leaders and constituents, exists. The goal is change in which the purpose of the leader and that of the constituent become enmeshed, creating a collective purpose. Empowered staff become critical thinkers and are active in their roles within the organization. A creative and committed staff is the most important asset that administrators can develop.[37]

Transformational leaders mobilize their staff by focusing on the welfare of the individual and humanizing the high-tech work environment. Experts favor a leadership style that empowers others and values collaboration instead of competition.[38] People are empowered when they share in decision making and when they are rewarded for quality and excellence rather than punished and manipulated. When the environment is humanized, people are empowered, feel part of the team, and believe they are contributing to the success of the organization. Leaders who share power motivate people to excel by inspiring them to be part of a vision rather than punishing them for mistakes.[39] In nursing, empowerment can result in improved patient care, fewer staff sick days, and decreased attrition. Nurses who are transformational leaders have staff with higher job satisfaction and who stay in the organization for longer periods.[40]

Nurse executives who like to feel in charge may feel threatened by the concept of sharing power with staff. So they need to be personally empowered to assist in the empowerment of others. They will have a sense of self-worth and self-respect and confidence in their own abilities. Bennis and Nanus believe the most important trait of successful leaders is having positive self-regard.[41] Self-regard is not, however, self-centeredness or self-importance; rather, leaders with positive self-esteem recognize their strengths and do not emphasize their weaknesses. A leader who has positive self-regard seems to create in others a sense of confidence and high expectations. Techniques used to increase self-worth include visualization, affirmations, and letting go of the need to be perfect.[42]

Through research and observations, Bennis defined four competencies for dynamic and effective transformational leadership: (1) management of attention, (2) management of meaning, (3) management of trust, and (4) management of self.[43] The first competency is the management of attention, achieved by having a vision or sense of outcomes or goals. Vision is the image of a realistic, attainable, credible, and attractive future state for an organization.[44] Vision statements are written to define where the healthcare organization is headed and how it will serve society. They differ from mission and philosophy statements in that they are more futuristic and describe where energies are to be focused.[45]

The second leadership competency is management of meaning. To inspire commitment, leaders must communicate their vision and create a culture that sustains the vision. A culture or social architecture as described by Bennis and Nanus is "intangible, but it governs the way people act, the values

> **People are committed to visions that are mutually developed, are based on a sense of quality, appeal to their values and emotions, and are feasible yet challenging.**

and norms that are subtly transmitted to groups and individuals, and the construct of binding and bonding within a company."[46] Barker believes that "social architecture provides meaning and shared experience of organizational events so that people know the expectations of how they are to act."[47]

Nursing leaders transform the social architecture or culture of healthcare organizations by using group discussion, agreement, and consensus building, and they support individual creativity and innovation. To do this, Barker believes that the nurse transformational leader will pay attention to the internal consistency of the vision, goals, and objectives; selection and placement of personnel; feedback; appraisal; rewards; support; and development.[48] For example, rewards and appraisals must relate to the goals, and the vision must be consistent with the goals and objectives. Most importantly, all the elements must enhance the self-worth of individuals, allow creativity, and appeal to the values of nurses. For many nurse leaders, these are new skills that will take time and support from mentors to develop.

Because vision statements are a new concept to many, nursing leaders should provide opportunities for staff to openly explore feelings, criticize, and articulate negative reactions. Face-to-face meetings between nursing leaders and staff are desirable because in reactions involving trust and clarity, memorandums and suggestion boxes are not adequate substitutes for direct communication.[49]

The third competency is the management of trust, which is associated with reliability. Nurses respect leaders whose judgment is sound and consistent and whose decisions are based on fairness, equity, and honesty. Staff can be heard to comment about leaders they trust with statements such as "I don't always agree with her decision, but I know she wants the best for the patients." Bennis believes that "people would much rather follow individuals they can count on, even when they disagree with their viewpoint, than people they agree with but who shift positions frequently."[50]

The fourth competency is management of self, which is knowing one's skills and using them effectively. It is critical that nurses in leadership positions recognize when they lack management skills and then take responsibility for their own continuing education. Incompetent leaders can demoralize a nursing unit and contribute to poor patient care. When leadership skills are mastered by nurse leaders, stress and burnout are reduced. Nurse leaders thus need to master the skills of leadership.[51]

Although effective leaders support shared power and decision making, they continue to accept responsibility for making decisions even when their decisions are not popular. Constituents like to have their wishes considered, but there are times when they want prompt and clear decisions from a leader. This is especially true in times of crisis.[52]

Transformational leaders are flexible and able to adapt leadership styles to the chaos and rapid change occurring in the current healthcare environment.

Differences Between Leadership and Management

Managers come from the "headship" (power from position) category. They hold appointive or directive posts in formal organizations. They can be appointed for both technical and leadership competencies, usually needing both to be accepted. Managers are delegated authority, including the power to reward or punish. A manager is expected to perform functions such as planning, organizing, directing (leading), and controlling (evaluating). Informal leaders, by contrast, are not always managers performing those functions required by the organization. Leaders often are not even part of the organization. Florence Nightingale, after leaving the Crimea, was not connected with an organization but was still a leader.

> **Zaleznik indicates that the manager is a problem solver who succeeds because of "persistence, tough-mindedness, hard work, intelligence, analytical ability, and, perhaps most important, tolerance and good will.**[53]

Managers focus on results, analysis of failure, and tasks—management characteristics that are desirable for nurse managers. Effective managers also need to be good leaders. Managers who are leaders choose and limit goals. They focus on creating spirit and, in doing so, develop committed constituents. Manager-leaders do this by seeking advice and solutions to problems. They ask for information and provide positive feedback. Leaders understand the power of groups. They empower their constituents, making their subordinates strong—the chosen ones, a team infused with purpose. Mistakes are tolerated by manager-leaders who challenge constituents to realize their potential.

Managers emphasize control, decision making, and decision analysis. As manager-leaders, they are concerned with modeling appropriate behavior as symbols of values and norms. Effective manager-leaders are technically capable and provide assurance in crises.

Managers focus inward but add the leadership dimension of connecting their group to the outside world, focusing intense attention on important issues. They escalate issues and complaints up the organization to be handled quickly and appropriately, rather than try to control them.[54]

Although managers are sometimes described in less glowing terms than leaders, successful managers are usually successful leaders. Leadership is a desirable and prominent feature of the directing function of nursing management.

Similarities Between Leadership and Management

Gardner asserts that first-class managers are usually first-class leaders. Leaders and leader-managers distinguish themselves beyond run-of-the-mill managers in six respects[55]:

1. They think longer term—beyond the day's crises, beyond the quarterly report, beyond the horizon.
2. They look beyond the unit they head and grasp its relationship to larger realities—the larger organization of which they are a part, conditions external to the organization, global trends.
3. They reach and influence constituents beyond their jurisdiction, beyond boundaries. Thomas Jefferson influenced people all over Europe. Gandhi influenced people all over the world. In an organization, leaders overflow bureaucratic boundaries—often a distinct advantage in a world too complex and tumultuous to be handled "through channels." Their capacity to rise above jurisdictions may enable them to bind together the fragmented constituencies that must work together to solve a problem.
4. They put heavy emphasis on the intangibles of vision, values, and motivation and understand intuitively the nonrational and unconscious elements in the leader-constituent interaction.
5. They have the political skill to cope with the conflicting requirements of multiple constituencies.
6. They think in terms of renewal. The routine manager tends to accept the structure and processes as they exist. The leader or leader-manager seeks the revisions of process and structure required by changing reality.

Good leaders, like good managers, provide visionary inspiration, motivation, and direction. Good managers, like good leaders, attract and inspire. People want to be led rather than managed. They want to pursue goals and values they consider worthwhile. Therefore they want leaders who respect the dignity, autonomy, and self-esteem of constituents.[56]

> **Effective nurse executives combine leadership and management.**

Mitchell describes five major requirements for every executive, implying that being an effective executive requires the attributes of a leader[57]:

1. Adjustment to a complex social environment of several or many units
2. Ability to influence and guide subordinates
3. Emotional and intellectual maturity as a preparation for leadership
4. Ability to think through and make decisions and to translate decisions into effective action
5. Capacity to see beyond the immediate or surface indications and, with experience, to acquire perspective

Effective nurse leader-managers will work to achieve these same requisites.

Leadership is a subsystem within the management system. It is included as an element of management science in management textbooks and other publications. In some, the term *leading* has replaced the term *directing* as a major function of management. In such a context, communication and motivation are elements of leadership (a concept that could be debated according to management theorists' philosophical bent).

Management includes written plans, clear organizational charts, well-documented annual objectives, frequent reports, detailed and precise job descriptions, regular evaluations of performance against objectives, and the administrative ordering of theory.[58] Nurse managers who are leaders can use these tools of management without making them a bureaucratic roadblock to autonomy, participatory management, maximum performance, and productivity by employees.

Leadership Versus Headship

A job title does not make a person a leader, nor does it cause a person to exercise leadership behavior over subordinates. This is as true of nurses as it is of personnel in industry or the military services. It is a mistake to refer to the dean of a college, a professor of nursing, a nurse administrator, a supervisor, a nurse manager, or any nurse as a leader by virtue of position. That person is in a headship position rather than a leadership one, because "leadership is more a function of the group or situation than a quality which adheres to a person appointed to a formal position of headship."[59] A person's behavior indicates whether that person also occupies a functional leadership position.

Gardner writes that not all people in positions of high status are leaders. Some are chief bureaucrats or custodians. Their high status does have "symbolic values and traditions that enhance the possibility of leadership" as people have higher expectations of people in headship positions.[60] Authority embodied in a title or position of headship is legitimized power; it is not leadership.[61]

Appointed heads are not selected by persons they direct. Appointed heads frequently work toward organizational goals while ignoring the personal goals of employees. Their authority comes from high in the organization and not from their influence within the group.

In cases in which heads are elected by the group, they keep their positions only as long as they satisfy the members' needs for affiliating with the organization. They are responsible only to the group, whereas the appointed head is usually responsible to both the appointive authority and the group. Nurses who are elected to chair committees or who preside over professional organizations will not be reelected unless they satisfy the members' needs.

> *Leadership is an attempt to influence groups or individuals without the coercive form of power.*

Appointed heads may lack the freedom to choose relationships with subordinates because their supervisors do not allow it. They have authority and power without being accepted by the group. If appointed nurse managers are allowed to and can exercise their leadership abilities, they can be accorded leadership status by the group. The nurse managers understand and motivate employees in order to be trusted by them.[62]

Preparation of Nursing Leaders

Gardner believes that 90% of leadership can be taught.[63] Education begins in basic nursing education programs. To develop risk-taking behaviors and self-confidence, students should be encouraged to create new solutions and to disagree and debate and should be allowed to make mistakes without fear of reprisal. Faculty should encourage and support students who exercise their leadership abilities in projects and organizations on campus and in the community.

When nurses graduate and enter the workforce, most are not ready to assume a leadership role. They require opportunities for self-discovery to understand their strengths and for skill building. This skill building occurs through on-the-job training, along with support from peers and mentorship from effective leaders. These mentors must be dynamic, not status quo–seeking role models who teach nurses how to preserve sameness. Tack writes that to be prepared for the future, leaders must be mentored by "those who see the world differently and project a dramatically different future, those who tend to shake things up rather than follow established precedents."[64]

Organizational managers, including nurse executives, teach managers the nature of leadership. They train nurse managers in leadership skills and put managers in the proper environment to learn leadership. This includes "starting up an operation, turning around a troubled division, moving from staff to line, working under a wise mentor, serving on a high-level task force and getting promoted to a more senior level of the organization."[65]

Nurse executives and managers should be trained to coach their constituents on leadership skills. Constituents can be trained to help managers in leadership. Leaders can listen and articulate, persuade and be persuaded, use collective wisdom to make decisions, and teach constituents to relate or communicate upward.

Gender Issues

Because most nurses are women, it is essential to understand gender issues. Research indicates that gender differences do exist in leadership styles and competencies.[66] Masculinity has been associated with being task oriented and using a direct approach for solving problems. Femininity has been characterized as being people oriented and supportive, sharing feelings, and caring for others.

"Transformational leadership is needed on gender issues related to nursing leadership."

Evidence-Based Practice 21-1

Desjardins and Brown conducted 2-hour interviews of 72 college presidents that included questions concerning, power, conflict resolution, and learning style. The findings indicated that most women practiced leadership in a care-connected style.[67] This orientation, first described by Gilligan, values intimacy and nurturing in interactions with others.[68] Most decisions made by men are in the justice and rights mode, first described by Kohlberg in his work on moral reasoning.[69] This style of decision making values autonomy, objectivity, and fairness.

Evidence-Based Practice 21-2

Rosener's research supports the thesis that leadership style is connected to gender issues. Rosener describes four major areas of difference in the women leaders whom she studied. First, these women tend to encourage participation; second, they share power and information more readily; third, they attempt to enhance the self-worth of others; and fourth, they energize others.[70]

It is important to remember that the modes and traits described by both researchers are gender related but not gender specific. Women and men fall into both modes, but more men are found in the justice and rights mode.[71] Rosener's work also indicates that men operate more often through management transactions, exchanging rewards for services rendered or punishments for poor performance. Men, she found, also work more out of the power of their positions.[72]

Evidence-Based Practice 21-3

Gender issues as they relate to leadership in healthcare organizations have not been well studied. Dunham and Klahefn found that male and female nurse executives are not more likely to exhibit transformational leadership rather than transactional leadership, which focuses more on day-to-day operations.[73] Borman's research on executives in healthcare organizations indicates that women, more than men, identify connections to others and flexibility as important characteristics of leaders.[74] The literature points out that flexibility may be a desirable attribute in a rapidly changing or restructured organization; therefore women may have an advantage over men.[75]

Gender differences in leadership style and competencies do not translate into one style being better than the other. However, if nurses are sensitized to gender differences, they will accept individuals for their unique leadership strengths instead of resisting them. This accepting atmosphere will encourage nurses (both men and women) to develop self-confidence and become strong leaders.

Nursing and Leadership Healthcare Policy

Nursing is conspicuous by its absence from lists of national leaders. National consumers do not perceive nurse leaders as having power. The healthcare system has failed to recognize nurses as professionals who have knowledge useful in creating solutions to complex problems. Cutler's perspective of nursing educators and nursing service personnel is that they have been the product of directive and authoritarian leadership.[76]

Historically, nurses have avoided opportunities to obtain power and political muscle. The profession now understands that power and political savvy will assist in achieving its goals to improve health care and to increase nurses' autonomy. Also, if the healthcare system is to be reformed, nurses must participate individually and collectively. Nurses need to find ways to influence healthcare policymaking so that their voices are heard.[77] Milio believes that nurses have the capacity for power to influence public policy and recommends the following steps to prepare[78]:

1. Organize.
2. Do homework. Learn to understand the political process, interest groups, specific people, and events.
3. Frame arguments to suit the target audience by appealing to cost containment, political support, fairness and justice, and other data relevant to particular concerns.
4. Support and strengthen the position of converted policymakers.
5. Concentrate energies.
6. Stimulate public debate.
7. Make the position of nurses visible in the mass media.
8. Choose the most effective strategy as the main one.
9. Act in a timely fashion.
10. Maintain activity.
11. Keep the organizational format decentralized.
12. Obtain and develop the best research data to support each position.
13. Learn from experience.
14. Never give up without trying.

Nurses in leadership positions are most influential.[79]

Buffering

Nursing leaders can act as buffers or advocates for nurses. In doing so, they protect constituents from internal and external pressures of work. Nurse managers can reduce barriers to clinical nurses completing their clinical work.

Buffering protects practicing clinical nurses from external health system factors, the healthcare organization, other supervisors and employees, top administrators, the medical staff, and themselves when their behavior jeopardizes their careers. Buffering is another facet of the theory of leadership related to management, and it requires leadership training.

The nurse practitioner, the extended-role nurse, staff nurses, and ancillary personnel can be protected by buffering action by nurse managers. Professional nurses do not want to have additional responsibilities delegated if they are already under severe pressure and stress. Delegation of decision making is power; delegation of work is drudgery. Professional nurses are there to motivate, not to dissatisfy.

Smith and Mitry suggest three methods of buffering, the benefits of which are improved performance, better morale, increased loyalty, a healthier organization, and respect for leaders[80]:

1. Coordinating work—that is, support services and standardized records
2. Insulating by intervening with pressure groups and creating unity of command
3. Evaluating the impingement

Management writers say there is a difference between leadership and managers, but their textbooks and writings on the subject all include leadership content. Professional nurses want to be led, not directed or controlled. Also, nurse managers can learn the concepts, principles, and laws that will assist them in becoming effective leader-managers.

Different situations require different leadership styles. The leader-manager assesses each situation and exercises the appropriate leadership style. Some employees want to be involved; others do not. There must be a fit between the leader and constituents. The leader demonstrates this by changing style and training others until a transition is made. A flexible leadership style is necessary and vital.

Transformational Leader as Coach

Coaching and mentoring are important skill sets for the transformational leader. Coaching denotes a way of being with others which provides opportunities to facilitate growth and development. Coaching requires exquisite communication skills that models ways of interacting and networking with others whereby those coached will find ready examples of best practices in working with others. Hill describes the predictable process of coaching, which includes the following[81]:

- Observing
- Examining coach motives
- Creating a discussion plan for the coaching session
- Initiating
- Providing and eliciting feedback and;
- Follow-up meeting

As a coach, observing behaviors and responding with insights and strategies will go further than "instructing" others on "what to do." Such will afford greater opportunities to learn and advance skills and opportunities. Porter-O'Grady and Malloch describe innovation coaching, stating the importance of creating the structure and content of the experience. Specifically, the following guidelines are given to facilitate this effort[82]:

- Setting the bar high.
- Being clear about who you are.
- Treating transformation as a mission, not a job.
- Exposing staff to different messages and different messengers.
- Creating an egalitarian organizational structure.
- Putting money where the ideas are.
- Letting the talented experiment.
- Allowing people to share in the fruits of their creativity.

Figure 21-1 outlines impediments to effective coaching, which includes use of power, problem solving, self-image, and knowledge. Figure 21-2 provides a model for considering coaching from a transformational perspective, illustrating driving forces, adaptation, and other contextual issues. [83]

FUTURE DIRECTION: QUANTUM LEADERSHIP

Porter-O'Grady and Malloch describe quantum leadership as new leadership for a new age. From a conceptual perspective, quantum theory considers the whole, integration, synthesis, relatedness, and team action. Figure 21-3 compares the Newtonian and the Quantum perspective. "Quantum theory has taught us that change is not a thing or an event but rather a dynamic that is constitutive of the universe."[84] Quantum leadership incorporates transformation, a dynamic flow that integrates transitions from work, rules, scripts, chaos, and loss. Adaptation considers such driving forces from sociopolitical,

| FIGURE 21-1 | IMPEDIMENTS TO EFFECTIVE COACHING |

Use of power

- Inadequate power
- Autocratic application of power
- Lack of empowerment
- Nonstrategic use of power

Self-image

- Poor self-esteem
- Unclear role
- Psychological flaws

Knowledge

- Undeveloped knowledge
- Learning needs
- Inexperience
- Lack of personal technique

Problem solving

- Inadequate worldview
- Intolerance of diversity
- No clear process
- Situational solutions

Source: Author.

| FIGURE 21-2 | INNOVATIVE AS A WAY OF LIFE. THE LEADER FOCUSES ON THE CENTRAL COMPONENTS OF PERSONAL TRANSFORMATION TO ENSURE EACH PERSON CAN EMBRACE CHANGE. |

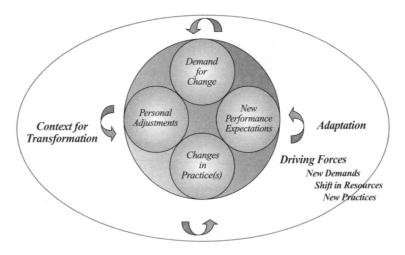

Source: Malloch, Porter-O'Grady. The quantum leader: Applications for the new world of work. (2005)

economic, and technical perspectives. The term *chaos* used in quantum leadership refers to the transitional period focused on relational and whole systems thinking as compared with separate components and linear thinking. Figures 21-4 and 21-5 provide a pictorial view of the conceptualization of transformation for quantum leadership. "New rules will apply in the new age."[85] Figure 21-6 outlines seven imperatives underscoring the need to consider quantum leadership for dramatic changes mandated in this new age.

FIGURE 21-3 | **CONCEPTUAL FOUNDATIONS**

Newtonian

- Mass production
- Compartmentalism
- Reductionism
- Analysis
- Discrete action

Quantum

- Envision the whole
- Integration
- Synthesis
- Relatedness
- Team action

Source: Author.

FIGURE 21-4 | **THE UNIVERSAL CYCLE OF TRANSFORMATION. THIS ILLUSTRATION SHOWS THE DYNAMIC AND INTERACTING FORCES OF TRANSFORMATION**

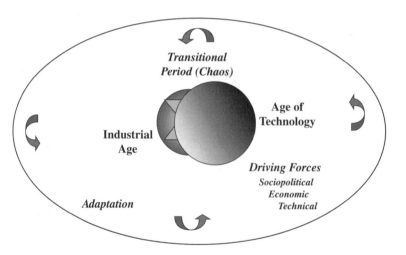

Source: Malloch, Porter-O'Grady. The quantum leader: Applications for the new world of work. (2005)

Evidence-Based Practice 21-4

In a systematic review, Wong and Cummings sought to describe finding of studies that examine the relationship between nursing leadership and patient outcomes. Only English research articles were reviewed, and data extraction and methodological quality assessment were completed with a final of seven quantitative research articles reviewed. The researchers discovered significant associations between positive leadership behaviors, styles, or practices and increased patient satisfaction and reduced adverse events. There were inconclusive findings related to leadership and patient mortality rates. The researchers concluded that their review suggested that an emphasis on developing transformational nursing leadership be pursued as an important organizational strategy to improve patient outcomes.[86]

FIGURE 21-5 UNIVERSAL DYNAMICS OF TRANSFORMATION. THIS ILLUSTRATION SHOWS THE CONTINUOUS CYCLE OF INTERACTING PROCESSES THAT ARE THE FOCUS OF THE TRANSFORMING WORK OF LEADERSHIP

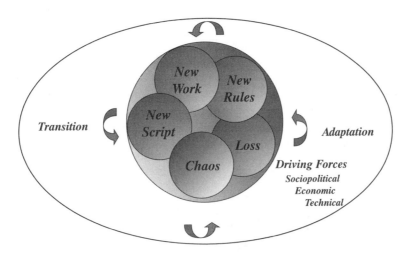

Source: Malloch, Porter-O'Grady. The quantum leader: Applications for the new world of work. (2005)

FIGURE 21-6 SEVEN NEW AGE IMPERATIVES

1. Open access to health information
2. Medicine/nursing based on genomics
3. Mass-customized diagnosis and treatment
4. User-specific insurance programs

5. Integration of allopathic and alternative therapies
6. Payment incentives tied to outcomes (quality)
7. Focused service settings for specific populations

Source: Malloch, Porter-O'Grady. The quantum leader: Applications for the new world of work. (2005)

SUMMARY

The theory of nursing leadership is a part of the theory of nursing management. Leadership is a process of influencing a group to set and achieve goals. There are several major theories of leadership. One of the earliest is the trait theory, which suggests that leaders have many intellect, personality, and ability traits. Trait theory has been succeeded by other leadership theories indicating that managers, including nurse managers, can learn the knowledge and skills requisite to leadership competencies.

Behavioral theories of leadership include McGregor's Theory X and Theory Y, Likert's Michigan studies, Blake and Mouton's Managerial Grid, and Lewin's studies.

Other studies of leadership focus on contingency-situational leadership styles and factors such as people, tasks, situations, organizations, and environment. Theorists include Fiedler; Hersey, Blanchard, and Johnson; Reddin; and Gardner. John W. Gardner's study of leadership includes the nature of leadership, identification of leadership tasks, leader-constituent interaction, and the relationship between leadership and power.

Bennis and Nanus define a theory of leadership they call transformational. This leadership method involves change in which the purposes of the leader and follower become intertwined. The effective leader creates a vision for the organization and then develops a commitment to the vision. Bennis and Nanus believe that the wise use of power is the energy needed to develop commitment and to sustain action.

Nurse managers should learn to practice leadership behaviors that stimulate motivation within their constituents, practicing professional nurses, and other nursing personnel. These behaviors include promotion of autonomy, decision making, and participatory management by professional nurses. These behaviors are facilitated by effective nurse manager-leaders.

Quantum leadership offers a new age perspective as one transforms and redesigns the workplace into a culture of greater safety and quality.

APPLICATION EXERCISES

Exercise 21-1

Identify a transformational leader in your clinical or work setting. What characteristics have you observed that sets this individual apart as someone making a difference in the work setting? What do others (on the unit, clinic, department) say about this individual? Is there agreement?

Exercise 21-2

Name a nurse you consider to be an outstanding leader and state why you consider him or her outstanding.

Exercise 21-3

Brower describes the leader in politics as a person of stature who can rally the people, a person with outstanding ability and character. He says there is an emotional bond between the leader and the led, a "bond which must exist between a leader and his people if either is to confront greatness."[87] He believes that the abrasive strains of television may have irreparably damaged the bond between leader and led. Television shows leaders in their weaknesses because it constantly focuses on them. It was once thought that a talent such as President Jefferson would freely rise to the top in a natural aristocracy. American leaders would be people of ability and morality; they would be wise and virtuous. According to Brower, "Leadership, a relationship, depends very much on the basis of current enthusiasm or negation. Indeed it cannot exist at all in this country without the consent of the governed. We may very well be short on leadership because we are short on ourselves."[88]

Assuming that the characteristics of leadership are applicable to occupations, government, business, industry, and service institutions and professions, list three characteristics described by Brower and apply them to nursing.

Exercise 21-4

Kurt Lewin suggests that there are three leadership styles: autocratic, democratic, and laissez-faire.

1. Which leadership style does your supervisor exhibit?
2. List three of his or her activities or decisions that illustrate the style.
3. How does your supervisor's leadership style affect your work and attitude?

Exercise 21-5

Gardner asserts that first-class managers are usually first-class leaders. He believes that leaders and leader-managers distinguish themselves beyond the general run of managers in six respects. Give brief examples of how nurses you know fit all or some of the six characteristics.

Exercise 21-6

From the theory of leadership described in this chapter, describe and discuss actual examples of leadership demonstrated by persons in your organization. Consider the following:

1. Gardner's nine tasks performed by leaders
2. A charismatic leader
3. A transforming leader
4. McGregor's Theory X and Theory Y
5. Likert's authoritative and democratic systems
6. Leadership style
7. The implications for staff development

Notes

1. Baldrige National Quality Program. (2003). *Criteria for performance excellence.* Gaithersburg, MD: National Institute of Standards and Technology.
2. Davenport, T., Delong, D., & Beers, D. (1998). Successful knowledge management projects. *Sloan Management Review, 1,* 43–57.
3. Heifetz, R., & Laurie, D. (2001). The work of leadership. *Harvard Business Review, 79,* 131–140.
4. Page, A. (Ed.). (2004). *Keeping patients safe, transforming the work environment of nurses.* Washington, DC: The National Academies Press.
5. Ibid.
6. Ibid.
7. Ibid., p. 136.
8. Ibid.
9. Gardner, 1986b, p. 15; Huxley, E. (1975). *Florence Nightingale.* New York: G. P. Putnam's Sons.
10. Gardner, 1986b, p. 15; Huxley, E. (1975). *Florence Nightingale.* New York: G. P. Putnam's Sons.
11. Holloman, C. R. (1986). Leadership or headship: There is a difference. *Notes & Quotes,* 4; Holloman, C. R. (1986). "Headship" vs. leadership. *Business and Economic Review, 34,* 35–37.
12. Lundborg, L. B. (1982). What is leadership? *Journal of Nursing Administration,* 32–33.
13. Gardner, 1986a, p. 6.
14. Holloman, 1986; Levenstein, A. (1985). So you want to be a leader? *Nursing Management,* 74–75; Jones, G. R. (1983). Forms of control and leader behavior. *Journal of Management,* 159–172; McGregor, D. (1966). *Leadership and motivation* (pp. 70–80). Cambridge, MA: MIT Press.
15. Merton, R. K. (1969). The social nature of leadership. *American Journal of Nursing,* 2614–2618.
16. McGregor, 1966, p. 73.
17. Talbott, C. M. (1971). Leadership at the man-to-man level. *Supplement to the Air Force Policy Letter for Commanders,* 13.
18. Mitton, D. G. (1969). Leadership: One more time. *Industrial Management Review,* 77–83.
19. Kilpatrick, J. (1974, February). Conservative view. *Sun-Herald* (Biloxi, MS), p. 4.
20. McGregor, 1966, p. 75.
21. Gardner, 1986b, 1986c, 1986d.
22. Gardner, 1986b, p. 7.
23. Gardner, 1986c.
24. McGregor, 1966, pp. 55–57.

25. Ibid., pp. 49–65.

26. Likert, R. (1967). *The human organization* (pp. 4–10). New York: McGraw-Hill.

27. The Grid synopsis was furnished courtesy of Scientific Methods, Inc., Box 195, Austin, TX, 78747.

28. Megginson, L., Mosley, D., & Pietri, P., Jr. (1989). *Management: Concepts and applications* (3rd ed., pp. 346–347, 352–353). New York: Harper & Row.

29. Phillips, J. S., & Lord, R. G. (1986). Notes on the practical and theoretical consequences of implicit leadership theories for the future of leadership measurement. *Journal of Management, 33.*

30. Ibid.

31. Fiedler, F. E. (1969). Style or circumstance: The leadership enigma. *Notes & Quotes,* 3; Megginson et al., 1989.

32. Hersey, P., Blanchard, K. H., & Johnson, D. E. (1996). *Management of organizational behavior: Utilizing human resources* (7th ed., pp. 134–135). Englewood Cliffs, NJ: Prentice Hall.

33. Reddin, W. J. (1970). *Managerial effectiveness* (p. 230). New York: McGraw-Hill; Hodgetts, R. M. (1986). *Management: Theory, process and practice* (4th ed., pp. 319–320). Orlando, FL: Academic Press.

34. Barker, A. M. (1991). An emerging leadership paradigm. *Nursing and Health Care,* 204–207.

35. Bennis, W., & Nanus, B. (1985). *Leaders: The strategies for taking charge* (p. 3). New York: Harper & Row.

36. Ibid., p. 15.

37. Lundeen, S. P. (1992). Leadership strategies for organizational change: Applications in community nursing centers. *Nursing Administration Quarterly,* 60–68.

38. Tack, M. W. (1991). Future leaders in higher education: New demands and new responses. *Phi Kappa Phi Journal,* 29–31; Desjardins, C., & Brown, C. O. (1991). A new look at leadership styles. *Phi Kappa Phi Journal,* 18–20.

39. Bennis & Nanus, 1985.

40. Medley, F., & Larochelle, D. R. (1995). Transformational leadership and job satisfaction. *Nursing Management,* 64JJ–64NN.

41. Bennis & Nanus, 1985, p. 57.

42. Barker, 1991.

43. Bennis, W. (1991). Learning some basic truisms about leadership. *Phi Kappa Phi Journal.*

44. Bennis & Nanus, 1985.

45. Barker, A. M. (1990). *Transformational nursing leadership: A vision for the future.* Baltimore: Williams and Wilkins.

46. Bennis & Nanus, 1985.

47. Barker, 1991, p. 207.

48. Ibid.

49. Gardner, 1986c.

50. Bennis, 1991, p. 24.

51. Campbell, R. P. (1986). Does management style affect burnout? *Nursing Management,* 38A–38B, 38D, 38F, 38H.

52. Gardner, 1986c.

53. Zaleznik, A. (1977). Managers and leaders: Are they different? *Harvard Business Review,* 68.

54. Zenger, J. H. (1985). Leadership: Management's better half. *Training,* 44–53.

55. Gardner, 1986a, p. 12.

56. Zenger, 1985.

57. Mitchell, W. N. (1968). What makes a business leader? *Notes & Quotes,* 2.

58. Zenger, 1985.

59. Holloman, 1969.

60. Gardner, 1986a, p. 6.

61. Ibid.

62. Holloman, 1986.

63. Gardner, 1986a.

64. Tack, 1991, p. 30.

65. Zenger, 1985.

66. Desjardins & Brown, 1991.

67. Ibid.

68. Gilligan, C. (1982). *In a different voice: Psychological theory and women's development.* Cambridge, MA: Harvard University Press.

69. Kohlberg, L. (1981). *The philosophy of moral development, moral stages and the idea of justice.* San Francisco: Harper and Row.

70. Rosener, J. (1990). Ways women lead. *Harvard Business Review, 1,* 19–24.

71. Desjardins & Brown, 1991.

72. Rosener, 1990.

73. Dunham, J., & Klahefn, K. A. (1990). Transformational leadership and the nurse executive. *Journal of Nursing Administration, 1,* 28–34.

74. Borman, J. S. (1993). Women and nurse executives: Finally, some advantages. *Journal of Nursing Administration, 1,* 34–40.

75. Helgesen, S. (1990). *The female advantage.* New York: Doubleday.

76. Cutler, M. J. (1976). Nursing leadership and management: An historical perspective. *Nursing Administration Quarterly, 1,* 7–19.

77. Murphy, N. J. (1992). Nursing leadership in health policy decision making. *Nursing Outlook,* 158–161.

78. Milio, N. (1984). The realities of policy making: Can nurses have an impact? *Journal of Nursing Administration, 1,* 18–23.

79. Ibid.

80. Smith, H. L., & Mitry, N. W. (1984). Nursing leadership: A buffering perspective. *Nursing Administration Quarterly, 1,* 45–52.

81. Hill, L. A. (2007). Coaching. Retrieved February 29, 2008, from http://www.harvardmanagementor.com/demo/plusdemo/coach/index.htm

82. Porter-O'Grady, T., & Malloch, K. (2004). *Quantum leadership: A textbook of new leadership.* Sudbury, MA: Jones and Bartlett Publishers.

83. Ibid., p. 61.

84. Porter-O'Grady, T., & Malloch, K. (2007). *Quantum leadership: A resource for healthcare innovation* (2nd ed.). Sudbury, MA: Jones and Bartlett Publishers.

85. Ibid., pp. 352–353.

86. Wong, C. L., & Cummings, G. G. (2007). The relationship between nursing leadership and patient outcomes: A systematic review. *Journal of Nursing Management, 15,* 508–521.

87. Brower, B. (1971, October 8). Where have all the leaders gone? *Life,* 708.

88. Ibid.

References

Aiken, L. (2002). Superior outcomes for magnet hospitals: The evidence base. In M. McClure & A. Hinshaw (Eds.), *Magnet hospitals revisited: Attraction and retention of professional nurses.* Washington, DC: American Nurses Publishing.

Herrin, D., Jones, K., Krepper, R., Sherman, R., & Reineck, C. (2006). Future nursing administration graduate curricula, part 2. *Journal of Nursing Administration, 36,* 498–505.

Kleinman, C. S. (2003). Leadership roles, competencies, and education, how prepared are our nurse managers. *Journal of Nursing Administration, 33,* 451–455.

Murphy, L. (2005). Transformational leadership: A cascading chain reaction. *Journal of Nursing Management, 13,* 128–136.

Thomas, J., & Herrin, D. (2008). The executive master of science in nursing program. *Journal of Nursing Administration, 38,* 4–7.

Upenieks, V. V. (2003). What constitutes effective leadership? Perceptions of magnet and nonmagnet nurse leaders. *Journal of Nursing Administration, 33,* 456–467.

22 CREATING A CULTURE OF MAGNETISM

Anita J. K. Langston, MSN, RN, ANP-BC, CCNS, CCRN
Robert W. Koch, DNS, RN

LEARNING OBJECTIVES AND ACTIVITIES

- Identify the eight domains of evidence for a culture of magnetism.
- Recognize the elements of the 14 forces of magnetism.
- Create effective methods of both vertical and horizontal communication.
- Distinguish between a flat organizational structure and the traditional vertical organizational structure.
- Collaborate in interdisciplinary groups to deliver effective patient care.
- Devise methods that foster the growth, professionalism, and autonomy of the direct care nurse.
- Develop a culture of inquiry, identifying and applying evidence-based practice in the clinical setting.
- Create an atmosphere of quality care and positive patient outcomes.

CONCEPTS

Magnet Recognition Program®, domains of evidence, forces of magnetism, transformational leadership, structural empowerment, autonomous nursing practice, professional practice models, Nursing Work Index, organizational culture.

QUOTE

There is no speed limit on the road to excellence.

—Anonymous

Introduction

The projected nursing workforce shortages as well as quality and safety issues in the healthcare industry are in the spotlight of public awareness. Solutions to address these issues are receiving much attention. One program discussed in this chapter addresses the creation of an organizational culture that promotes quality patient outcomes using evidence-based practice to achieve above benchmark results. The Magnet Recognition Program®, administered through the American Nurses Credentialing Center (ANCC), provides the designation of "magnet" to facilities that have met the standards of the program. The Magnet Recognition Program measures nursing quality indicators and patient outcomes based on the American Nurses Association's (ANA) *Scope and Standards for Nurse Administrators* to identify best nursing services and quality patient outcomes.[1]

HISTORICAL PERSPECTIVE

The Magnet Recognition Program began when the American Academy of Nurses formed a task force in the early 1980s to address the nursing shortage in the United States at that time. One member of this task force was Dr. Mabel Wandelt, a professor at the University of Texas at Austin. She noted that certain facilities had no difficulty in attracting and retaining qualified nurses, despite a nursing shortage.[2] This observation led to the research study to identify institutions that could attract and retain nurses and the factors related to that achievement. This hallmark study was conducted by McClure and Hinshaw at 41 hospitals of different sizes from eight regions of the United States.[3] These hospitals were predominantly private, nonprofit organizations, and all were affiliated with an educational program of nursing. Groups of nursing directors and groups of staff nurses were each interviewed and asked key questions about the elements of their workplace that made it a good place to work. Interestingly, the findings indicated key features important for both the nursing directors and the staff nurses. These predominant features existed in these facilities despite the size of the organization or the region of the country. Elements such as quality of leadership, educational opportunities, and working as teams were strong factors identified. Other elements identified are presented under the categories of administration, professional practice, and professional development and published in *Magnet Hospitals: the Attraction and Retention of Professional Nurses* in 1983.[4]

Further research and studies on these facilities added to the body of knowledge first established by the American Academy of Nurses' task force. Marlene Kramer and Claudia Schmalenberg in addition to others on their research team, conducted six different studies beginning in 1985 to substantiate the characteristics of the organizational culture in magnet facilities. In their study, 279 staff nurses were given a list of 37 items that were deemed necessary in the delivery of quality nursing care. The original list of 65 items was pared down to 37 and is currently known as the Nursing Work Index. Additional research in this area led to the identification of eight essentials of magnetism[5]:

1. Working with other nurses who are clinically competent
2. Good nurse–physician relationships and communication
3. Nurse autonomy and accountability
4. Supportive nurse manager-supervisor
5. Control over nursing practice and practice environment
6. Support for education (in-service, continuing education, etc.)
7. Adequate nurse staffing
8. Concern for the patient is paramount.

The Magnet Hospital Recognition Program for Excellence in Nursing Services was approved by the ANA Board of Directors in late 1990 and administered by the newly formed ANCC, a subsidiary of ANA. The purpose of the program was to officially recognize what is now referred to as magnet hospitals, which are healthcare facilities that successfully recruit and retain nurses in a supportive environment. A pilot study, conducted in five facilities, led to the first award of magnet hospital designation to the University of Washington Medical Center in Seattle in 1994.

The magnet program's link to quality patient care with nursing excellence has catapulted magnet facilities to an esteemed place in the healthcare industry and in their communities. Presently, there are over 275 magnet facilities in over 45 states in the United States, New Zealand, and Australia.[6]

EVIDENCE AND OUTCOMES

Health care is now focused on evidence and outcomes. This has prompted a series of scholarly investigations that focus on the extent to which magnet facilities promote quality patient care and foster positive work environments for nurses. For example, magnet facilities experience less professional burnout among professional nurses.[7] Patient-related outcomes in magnet facilities have been compared with outcomes of patients in nonmagnet facilities. One study indicated that magnet hospitals had a 4.6% lower mortality rate.[8] One contributing factor to this success is that magnet hospitals have a significantly higher ratio of registered nurses (RNs) to patients than their nonmagnet peers.

Furthermore, 43% of nurses in ANCC magnet facilities consider the quality of care in their facility as excellent, compared with 10% of nurses in a national sample.[9] Nurses in ANCC magnet facilities report significantly higher rates of autonomy and control of the practice environment and participation in policy decisions. Magnet hospital nurses also report the presence of a powerful chief nursing office that provides the support and resources needed to deliver quality care.

Kosel and Olivo reported a positive correlation between employee satisfaction and customer satisfaction in magnet facilities. Job satisfaction for nurses equates with the desire to provide quality nursing care in a supportive environment. Facilities that recognize this key component enjoy higher patient satisfaction scores, higher percentage of the healthcare market share, and a reduction in RN turnover and vacancy numbers as well as positive patient outcomes.[10]

Finally, even more direct benefits can be seen when a healthcare agency secures magnet status. Studies indicate that the facilities achieving this award show decreased lengths of patient stay, fewer adverse patient outcomes, a reduction in RN turnover, and a reduction in the cost for marketing to attract nurses.[11] Each of these variables has significant impact on a hospital's "bottom line."

SELF-ASSESSMENT OF THE ORGANIZATION

The initial steps in the magnet journey begin with a thorough evaluation of the organization to determine readiness. Through this activity, leaders in the nursing organization understand the strengths, weakness, and opportunities that must be considered in transformation of the nursing organization. Organizations recognizing the benefits of the magnet hospital designation and desiring to embark on the journey begin with a self-assessment of the organizational culture and perform a gap analysis.

Current criteria for potential organizations include specific requirements for the chief nursing officer (CNO), who must hold a Master's degree. Either the baccalaureate or master's degree must be in nursing. Additionally, the organization must show evidence that the ANA's *Scope and Standards for Nurse Administrators* is being implemented in all areas in which nursing is practiced. One criterion indicates that the nursing organizations must be in compliance with all local, state, and federal regulatory guidelines.

Data collection on nurse-sensitive quality indicators must occur at the unit and organizational level. A method must be established for nurses to provide feedback without fear of retribution, and the organization cannot have a record of an unfair labor practice involving a nurse within the previous 3 years upon application.

To focus only on the goal of magnet designation and not create a culture that fosters healthy work environments in which evidence-based practice creates positive patient outcomes is a mistake. The creation of a sustainable culture that is constantly evaluating and evolving takes the investment of time and patience. Resources can be found on the ANCC website: http://www.nursecredentialing.org to assist in the self-assessment process.

Organizations may be surprised to learn that the perceptions of the staff nurse are markedly different from that of leadership. Discovering this at the beginning of the journey can allow time for organizational leaders to improve communication, mentor staff nurses into positions of shared decision making, and cultivate a healthy work environment. Participation in such surveys may be encouraged and rewarded with an extra educational day or prize drawings.

Although survey responses should always ensure the anonymity of the staff nurse, they should also include a method to compare the responses of each nursing unit. Evaluation of the strengths and weaknesses of the organization on a unit level provides a basis for a focused effort to duplicate what works well. Facilities awarded the magnet designation are able to demonstrate characteristics of a magnet culture throughout the organization, not just on one or two premier units.

THE MAGNET MODEL

With the exponential growth of the magnet program, ANCC recognized the need to fine tune the appraisal and application process. Through the conduction of a statistical analysis on the previous 165 sources of evidence required for submission and utilizing a panel of experts on magnet facilities, changes were made and unveiled in 2008. ANCC now has a model representative of the characteristics of a magnet facility and clearly demonstrates the five areas that any organization aspiring to magnet status must address. The Magnet Model® consists of these five areas:

1. Transformational leadership
2. Structural empowerment
3. Exemplary professional practice
4. Knowledge, innovation, improvements
5. Empirical quality outcomes

Within this model, the eight domains of evidence can be found. The traditional 14 forces of magnetism remain as the core of the program but are now organized in a clear manner:

- Force 1: Quality of nursing leadership
- Force 2: Organizational structure
- Force 3: Management style
- Force 4: Personnel policies and programs
- Force 5: Professional models of care
- Force 6: Quality of care
- Force 7: Quality improvement
- Force 8: Consultation and resources
- Force 9: Autonomy
- Force 10: Community and the healthcare organization
- Force 11: Nurses as teachers
- Force 12: Image of nursing
- Force 13: Interdisciplinary relationships
- Force 14: Professional development

TRANSFORMATIONAL LEADERSHIP

The term *transformational leadership* has been in the literature for the past 30 years. James Burns describes characteristics of transformational leadership in the study from 1978. According to Burns, transformational leadership involves a relationship between the leader and the follower, in which there is an investment to work together to further common goals. Successful leaders can recognize the wants and needs of the follower, combine these with their own needs, and reach goals in a manner that satisfies the values and motivations of both.[13] The need for the healthcare industry to undergo transformation is apparent during the age of rapidly evolving healthcare technology. Nursing shortage in the clinical setting as well as the academic setting is corresponding with an aging population explosion. As magnet hospitals address the issues facing all healthcare organizations, proactive leadership that is visionary can play a role in maintaining the culture of magnetism. Hospitals on the journey will be able to stay on the pathway toward excellence.

Provision of excellent nursing care, ensuring positive patient outcomes, and supporting an environment of evidence-based practice will always be priorities in magnet hospitals. The quality of nursing leadership is considered a key element in moving an organization in a forward motion. Transformational leadership establishes relationships and engages others to work together to achieve common goals. In contrast, the goal in transactional leadership is not a shared phenomenon, and the transaction between leader and follower generally results in a quid pro quo relationship: "If you do this for me, I will do this for you." Transactional leadership fails if one of the parties is thought not to fulfill their end of the bargain. The rewards are characteristically extrinsic, such as the paycheck, bonus check, or a better schedule.[14]

Five transformational stages and practices as defined by Henriksen, Keyes, Stevens, and Clancy are (1) recognizing a need for a change, (2) developing a vision, (3) developing commitment and trust, (4) implementing change, and (5) sustaining the change. Transformation within an organization requires leadership with a vision and a plan to enact the vision. Sustainable transformation occurs when change happens in phases, such as described by Henriksen et al.[15] These five stages are discussed further below.

STRUCTURAL EMPOWERMENT

Eight Domains of Evidence: Leadership

Force of Magnetism: Quality of Nursing Leadership

The characteristic of having strong, quality nursing leadership has been identified as a key in the ability to attract and retain nurses, from the first studies of magnet hospitals[16] to ongoing research on current magnet facilities. Leadership in these organizations was frequently described as "listening" and responsiveness to the voice and needs of the direct care nurse.[17] Skillful leadership that can be considered transformational requires a formal vision for the direction in which the organization aspires.

Quality nursing leaders have the tools necessary to promote change and cultivate the relationships in the executive level administration, in middle managers, and in the direct care nurses. Unfortunately, many nursing leaders obtain their administrative position based on proficient clinical skills and are never exposed to leadership skill development. Educational preparation for a leadership role is ideally obtained in academic graduate-level nursing programs.

Organizational structures should include providing the support necessary for the leadership to obtain graduate level degrees. However, leadership skill development can also be derived from focused leadership programs. Many external leadership programs are available for this, but some organizations establish their own leadership institutes.

For example, Tennessee currently enjoys collaboration with the Tennessee Center for Nursing and the University of Tennessee-Knoxville School of Nursing in providing a 4-day program entitled the Tennessee Leadership Institute for Nursing Excellence. Organizations within the state may nominate qualified candidates and then provide support in transportation costs and salary for the individual. Lodging, meals, and the cost of the program are provided by the leadership institute.

The University of Pittsburgh Medical Center recognized a need for transformation in their large healthcare organizational system. Realizing that each facility operated singly and did not interact as a system in a cohesive manner, the organization developed a Transformational Model for Professional Practice in Healthcare Organizations®. This model was developed by the Beckwith Institute for Innovation in Patient Care.[18] The Beckwith Institute for Innovation in Patient Care is part of the University of Pittsburgh Medical Center and provides services for the organization and others wishing to use its consulting services. Part of this program includes the Beckwith Leadership Fellows Program, which provides educational support as well as mentorship in leadership development.[19]

Recognizing a Need for Change   Nursing leaders of healthcare organizations should be able to objectively evaluate the climate of their system and evaluate if it can meet the needs of its consumers. The Institute of Medicine's *Report on Patient Safety* and similar reports, which highlight the need for improvement in the provision of a safe healthcare environment, are part of the public domain and place a spotlight on each healthcare organization. The difficulty lies in convincing other key decision makers in the organization to commit to the financial investment required to make significant organizational changes. The CNO must command the respect of the executive leadership and demonstrate competency in leadership skills.

Developing a Vision   A vision of the future and what the healthcare organization aspires to is guided by the nursing executive team and shared with all stakeholders. By providing a clear, positive vision of the future, healthcare workers are energized and inspired. "They provide a new sense of direction, give new meaning to the work, and collectively raise consciousness levels in terms of being part of a worthwhile enterprise."[20] The healthcare organization's strategic plan and the nursing's strategic plan for the future should be congruent with this vision and in alignment with each other. The CNO and the executive nursing leadership are responsible for guiding the healthcare organization to excellence in patient care services.

Developing Commitment and Trust   There is a relationship between organizational commitment and the type of leadership within the organization.[21] Creating a culture that has a vision of excellence in the delivery of patient care services requires action to support the vision. Communication to healthcare workers needs to be clear, consistent, and two-way. Sharing with the healthcare team a vision for the future should be followed with shared decision-making strategies to achieve the vision. Listening and responding to those that are responsible for the delivery of care is essential in the development of commitment and trust. Organizational commitment is directly related to acceptance of the organization's goals and the empowerment of the direct care nurse.[22]

Trust is cultivated and requires time to develop. Concern for the patient is paramount in magnet facilities and can be demonstrated with every organizational purchase, change in structure, and formulation of organizational policy. An organization that is perceived as placing the needs of the patient first will receive the commitment and trust of the healthcare worker and community.

Force of Magnetism: Management Style

Management style in magnet facilities is considered participative. Direct care nurses at all levels have a voice in the delivery of nursing care and the programs and policies affecting them. This can be facilitated through formal and informal means. Staff nurse participation on the unit and in organizational councils is supported by management through scheduled time away from patient care responsibilities. Direct care nurses without experience in committee dynamics may need encouragement and guidance to be effective council members. Nursing surveys are an effective method to obtain feedback from staff nurses and should have provisions of anonymity to ensure honesty in responses. Informal solicitation of suggestions for improvement can relay to the staff nurse that their opinions matter. Action in response to nurse feedback is imperative, and examples of changes that resulted from this feedback should be readily available.

Leadership should make a dedicated effort to be visible and accessible to nurses on all shifts. This can require innovation and may be achieved differently with each organization, depending on the size and structure. Nursing directors are known by their staff and create opportunities to develop relationships. Creation of an open door policy can allow staff to feel at ease in bringing up work-related issues that have potential to escalate if not addressed at the onset.

Communication between management and nursing staff is essential to achieve commitment to the organization and to establish a sense of partnership. Communication is considered vertical when it comes only from the upper level administrators, such as in the announcement of new policies in a staff meeting. This can be perceived as a paternalistic atmosphere and is not conducive to participative management. Horizontal communication is the dissemination of information through unit and organizational councils.

An example of the horizontal communication method is when a nursing unit representative on the quality care committee shares a change in policy with coworkers on the unit. Communication should include not only issues that directly concern the nursing unit but should also include the organization as a whole. Expansion and renovation plans, changes in the organizational structure, and plans for future programs need to be relayed to each member of the organization.

Common communication methods are newsletters, staff meetings, memos on bulletin boards, and regular rounding on the clinical units. Effectiveness of rounding by nursing administration depends on the method used and also on the action resulting from this interaction. During rounds on nursing units, nursing directors may ask the direct care staff a question as simple as "What do you need to provide the best patient care possible today?" Responses can vary from the easy fix, such as "an extra linen cart at the end of the hall" to the more difficult response such as "more support staff." Regardless, genuine concern from nursing directors and communication on what can or cannot be done is an important feature to successful rounding.

With present information technology, providing e-mail access to all employees is now a standard practice. In consideration for the variances in technological knowledge of the multigenerational workforce, support should include the provision of basic computer classes for those without previous exposure to electronic mail. Electronic communication allows information to be readily available in the quickest manner possible. It supports communication with nursing staff of the frequently forgotten off-shift hours of nights and weekends. The intranet, the in-house server, provides a new method to post memos, provide access to staff meeting minutes, and links to the internet. Unit councils in some facilities have created websites for their particular nursing unit. In doing so, team camaraderie is encouraged, communication is improved, and ultimately the quality of patient care is enhanced. Innovations such as these must have the support of nursing management to exist.

As mentioned, there are not always easy answers as barriers arise to the provision of quality nursing care, but shared decision making allows those closest to the problem to become a part of the solution. Ensuring that staff nurses take part in the decision-making process at varied levels in the organization is one component of the core competencies of the nurse administrator.[23]

Eight Domains of Evidence: Resource Utilization and Development

Force of Magnetism: Organizational Structure

Magnet facilities contain organizational structures that are decentralized and rely heavily on unit-based, shared decision-making councils. This is characterized by an organizational structure that has a more horizontal dimension rather than vertical. The organizational structure is flexible and responsive to changes. Shared decision making, along with the support of the organization to develop professionally, results in the empowerment of the nurse and job satisfaction.[24]

Traditional healthcare organizations operate with the administration and management leaders controlling and wielding power. The opinion of the staff nurse was unimportant and not seriously evaluated for worth. Research indicates it is the opinion and suggestions of the person most actively involved in the delivery of care that can pinpoint areas requiring improvement.

Implementing Change Organizational restructuring in the early 1990s occurred as the response to fiscal decision making.[25] Key decision makers were all at the executive level and did not always include nursing at the table. This resulted in more responsibilities for middle management, sometimes doubling their area of unit coverage, and either the elimination of jobs or increased work loads for clinical experts and educators. Decision makers were not close to the front line and often had differences of perception with the direct care staff. Among the recommendations of the Institute of Medicine in their report, *Keeping Patients Safe*, are suggestions to include the direct care workers in workplace decision making and to have leadership invite the direct care staff in organizational councils and committees.

Creating a learning environment in which healthcare workers can learn methods to create new solutions to problems encountered is another recommendation of the Institute of Medicine report. Seeking to apply evidence-based practice to achieve positive patient outcomes requires a systematic approach many leaders have never used before. Collaboration with all disciplines and involvement in patient care delivery is essential to achieving positive patient outcomes.

Sustaining the Change Organizational structures include systematic monitoring and periodic evaluations of outcomes. A continuation of communication keeps all stakeholders aware of progress toward the vision. Recognition of the positive results from changes put into place fortify those involved in the change process. The direct care staff feel supported as they recognize the need to embrace the organizational changes. A sustainable change becomes part of the culture of the organization and expectations of delivering quality patient care are part of the day-to-day mindset. Policies of the organization ensure shared decision making occurs and facilitates involvement of the direct care staff. Once this occurs, the organization can operate smoothly even as leadership may change.

Force of Magnetism: Professional Development

The professional growth and development of the nursing staff is considered a priority of the organization. Evidence of this support is seen for the direct care nursing staff as well as the administrative nursing staff. Quality orientation programs should be flexible enough to meet the individual needs of a diverse nursing population. The current multigenerational workforce has varied learning styles and needs. Nursing educators construct orientation and in-service programs to accommodate this variety.

In-service educational programs need to be developed based on a needs assessment and evaluated for effectiveness. Consideration for off-shift nursing staff is apparent when scheduling in-service programs. Many facilities hire specific nursing educators for the night or weekend shifts. As evidence of program availability, leaders submit records of attendance demonstrating unit participation.

Effective programs to develop clinical competency are in place, utilized by the nursing staff and supported with both fiscal resources and time allotment to complete. A program such as a clinical ladder, which rewards the professional development of the direct care nurse, is one example. Control over the design and decisions of who is allowed to progress on the ladder should be done by a team of nursing peers. Design of clinical ladder programs by the nurses who are affected by it results in a higher participation rate of the nursing staff.

Clinical ladder programs that are extremely labor intensive with little rewards will not encourage nurses to grow in clinical competency. Research studies done by Kramer and Schmalenberg[26] identified working beside nurses who are clinically competent as one of the eight essential elements of magnetism. An aggressive campaign and financial support for specialty certification is recommended as another method to further professional development.

Many nurses desire and plan to obtain specialty certification, but constraints on time, fear of failure, and lack of financial resources to purchase study material and to pay exam fees become obstacles. Providing methods to overcome such obstacles indicate to the nursing staff that the organization is supportive and will recognize the individual efforts of nurses to obtain specialty certification. Certification study courses, exam study material, and payment of testing fees are provided to the nursing staff as benefits by many organizations. Progression on the clinical ladder, bonus pay, and recognition programs are a few methods used to reward the nurse successful in achieving certification. Some nurses are also given extra professional development days to maintain certification.

Recognition for educational advancement is evident and promoted. Tuition reimbursement programs encourage nurses to obtain baccalaureate and master's level degrees in nursing. Research has indicated that nursing care provided by BSN-prepared nurses is linked to a decrease in negative patient outcomes and mortality.[27] Healthcare facilities wishing to obtain a magnet designation must make this a priority in hiring practices and in the support of nursing staff currently employed. The percentage of nurses taking advantage of such programs is an indicator if the tuition reimbursement program is equitable and effective.

Management staff is noted for the flexibility in staff schedules to allow for nurses to attend classes. Partnerships with community academic programs can lead to innovative methods for nurses to attend class. Organizations can provide space and time for nurses to attend classes on-site. Once academic advancement is completed, magnet organizations recognize achievements in clinical ladder advancement or in job promotion.

The creation of a learning environment requires the example set by the leadership in the organization. Furthering a nursing degree, obtaining a specialty certification, and attending professional development courses are expected of all nursing leadership, including the CNO, in a magnet organization. This is reflected in each job description and performance evaluation. In addition, the placement of advanced practice nurses (APNs) within the organization allow for direct nursing staff to have opportunities to observe role models and to develop mentoring relationships. Mentoring relationships provide encouragement of direct care nursing staff to attend local professional organization programs. Organizational support of professional development is also evident when nurses are given financial support and time off to attend regional, state, and national nursing programs.

Force of Magnetism: Image of Nursing

Magnet facilities recognize nursing services as a valuable contributor to the organization. The CNO is integral in the formulation of the strategic plan for the organization and has influence with the highest decision-making body. This can be seen in a variety of ways, but frequently the CNO is the leader in both the development and the implementation of organizational changes. Opinions of executive nursing leadership is valued and sought out, seen by the inclusion on the organization's executive committees. The CNO is known for strong quality leadership and willing mentors.

Nursing is favorably spoken of by other departments and disciplines and noted for the excellence in providing patient care services. Nurses are considered integral in the success of the organization and are participants in many interdisciplinary committees. Nurses in nontraditional roles not under nursing services are valued and are contributors in decision making. Nurses are considered assets in roles such as informatics, resource analysis, human resources, organizational performance, and risk management.

Organizational marketing strategies include positive nursing images. Announcements of individual nurse's achievements are made within the organization and in the community. Nursing services are featured on the public website for the organization. The community recognizes that nurses provide excellent patient care in this organization.

Force of Magnetism: Policies and Programs

Magnet organizations rely on the combination of many factors to attract and retain nurses while providing excellent patient care. Competitive salaries and benefits are components. Appropriate compensation is used to reward all levels of nursing, and systems are in place to promote advancement within the profession.

Organized programs to recruit nurses to the facility and to retain the ones already present are designed with the assistance of the direct care staff. Effective recruitment and retention programs do not rely heavily on sign-on bonuses. Programs designed with the collaboration of nursing, finance, and human resources assess the trends of the workforce and current status of the nursing staff, rely on the input of the direct care nurse, and then target specific demographics for recruitment.

The goal of the organization may be to create a more culturally diverse workforce that mirrors the population of the community served. Active campaigning in this population is then needed. Targeting local high school populations to enhance the desire to enter a healthcare profession and offering a "shadow a nurse" type of program are effective methods. Collaborating with local schools of nursing to offer clinical sites, extern programs for student nurses to work, and participating in career fairs is standard practice.

Creating a healthy work environment is a very effective, specific component in retaining nurses. Policies are in place to ensure intolerance for any type of harassment, discrimination, or retribution for whistle-blowing/reporting of errors. Many organizations strive for a "no-blame" culture to encourage the reporting of any medical or practice near-misses or errors. Examining the cause of the error is then the focus and serves to create solutions.

Recognition of the aging workforce creates opportunities to reconfigure workspace accordingly. Computer and cardiac monitor screens can use large fonts and symbols, ergonomic chairs and keyboards, and the use of patient lift devices to encourage older nurses to remain at the bedside.

Many methods may be used to evaluate job performance. Self-assessment and peer review are part of the performance appraisal, and 360-degree evaluations are used when appropriate. Nurses may voice discomfort when assigned the task of self-assessment and peer review but can be mentored in these tasks, acknowledging that this is a part of professionalism. Peer review may be conducted in the manner of chart audits, participation in councils that review applications for clinical ladder advancement, or in a more formal system of evaluation. Professional standards are part of the performance evaluation and promotion of career development is present.

Goal setting is a common method used to promote professional development and encourages discussion in how to accomplish meeting such goals. Appropriate use of 360-degree evaluations is important in leadership positions. Nurses in leadership roles may conduct performance evaluations on themselves and then seek out evaluations from those that they lead, their peers, and their supervisor.

The nurse staffing system throughout the facility is based on ANA's *Principles of Nurse Staffing*. Direct care nurses are actively involved in designing staffing plans that meet the needs of the patient. Flexibility is expected and allows adjustments based on patient acuity and illnesses of staff. The state's nurse practice act is followed with all staffing plans, which includes appropriate delegation to, and supervision of, any unlicensed personnel.

Force of Magnetism: Community

Facilities with the magnet designation are partners with the community they serve, working together to address their healthcare issues. The community has a sense of this partnership and will form alliances that are mutually beneficial. Such involvement can be found with nurse executives serving on community-based committees and boards as well as with the individual participation in interest groups.

The facility may provide space needed for community meetings and classes. Many support groups and disease awareness organizations require donated space for educational lectures and group meetings. Nurses within the organization may be contacted to provide lectures or lead discussions on their specialty area of nursing. The organization may sponsor or plan a community health fair, using volunteers from the nursing staff to provide health screening. Organizations frequently compensate volunteers with salary for this commitment.

Recognition and encouragement from the organization for community involvement is demonstrated in the flexibility allowed in scheduling time off and in the performance evaluations or career ladder advancement, which rewards such participation. There is acknowledgment for community involvement on a personal level, even when not directly in the field of health care. Job descriptions for nursing leadership frequently have a component related to community involvement. Organizational newsletters and award ceremonies may be used to recognize the community involvement of the nurse.

Collaboration with the area's healthcare organizations, community-based organizations, and institutions synergize the effort to improve healthcare for the community. Health promotion programs, emergency preparedness, and healthcare literacy may be addressed by such collaboration. The facility can demonstrate dedicated resources to support community involvement. This can be financial but can also be in material and human resources. There is a system in place to evaluate the outcomes of such community programs. Evaluation for effectiveness is a necessary piece for any type of program and will be used to make appropriate changes.

EXEMPLARY PROFESSIONAL NURSING PRACTICE

Eight Domains of Evidence: Professional Practice Model

Force of Magnetism: Models of Care

The concept of a professional practice model is the description of how nursing care is delivered. An emphasis is placed on the theoretically based nursing practice model instead of a care delivery model designed for cost benefits.[28] As nursing has evolved and redefined the role of the RN, models of care have also changed. In the culture of evidence-based practice, nursing is forced to examine models of care to determine if research supports it, if positive patient outcomes result from it, and if it meets the needs of both the nurse and the consumer (patient). Organizations are moving away from the one-size-fits-all mentality and recognizing more than one model of care may be necessary within one organization. Involving direct care nurses in the process of selecting or developing a professional practice model allows for those with the unique knowledge of a clinical unit to have control over the method of care delivery. A variety of care models used within one organization is often seen, with each unit selecting the most effective for their patient population. Information and educational support on various types of professional models of care should be found in professional specialty organizations, national guidelines, and in state or federal regulations. An example of this being utilized is seen in the American Association of Critical Care Nurses' *Synergy Model of Care* within the critical care units. Nurses interviewed in these units should be acutely aware of the model of care being used, can provide examples of its use, and should be able to reference American Association of Critical Care Nurses as the organization promoting it.

Two of the aforementioned eight essentials of magnetism are control of and over nursing practice and perceived adequacy in staffing.[29] Both of these characteristics play a part in designing a professional practice model. Control over nursing practice should not be considered synonymous with autonomy. Autonomy is more closely related to the practice of the individual, the nurse making clinical practice decisions regarding the care of the patient. Nursing having control over the practice of nursing involves the organization as a whole and includes decisions in the method of delivery of nursing care. Nursing having control of the nursing practice and the practice environment is one of the key components of ANA's *Scope and Standards for Nurse Administrators*.[30]

Evidence-Based Practice 22-1

Ingersoll, Witzel, and Smith describe the importance of relating the professional practice model to the mission, values, and vision of the organization. Each component of the practice model should be a reflection of the mission and values of the organization. The performance appraisal of the individual nurse evaluates how these values are demonstrated in practice. The competencies required to advance on a clinical ladder program are "consistent with, and supportive of the professional practice model designed to guide clinical practice and administration of nursing services."[31] Organizations in research studies that score high in nurses' perception of control over the practice of nursing frequently have structures in place to ensure nurses are included in decisions related to their practice. This is an example of shared governance or participative management.[32]

Primary nursing, family-centered care, team nursing, district, and holistic nursing are a few of the models of care used in the past and remain in use today. Through the evidence of research, nursing has discovered the value of having the RN at the bedside. Models of care that moved the RN further away from direct patient care and into a more supervisory role had fewer positive patient outcomes. Using a skill mix that had a large percentage of unlicensed assistive personnel prevented the RN from direct patient observation. More failure to rescue was observed and nurse satisfaction lessened.[33] Magnet facilities not only make a concerted effort to return the RN to the patient bedside but also to provide the RN with support for educational growth and the resources needed for quality nursing care delivery.

Each organization has the responsibility to comply with the state's nurse practice act when considering the delivery of nursing care. As nurses become more and more mobile, perhaps moving from the area of educational preparation, knowledge about the specific nurse practice act for the state in which they are currently employed is imperative. Organizations use the orientation process of new hires to provide information about regulatory statutes, but an annual educational program is needed as well. Links to the nurse practice act on the intranet site is done by some organizations; on-line self-learning modules have also been done. Responsibility to remain updated on regulatory statutes of one's profession rests on the individual, but the organization has the responsibility to ensure that nurses are current on this information.

Staffing ratios and skill mix are topics of much discussion in the clinical setting and in the administrative board room. Administrators looking at financial budgets require nurse managers to be accountable for the largest financial expenditure, nursing salaries. Some financial analysts believe that if nurses "worked smarter" they could provide care to 10 to 12 patients on a medical-surgical floor. Research has clearly indicated that nursing care provided by RNs with smaller patient assignments reduces the incidences of negative nurse-sensitive outcomes and patient mortality.[34]

Is there a magic nurse-to-patient ratio required of magnet hospitals? The answer is no, but magnet facilities have methods in place, with nursing involvement, that ensure the needs of the patient unique to each clinical unit are met and provided for by the one most qualified to give it. Nurses in the clinical setting are aware that numbers do not always reflect the work of the nurse. Several methods to measure patient acuity level have surfaced, each with good and bad characteristics. A flexible staffing matrix, allowing for the nurse in charge to make changes as needed and to best serve the patient, is essential.

Eight Domains of Evidence: Safe and Ethical Practice

Force of Magnetism: Nurses as Teachers

Part of the professional growth and development of nurses include opportunities, expectations, and support for nurses to practice the role of teacher. The incorporation of teaching is part of job descriptions for all level of nurses and in performance evaluations. Patient education is valued and expected to be interdisciplinary, demonstrated through documentation, and evaluated for outcomes.

Patients and their families receive education that is holistic and individualized to meet their cultural, spiritual, and emotional needs. Assessment of the learning needs of the community in which the facility operates is apparent in the patient educational programs that are designed. For instance, if the facility is serving a population demographic that has a large percentage of people speaking only Spanish, then written educational materials should be available in that language.

Nurses performing as teachers will be seen not only in patient education but during the interaction with fellow nurses and nursing students. Nurses in roles of preceptors, adjunct faculty, and mentors can be demonstrated at all levels in the organization. Direct care staff, nurse managers, directors, and nurse executives are involved in the provision of learning opportunities to a variety of undergraduate nursing students as well as graduate students.

APNs are actively involved in teaching within the clinical setting, taking advantage of teachable moments at the bedside. APNs are also available as preceptors for graduate nursing students.

Collaborative partnerships with academic institutes in the community are mutually beneficial. As partners in combating the nursing shortage, some magnet organizations supply faculty, along with their salary, to local schools of nursing. This allows nursing programs to accept more qualified candidates into nursing programs. Clinical experiences may be held during evenings and weekends.

Dedicated nursing units have been formed in which nursing staff volunteer to serve as the clinical instructor for the partnered nursing program. The nursing staff receives training and instruction in educational methods, and the nursing program has a clinical unit of nursing staff dedicated to providing valuable learning experiences for their students. Innovative clinical opportunities allow nursing schools to ensure quality experiences for their students and the professional growth of the nursing staff.

Force of Magnetism: Interdisciplinary Relationships

Nursing is one component of the healthcare team and is valued by other disciplines within the organization for the expertise it provides. Likewise, nursing recognizes the contributions made by other essential professions. Interdisciplinary relationships are collaborative and positive. Evidence of this relationship exists in interdisciplinary councils, committees, and projects that exist to further the organizational vision of excellence in patient care services. Organizational policies mandate the varied membership of such shared governance councils and committees. Formulation of clinical care guidelines and the approval of patient care policies are done with multiple contributors from across the organization.

Input from all professional disciplines is received with respect of and acknowledgment for its unique perspective. Interdisciplinary patient care rounding is one method in which professionals meet to discuss patient goal setting and has been successful in shortening the length of stay for the patient.[35] Some organizations include the patient and family in interdisciplinary rounds to discuss the progress of the patient. Grand rounds is another venue in which a number of disciplines can interact and present a case study to the healthcare team members for educational purposes.

Documentation in an electronic format can now facilitate interdisciplinary participation in data collection, assessment, goal setting, and evaluation of the patient. Many organizations have one format for the documentation of patient education. With the ability of multiple professions accessing this one format, knowledge is easily shared and patient education can be reinforced by each discipline.

Conflict management strategies are in place and methods to resolve issues are clear to all members of interdisciplinary committees and councils. Support is provided to team leaders in group management techniques through educational programs, role modeling behavior, and mentoring.

Force of Magnetism: Quality of Care (Safe and Ethical Practice)

Facilities on the magnet journey address patient safety issues that are of concern to all of the healthcare industry. Healthcare organizations may feel pressure to select measures that are proven to be efficient or cost saving but may impinge on the goal of patient safety.[36] Magnet facilities place patient safety above all other goals and have the methods to assess, design, implement, and evaluate safety programs. Such programs rely on the input from multiple disciplines to address methods and policies that ensure a safe patient care and environment.

Contributions from nurses at all levels are used to develop innovative patient safety programs. Evidence that patient safety outcomes have improved by such programs can be demonstrated. This safety-conscious attitude is imparted to every employee in the organization, and individual accountability for patient safety is present. The organization recognizes and addresses the need for employee safety as well. Programs to address such issues may be unique for the needs of the organization but include violence in the workplace and facility access.

Methods to report unsafe or incompetent practices are in place and are nonpunitive. Nurses have a recourse that can be used when encountering immediate issues concerning unsafe practice of a peer or of a physician.

The ANA's *Code of Ethics for Nurses* is followed throughout the organization. Nurses are provided education and support in using this code of ethics in their practice. There is access to members of the ethics committee for formal and informal consultation. Examples can be found of how these ethical principles are implemented. Privacy of the patient and the staff is protected with formal policies. Consequences for any breach in confidentiality are clear within this policy and are executed after the appropriate investigation.

The patient's bill of rights and the ANA's *Bill of Rights for the Registered Nurse* are utilized by the organization. The patient's bill of rights informs the patient and family of the right to participate in their healthcare treatment choices. The ANA's *Bill of Rights for the Registered Nurse* seeks to inform the nurse of the right to deliver quality nursing care in a safe environment.

Eight Domains of Evidence: Autonomous Practice

Force of Magnetism: Autonomy

The presence of autonomy is one of the characteristics first identified in the original magnet hospitals in the early 1980s,[37] yet confusion over the meaning of autonomy and how it is perceived in the clinical setting continues today. Autonomy and accountability are also identified as one of the eight essential elements of magnetism,[37] and research indicates that it is positively correlated with job satisfaction and patient satisfaction.[38,39]

During the research study conducted by Aiken, Sloane, Lake, Sochalski, and Weber[40] on dedicated AIDS units, they noted that these units were designed by the nurses practicing in them. The researchers considered this control over the practice of nursing care a key to the positive outcomes experienced. In the white paper from Volunteer Hospitals of America Research Series, *The Business Case for Workforce Stability*, researchers found that giving employees more opportunities for input and using their feedback to make changes increased job satisfaction and correlated with growth in revenue.[41]

Evidence-Based Practice 22-2

One official definition of autonomy is "socially granted and legally defined freedom to make practice decisions without technical evaluation from sources outside the profession."[42] Nurses interviewed by Kramer et al.[43] define clinical autonomy as "the freedom to act based on what you know in the best interests of the patient, to make independent clinical decisions in the nursing sphere of practice and interdependent decisions in those spheres where nursing overlaps with other disciplines."

The practice of autonomy is expected in any profession, including nursing. Nurses no longer bear the task of only following physician orders. Professional autonomy and accountability dictates that the nurse exercises judgment derived from professional education, clinical expertise, and the ethical desire to provide quality nursing care.

Nurse administrators are charged by the ANA's *Scope and Standards for Nurse Administrators* to provide the RN the tools and environment conducive to achieving autonomy in nursing practice.[44] Empowerment to provide nursing care in a safe and competent manner relies on an organization that values nursing judgment and encourages interdisciplinary collaboration. Clinical competence is enhanced by supportive nursing management in an organization that is not punitive if a mistake occurs.

Nurses are confident that they are supported in making clinical decisions. If the nurse does make an error in judgment, focus is on gaining expertise and analyzing the decision-making process, not on punishment for decision making. Competence is a precursor to autonomy, and working beside nurses who are clinically competent was also identified as one of the eight essential elements of a magnet facility. (Figure 22-1) Formal and informal encouragement of professional development is seen in tuition reimbursement programs, clinical ladder programs, rewards for certification, and active membership in professional organizations.

Magnet facilities are able to demonstrate autonomous nursing practice on multiple levels. Nursing administrators are empowered to make the organizational decisions concerning nursing. Strong, competent leadership is essential to establishing the culture of autonomous nursing practice. Nursing as a body is recognized in the organization to have a value in decision making. APNs have the authority to practice within the scope of practice regulated by the state, and direct care nurses have the freedom to act on knowledge and guidelines set forth by their professional organization or specialty.

APNs contribute to the autonomy of the direct care nurse when the role of the APN is structured to be a clinical advisor or role model.[45] When the APN is involved in compliance issues or multiple projects instead of as the unit clinical expert, staff nurses do not feel the support needed to grow in their own expertise. Having access to clinical experts at the bedside can stimulate questions and answers regarding complex issues nurses face daily. Immediate feedback by the APN is an effective method in changing practice.

Evidence-Based Practice 22-3

Kramer et al.'s 2007 study[45] indicates the renegotiation of the scope of practice as one of the structures that enables autonomy. In short, nurses are expected to practice in a culture that is different from the one taught in years gone by. Rapid response teams are one example in which nurses rapidly assess a patient in need of immediate attention and provide care as needed. Frequently, such teams are composed of APNs, but not always. Nurses with the clinical expertise and knowledge can fill this role, along with other team members.

Organizational support for nurses to practice with autonomy is evident in the facility's mission, values, job descriptions, policies, and procedures. It also ensures accountability for autonomous practice with performance evaluations. In an organization with shared decision making, nurses' participation allows nurse control over their practice. Attending a national professional conference and returning to put new evidence-based nursing interventions into practice is an indicator of practicing with autonomy.

Research studies indicate that nursing units with a higher degree of perceived nurse–physician collaboration also experience a higher degree of nursing autonomy.[46,47] Fostering collaborative

FIGURE 22-2	TOOLS NEEDED FOR CLINICAL COMPETENCE

- Internet and medical library access to research professional journals, databases, and national guidelines
- Support, financially and with time off, to participate in professional organizations
- Support in obtaining and maintaining specialty certification, financially and with educational programs
- Leadership examples in specialty certification and in membership of professional organizations
- Access to clinical experts at the bedside
- Opportunities to participate in shared decision making

Source: Author.

nurse–physician relationships is the responsibility of nursing management. Establishing clear communication and having mutual respect for each other's clinical expertise is essential. Interdisciplinary work groups in which representatives from nursing and medicine strive to achieve the common goal of using best practice as supported by research is an effective method.

Organizations are responsible for maintaining this culture of mutual respect by having policies and procedures in place to deal with disruptive behavior by the physician or by the RN. No tolerance for unprofessional behavior should be clear and demonstrated in practice.

Evidence of a peer-review process is present in magnet facilities. Peer review can be an intimidating idea for the direct care nurse. Mentorship in this process is helpful and can demonstrate effective professional development of both those providing the evaluation and in those receiving the evaluation. Some facilities use peer review in the performance evaluation process done annually, whereas others have direct care nurses routinely conduct chart audits year-round.

One organization described a communication system of immediate feedback for nurses using individual mailboxes on the nursing unit. The nurse can share information in a nonthreatening manner about any problems encountered by the next nursing shift. Peer review can also be facilitated with direct care nurses taking part in the interview process for new hires. Hiring nurses who are willing to be accountable for autonomous nursing practice builds a team with the spirit of "patients' needs come first" attitude. With this spirit, team members naturally assist in patient care if the primary nurse is busy with another task. Any method of peer review, done in the spirit of developing professional growth, is an essential tenet to a profession.

Force of Magnetism: Consultations and Resources

The practice of nursing is supported through the availability of clinical experts. The scope of practice of the APN is defined by the state's nurse practice act, but the role is specified in the job description by the organization. The APN may serve as the change agent to energize the practice environment and ensure that policy changes are disseminated and clearly understood. APNs may be utilized to facilitate unit-based journal clubs, multidisciplinary patient rounds, grand rounds, or nursing research at the bedside.

Active participation in both community and professional nursing organizations is encouraged by the organization. Results from such participation are reflected in the nursing care at the bedside. Collaborations with local educational institutions result in mutually beneficial relationships. There are internal and external resources available to support the use of consultants and knowledgeable experts.

Eight Domains of Evidence: Research and Evidence-Based Practice

Force of Magnetism: Quality of Care

The organization actively seeks to develop an atmosphere of learning and will base decisions concerning patient care on research or best evidence. There is an infrastructure dedicated to supporting the direct care nurse to grow in the skills needed to read, evaluate, and apply nursing research. The direct care nurse is active in questioning current nursing practice and seeks to apply best practice to the clinical setting. To support this learning culture, experts must be available for mentoring and educational programs are available to cultivate the researcher at the bedside. There is a clear delineation between what constitutes nursing research and quality improvement projects. The facility will have nursing representatives on the institutional review board, and nurses are aware of issues concerning the protection of the patient when conducting research.

There is a dedicated budget for nursing research that reflects both current and future projects. The direct care nurse has access to electronic professional nursing journals and an in-house medical library. Examples can be demonstrated in which current research has resulted in a change in the practice of nursing.

Organizations designated as a magnet facility are in a continual mode of quality improvement, including the quality of patient care delivery and the work environment. There is an organized method to assess the need for improvement in both of these areas as well as interdisciplinary participation in the design of new programs. Nurse-sensitive outcomes are used to track and compare data from other like organizations.

The direct care nurse is active in this process through data collection, participation in the design of quality improvement projects, and dissemination of information. Communication regarding the outcomes of quality improvement projects can be done on a regular schedule, such as monthly or quarterly dashboards. The direct care nurse is well versed in reading such reports, and dashboards are frequently posted in public view. Striving for excellence is easier when there are specific goals, such as zero incidences of nosocomial pressure ulcers, and pride in achievement results when the goal is met. Involving the direct care staff in unit assessment to select a quality improvement project encourages nurses to change old habits and work together as a team to strive for excellence in patient care. Peer pressure is effectively used to ensure compliance in behavioral changes. Mentoring nurses in this process may be necessary and can be done by the APN for the unit or the nurse manager.

Eight Domains of Evidence: Quality Processes

Force of Magnetism: Quality of Care

One of the most key features of magnet hospitals is the ability to attract and retain nurses. Research studies have indicated that nurses want to work in an environment that fosters an atmosphere in which quality nursing care can be delivered. Nurses perceive that they are providing quality nursing care and would recommend family and friends to use the facility for their health care.[48,49] To establish this atmosphere there must be infrastructures within the organization that are used to develop, administer, monitor, and evaluate the quality of patient care. Leadership is very involved in this process along with direct care staff. Emphasis on the quality of care is noted within the mission statement of the organization and will have a place in the vision/strategic plan for the future.

Unit councils and organizational councils with interdisciplinary membership are actively engaged in creating policies and procedures that reflect best practice. The nursing process is operationalized throughout the organization. Human and material resources, along with fiscal support, are adequate to provide quality care.

Organizations wishing to document nurses' perception of the quality of care use a survey tool as a method of measurement. The perception of quality in nursing care is documented as well as nurse-sensitive patient outcomes. Data collected need to be calculated on a unit basis and then compared with like units across the nation. The use of a national database is required for this type of comparison. Many organizations use the National Database on Nursing Quality Indicators®, a repository of nursing-sensitive indicators, which was formed by the ANA and is currently administered through the University of Kansas, School of Nursing. However, other national databases may be directed by professional specialty organizations or by private institutions. Comparison of this information with like patient care units across the nation allows the organization to identify areas needed for improvement.

Eight Domains of Evidence: Outcomes

The added dimension of the eighth domain of evidence brings into focus the need to measure the effectiveness of clinical practice and programs. Outcome measurement demonstrates indications for changes in practice and can be used for objective evaluations. More magnet facilities are undergoing a redesignation process that has been similar to the original application. An expectation for growth on the journey to nursing excellence is now part of this evaluation process. Examples can be centered on patient outcomes in addition to outcomes from the professional development of nurses.

SUMMARY

"Described as the heart of the Magnet Recognition Program®, the Forces of Magnetism may be thought of as attributes or outcomes that exemplify excellence in nursing. The full expression of the current 14 Forces of Magnetism is the requirement for designation as a Magnet facility and embodies a professional environment guided by a strong and visionary nursing leader who advocates and supports excellence in nursing practice."[50]

APPLICATION EXERCISES

Exercise 22-1

A small rural 50-bed hospital is interested in attaining magnet recognition. Is this a feasible goal for a healthcare institute of this size? Why or why not? What factors should leaders in this hospital consider before embarking on the magnet journey?

Exercise 22-2

Complete a self-assessment to determine a gap analysis for achieving magnet recognition in the hospital which you are employed or in which you are student. Use the Staff Nurse Self-Assessment Survey in Figure 22-1 to guide your assessment.

Exercise 22-3

Consider the last time either you or a family member/friend was a patient in a hospital. If the facility was magnet designated, how did this affect the delivery of patient care? If the facility was nonmagnet designated, how did this affect the delivery of patient care?

Notes

1. American Nurses Credentialing Center (ANCC). (2007). *What is the magnet recognition program?* Retrieved January 30, 2008, from http://www.nursecredentialing.org/magnet/index.html

2. McClure, M. L., & Hinshaw, A. S. (Eds.) (2002). *Magnet hospitals revisited: Attraction and retention of professional nurses.* Washington, DC: American Nurses Publishing.

3. Ibid.

4. McClure, M. L., Poulin, M. A., Sovie, M. D., & Wandelt, M. A. (1983). *Magnet hospitals: Attraction and retention of professional nurses.* American Academy of Nursing Task Force on Nursing Practice in Hospitals. Kansas City, MO: American Nurses Association.

5. Kramer, M., & Schmalenberg, C. (2002). Staff nurses identify essentials of magnetism. In M. L. McClure & A. S. Hinshaw (Eds.), *Magnet hospitals revisited: Attraction and retention of professional nurses* (pp. 25–59). Washington, DC: American Nurses Publishing.

6. Ibid., ANCC, 2007.

7. Aiken, L. H., & Sloane, D. M. (1997). Effects of organizational innovations in AIDS care on burnout among urban hospital nurses. *Work and Occupations, 24,* 453–478.

8. Aiken, L., Smith, H., & Lake, E. (1994). Lower Medicare mortality among a set of hospitals known for good nursing care. *Medical Care, 32,* 771–787.

9. Aiken, L. H., Havens, D. S., & Sloane, D. M. (2000). The magnet nursing services recognition program: A completion of successful applicants with reputational magnet hospitals. *American Journal of Nursing, 100,* 146–153.

10. Kosel, K. C., & Olivo, T. (2002). *The business case for workforce stability.* Voluntary Hospitals of America, available at https://www.vha.com/news/release/public/02111_summary. Accessed July 21, 2008.

11. Tuazon, N. (2007). Is magnet a money-maker? *Nursing Management,* June, 24–31; University of Pittsburgh Medical Center, (2008). Beckwith Fellows Leadership Program. Retrieved January 3, 2008, from http://www.beckwithinstitute.org/Fellows.htm

12. Ibid., ANCC, 2007.

13. Burns, J. M. (1978). *Leadership.* New York: Harper & Row.

14. Henriksen, K., Keyes, M., Stevens, D., & Clancy, C. (2006). Initiating transformational change to enhance patient safety. *Journal of Patient Safety, 2,* 20–24.

15. Ibid.

16. Ibid., McClure et al., 1983.

17. Ibid.

18. Wolf, G., Hayden, M., & Bradle, J. (2004). The transformational model for professional practice: A system integration focus. *Journal of Nursing Administration, 34,* 180–187.

19. University of Pittsburgh Medical Center, 2008.

20. Ibid., Henriksen et al., 2006.

21. Leach, L. (2005). Nurse executive transformational leadership and organizational commitment. *Journal of Nursing Administration, 35,* 228–237.

22. McDermott, K., Spence Laschinger, H. K., & Shamian, J. (1996). Work empowerment and organizational commitment. *Nursing Management, 27,* 44–48.

23. American Nurses Association (ANA). (2004). *Scope and standards for nurse administrators* (3rd ed.). Washington, DC: Author.

24. Upenicks, V. (2003). Nurse perceptions of job satisfaction and empowerment: Is there a difference between nurses employed in magnet versus non-magnet hospitals? *Nursing Management, 34,* 43–44.

25. Duffy, J., Baldwin, J., & Mastorovich, M. (2007). Using the quality-caring model to organize patient care delivery. *Journal of Nursing Administration, 37,* 546–551.

26. Kramer & Schmalenberg, 2002.

27. Aiken, L. H., Clarke, S. P., Cheung, R. S., Sloane, D. M., & Silber, J. H. (2003). Educational levels of hospital nurses and surgical patient mortality. *Journal of American Medical Association, 290,* 1617–1623.

28. Ibid., Duffy et al., 2007.

29. Aiken, L. H., Clarke, S. P., Sloane, D. M., Sochalski J. & Silber, J. H. (2002). Hospital nurse staffing and patient mortality, nurse burnout, and job dissatisfaction. *Journal of American Medical Association, 288,* 1987–1993.

30. Ibid., ANA, 2004.

31. Ingersoll, G., Witzel, P., & Smith, T. (2005). Using organizational mission, vision, and values to guide professional practice model development and measurement of nurse performance. *Journal of Nursing Administration, 35,* 86–93.

32. Arford, P., & Zone-Smith, L. (2005). Organizational commitment to professional practice models. *Journal of Nursing Administration, 35*, 467–472.

33. Ibid., Aiken et al., 2002.

34. Ibid., Aiken et al., 2003.

35. Dutton, R., Cooper, C., Jones, A., Leone, S., Kramer, M., & Scalea, T. (2003). Daily multidisciplinary rounds shorten length of stay for trauma patients. *Journal of Trauma-Injury Infection & Critical Care, 55*, 913–919.

36. Institute of Medicine. (2004). *Keeping patients safe: Transforming the work environment of nurses.* Washington, DC: National Academy Press.

37. Ibid., McClure et al., 1983.

38. Ibid., Aiken et al., 2002.

39. Ibid., Aiken et al., 2002.

40. Aiken, L. H., Sloane, D. M., Lake, E. T., Sochalski, J., & Weber, A. (1999). Organization and outcomes of inpatient AIDS care. *Medical Care, 37*, 760–772.

41. Kosel & Olivo, 2002.

42. McKay, P. (1983). Interdependent decision making: Redefining professional autonomy. *Nursing Administration Quarterly, 7*, 21–30.

43. Kramer, M., Maguire, P., Schmalenberg, C., Andrews, B., Burke, R., Chmielewski, L., Donohue, M. T., Ellsworth, M., Poduska, D., Smith, M. E., Tachibana, C. (2007). Excellence through evidence: Structures enabling clinical autonomy. *Journal of Nursing Administration, 37*(1), 41–52.

44. Ibid., ANA, 2004.

45. Ibid., Kramer et al., 2007.

46. Manojlovich, M. (2005). Linking practice environment to nurses' job satisfaction through nurse-physician communication. *Journal of Nursing Scholarship, 37*, 367–371.

47. Rosenstein, A. H. (2002). Nurse-physician relationships: Impact on nurse satisfaction and retention. *American Journal of Nursing, 102*, 26–34.

48. Ibid., Kramer et al., 2002.

49. McLure & Hinshaw, 2002.

50. Ibid., ANCC, 2007.

References

Aiken, L. H. (2002). Superior outcomes for magnet hospitals: The evidence base. In M. L. McLure & A. S. Hinshaw (Eds.), *Magnet hospitals revisited: Attraction and retention of professional nurses* (pp. 61–81). Washington, DC: American Nurses Publishing.

Aiken, L. H., Clarke, S. P., Sloane, D. M., Sochalski, J. A., Busse, R., Clarke, H., et al. (2001). Nurses' report on hospital care in five countries: The ways in which nurses' work is structured have left nurses among the least satisfied workers, and the problem is getting worse. *Health Affairs, 20*, 43–53.

Aiken, L. H., & Sloane, D. M. (1997). Hospital nurses' occupational exposure to blood: Prospective, retrospective, and institutional reports. *American Journal of Public Health, 87*, 103–108.

American Association of Critical Care Nurses. (2002). *Safeguarding the patient and the profession: The value of critical care nurse certification.* Retrieved June 16, 2003, from http://www.aacn.org

American Nurses Association Policy Series. (1998). Looking for quality patient outcomes the American Nurses Credentialing Center's Magnet Recognition Program recognizes excellence. *Nursing Trends and Issues, 3*, 1–6.

Buerhaus, P. I., Staiger, D. O., & Auerbach, D. I. (2000a). Implications of an aging registered nurse workforce. *The Journal of the American Medical Association, 283*, 2948–2954.

Buerhaus, P. I., Staiger, D. O., & Auerbach, D. I. (2000b). Policy responses to an aging registered nurse workforce. *Nursing Economic$, 18*, 278–286.

Commission on Workforce for Hospitals and Healthcare Systems. (2002). *In our hands: How hospital leaders can build a thriving workforce.* Chicago: American Hospital Association.

Department of Health and Human Services, Bureau of Health Professions. (2000). *The registered nurse population: National sample survey of registered nurses* (4th ed.). Washington, DC: U.S. Government Printing Office.

Department of Health and Human Services, Health Resources and Services Administration, Bureau of Health Professions, National Center for Health Workforce Analysis. (2002, July). *Projected supply, demand, and shortages of registered nurses: 2000–2020.* Retrieved November 13, 2002, from http://bhpr.hrsa.gov/oldhealthworkforce/rnproject/report.htm

Drugger, B. (1998). Magnet recognition, JCAHO commendation, and shared governance. *Journal of Shared Governance, 4*, 11–15.

Havens, D. S. (2001). Comparing nursing infrastructure and outcomes: ANCC Magnet and nonmagnet CNEs report. *Nursing Economic$, 19*, 258–266.

Herrin, D. M. (1994). Linking management and advance practice at the department level: A collaborative leadership model. *Aspen's Advisor for Nurse Executives, 9*, 6–9.

Joint Commission on the Accreditation of Healthcare Organizations. (2002). *Health care at the crossroads: Strategies for addressing the evolving nursing crisis.* Retrieved November 3, 2002, from http://jcaho.org/news+room/news+release+archives/health+care+at+the+crossroads.pdf

Kaldenberg, D. O., & Regrut, B. (1999). Do satisfied patients depend on satisfied employees? *The Satisfaction Report*, Press Ganey (3).

Laurent, C. L. (2000). A nursing theory for nursing leadership. *Journal of Nursing Management, 8*, 83–88.

Monarch, K. (2002). The mark of excellence: The ANCC Magnet Nursing Services Recognition Program. *Maryland Nurse, 4*, 12–15.

Morrison, R. S., Jones, L., & Fuller, B. (1997). The relation between leadership style and empowerment on job satisfaction of nurses. *Journal of Nursing Administration, 27*, 27–34.

Nelson, J. W. (2002). The empirical relationship of primary nursing and organizational commitment. *Creative Nursing, 8*, 13–16.

New law, JCAHO report recognizes success of magnet concept. (2002). *American Nurse, 34*, 16.

Schmieding, N. J. (n.d.). Ida J. Orlando. Retrieved November 6, 2002, from http://www.uri.edu/nursing/schmieding/Orlando/

Sochalski, J. (2001). Quality of care, nurse staffing, and patient outcomes. *Policy, Politics, & Nursing Practice, 2*, 9–18.

Spence Laschinger, H. K., Finegan, J., Shamian, J., & Wilk, P. (2001). Impact of structural and psychological empowerment on job strain in nursing work settings: Expanding Kanter's model. *Journal of Nursing Administration, 31*, 260–272.

Staiger, D. O., Auerbach, D. I., & Buerhaus, P. I. (2000). Expanding career opportunities for women and declining interest in nursing as a career. *Nursing Economic$, 18*, 230–236.

Trossman, S. (2002). Nursing magnets: Attracting talent and making it stick: Magnet hospitals help stem the nursing shortage with better recruitment and retention. *Nevada RNformation, 11*, 21.

Wilson, B., & Spence Laschinger, H. K. (1994). Staff nurse perception of job empowerment and organizational commitment: A test of Kanter's theory of structural power in organizations. *Journal of Nursing Administration, 24*, 39–47.

23 MANAGING A CULTURALLY DIVERSE WORKFORCE

Francine Mancuso Parker, RN, MSN, EdD
Jeanne-Marie Tapke, RN, MSN, SPHR

LEARNING OBJECTIVES AND ACTIVITIES

- Appreciate the value of culturally diverse recruitment and retention strategies.
- Describe nurse leader and manager behavioral characteristics necessary to manage a culturally diverse workforce.
- Identify aspects of magnet hospitals that maximize effective management of a culturally diverse workforce.
- Be aware of generational differences within the nursing workforce.
- Value the impact and strength of a diverse workforce on the healthcare environment.
- Integrate principles of cultural competency throughout healthcare environment.
- Appreciate the importance of relationship building.

CONCEPTS

Workforce diversity, cultural sensitivity, cultural competence, interview, transformational leadership, magnet credentials, professional environment, ethical environment, collaboration, autonomy and empowerment

QUOTE

You can't be what you can't see.

—Marian Wright Edelman

Introduction

A culturally diverse workforce, an unrelenting nationwide nursing shortage, increased work loads, healthcare restructuring, downsizing, and cost containment present a daunting challenge to nurse executives in regards to retaining a committed workforce.[1] With national nurse turnover rates hovering above 20%, it is imperative that quality, competent nurses be recruited and, once in the system, measures to promote job satisfaction and retention be initiated.[2] Increased work loads, mandatory overtime, work environment stress, and increased nurse-to-patient ratios loom heavy and are contributing factors to dissatisfaction, turnover, and nurses leaving the profession.[3] Shaver and Lacey add that short staffing equivocates with decreased job satisfaction.[4]

Benefits of a culturally diverse workforce are reported in the literature and include improved quality of patient care, increased patient safety and satisfaction, and increased patient and nurse satisfaction.[5] Nurses who report high levels of satisfaction in the work environment identify positive characteristics such as increased autonomy, clinical ladder advancement, and participatory decision-making and ethical practices. When nurses feel valued and are given recognition for their work, job satisfaction increases.[6]

It is well documented that nurse job satisfaction is the strongest predictor of intent to stay or leave the job. Increasingly, nurses nationwide are reporting increased stress and dissatisfaction with their profession.[7] Research findings support that autonomy, task orientation, and work pressure experienced by nurses are related to stress and dissatisfaction. Positive experience related to these factors is important in increasing job satisfaction, retaining nurses, and decreasing turnover. Achieving magnet hospital status is not a goal or economically feasible for various hospitals. However, it would be helpful to look at the criteria and standards required for accreditation, including the management practices of these facilities, because these organizations have documented positive retention and outcomes.[8] An assumption of strategic human resource development for managing a culturally diverse workforce is improved organizational performance, which requires understanding of and integration with the organization's strategic objectives. An additional assumption, nurse executives and managers must understand current and future needs of nursing within the organization.[9] The nursing process is a proven method for analysis and decision making and is recommended for use here. Figure 23-1 provides an outline of the process.

Roy describes the process as a problem-solving approach for gathering data, identifying the capacities and needs of the human adaptive system, selecting and implementing approaches, and evaluating the outcome.[10] The process is cyclical, overlapping, and interrelated. Within this framework, the manager evaluates resource development related to staffing, training and development, performance appraisal, compensation, safety and health, labor relations, managing change and culture, work, and organizational design.

Nurse executives, front-line managers, and human resource professionals must use innovative strategies to manage a diverse, culturally competent workforce.

A CULTURALLY DIVERSE WORKFORCE: RECRUITMENT ISSUES

Culture has many implications in the workforce. It can be described as the sum total of socially transmitted behavioral patterns, including the arts, beliefs, values, customs, and life-ways and other products of human work and thought of a population of people that focus on their worldview and decision making. Nurse administrators must be sensitive to the many nuances of culture and its meanings for those providing care.[12]

Studer, a performance excellence consultant for the healthcare industry, states, "It all starts with the selection and the first 90 days."[13] The most elaborate recruitment strategies will not prove financially effective if the organization cannot retain valuable employees. The goal of providing the right number of highly skilled nurses is intimately woven into nurse retention considering cultural sensitivity and

FIGURE 23-1	OUTLINE OF THE NURSING PROCESS

Assessment of behavior: Gathering data about the behavior needed by an individual in the organization and position

Assessment of stimuli: Identification of influencing internal and external stimuli. Stimuli are classified as

1. Focal—those most immediately confronting the person

2. Contextual—all other stimuli present that are affecting the situation

3. Residual—those stimuli whose effect on the situation are unclear

Nursing diagnosis: Formulating statements that interpret data about the adaptation, including behaviors

Goal setting: Establishing behavioral outcomes

Intervention: Determining how to attain goals

Evaluation: Judging the effectiveness of the intervention in relation to the behavior after the intervention in comparison with the goal established[11]

Source: Author.

cultural competence as essential to nurse retention. Based on an assessment of each unit or department for characteristics such as size and general patient acuity, and cultural issues, an individualized plan for recruitment should be devised. Nurse staffing needs are more effectively served if a formal nurse recruitment plan is developed. Nurse leaders, hospital administrators, human resource staff, and marketing often collaborate to create the best recruitment plan. This is a proactive measure by nurse leaders and managers to minimize emergency measures for nurse recruitment. It systematically determines current nursing needs, predicts future needs, establishes recruitment objectives, identifies matching strategies for realizing these objectives, executes the plan, and evaluates its success. The same marketing principles apply whether you are targeting patients or staff. You must identify your audience, develop a targeted message, choose the appropriate vehicle to deliver that message, and measure results. This is particularly important when considering the cultural make-up of the community and nursing unit or department.

Creative collaboration within the community is a proven successful strategy for recruitment of a culturally sensitive workforce. Nurse leaders becoming involved in colleges of nursing, career planning workshops, job fairs, and speaking bureaus provide excellent opportunities to promote both the profession and organization for recruiting purposes.

Behavioral Interviewing: Cultural Sensitivity Issues

The best way to determine how an employee will conduct themselves in a future job is by looking at past behaviors.[13] The behavioral interview technique is used by managers to evaluate a candidate's experiences and behaviors to determine their potential for success. The interviewer identifies desired skills and behaviors and then structures open-ended questions and statements to elicit detailed responses.

Managers that use behavioral interviewing have predetermined, through a detailed analysis of the position, the skill sets required to be successful in the position. In addition to the specific clinical skills necessary for patient care, desirable qualities and leadership skills might include motivation, cultural sensitivity, cultural competence, communication, interpersonal skills, planning and organization, critical-thinking skills, team-building skills, and the ability to influence others. Conducting a position analysis requires a manager to reflect on questions such as: What are the necessary skills to do this job? What makes a successful candidate? What would make an unsuccessful candidate? Why have nurses left this position previously? What is the most difficult part of this job? What does it mean to be culturally sensitive in this position? How can cultural competence be determined in this position?

Interviewing is a two-way process. Figure 23-2 outlines examples of behavioral-based interview questions that can be useful in the interview process. The candidate gains an understanding of the priorities for the unit and department by the content of questions asked. This is an excellent opportunity to introduce the core values and performance standards of the unit and organization. The questions should reflect current goals and initiatives, with emphasis on cultural sensitivity. For example, quality and patient safety initiatives, evidence-based practice, interdisciplinary collaboration, theory-based nursing, and research initiatives as well as culturally sensitive issues can be the focus of the interview. The interviewer also gains insight to the priorities of the interviewee by the questions asked.

Peer Interviewing: Cultural Sensitivity Issues

Peer interview is a process that allows staff to participate in the evaluation and hiring of potential candidates. Capable interviewing teams are representative of the organization, work group, or position being filled. Culturally competent peers generally provide a level of sensitivity and may be able to identify peers who may not be reflective of the organization's goals. It is important for the nurse administrator to seek medium to high performers who reflect diversity in age, race, ethnicity, and gender and also of thought and maturity. Success of the team lies in training, which focuses on understanding the

| FIGURE 23-2 | BEHAVIORAL-BASED INTERVIEW EXAMPLES |

- Describe a time when you had too many things to do and were required to prioritize tasks.
- Describe a time when you were culturally sensitive to a patient you cared for.
- Identify a time when you had to make a quick, critical decision.
- Give me an example of a time when you used your critical thinking to solve a problem.
- Describe a situation in which you were able to use persuasion to successfully convince someone to see things your way.
- Describe a time when you were faced with a stressful situation that required your coping skills.
- Give an example of a time when a goal you set was successfully achieved.
- Describe a time when you set your goals too high or too low.
- What is your experience with delegation?
- Has there been a time when you had to follow a policy with which you did not agree?
- What is your personal approach to dealing with conflict?
- Tell me about a time you were able to effectively interact with a coworker even when that person may not have liked you (or vice versa).
- Describe a difficult decision you have had to make in the last year.
- Talk to me about a circumstance when something you tried to accomplish failed.
- Give me an example of when you took the lead in solving a problem.
- Give me an example of a time when you motivated others.
- Describe a time when you anticipated potential problems and developed preventive measures.
- Talk about a time when you were required to make an unpopular decision.

Source: Author.

selection process. This type of preparation can be achieved by internal or external facilitators.[14,15] Determining the degree of cultural sensitivity is also an important factor in the peer interview process.

The manager generally conducts the first stage of interviewing and presents peer-interviewing teams with candidates they would likely hire. Candidates should be informed of the peer process so they can be prepared for a possible new experience. There are advantages and disadvantages to this procedure. This process is time consuming and can be difficult if there are several well-qualified candidates applying for a position. Although it is useful in some situations, it is less efficient in others. For example, if the vacancy being filled is due to a termination that some staff disagreed with, then the process will be more difficult. Gains are that some key employees will have had contact with the new hire and some level of confidence in their ability. Participation in peer review allows employees to have ownership in the process and accountability that the new hire is successful. Managers must trust their employees' decisions and support a candidate that is recommended. Figure 23-3 outlines strategies for recruitment.

Laws That Impact the Hiring Process: Consideration for Cultural Sensitivity

Title VII is a provision of the Civil Rights Act of 1964 that prohibits discrimination, in virtually every employment circumstance, based on race, color, religion, gender, pregnancy, or national origin. In general, Title VII applies to employers with 15 or more employees.

| **FIGURE 23-3** | **STRATEGIES FOR RECRUITING NURSING STUDENTS FOR A CULTURALLY DIVERSE WORKFORCE** |

1. Form a committee to create a plan.
   a. Include clinical nurses
   b. Set goals
   c. Create a management plan for each goal

2. Obtain recruitment materials from organizations. Note the level of cultural sensitivity. Consider materials from the National League for Nursing, American Nurses Association, the American Organization for Nurse Executives, National Student Nurses Association, American Association of Colleges of Nursing, and state and local agencies

3. Prepare additional culturally sensitive materials (e.g., news stories from newspapers, TV, and radio; posters for school; speakers' bureau, tours).

4. Coordinate with other nurse education programs and prospective employers of nurses. How is cultural competency addressed?

5. Prepare and offer consultation programs for junior and senior high schools; consider cultural sensitivity issues.

6. Coordinate activities of recruiters in school of nursing. How is culture addressed with regards to written materials?

7. Involve community agencies in recruitment efforts.

8. Evaluate results accomplished from steps 1–7.

9. Do work-study programs (e.g., cooperative education, high schools with employer, high schools with school of nursing).

Source: Author.

The purpose of Title VII protection is to "level the playing field" by forcing employers to consider only objective, job-related criteria in making employment decisions. The above classes of individuals are considered "protected" under Title VII because of the history of unequal treatment identified in each class.

Title VII must be considered when reviewing applications or resumes (i.e., by not eliminating candidates on the basis of a "foreign" last name), when interviewing candidates (i.e., by asking only job-related questions), when testing job applicants (i.e., by treating all candidates the same and ensuring that tests are not unfairly weighted against any group of people), and when considering employees for promotions, transfers, or any other employment-related benefit or condition. For intentional discrimination, employees may seek a jury trial, with compensatory and punitive damages up to the maximum limitations established by the Civil Rights Act of 1991.

The Equal Pay Act is an amendment to the Fair Labor Standards Act that prohibits employers from discriminating between men and women by paying one gender more than the other "for equal work on jobs the performance of which requires equal skill, effort, and responsibility, and which are performed under similar working conditions."[15]

The Age Discrimination in Employment Act of 1967 and the 1990 Americans with Disabilities Act are federal antidiscrimination laws that prohibit private employers, state and local governments, employment agencies, and labor unions from discriminating against qualified individuals for age or disabilities in job application procedures, hiring, firing, advancement, compensation, job training, and other terms, conditions, and privileges of employment.

On-Boarding: Implications for Cultural Competence

The process for new employee orientation and mainstreaming is often referred to as "employee on-boarding." Keeping in mind that you never get a second chance to make a first impression, nurse managers should make absolutely sure that new hires feel welcomed, valued, and prepared for what lies ahead during the new employee orientation or on-boarding process. Welcoming the whole person, rather than just a set of job functions, helps new hires more quickly assimilate to the unit and organizational culture.

Good on-boarding programs are still the exception not the rule. The first 30, 60, and 90 days of an employee's tenure with an organization are absolutely vital, yet on-boarding is one of the least developed talent management functions. It is very difficult to recover from a poor initial experience. The most difficult process of all is socialization, or how the employee gets to know the culture, informal structure, and operating norms of the new environment. Without this knowledge and understanding, the time to competency for new employees may be increased. Determining cultural sensitivity during this first 30, 60, and 90 days is imperative to retaining a culturally competent, committed workforce.

A key part of individualized on-boarding is an inclusive plan that addresses who, what, when, where, and how the process progresses. Some important things to consider are as follows:

1. Timely access to critical systems such as intranet, pixis, or key cards
2. Introducing to employees who have successfully integrated in the last year
3. Designating an appropriate mentor
4. Providing face-to-face feedback within the first several weeks
5. Developing a plan to appropriately address identified issues

If a candidate knows that necessary resources and support are available to carry out the responsibilities of the position being sought, confidence in his or her ability to achieve organizational goals will be realized. Cultural sensitivity is key to successful on-boarding.

Mentoring is an important success factor in nursing, particularly with new nurse hires. A mentor is an individual, usually older, always more experienced, who helps and guides another individual's development. Culturally sensitive mentors are critical to a greater sense of comfort and confidence in new hires. A mentor's responsibilities may include facilitating internal introductions, which could help the new hire build strong networks. Showing the new hire available resources, providing understanding of internal politics, communication issues, and how to tackle problems that might arise are valuable mentor activities. This guidance is not done for personal gain. In an on-boarding process mentors are usually not a new employee's preceptor, but one who helps the new nurse understand "how things are done here."

LEADER AND MANAGER CHARACTERISTICS THAT SUPPORT RETENTION

Research over the past decade has reported strong linkage between nurse satisfaction, productivity, and retention.[16] Effective management and leadership is a formidable catalyst for a successful linkage. Open communication, a supportive environment, and adequate resources for effective and safe patient care delivery are critical factors under a nurse managers' purview. Boyle conducted a study with staff nurses, reporting a positive correlation with an environment in which the manager promoted open dialogue and shared decision making, which in turn contributed to job satisfaction and commitment to the organization.[17] A participatory management style was found to promote nurse retention. However, a successful nurse manager is realistic and aware of the multiple stressors and arduous challenges accompanying leading a culturally diverse workforce in these trying times of short staff, increased turnover, and unprecedented nurse-to-patient ratios. What has not changed is consumer demand for safe, efficient, and culturally sensitive care delivery.

How effective the nurse manager is or is perceived to be by the staff has tremendous impact on the functioning of the work unit.[18] "Staff nurses are more likely to respond favorably to role models that demonstrate integrity and strong ethical and moral values."[19] Behaviors of the successful manager match words spoken. Strategizing to offset the factors influencing a high rate of turnover is an essential attribute for the nurse manager. If nurses observe their manager engaging in administrative negotiation to decrease work load, decrease nurse-to-patient ratios, accommodate flexible schedule requests, and reduce environmental stress, they are more likely to view the manager positively.

Savvy leaders and managers collaborate with schools of nursing to facilitate positive clinical learning experiences for students. The perceptive nurse manager realizes the recruiting possibilities and benefits from creating a positive learning environment. It is the responsibility of the manager to mentor, role model, and educate staff on the crucial nature of these relationships and participate in ensuring an optimal encounter with nursing students.

Adams and Bond studied over several years multiple organizations and various nurse workforces and determined that "relative staff stability ... associated with a positive ethos of nursing care, which embraced the elements of innovation, research-based practice, an interest in staff development, and patient and family involvement in care decisions."[20] To actualize these concepts into action is a call to ensure the nursing workforce has time to research and time to interact with patients and family members beyond clinical skill implementation. A reasonable response to this action would be an adequate number of proficient nurses empowered to practice autonomously and as a team member in meeting patient care outcomes. Nursing executives and managers must be a strong voice for the workforce at the corporate table in articulating reasonable and appropriate staffing levels, nurse-patient ratios, and safe work loads.

Leading and Managing a Diverse Nurse Workforce: Generational Differences

Generational diversity may contribute to workplace conflict if the qualities and differences are not recognized and appreciated.[21] Younger nurses, those born between 1965 and 1980, referred to as Generation X, or those born between 1981 and 1999 and referred to as Generation Y, place high value on personal time and interests. This generation is "flexible, adaptable, techno literate, independent, entrepreneurial."[22] Younger nurses are less apt to stay in a work environment that does not meet their needs or does not afford the "working hard" and "playing hard" philosophy characteristic of the new generation of nurses who balance personal and professional interests. Thus working overtime, pulling extra shifts, and coming in on days off may not occur with frequency among young nurses. Many younger nurses will seek a variety of experiences, readily change jobs, and, if not satisfied, leave nursing if personal and professional needs are not met.[23] Nurse managers must be flexible in their scheduling approach with the younger nurse who wants stability, particularly if motherhood and advanced education are part of the equation.

Retaining the seasoned, more mature nurse becomes as critically important as recruiting from the younger generation in the wake of the nursing shortage. The decision of a mature Baby Boomer nurse (born between 1946 and 1964) may be influenced by factors reflective of one nearing retirement (i.e., salary, pension, rank in staff assignment).[24] Although computer skills may be a weakness for some, a strong work ethic is a desirable characteristic of many older nurses.[25] Retaining the older nurse provides wisdom and years of experience that deserve appreciation and valuing as well as recognition with commensurate financial rewards for loyalty and longevity. There is a shortage of nursing faculty with a not so bright outlook for this trend to reverse in spite of legislative initiatives at the federal and some states level.[26] Competition for clinical learning experiences adds to the problem of not enough resources to accommodate the number of nursing program applicants. However, recruitment initiatives must be innovative to replenish the aging, retiring workforce. Another option, according to Cyr, is to entice nurses nearing retirement to continue working.[27]

Intensified recruitment strategies targeting quality students are necessary to reverse the probability of a major nursing workforce, as well as nursing faculty, shortage in the coming years. Regardless of age, retaining nurses may be a function of showing appreciation, promoting autonomy and cultural sensitivity, providing a positive work environment where healthy relationships are fostered, and consistent and deliberate recognition of nurse work efforts. Figure 23-4 outlines strategies that may be useful for retaining the Baby Boomer nurse and the Generation X or Y nurse.

Human resource development strategies for recruiting, retaining, and satisfying the nursing workforce targets two generations with distinct characteristics and differences. Wieck, Prydun, and Walsh determined that leadership traits valued by younger nurses included honesty (the highest ranking trait), nurturing attitude, supportive, approachable, and team players.[28] The older generation nurses noted the same attributes, with the addition of fairness and integrity as valued traits in a leader.

Cultural and Diverse Workforce Issues

Today's healthcare industry challenges the nursing workforce to be technologically savvy, professionally adept, and clinically competent in the midst of a growing culturally diverse patient and staff workforce. With one in four individuals representative of an ethnic minority group in the United States today, the total exceeds 75 million.[29] The challenge incumbent upon the nursing profession is to deliver safe, excellent, competent care while respecting the various patient customs, languages, religions, and health practices. "Culturally competent individuals value diversity and respect individual differences regardless of one's race, religious beliefs, or ethnocultural background."[30] The American Organization of Nurse Executives "recognizes that the success of nursing leadership is dependent on reflecting the diversity of the communities nurses serve."[30] Figure 23-5 describes this principle.

Just as the expectation is that the healthcare professional will be sensitive to the cultural influences of those for whom they care, the nurse administrator must also be culturally sensitive in recruitment, hiring, and retention strategies. It is important to increase one's cultural awareness and sensitivity, because culture is largely unconscious and can be powerfully influential in communication, decision making, and handling conflict.

Terms such as cultural awareness, cultural sensitivity, cultural competence, and cultural skill are often included in discussions of cultural diversity and are at times used interchangeably.[31] Jeffreys describes cultural awareness as a process where one becomes sensitive to others by first engaging in self-awareness of personal biases and the impact of these biases on perceptions of culturally different

---

FIGURE 23-4 | **USEFUL STRATEGIES FOR RETAINING THE BABY BOOMER NURSE AND THE GENERATION X OR Y NURSE**

Retaining the Baby Boomer Nurse	Retaining the Generation X or Y Nurse
Creative scheduling, i.e., job sharing	Predictable, stable schedule
Competitive salary	Competitive salary
Retirement and pension	Facilitate autonomy and decision making
Curtail physical work	Performance-based awards
Preceptor and mentor role	Continuous learning
Innovative work environment (Beatty & Burroughs, 1999)	Technologically savvy: allow to share expertise
Education and training	Active learning methods: visual (Clark, 2009)

Source: Author.

FIGURE 23-5	GUIDING PRINCIPLE 1: HEALTHCARE ORGANIZATIONS WILL STRIVE TO DEVELOP INTERNAL AND EXTERNAL RESOURCES TO MEET THE NEEDS OF THE DIVERSE PATIENT AND WORKFORCE POPULATIONS SERVED.

1. Designate fiscal resources to develop programs and policies to meet the needs of diverse patient populations served.

2. Establish system processes to ensure the needs of all patient populations are met.

3. Include members from the local community with diverse backgrounds in organizational planning processes.

4. Educate the community on the importance of collecting data, including patient and workforce race, ethnicity, and primary language spoken, for use in improving patient safety and quality.

5. Develop processes and policies to ensure that non–English speaking and limited English proficiency patients will be ensured of access to interpretive services and written translated patient education materials and documents.

6. Implement processes to promote both the consistency of quality of care across various patient populations, and a balance in demographics between the patient and the workforce populations.

7. Execute employment recruitment plans and strategies to attract a workforce that is reflective of the populations served.

8. Train staff members in the importance of understanding the diversity of the patient population served and provision of culturally competent care.

9. Support staff members in obtaining training and education in healthcare interpretation.

Source: Author

individuals.[32] Purnell and Paulanka describe cultural awareness as a greater appreciation of the external signs of diversity, including arts, music, outward appearance, and physical features.[33] Personal attitudes and increasing awareness of one's own communication patterns so as not to offend someone from a different cultural background are hallmarks of cultural sensitivity. When one increases cultural sensitivity, it is with the expectation that this will facilitate cultural competence. The characteristics of cultural competence as described by Purnell and Paulanka have implications for the nursing workforce.[34] Figure 23-6 outlines strategies for promoting cultural competency.

Practicing cultural competence is essential in promoting a unified work environment given the diversity of our workforce and patient population. A U.S. census report is compiled every 10 years. The 2000 U.S. Census indicates the following population statistics[35]:

- 75.1% Whites
- 12.5% Hispanic/Latino
- 12.3% Black/African-American
- 0.9% Native American or Alaskan Native
- 3.6% Asian
- 0.1% Native Hawaiian or other Pacific Islanders
- 5.5% some other race
- 2.4% two or more races

| FIGURE 23-6 | STRATEGIES FOR PROMOTING CULTURAL COMPETENCE |

1. Developing an awareness of one's own existence, sensations, thoughts, and environment without letting them have an undue influence on those from other backgrounds.

2. Demonstrating knowledge and understanding of the client's culture, health-related needs, and culturally specific meaning of health and illness.

3. Accepting and respecting cultural differences.

4. Not assuming that the healthcare provider's beliefs and values are the same as the client's.

5. Resisting judgmental attitudes such as "different is not as good."

6. Being open to cultural encounters.

7. Being comfortable with cultural encounters.

8. Adapting care (communication, decision making, conflict resolution) to be congruent with the client's culture.

9. Cultural competence is a conscious process and not necessarily linear.

Source: Author.

MAGNET HOSPITALS: IMPLICATIONS FOR A CULTURALLY SENSITIVE WORKFORCE

In the early 1980s, amidst a nationwide nurse staffing crisis, the American Academy of Nurses identified a number of hospitals that demonstrated a better-than-average ability to attract and retain professional nurses. They also studied factors associated with higher staff retention rates. The term *magnet* came into popular use to refer to hospitals that had these characteristics. A decade later, in 1994, the American Nurses Credentialing Center, a subsidiary of the American Nurses Association, developed a formal Magnet Recognition Program. In the last decade, important research has been undertaken to determine the correlation with magnet hospitals and nurse satisfaction. Nurse autonomy and effective nursing leadership are consistently reported as factors contributing to nurse satisfaction within magnet hospitals.[36] Nurses are given consistent recognition for their efforts; education is valued in staff nurses and they are appreciated for excellent patient care and professional contributions to the unit and organization.[37]

Magnet hospitals create a work environment where nurses are empowered to be autonomous in decision making and collaborative in multidisciplinary interactions. "A learning environment is created as nurses question old ways and find new solutions to old questions"[38] Empowered nurses in turn empower colleagues and staff to become team players in patient care delivery. Empowered nurses inspire patients to accept responsibility for individual health promotion and needs. Through literature searches for best practice, nurses willingly share evidence-based research for optimal patient care delivery interventions. Legitimate power is operationalized in planning, implementing, and evaluating patient care.[39]

Building Healthy Relationships

Building healthy personal and professional relationships takes hard, conscious, persistent work but is a necessary endeavor to create a positive, safe, professional work environment. Patience, tolerance, acceptance of others, and the ability to forgive are just a few of the traits one must possess if healthy, pro-

Evidence-Based Practice 23-1

Upenieks used an exploratory descriptive design to research perceived valuable leadership qualities among two magnet and two nonmagnet hospitals' nursing leaders. Magnet nurse leaders disclosed being honest, supportive, visible, accessible, effective communicator, advocate, and business savvy as their leadership attributes. Promoting an autonomous climate for nursing practice markedly contributed to nurse satisfaction on the job. "Most (86%) supported an autonomous climate and stated that nurses prefer to have control over their practice environments and accountability in decision making. They also professed supporting nurses in their self-governing decision making." Leadership qualities reported by nonmagnet leaders included self-assuredness, flexible, fair, visionary, accessible, knowledgeable, and credibility. Strong nurse–physician relationships exemplifying collaboration and sense of team were characteristics described as important among magnet and nonmagnet leaders.[40]

Organizational infrastructures necessary to support a successful, professional climate included

- Avenues for professional development through clinical ladders, continuing education, or higher education
- Autonomous work environment exemplifying participatory management style
- Adequate professional nursing staff
- Monetary compensation and rewards for nursing workforce
- Adaptive, creative, flexible scheduling
- On campus, extended child care services if 12-hour shift work continues.[41]

ductive interpersonal relationships are to be achieved. However, to develop healthy relationships with another, one must first have a good relationship with himself or herself. This concept translates to the ability to fail successfully, set personal and professional goals, appreciate oneself and others, and, among all else, be passionate about work undertaken.

Essential human relations skills include tact, diplomacy, understanding, honesty, objectivity, consideration, and motivation. Internalizing these character traits where they become part of who you are can improve the quality of your relationships with your peers, members of the healthcare team to whom you delegate and physicians. Develop self-confidence, self-control, and integrity. Do you communicate what you mean to say? Does what is on the outside match what is on the inside?

In the often chaotic, fast-paced, stressful healthcare environment, it can become easy to lose the human touch of kindness and civility. Basic behaviors such as offering praise and positive reinforcement should replace criticism and sarcasm. Challenge yourself not to react to harsh words or criticism from another; rather take a deep breath, regroup, and respond to the individual in a rational, even-toned voice. Challenge yourself to recognize that often those who appear the most "unlovable" are the ones who need love and attention the most. This applies to the unruly, difficult patient who is overly demanding as well as the nursing assistant who defies a simple delegated task.

Pay attention to the clues that are subtly and not so subtly transmitted from those that are in need. Any problem is best approached with straightforward, objective language. Describe the problem as you see it in a neutral tone of voice, attacking the problem, not the person. For example, say you delegated a task to a nursing assistant who did not perform a task as you instructed and is sitting at the nurses' station reading a magazine. An appropriate reaction might be, "Miss T, for the patient in room 111 to receive the best care . . . it is important for him to be ambulated 3 times a day as the physician ordered and I need for you to complete this now." Follow this with a simple "thank you." Of course, in an ideal healthcare world, all interactions would be this simple and flow this smoothly. Yet the reality is nursing functions in a complex, technology-driven environment, taking care of high acuity patients with a diverse, culturally blended workforce. Add to the mix family members who have access to any medical condition, procedure, or intervention through the Internet and are scrutinizing nurse actions and interactions.

Nurses can improve communication and relationships by a willingness to be open to the opinions, views, and perspectives of others. Baby Boomers must be willing to embrace evidence-based best practice research Generation X or Y nurses bring to the healthcare environment. The younger nurse must be respectful of the seasoned nurse and embrace their wisdom from decades of clinical experience. When one is willing to entertain views different from his or her own, a window of opportunity is opened for growth, shared decision making, and insight.[42]

SUMMARY

The evidence is clear: Managing a generational and culturally diverse workforce in the midst of a critical nursing shortage poses a daunting challenge for nursing administration and human resource professionals. Aggressive recruitment strategies are necessary to offset the mass of retiring nurses in the coming years. Creative retention initiatives must be instituted to improve nurse satisfaction and reduce the high cost of turnover. Transformational leadership style has merit for guiding the nursing workforce through difficult times within the healthcare industry. A nurse leader who is inspiring, visionary, creative, and in touch with the needs of the workforce is more likely to engender commitment to the work unit and organization. Generational differences among the nurse workforce are a consideration when planning and implementing retention strategies to increase job satisfaction, which ultimately positively impacts patient care outcomes.

APPLICATION EXERCISES

Exercise 23-1

F. T. has assumed a newly formed clinical nurse specialist position in a large academic acute care hospital. Primary responsibilities of the role include updating the current recruitment program for nursing, creating innovative strategies to increase retention and decrease turnover, and developing an on-boarding program for new registered nurse graduates.

Help F. T. devise a working plan for proceeding with the initiatives to be undertaken. Include human and fiscal resources needed for the successful completion of this role. Questions to consider:

1. What are the culturally sensitive issues that need to be addressed?
2. How would cultural competency testing be approached?
3. What information does F. T. need to begin?
4. What data, if any, should be collected?
5. What short-term challenge is F. T. likely to face as he begins to develop a plan of action?
6. What leadership skills can F. T. use to facilitate a successful outcome?

Exercise 23-2

Joan W., a nurse manager for 3 years, is considering returning to a staff RN position due to the stress associated with running a busy medical surgical unit. Turnover and work load rates are high with unprecedented nurse-patient ratios. The staffs' unhappiness is evident and has even been brought to her attention by patient family members. Joan's management style is proving ineffective, and she has little guidance from nursing administration as to how to change the situation. What steps could nursing administration take to be supportive of Joan, possibly reversing her decision to leave the nurse manager role?

Notes

1. Jones, C. B., & Gates, M. (2007, Sept.). The costs and benefits of nurse turnover: A business case for nurse retention. *The Online Journal of Issues in Nursing* [serial online], *3*.

2. Peterson, C. A. (2001). Nursing shortage: Not a simple problem—no easy answers. *Online Journal of Issues in Nursing, 6*, 1–14.

3. Jones & Gates, 2007; Aiken, L. H., Clarke, S. P., Sloane, D. M., Sochalski, J., & Silber, J. H. (2002). Hospital nurse staffing and patient mortality, nurse burnout, and job dissatisfaction. *Journal of the American Medical Association, 288*, 1987–1993; Shaver, K. H., & Lacey, L. M. (2003). Job and career satisfaction among staff nurses. *Journal of Nursing Administration, 33*, 166–172; Cline, D., Reilly, C., & Moore, J. F. (2003, Oct.). What's behind RN turnover? *Nursing Management* [serial online], *10*.

4. Shaver & Lacey, 2003.

5. Jones & Gates, 2007.

6. Strachota, E., Normandin, P., O'Brien, N., Clary, M., & Krukow, B. (2003). Reasons registered nurses leave or change employment status. *Journal of Nursing Administration, 33*, 111–117; Upenieks, V. (2003a). Nurse leaders' perception of what compromises successful leadership in today's acute inpatient environment. *Nursing Administration Quarterly, 27*, 140–153.

7. Atencio, B. L., Cohen, J., & Gorenberg, B. (2003). Nurse retention: Is it worth it? *Nursing Economic$, 21*, 262–268, 299.

8. Ibid., p. 266.

9. Schuler, R. S., & Jackson, S. E. (2006). *Strategic human resource management.* Malden, MA: Blackwell Publishing.

10. Roy, C. (1991). Senses. In C. Roy & H. Andrews (Eds.), *The Roy adaptation model: The definitive statement* (pp. 165–189). Norwalk, CT: Appleton & Lange. Retrieved March 18, 2008, from http://www.bc.edu/schools/son/faculty/theorist/Roy_Adaptation_Model.html

11. U.S. Census Bureau. (1999). *Statistical abstracts of the United States* (p. 132). Department of Records, Washington, DC.

12. Studer, Q. (2003). *Hardwiring excellence.* Gulf Breeze, FL: Fire Starter Publishing.

13. Klehe, U.-C., & Latham, G. (2006). What would you do—Really or ideally? Constructs underlying the behavior description interview and the situational interview in predicting typical versus maximum performance. *Human Performance, 19*, 357–382, 2006; Frase-Blunt, M. (2001). Peering into an interview. *HR Magazine, 46*, 71–77.

14. Ibid., Studer, 2003.

15. Equal Employee Opportunity Commission. Retrieved on March 18, 2008, from http://www.eeoc.gov/policy

16. Boyle, D. K. (1999). Managers' leadership and critical care nurses' intent to stay. *American Journal of Critical Care, 8*, 361–371.

17. Shabbrook, P., & Fenton, K. (2002). A strategy for improving nurse retention and recruitment levels. *Professional Nurse, 17*, 534–536.

18. Fletcher, C. E. (2001). Hospital RN's job satisfactions and dissatisfactions. *Journal of Nursing Administration, 31*, 324–331.

19. McGuire, E., & Kennerly, S. M. (2006). Nurse managers as transformational and transactional leaders. *Nursing Economic$, 24*, 179–185.

20. Adams, A., & Bond, S. (2003). Focus on staff stability: Its role in enhancing ward nursing practice. *Journal of Nursing Management, 11*, 284–286.

21. Scott, D. E. (2007). The generations at work: A conversation with Phyllis Kritek. *American Nurse, 39*, 7.

22. Shader, K., Broome, M. E., Broome, C. D., West, M. E., & Nash, M. (2001). Factors influencing satisfaction and anticipated turnover for nurses in an academic medical center. *Journal of Nursing Administration, 31*, 210–216.

23. Kupperschmidt, B. R. (1998). Understanding Generation X employees. *Journal of Nursing Administration, 28*, 36–43; Strachota et al., 2003; Shader et al., 2001.

24. Kleinman, C. S. (2004). Leadership and retention: Research needed. *Journal of Nursing Administration, 34*, 111–113.

25. Letvak, S. (2002). Retaining the older nurse. *Journal of Nursing Administration, 32,* 387–392.

26. U.S. General Accounting Office. (2001). *Report to the Chairman, Subcommittee on Health, Committee on Ways and Means, House of Representatives: Nursing workforce, emerging nurse shortages due to multiple factors.* Washington, DC: U.S. General Accounting Office. Nurse Reinvestment Act, 2002.

27. Cyr, J. P. (2005). Retaining older hospital nurses and delaying their retirement. *Journal of Nursing Administration, 35,* 563–567.

28. Wieck, K. I., Prydun, M., & Walsh, T. (2002). What the emerging workforce wants in its leaders. *Journal of Nursing Scholarship, 34,* 283–288.

29. Clark, C. C. (2009). In press. *Creative nursing leadership & management.* Sudbury, MA: Jones and Bartlett Publishers.

30. Jeffreys, M. R. (2005). Clinical nurse specialists as cultural brokers, change agents and partners in meeting the needs of culturally diverse populations. *Journal of Multicultural Nursing and Health, 11,* 41–48.

31. Purnell, L. D., & Paulanka, B. J. (2005). *Guide to culturally competent health care.* Philadelphia: F.A. Davis.

32. American Organization of Nurse Executives. (2007). *AONE position statement and guiding principles for diversity in health care organizations: The American Organization of Nurse Executives nurse recruitment & retention study executive summary.* Scottsdale, Arizona: HSM Group.

33. Ibid., Jeffreys, 2005.

34. Ibid., Purnell & Paulanka, 2005.

35. Ibid.

36. U.S. Census Bureau. (2000). Retrieved March 13, 2008, from http://www.census.gov

37. Upenieks, V. (2003b). Recruitment and retention strategies: A magnet hospital prevention model. *Nursing Economic$, 21,* 7–13, 23.

38. Aiken, L., Havens, D., & Sloane, D. (2000). The magnet nursing services recognition program: A comparison of two groups of magnet hospitals. *American Journal of Nursing, 100,* 26–35; Upenieks, V. (2003c). The interrelationship of organizational characteristics of magnet hospitals, nursing leadership and nursing job satisfaction. *Health Care Manager, 22,* 83–98.

39. Thyer, G. L. (2003). Dare to be different: Transformational leadership may hold the key to reducing the nursing shortage. *Journal of Nursing Management, 11,* 73–79.

40. Porter-O'Grady, T. (2001). Is shared governance still relevant? *Journal of Nursing Administration, 31,* 468–473.

41. Ibid., Upenieks, 2003c, p. 10.

42. Upenieks, V. V. (2003d). What constitutes effective leadership? *Journal of Nursing Administration, 33,* 456–467.

References

Bass, B. M., & Avolio, B. J. (1990). *Developing potential across a full range of leadership: Cases on transactional and transformational leadership.* Mahwah, NJ: Lawrence Erlbaum Association.

Beatty, P. T., & Burroughs, L. (1999). Preparing for an aging workforce: The role of higher education. *Educational Gerontology, 25,* 595–611.

Buchan, J. (1999). Still attractive after all these years? Magnet hospitals in a changing health care environment. *Journal of Advanced Nursing, 30,* 100–108.

Force, M. V. (2005). The relationship between effective nurse managers and nursing retention. *Journal of Nursing Administration, 35,* 336–341.

Hart, K. A. (2006). *The aging workforce: Implications for recruiters.* Retrieved on July 21, 2008 from http://www.hodes.com/publications/talentmatters/aarchives/hcmatters_julo6.asp

Hayhurst, A., Saylor, C., & Stuenkel, D. (2005). Work environmental factors and retention of nurses. *Journal of Nursing Care Quality, 20,* 283–288.

Joint Commission on Accreditation of Healthcare Organizations. *Health care at the crossroads: Strategies for addressing the evolving nursing crisis.* Retrieved March 4, 2008, from http://www.jointcommission.org/NR/rdonlyres/5C138711-ED76-4D6F-909F-B06E0309F36D/0/health_care_at_the_crossroads.pdf

Kennerly, S. (2000). Perceived worker autonomy: The foundation for shared governance. *Journal of Nursing Administration, 30,* 611–617.

Kleinman, C. (2004). The relationship between managerial leadership behaviors and staff nurse retention. *Hospital Topics: Research and Perspectives on Healthcare, 82,* 2–9.

Laschinger, H. K. S., Shamian, J., & Thomson, D. (2001). Impact of magnet hospital characteristics on nurses' perceptions of trust, burnout, quality of care, and work satisfaction. *Nursing Economic$, 19,* 209–219.

Leach, L. S. (2005). Nurse executive transformational leadership and organizational commitment. *Journal of Nursing Administration, 35,* 228–237.

Lundgren, S. M., Nordholm, L., & Segesten, K. (2005). Job satisfaction in relation to change to all-RN staffing. *Journal of Nursing Management, 13,* 322–328.

Makinen, A., Kivimaki, M., Elovainio, M., Virtanen, M., & Bond, S. (2003). Organization of nursing care as a determinant of job satisfaction among hospital nurses. *Journal of Nursing Management, 11,* 299–306.

Mills, A. C., & Blaesing, S. L. (2000). A lesson from the last nursing shortage. *Journal of Nursing Administration, 30,* 309–315.

Newhouse, R. P., Hoffman, J. J., & Hairston, D. P. (2007). Evaluating an innovative program to improve new nurse graduate socialization into the acute healthcare setting. *Nursing Administration Quarterly, 31,* 50–60.

Ribelin, P. (2003, Aug.). Retention reflects leadership style. *Nursing Management* [serial online], 8.

Colakogl, S., Lepak, D. P., & Hong, Y. (2006). The new world of work and organizations. *Human Resource Management Review, 16,* 209–218.

Note: Page numbers followed by f denote figures.

A

AACN (American Association of Colleges of Nursing), 23, 465, 613, 614
Academic Center for Evidenced-Based Practice, 9
Accelerating Quality Improvement in Health Care: Strategies to Speed the Diffusion of Evidenced-Based Innovations, 9
Accountability
  autonomy and, 208–209
  shared governance and account-abilities
    of management, 206–207
    of practice, 206
    for quality, 206
ACE star model of evidenced-based practice, 123
Achievement orientation, 57f, 58
Ackoff, R.L., 304–305
ADA (Americans with Disabilities Act), 461f, 607, 671
Adams, A., 672
Adams, R., 353
Adaptability, 57f, 58
ADN (associate degree in nursing), 239
Advance directives, 82–83
  durable power of attorney for health care, 83
  living will, 83
Advanced practice nurses (APNs), 465, 652
Age Discrimination in Employment Act (1967), 461f, 671
Agency for Healthcare Research and Quality (AHRQ), 11
  definition of medical errors, 473
  nurse turnover and quality care, 271–272
  patient safety indicators, 11–12
  quality indicators, 11
  website, 17
Agor, W.H., 145, 146
AIDA mnemonic, 159
Aiken, L.H., 271, 657
Albrecht, K., 108–109
Alderfer, Clayton, 414
Alward, R.R., 353
American Academy of Nursing, 350, 516, 644
American Association of Colleges of Nursing (AACN), 23, 465, 613, 614
American Association of Critical Care Nurses, 7
  Healthy Work Environments, 113–114

Standards for Establishing and Sustaining Healthy Environments, 8
  Synergy Model of Care, 654
  website, 17
American College of Surgeons, 463–464
American Health Information Management Association, 412
American Hospital Association (AHA), 17, 459
American Nurses Association (ANA)
  Bill of Rights for the Registered Nurse, 271f, 657
  Code of Ethics for Nurses with Interpretive Statements, 458, 479, 657
  components of professional nursing practice environ-ment, 22–23
  description of a standard, 474–475
  Guidelines for Review of Nursing Care at the Local Level, 542
  mandated nurse-staffing ratios, 354
  nurse's control over their work environment, 93
  Nursing Scope and Standards of Practice, 550
  Nursing's Social Policy Statement, 458
  Principles of Nurse Staffing, 653
  research and professional sup-port, 63
  Scope and Standards for Nurse Administrators, 21–23, 25, 25f, 75–76, 209, 336, 458, 503, 516, 554, 643, 645, 654, 657
  Standards of Clinical Nursing Practice, 336, 503, 554
  support for database develop-ment, 10
American Nurses Association Political Action Committee, 459
American Nurses Credentialing Center Magnet Recognition Program, 21, 25, 25f, 104, 147, 237, 350, 516, 643, 644, 676
American Organization of Nurse Executives (AONE), 7, 23
  cultural competence, 674
  change management compe-tencies, 103
  evidenced-based practices, 280

factors to improve workplace initiatives, 8
future of client care, 593
Healthy Work Environments, 170–171
leadership, 407, 595
mandated ratios, 360
Nurse Executive Competencies, 184–185, 186f, 187f, 481–482
Nurse Leader-Patient Safety Competency Model, 226–227f, 227f, 228f
Political Action Committee, 459
research and professional sup-port, 62–63
Role of the Nurse Executive in Patient Safety: Guiding Principles Toolkit, 226
Transforming Care at the Bedside (TCAB), 8
American Society for Testing and Materials, 412
Americans with Disabilities Act (ADA) (1990), 461f, 607, 671
ANA. *See* American Nurses Association (ANA)
ANCM (Attending Nursing Caring Model), 35
Andragogy and HRD, 276–277
Anticipatory principle, 106
AONE. *See* American Organization of Nurse Executives (AONE)
APNs (advanced practice nurses), 465
Appreciative inquiry, 106
Argumentation and Debate, 109
Arousal-activation theory, 414
Artifacts, of organizational culture, 223, 223f
Assault and battery, 478–479
Assessment center process, recruit-ment, 266, 268
Associate degree in nursing (ADN), 239
Assumptions, of organizational cul-ture, 223, 223f
Attending Nursing Caring Model (ANCM), 35
Audits
  evaluation, 536–537
  Orem's nine categories of self-care requirements, 536
  outcome criteria/variables, 537
  Phaneuf audit, 536
  Quality Patient-Care Scale, 536
Auger, J.A., 352, 353
Authenticity, 109

Autonomy, 77, 79–80, 200–202
  and accountability, 208–209
    of management, 206–207
    of practice, 206
    for quality, 206
  autonomous practice, 657–659
    consultations and resources, 659
    evidenced-based practice, 658
    tools needed for clinical competence, 658f
  in human resource development, 276
Aydelotte, M.K., 336, 337

B
Baby Boomer Nurses
  embracing evidenced-based best
    practice research, 678
  retention of, 674, 674f
Bachelor of science in nursing (BSN)
    degree, 239
Bailey, M., 172
Baker, H.K., 156
Balancing measures, 500
Baldwin, J., 517
Barker, A.M., 628
Barnard, CI, 168
Batalden, P.B., 533, 533f, 535
Beckham, J.D., 300
Beckwith Institute for Innovation in
    Patient Care, 648
Behavioral goals and change, 65–66, 66f
Behavior-Anchored Rating Scales
    (BARS), 571
Behaviors, organizational culture, 223,
    223f
Benchmarking
  quality management, 512
  and six sigma strategies, 412, 413f
  standards of care, 511
  standards of practice, 511–512
  structure standards, 511
Beneficence, 77, 80
Benne, K.D., 218–219f
Benner, P., 579
Bennis, W., 627, 628
Bentham, Jeremy, 76
Beth Israel Hospital, Boston, model of
    nursing care, 64f
Beyers, M., 124, 310
Bill of Rights for the Registered Nurse,
    271f, 657
Birnbaum, D., 570
Blake and Mouton's Managerial Grid,
    624–625, 627
Blanchard, K.H., 626
Bond, M., 127
Bond, S., 672
Borman, J.S., 632
Bosses, best and worse, 61–62, 61–62f
Boulding, K.E., 30
Boulet, J.R., 600
Bower, K., 39–40, 41
Boyle, D.K., 672
Brainstorming, 537–538
Bright Corridor, 561
Brown, R.V, 140
Brown-Stewart, P., 266
Brunton, G., 466
BSN (bachelor of science in nursing), 239

Budgeting principles
  approaches
    break-even analysis, 380f
    fixed budgeting, 380
    flexible budgeting, 380
    program budgeting, 380
    zero-based budgeting, 379
  budget stages, 372f
    cost factors, 373, 374f
    execution stage, 373
    expense budgeting, 373–374
    expenses, 373
    formulation stage, 372–373
    review and enactment stage, 373
  capital budget, 388–391, 389f
    capital equipment, 390–391, 390f
    optimal capital allocation, 391
    strategic capital-building budget,
      390–391
  controlling process
    monitoring the budget
      accounting system report, 393,
        394f, 395f, 396f
      objectives, 393
      rollover funds, 394
    overview, 392
  cost centers, managing
    cost center reports, 373
    overview, 371
    relationship of budget and objec-
      tives, 371–372
  definitions
    average daily census, 379
    budget, 377
    caregiver, 379
    case mix, 379
    fiscal year, 379
    hours of care, 379
    patient days, 378–379, 378f
    revenue, 377
    revenue budgeting, 377–378
    year to date, 379
  evidenced-based practice, 401
  introduction, 369
  managed care
    health care cost coalitions,
      400–401
    health maintenance organizations,
      399–400
    health promotion and wellness
      programs, 401
    hospital physician organizations,
      401
    overview, 398
    preferred provider organizations,
      400
    provider-sponsored organizations,
      401
    prudent buyer systems, 401
  management implications, 401
  motivational aspects
    cutting the budget, 396–397
    legitimate budget activities, 397
  operating or cash budget
    described, 381
    developing, 382–383
      adjustment explanation, 383f
      budget worksheet, 382f
    negative cash flow, 381–382

performance budgeting, 391–392
  personnel budget, 383–387
    calculating, 384–385, 385f
    data collection, 386
    decisions to be made, 386
    new position requisition, 385f
    nonproductive full-time equiva-
      lents (FTEs), 386–387
    patient-acuity rating system
      budget, 383–384, 384f
    strategies to reduce overages, 386
  procedures, 370–371
  product evaluation
    checklist, 388f
    committee, 387–388
  purpose of the nursing budget, 370
  reimbursement
    based on clinical performance, 398
    U.S. health care system, 398, 399f
  revenues, 392
  summary, 401–402
  supplies and equipment, 387
  types of budgets
    cost-benefit analysis, 381
    cost-to-charge ratios, 381
    operating, 381
  types of expenses/costs
    activity-based costing, 377
    chart of accounts, 376
    cost accounting, 375
    cost of nursing care, 376–377
    direct and indirect, 375
    financial accountability, 376
    fixed, 374
    inventory and cost transfer, 376
    service units, 375
    sunk, 375
    unit of service, 375–376
    variable, 374–375
Bulmer, J.M., 597
Bureaucracy, 188f
  Hall's study of ten organizations,
    189–190
  professionalism and bureaucracy,
    189f
  strong points of bureaucratic organi-
    zations, 188
  term, 188
Burns, James, 647
Business Case for Workforce Stability,
    657
Butler, Samuel, 368

C
California Department of Nurse Execu-
    tives, mandated ratios, 360
Care delivery, managing the process of
    benchmarking and six sigma strate-
      gies, 412, 413f
  checklist for assessing job satisfac-
    tion, 425–426
  delegating, 409
  directing and nursing administration
    activities related to, 408f
    effective directing, 408–409
    major elements of, 407
    properties of a positive work envi-
      ronment, 408
    qualities of a good leader, 408

evidenced-based practice, 421
future goals worksheet, 423f
goal evaluation checklist, 423f
introduction, 407
management by objectives (MBO)
  description of, 409–410
  process
    discussing the goals: first meet-
      ing, 410
    learning the process, 410
    management by results,
      411–412
    organizational development,
      412
    problems with, 411–412
    taking action, 411
motivation, enhancing
  building self-esteem, 420
  career planning, 419
  effective communication, 419
  encouraging self-actualization,
    420–421
  endorsing teamwork, 420
  other activities to stimulate moti-
    vation, 421
motivation theories
  content theories, 413–414
  described, 412–413
  Maslow, 413–414
    hierarchy of needs, 416–417
    holistic-dynamic theory,
      415–416
    prerequisites to satisfying needs,
      416
  process theories
    arousal-activation theory, 414
    equity theory, 415
    expectancy-valence theory, 415
    intention-goal theory, 415
  questions to consider, 413
  usefulness to nurse managers, 417
nurse as knowledge worker, 417–418
science of human behavior: Theory
  X and Theory Y, 418–419
summary, 421–422
Career planning, 419
  career ladders and career develop-
    ment programs, 273–274,
    274–275f
  job variety and job sharing, 275
CareMaps, 38–39
Carondelet/St. Mary's Hospital and
  Health Center model, 39
CASH system. See Complex adaptive
  systems (CAS)
CASH system (PCS), 352
Catherine McAuley Health System, 238
Cavanaugh, D.E., 302
Center for Case Management's model,
  38–39
Center for Health Design, website, 17
Center for Medical Home
  Improvement, website, 17
Centers for Medicare & Medicaid
  Services, 464
  Cost Report, 375
  hospital select indicator rates, 534
  legal requirements, 336
Central tendency, 537, 572

Certification, 26, 465, 466
Certification and Regulation of
  Advanced Practice Nurses,
  465
Chain of command, 188f
Change. See also Creativity and innovation; Critical thinking
  adding the evidence
    ACE star model of evidenced-
      based practice, 123
    evidenced-based decision making,
      122–123
    planning, 123–124
    windows of opportunity, 124
  change agent
    examples of the application of
      change theory, 120
    the nurse as, 119–120
  change theory
    comparison of theories, 117f
    Havelock's theory, 116
    Lewin's theory, 115
    Lippitt's theory, 116–117
    new management theory
      incremental change, 118
      leadership skills for change, 119
      seven steps to being the best, 119
      steps in the process, 119
      transformational change,
        118–119, 120
    Reddin's theory, 114
    Roger's theory of change, 115–116
    Spradley's model, 117–118
    tipping point, 118
  collection and development of data,
    122
  evidenced-based practice, 121, 128
  introduction, 103–104
  need for change, 113–114
    changing values of nurses, 113
    framework for, 113–114
    need for nurses' continuing educa-
      tion, 113
    nurse managers, 113
    reasons for designing orderly
      change, 112–113
    structural change, 113
  resistance to, 120–121
  strategies to overcome obstacles to
    change, 122
  summary, 128–129
  training and education
    anticipating potential failures,
      126–127
    communications, 125–126
    critical thinking, 125
    implementation science, 127
    organizational environment, 126
    rewards, 125
    using groups as change agents, 125
  values and beliefs, 121–122
Change agent role, 595
Change catalyst, 57f, 59
Charismatic leaders, 623
Child Labor Provisions, 461f
Churchill, Winston, 2, 608
CINAHL (Cumulative Index to
  Nursing and Allied Health
  Literature), 602

Civil law. See Legal issues
Civil Rights Act (1964), 459–460
  termination of employees, 278
  Title VII, 670–671
Civil Rights Act (1991), 671
Clancy, C., 647
Clancy, T.R., 327
Clarity, 109
Clarke, S.P., 366
Clifford, Joyce, 64f
Clinical decision-making
  cost-benefit analysis, 141f, 144
  decision-tree model, 140
  descriptive model, 140
  normative model, 139–140
  the patient's decision-making
    activity, 139
  prescriptive decision theory, 144
  steps in the decision-making process,
    141f
    1. establish goals and objectives,
      142
    2. identify the problem, 142
    3. develop plausible solutions,
      142–143
    4. evaluate all alternatives, 143
    5. selecting the problem, 143
    6. implement solution, 143
    7. follow-up, 143
  strategic model, 141–142
Clinical microsystems, 498–499, 499f
Clinical nurse
  the generalized clinical nurse (GCN),
    562–563f
  leader role, 614
  performance standards for, 554,
    555–556f
Clinical practice management
  case management models
    Carondelet/St. Mary's Hospital
      and Health Center model, 39
    Center for Case Management's
      model, 38–39
    factors related to case management
      case managers at Hennepin County
        Medical Center, 39–40
      clinical and management skills of
        nurses, 40
      contracts for clients' services, 40
      critical path technique, 40
      matrix management model, 40
      outcome-based nursing practice,
        41
      reasons for implementing case
        management, 41
    nursing theory in professional
      practice
      Johnson's theory, 37
      Newman's theory, 37
      Orem's theory of self-care, 36
      Peplau's theory, 37–38
      Roy's theory, 36–37
      Watson's Theory of Caring, 35
    overview, 35
Cliska, D., 466
"Clockware," 5
CNO (chief nursing officer), 645, 652
Coaching
  job descriptions, 565–566

Coaching—*(continued)*
transformational
impediments to effective coaching, 635f
leader as coach, 634
model for, 635f
COBRA (Consolidated Omnibus Budget Reconciliation Acts), 462f
Cochrane database, 602
Cochrane Handbook, 123
Codman, Ernest, 463
Coefficient of determination *(r²),* 537
Coercion, 110
Cohen, Michael Henry, 549–550
Cohesion or norming phase, groups, 220
Coleman, D., 611
Collaborative decision-making. *See also* Communication; Communication media
clinical decision-making
cost-benefit analysis, 141f, 144
decision-tree model, 140
descriptive model, 140
normative model, 139–140
the patient's decision-making activity, 139
prescriptive decision theory, 144
steps in the decision-making process, 141f
1. establish goals and objectives, 142
2. identify the problem, 142
3. develop plausible solutions, 142–143
4. evaluate all alternatives, 143
5. selecting the problem, 143
6. implement solution, 143
7. follow-up, 143
strategic model, 141–142
consensus building, 145
definition, 138
evidenced-based practice, 148, 172
the future
managers, 171–172
organizational best practices
employee attitude surveys, 171
a good communication system, 171
six critical factors, 170–171
people as capital, 170
technology, 172
improving decision making, 145
introduction, 137–138
issues in decision making, 144–145
organizational *vs.* personal decisions
decision analysis, 147
professional autonomy, definitions of, 147–148
shared governance, 148
pitfalls in making good decisions, 138–139
problem-solving process
shared problem solving, 149–150
steps in the process, 149
role of intuition
critical thinking and, 145
intuitive nurses, 145–146
left-brain activities, 145

Myers-Brigg type indicator, 145
where intuitive ability functions best, 145
summary, 173
Collaborative governance, 207
Collaborative patient management model, 236
Collective bargaining
agreements, 85
arbitration, 90
defined, 85–86
grievance procedures, 88, 89f
issues: ethical considerations, 86–87
job security and, 94
mediation, 90
process, 87–88
purpose of today, 84–85
supervisory influence, 90–91
unionization
advantages of, 91–92
disadvantages of, 92–93
strikes, 93
vulnerability, 93–94
Columbia/HCA Healthcare Corp. v. Eighth Judicial District Court, 488
Combination of methods, 110
Commission for Administration Services in Hospitals (CASH), 352
Commitment, nurse executive role and, 199–200
Committee on Reviewing Evidence to Identify Highly Effective Clinical Services, 516–517
Committees
effectiveness of, improving, 216–217f
ethics committees
ANA Committee on Ethics guidelines, 80–81
establishing ethics committees, 82
responsibilities, 79
evaluating meeting effectiveness, 217f
functional roles of group members, 218–219f
organization of, 215–216, 215f
purposes of, 215
standards for evaluating, 214f
types of, 214
Communication. *See also* Collaborative decision-making; Communication media
climate for, 151
and conflict management, 156
cultural agendas, 151–152
difficult conversations, 155–156
direction, 154
effective, motivation and, 419
effective climate for, 152
elements of, 150–151
evidenced-based practice, 155
feedback
evidence on, 154
improved performance and, 155
influence on behavior and, 154
information, 154
introduction, 150
listening
causes of poor listening, 158–159

Crucial Conversations, 160–161
effective listening, 157–158
encouraging people to listen, 159–160
good listeners, 160
mnemonics, 159–161
power listening tools "AMPP," 160–161
providing information, 160
techniques to improve, 159
negotiation
introduction, 156–157
principles of, 157
steps in the process, 157
open-door policy, 153
organizational structure and, 204–205
as perception, 153–154
three basic principles of, 151
Communication media
electronic, 169
interviews, 165
managers, 161–162
meetings, 161
oral communication
face-to-face communication, advantages of, 163
presenting an effective speech, 163–164
techniques for effective public speaking, 164–165f
organizational publications, 168–169
questions, 162–163
written communication
material of, 165–166
rules to follow when writing, 166, 167f
written reports, 166, 168
Communications software, 440
Community-based nursing centers model, 235
Compensation programs, 576–578, 576f
Competence, 77
Complementary personnel, 342
Complex adaptive systems (CAS), 4
"clockware," 5
how complexity science may improve organizations, 6–7
macro-, micro-, and mesosystems as CAS, 6
natural and human systems properties, 6
paradoxical questions, 5–6
placing your group at the edge of chaos, 5–6
principles, 5
"swarmware," 5
working in CAS, 7
Computer technology terms, 449–451
Concepts and theories, professional practice. *See also* Management, historical perspective; Nursing management
evidenced-based practice, 42
introduction
core competencies, educating health care professionals, 20–21

IOM reports, 19–20
needed changes to the health care system, 20
the nurse administrator
certification, 26
described, 23
level of nursing administrative practice
nurse executive, 23–24
nurse manager, 24
standards of practice, 24–25
standards of professional performance, 25
magnet recognition program and scope and standards, 25, 25f
qualifications of, 25–26
patient outcomes in human relations management, 41
professional practice model of nursing
differentiated nursing practice, 22
interdisciplinary collaboration
ANA, components of professional nursing practice environment, 22–23
characteristics of, 22
Pew Health Professions Commission study, 22
magnet recognition programs, 21
preceptorships and residencies, 21
scope and standards for nurse administrators, 23
summary, 41–42
theory, concepts, and principles
critical theory *versus* critical thinking, 29–30
general systems theory, 30–32
the animal level, 31–32
an open system or self-maintaining structure: the cell, 30–31, 31f
the clockwork, 30
the framework, 30
the genetic-societal level, 31
the human level, 32
the level of social organization, 32
summary, 32
the thermostat, 30
transcendental systems, 32
overview, 29
Confidentiality, 77
Conflict management, 57f, 59–60, 60f, 65, 200
in a diverse workforce
active listening, 282
antecedent sources of, 281
assessing conflict, 280–281
characteristics of conflict, 280
conflict: beliefs, values, and goals, 281–282
introduction, 280
resolving conflict through negotiation, 282–283
results of conflict resolution, 283
stress and conflict, 281
through effective communication, 282
Conflict of storming phase, groups, 220

Congressional model of shared governance, 206
Conlin, G., 604
Connor, R.J., 350–351
Consent, 77
Consent to Medical Treatment Act (Texas), 83
Consolidated Omnibus Budget Reconciliation Acts (COBRA), 462f
Constructive principle, 106
Context
complex adaptive systems (CAS), 4
establishing informal groups, 4–5
ordinary/extraordinary management, 4
in organizational structure, 192–193, 193f
1980s approach to strategy, 4
Contingency theory, 193
Control charts, 539, 540f
Cooper, D.C., 597
Cooperrider, David, 106
Coordination, 188f
Corporate liability
board of directors, 480
corporate negligence, 480
credentialing liability, 480–481
respondeat superior, 480–481
Correlation, 537
Cost-benefit analysis, 141f, 144
Councilor model of shared governance, 206
Counseling, job description
directive approach, 567
elective approach, 567
importance of, 567
interviews, 566
nondirective approach, 567
Creative Health Care Management, 240
Creativity and innovation. *See also* Change; Critical thinking
creative problem solving theories
Drucker, 107
Godfrey, 106
Lattimer and Winitsky, 106
creativity
establishing a climate for, 104–105
metamanagement
definition of, 105
principles of appreciative inquiry, 106
task-related actions for nurses, 105–106
creativity in the workplace
creative individuals, 107
develop a model of shared governance, 108
hire creative people, 108
managing and nourishing creativity, 107–108
definition of, 104
managing creativity, 127–128
social intelligence
Albrecht's model, 108–109
nourishing behavior, 108
principles of perception related to change, 108
toxic behavior, 108
summary, 129

Credentialing liability, 480–481
Credentialing of individual practitioners
advanced practice registered nurses, 465
certification, 466
evidenced-based practice, 466
licensure defined, 464
National Council of State Boards of Nursing (NCSBN), 464, 465
nursing licensure/credentialing NCLEX-RN, 465
Nurse Practice Acts, 464–465
Critical path technique, 40
Critical thinking. *See also* Change; Creativity and innovation
activities and strategies for promoting, 111f
applications of, 110–111
and clinical reasoning, 110
complex adaptive systems, 110–111
concept analysis, 110
critical theory *vs.* critical thinking, 29–30
the ideal critical thinker, 109
methods of, 109–110
term, 109
uses for, 109
Crockett, C., 600, 601
Croke, E.M., 473
Crosby, Philip B., 527–530
four absolutes of quality, 528f
Quality Management Maturity Grid, 529f
Crosby, Phillip, 288
Crossing the Quality Chasm (2001), 7, 9, 114, 224, 225f
Cross-training model, staffing and scheduling, 348
Csikszentmihalyi, Mihaly, 592
Cultural competence, in human resource development, 279–280
Culture. *See* Organizational culture
Culture and climate, quality management, 530–531, 531f
Cummings, G.G., 636
Cumulative Index to Nursing and Allied Health Literature (CINAHL), 602
Curtin, Leah, 82
Curtin, L.L., 358
Curtis, B., 600, 601
Customary practice. *See* Standard of care
Customers, quality management, 530
Cutler, M.J., 633
Cyclic scheduling, 343f, 345

D
Darling, L.A.W., 277
Darling v. Charleston Community Hospital, 480
Data analysis, quality management
brainstorming, 537–538
control charts, 539, 540f
Delphi method, 538
fishbone cause-and-effect diagram, 541
histogram or bar chart, 541, 541f
nominal group technique, 538

Data analysis, quality management—
(continued)
Pareto diagram, 542, 542f
prioritization matrix, 538–539, 538f
process flowchart, 540, 540f
run chart of trend chart, 539, 539f
Data management in health care. *See
also* Information manage-
ment and technology
database management, 440–441, 441f
data cleansing, 433–434
data mining, 433
definition of data, 430
definition of information, 430–431
educating staff, 432–433
evidenced-based practice, 432
examples of data and information,
432f
"relational databases," 433
system prompts, 433
verification techniques, 433
Davies, Robert, 161
Davis, A.J., 79
Davis, D.L., 357
Davis, Gray, 354
Debate, 109
Decentralization, role of the nurse
executive and, 197, 198f
communication and decentralization, 205
decentralization with participatory
management, 203–204
Decentralized structure, 196–197, 197f,
198f
Decision making, staffing and
scheduling
evidenced-based practices, 361
mandated ratios, 360
Society for Health Systems approach,
360–361
Decision-making ability, 77
Decision-tree model, 140
Dee, V., 352, 353
Defamation, 478
del Bueno, D.J., 266
Delegating, 409
Delegation, 188f
Delphi method, 538
DeMarco, R., 604
Deming, W. Edwards, 524–527
application of Deming's theory,
525–526
Deming's 14 points, 525f
performance appraisals, 573
variation
causes, 526–527
concept, 526
Deming (Shewhart) APCD cycle,
526, 527f
Department of Health and Human
Services (DHHS), 459
Derdiarian, A.K., 46
Descriptive model, 140
Desktop publishing, 441–442, 442f
Developing others, 57f, 59
DHHS (Department of Health and
Human Services), 459
Differentiated nursing practice, 22,
239–240, 240f

Dillon, G.F., 600
Directing, nursing administration
activities related to, 408f
effective directing, 408–409
major elements of, 407
properties of a positive work envi-
ronment, 408
qualities of a good leader, 408
Discovery, ACE star model, 123
Discrimination in Employment Act,
278
Disraeli, Benjamin, 618
Diversity in the workforce. *See* Man-
aging a culturally diverse
workforce
Dixon, N., 215
DMAIC Mnemonic, 412
Dobbins, M., 466
Documentation, risk management and,
485–486, 487f
Donabedian model, 529–530
Donovan, H.M., 307
Dossey, B.M., 77
Dowling, G.F., 40
Dreyfuss Model of Skills Acquisition,
579
Drucker, Peter, 494
change, 122
definition of knowledge worker, 417
MBO and, 409–410
postmodern organization, 27
strategies for innovation, 107
windows of opportunity, 124,
310–311
Duchene, P., 353
Duffy, J.R., 517
Dunham, J., 632
Dunphy, D.C., 118
Durable power of attorney for health,
83
Dworkin, R., 78

E

East, D., 599
Edelman, Marian Wright, 666
Education. *See* Nursing staff educator;
Training and education
EEOC (Equal Employment
Opportunity Commission),
459, 460
Ehrat, K.S., 303
Eisenhower, Dwight, 406
Eldridge, L., 88
Electronic media, 169
Emotionally intelligent leadership
best and worse bosses, 61–62, 61–62f
emotional competencies
constituting emotionally intelli-
gent leadership, 56, 57f,
58–60
developing, 65–66, 66f
development of, 54
Joe, quality manager, 54f, 55–56
Tiffany, new nurse manager, 53f, 55
Victoria, remote nursing agency
director, 59–60, 60f, 65
18 work competencies, 54–55, 55f
emotional intelligence
definition of, 52

framework
dimensions of, 51f, 52–53
relationship management, 53
self-awareness, 52–53
self-management, 53
social awareness, 53
genetic component of, 52
at work, 64f
evidenced-based practice, 67
introduction, 51–52
research and professional support
American Nurses Association
(ANA), 63
American Organization of Nurse
Executives, 62–63
areas of need for emotionally intelligent leadership, 63–64
foundations and government
agencies, 63
research on hospital nursing, 63
role of the academic partner, 611
summary, 67
Empathy, 57f, 58, 109
Empowerment, in HR development,
276
End-of-life care, 79
Entrepreneurship, 205f
Equal Employment Opportunity Commission (EEOC), 459, 460
Equal Pay Act (1963), 461f, 671
Equity theory, 415
ERG theory of Alderfer, 414
Esteem needs, 416, 417
Ethical nurse leadership
collective bargaining
agreements, 85
arbitration, 90
defined, 85–86
grievance procedures, 88, 89f
issues: ethical considerations,
86–87
job security and, 94
mediation, 90
process, 87–88
purpose of today, 84–85
supervisory influence, 90–91
unionization
advantages of, 91–92
disadvantages of, 92–93
strikes, 93
vulnerability, 93–94
developing a health care ethics program
elements of, 78
ethics committees' responsibilities,
79
history of, 78–79
performance improvement indicators, end-of-life care, 79
evidenced-based practice, 78, 81
GoodWork Project, 94
implications for managing a clinical
practice
advance directives, 82–83
durable power of attorney for
health care, 83
living will, 83
ANA Committee on Ethics guidelines, 80–81

creating a moral space to preserve integrity, 82
denial of pain medication, 81–82
establishing ethics committees, 82
ethical boundaries in nurse-patient relationships, 81
ethics in business, 83–84
four ethical principles
autonomy, 79–80
beneficence, 80
justice, 80
nonmaleficence, 80
issues directly related to providing patient care services, 79
other ethical issues, 80
values-based management, 82
introduction, 75
professional ethics and integrity
Center for Ethics and Human Rights, 75
Code of Ethics for Nurses with Interpretive Statements, 75
ethical principles, 76
ethical terms, 77–78
ethical theories, 76–77
holistic ethics, 77
Scope and Standards for Nurse Administrators, 75–76
summary, 95
Euthanasia, 77
Evaluation
departmentation, 243f
goal evaluation checklist, 423f
mission statements, 294f
objectives, 302f
philosophy, 297f
planning, 317f
as a process of health policy, 457–458
product evaluation
checklist, 388f
committee, 387–388
Evaluation, ACE star model, 123
Evaluation of operations and care delivery systems
controlling techniques
benchmarking
quality management, 512
standards of care, 511
standards of practice, 511–512
structure standards, 511
Gantt charts, 507–508, 509f, 510f
nursing operating instructions, 507, 508f, 509f
nursing rounds, 506–507, 507f
program evaluation and review technique (PERT), 510–511
evaluation as a function of nursing management, 496
evidenced-based management, 512
evidenced-based practice, 517
the future, 516–517
introduction
control processes, 496, 497f
Fayol's elements of management, 496f
Urwick's principles of controlling, 496
master control plan, 512, 513–515f

measuring productivity
operational plan, 505–506f
overview, 504–506
operations management
introduction, 496–497
organizational transformation
clinical microsystems, 498–499, 499f
horizontal v. vertical hierarchy, 498
quantum characteristics for organizational leaders, 498
quality awards
nursing excellence, 516, 517f
organizational excellence, 512, 516
standards
external, 503–504
internal, 503
performance, 504
summary, 518
systems thinking
evaluation by root analysis, 500–501, 501f
introduction, 499–500
management tools: measurement issues, 500
management tools: performance issues
approaches to controls, 502
control functions, 502–503
controlling mechanisms, 502
elements of controls, 502
self-control, 501–502
task analysis and quality control, 503
Evidenced-based practice, 9. *See also under* specific topics
ACE star model, 123
evidenced-based decision making, 122–123
evidence summary, 123
Evidenced-based strategic planning
"balanced scorecard," 326–327
evidenced-based practice, 327–328
successful planning, 327
Expectancy theory, 553
Expectancy-valence theory, 415
Expert nurse witness, 476
case study, 476–477
functions of, 476
Extranets, 434

F

Facilitator role, 594
Facione, P.A., 109
Fair Labor Standards Act (FLSA), 461f, 671
False imprisonment, 478
Family and Medical Leave Act (FMLA) (1993), 461f
Fayol, Henri, principles of management, 26–27, 186, 496f
Federal laws, worker protection, considerations, 461–462f
Feedback
evidence on, 154
improved performance and, 155
influence on behavior and, 154

performance appraisal, 565
timely, 57f, 59
Feminist ethics, 77
Fieldler, F.E., 626
Fifth Discipline, The, 499
Fineout-Overholt, E., 122
Finkelman, A., 602
First impression error, performance appraisal, 572
Fishbone cause-and-effect diagram, 541
Fitzgerald, F. Scott, 548
"Five Ps" categories, 541
Fixed-ratio staffing: The California experience, 354
Flextime, 347–348
Float personnel, 342
Floyd, J.A., 603
FLSA (Fair Labor Standards Act), 461f, 671
FMLA (Family and Medical Leave Act), 461f
Follett, Mary Parker, 26
Forming or orientation phase, groups, 220
"Four Ms" categories, 541
14 forces of magnetism, 517f
Frankel, A., 500
Freely, A.J., 109
Friedman, M.G., 554
Friesen, M., 225
Full-time equivalents (FTEs), nonproductive, 386–387
Full-time nursing personnel, 342
Functional authority, 195
Functional departmentation, 244
Future goals worksheet, 423f

G

Gaebler, T., 383
Gain sharing, 205–206f
Galbraith, M.W., 598
Galvin, E.A., 603
Gantt, Henry L., 507
Gantt charts, 507–508, 509f, 510f
Gardner, Howard, 74, 94
definition of charisma, 623
definition of leadership, 621
leadership studies, 622–623
qualities of leadership, 630, 631
GCN (Generalized clinical nurse), 562–563f
Gender issues, in leadership, 632
Generalized clinical nurse (GCN), job description, 562–563f
General systems theory, 30–32
the animal level, 31–32
the cell, 30–31, 31f
the clockwork, 30
the framework, 30
genetic-societal level, 31
human level, 32
level of social organization, 32
the thermostat, 30
Generation X or Y nurse, retention of, 673–674, 674f
Genetic screening, risk assessment and, 491
Gerner v. Long Island Jewish Hillside Medical Center, 486

Goal evaluation checklist, 423f
Godfrey, R.R., 106
Goethe, 18
Goldsmith, S., 614
Goleman, D., 604
GoodWork Project, 94
Grace Reynolds Application and Study
  of PETO (GRASP) system,
  352, 361
Grasmick, L.L., 594
GRASP system, 352, 361
Greenhalgh, T., 111
Greenhouse, P., 235
Grimes, A.J., 29
Group practice model of care, 238–239
Groups
  as change agents, 125
  discussion, 109
  establishing informal groups, 4–5
  functional roles of group members,
    218–219f
  group cohesiveness, 221
  group dynamics, 218–220
  group leaders, 220
  Groupthink, 222–223, 222f
  phases of groups, 220–221
  placing your group at the edge of
    chaos, 5–6
  selected group techniques, 221–222f
  using groups as change agents, 125
Groupthink, 145, 222–223, 222f
*Guidelines for Review of Nursing CAre
  at the Local Level,* 542
Guzzetta, C.E., 77

H

Haase-Herrick, K., 601
Hall, R.H., 189
Hammond, H., 36
Hampton, D.R., 282
Hanley, D., 604
Hannah, K.J., 91
Hanson, R.L., 354–357
Hansten, R.I., 409
Havelock's theory of change, 116
Hawkins, R.E., 600
Hawthorne studies, 27, 218
Hay Job Evaluation System, 561
Hayward, S., 466
Headship v. leadership, 630–631
Health care cost coalitions, 400–401
Health Insurance Portability and
  Accountability Act (HIPAA),
  436, 445f
Health maintenance organizations
  (HMOs), 399–400
Health policy, laws, and regulatory issues
  credentialing of individual practitioners
    advanced practice registered
      nurses, 465
    certification, 466
    evidenced-based practice, 466
    licensure defined, 464
    National Council of State Boards
      of Nursing (NCSBN), 464,
      465
    nursing licensure/credentialing
      NCLEX-RN, 465
    Nurse Practice Acts, 464–465

Department of Health and Human
  Services (DHHS), 459
  federal and state health insurance
    Medicaid, 463
    Medicare, 462–463
  federal and state labor laws
    Equal Employment Opportunity
      Commission (EEOC), 459,
      460
    litigation examples, 460, 462
    summary of, 461–462f
    Title VII, Civil Rights Act (1964),
      459–460
  health policy
    as an entity, 456
    definition of, 456
    issues for the United States, 456f
    as a process, 456–458
      adoption, 457
      evaluation, 457–458
      formation, 457
      implementation, 457
      problem identification and
        agenda setting, 457
    introduction, 455–456
    nurses and public policy
      addressing pressing issues,
        458–459
      legitimate power, 458
      policy process, 458
      sources of power, 458f
    regulatory issues, Joint Commission
      on Accreditation of
      Healthcare Organizations
      (JCAHO), 463–464
    summary, 466
Health promotion and wellness pro-
  grams, 401
Healthy Work Environments, 170–171
Helper model of care, 238–239
Helton, B.R., 563
Hennepin County Medical Center,
  39–40
Henrikson, K., 647
Henry, B.J., 141
Herkimer, A.G.,Jr., 377
Hermeneutics, 29
Hersey, P., 626
Herzberg, Frederick, 414
Hierarchical structure, 194–196, 195f
Hierarchy of prepotency, 416
High Point Regional Health Center, 236
Hill, L.A., 634
Hinshaw, A.S., 643
HIPAA (Health Insurance Portability
  and Accountability Act)
  (HIPAA), privacy and secu-
  rity
  concerns, 436, 445f
Histogram or bar chart, 541, 541f
HMOs (health maintenance organiza-
  tions), 399–400
Hodgetts, R.M., 294
Hoffart, N., 237
Holistic ethics, 77
Holmes, Oliver Wendell, Jr., 454
Holt Companies, 82
Hospital at home model of nursing
  practice, 236

Hospital information systems, 437f
  administrative, 437f, 439
  clinical, 437f, 439–440
  implementing, 437, 438f, 439
Hospital physician organizations, 401
Hours per patient day (HPPD),
  356–357
Houston, Sam, 623
HRD. *See* Human resource development (HRD)
Human resource development (HRD)
  andragogy and HRD, 276–277
  assigning, 270
  career planning
    career ladders and career develop-
      ment programs, 273–274,
      274–275f
    job variety and job sharing, 275
  conflict management in a diverse
    workforce
    active listening, 282
    antecedent sources of, 281
    assessing conflict, 280–281
    characteristics of conflict, 280
    conflict: beliefs, values, and goals,
      281–282
    introduction, 280
    resolving conflict through negotia-
      tion, 282–283
    results of conflict resolution, 283
    stress and conflict, 281
    through effective communication,
      282
  cultural competence, 279–280
  empowerment and autonomy, 276
  introduction, 261, 275–276
  job promotion and advancement,
    277
  job termination
    disciplinary action, 278
    layoffs, 278–279
    necessity for, 277
    poor performance, 278
    specific legal guidelines, 277–278
    termination for cause, 278
  recruitment
    assessment center process, 266,
      268
    interview, 265–266
      candidates questions and inter-
        viewing tips, 266f
      guide, 266f
      illegal questions, 266f
      responsibilities, nurse executive
        and candidate, 267f
    marketing, 264–265, 265f
    nurse recruiter, 264
    recruiting nurses into employment
      goal in recruiting, 262
      opportunities for work-life bal-
        ance, 264
      providing up-to-date technol-
        ogy, 264
      room for advancement, 264
      strategic planning for, 263
    recruiting students into nursing,
      261–262, 263f
      evidenced-based practice, 262
    search committee, 269, 269f

retention
  ANA Bill of Rights for Registered
    Nurses, 271f
  introduction, 271
  job expectations and satisfaction,
    272
  strategies
    management education, 272
    nurse retention coordinator, 272
    retaining the older worker, 273
  turnover, 271–272
  selecting, 270
  self-awareness and lifelong learning,
    276
  summary, 283
Human Side of Enterprise, 418
Huston, C.J., 593
Huxley, Thomas, 260

I

Imig, S.I., 348
Immigration Reform and Control Act,
  461f
Inactivism, 304–305
Incident/occurrence reporting
  dos and don'ts of, 488f
  preparation of, 488
  use of, 487
Individual decisions, 109
Influence, 57f, 59
Information management and technology
  computer networking
    extranets, 434
    Internet
      continuing education online,
        436
      creating and maintaining web-
        sites, 435–436
      electronic medical records, 436
      key points in searching the
        Internet, 435
      privacy and security concerns,
        436
    intranet, 434
    introduction, 434
    local area networks (LANs), 434,
      440
    virtual private networks, 435
    wide area networks (WANs), 434
    wireless, 435
  computer technology terms, 449–451
  data management in health care
    data cleansing, 433–434
    data mining, 433
    definition of data, 430
    definition of information,
      430–431
    educating staff, 432–433
    evidenced-based practice, 432
    examples of data and information,
      432f
    "relational databases," 433
    system prompts, 433
    verification techniques, 433
  ethical, legal, and security issues,
    444–445
    guidelines to minimize risk, 445f
    key components of HIPAA, 436,
      445f

future trends
    ubiquitous computing, 446, 446f
    virtual reality (simulation), 446
  hospital information systems, 437f
    administrative, 437f, 439
    clinical, 437f, 439–440
    implementing, 437, 438f, 439
  Information Systems (IS) depart-
    ment, 430
  introduction, 429–430
  nursing informatics role in health
    care, 430, 431f
  nursing management applications
    computer applications, 443
    management of human resources,
      444, 444f
    nursing management minimum
      data set (NMMDS), 443–444
  software, general applications
    communications, 440
    database management, 440–441,
      441f
    personal digital assistants (PIAs),
      443
    personal information manager
      (PIM), 443
    spreadsheets, 442–443
    word processing and desktop pub-
      lishing, 441–442, 442f
  summary, 446–447
Information Systems (IS) department,
  430
Informed consent, 77
Ingersoll, G., 654
Initiative, 57f, 58
Inspirational leadership, 57f, 59
Institute for Healthcare Improvement,
  108, 238
Institute for Healthcare Quality, 11
Institute of Medicine (IOM)
  Committee on Reviewing Evidence
    to Identify Highly Effective
    Clinical Services, 516–517
  Crossing the Quality Chasm (2001), 7,
    9, 19–20, 114, 224, 225f
  definition of quality, 602
  *To Err is Human: Building a Safer
    Health System (1991),* 7, 19,
    191, 224, 224f, 398
  factors of problematic leadership,
    619
  IOM core competencies, 602, 603f
  Keeping Patients Safe, 7, 28, 224, 225f,
    650
  Knowing What Works in Healthcare,
    516–517
  medical errors, 471
  Quality Initiative, 11
  Report on Patient Safety, 648
Integration, 123
  vertical *vs.* horizontal, 202, 203f
Intentional torts. *See under* Legal issues
Intention-goal theory, 415
Interactivism, 305
Interdisciplinary collaboration
  characteristics of, 22
  components of professional nursing
    practice environment (ANA),
    22–23

Pew Health Professions Commission
    study, 22
  International Review, The, 479
Internet. *See also* Information manage-
    ment and technology
  continuing education online, 436
  creating and maintaining websites,
    435–436
  electronic medical records, 436
  key points in searching the Internet,
    435
  privacy and security concerns, 436
Internship programs, 340
Interquartile range, 537
Interview, recruitment, 265–266
  candidates questions and interview-
    ing tips, 266f
  guide, 266f
  illegal questions, 266f
  responsibilities, nurse executive and
    candidate, 267f
Interviewing, performance appraisals
    and job descriptions, 567–568
Interviews, 165
IOM. *See* Institute of Medicine (IOM)
IS (Information Systems), 430

J

Jackson, M., 409
Jacoby, K., 599
JCAHO. *See* Joint Commission on
    Accreditation of Healthcare
    Organizations (JCAHO)
Job enrichment, 205f
Job evaluation
  Hay Job Evaluation System, 561, 563
  work classification, 563–564
Job promotion and advancement, 277.
    See also under Performance
    appraisal
Job satisfaction, checklist for assessing,
    425–426
Job security, collective bargaining, 94
Job termination
  disciplinary action, 278
  layoffs, 278–279
  necessity for, 277
  poor performance, 278
  specific legal guidelines, 277–278
  termination for cause, 278
Johns Hopkins Medical Center, 9, 236
Johnson, D.E., 626
Johnson, J.E., 321
Johnson, K., 352
Johnson, M., 10
Johnson Behavioral System Model, 352
Johnson's theory, 37
Joint Commission on Accreditation of
    Healthcare Organizations
    (JCAHO), 11, 78, 412,
    463–464
  definition of licensed independent
    practitioners, 481
  disclosure of sentinel events, 485
  external standards, evaluation of
    health care, 336, 503
  incident reporting, 488
  integration of risk management and
    quality assurance, 484–485

Joint Commission on Accreditation of
Healthcare Organizations
(JCAHO)—*(continued)*
National Patient Safety Goals
(NPSGs), 534, 535
quality data collection for measurement, 535
staffing, 336, 338
use of restraints, 478
Juran, Joseph, 527, 528f
Justice, 80

K

Kanter, R.M., 145, 155, 233
Kaplan, R.S., 326, 327, 613
Keegan, L., 77
Keeping Patients Safe (IOM), 7, 28, 224,
225f, 650
Kelly, K., 5
Kennedy, W.R., 560
Kenner, C., 602
Keyes, M., 647
Keynes, John Maynard, 428
King, I.M., 291–292
Kinlein, M.L., 292
Kirkpatrick, D.L., 552
Klahefn, K.A., 632
Knowing What Works in Healthcare,
516–517
Knowledge worker, nurse as, 417–418
Knowles, Malcolm, 276
Koontz, H., 307, 496
Kopelman, R.F., 553
Kosel, K.C., 645
Kotzabassaki, S., 36
Kramer, Marlene, 644, 651, 657
Kruger, N., 604
Kuehl, Sheila, 354

L

Lake, E.T., 657
Lancaster, J., 140
Lancaster, W., 140
LANs (local area networks), 434, 440
Lattimer, R.L., 106
Laws. *See* Health policy, laws, and regulatory issues
Leader Behavior Description
Questionnaire, 625
Leader role, 595
Leadership. *See also* Emotionally intelligent leadership
definitions of, 620–621
effective, 621
evidenced-based practice, 632
future direction: quantum leadership, 634–635
conceptual foundations, 636f
seven new age imperatives, 637f
universal cycle of transformation,
636f
universal dynamics of transformation, 637f
gender issues, 632
history, 620
introduction
problematic leadership, 619
recommendations for nurse leaders, 619–620
transformational leadership, 619

leader-constituent interaction, 623
behavioral theories
Blake and Mouton's Managerial
Grid, 624–625
Lewin's studies, 625
Likert's Michigan studies, 624
McGregor's Theory X and
Theory Y, 623–624
problems with leadership questionnaires, 625–626
leadership *vs.* headship, 630–631
nursing and leadership health care
policy
buffering, 633–634
steps to prepare for, 633
preparation of nurse leaders, 631
style
Fielder's contingency model of
leadership effectiveness, 626
life cycle theory of Hersey,
Blanchard, and Johnson, 626
Reddin's three-dimensional theory
of management, 627
summary, 637–638
theories
Gardner's studies, 622–623
trait theory, 621–622
transformational
competencies for dynamic and
effective leadership
management of attention, 628
management of meaning, 628
management of self, 629
management of trust, 629
definition of, 627
empowerment of others as goal,
627–628
leadership and management
differences between, 629
similarities between, 630
transformational leader as coach, 634
impediments to effective coaching,
635f
model for transformational coaching, 635f
transforming leaders, 623
variables involved in, 621
Leapfrog Group, 11
Legal issues. *See also* Health policy,
laws, and regulatory issues;
Risk management
civil law
definition of, 472
intentional torts
assault and battery, 478–479
defamation, 478
definition of, 477
false imprisonment, 478
unintentional torts
expert nurse witness, 476
case study, 476–477
functions of, 476
medical malpractice
definitions of, 472–473
key areas for nursing negligence, 473–474
Monk v. Doctor's Hospital, 473
National Practitioner Data
Bank, 2005 reports, 474f,
475f

patient falls and medication
errors, 474
statistics, 473
strategies to reduce claims,
490f
medical malpractice tort reform, 477
negligence, 472
patient safety and the tort system, 477
standard of care
definition of, 474–475
or "customary practice,"
475–476
corporate liability
board of directors, 480
corporate negligence, 480
credentialing liability, 480–481
respondeat superior, 480–481
criminal law, 479
and ethical issues, staff development,
601
introduction, 471–472
nurses and the litigation process,
482, 483f
other areas of liability
floating, 482
following the chain of command,
482
inadequate staffing, 481–482
supervisor liability, 481
summary, 491
Lemin, B., 502
Leniency/stringency error, performance
appraisal, 572
Leonard, M., 500
Levenstein, A., 155
Levinson, H., 107
Levi Strauss & Co., 82
Lewin, Kurt
force field analysis, 357
leadership studies, 625
theory of change, 115
Libel, 478
Licensed independent practitioners,
481
Life cycle theory of Hersey, Blanchard,
and Johnson, 626
Likert, R., 624
Lindberg, C., 5, 6
Line authority, 188f
Line functions, 195
Linkow, P., 531, 531f
Lippitt's theory of change, 116–117
Listening
causes of poor listening, 158–159
Crucial Conversations, 160–161
effective listening, 157–158
encouraging people to listen,
159–160
good listeners, 160
mnemonics, 159–161
power listening tools "AMPP,"
160–161
providing information, 160
techniques to improve, 159
Litigation process, nurses and, 482, 483f
Living will, 83
Lloyd Noland Hospital v. Durham, 473
Local area networks (LANs), 434, 440

Locke, Edwin, 415
Locke, John, 76
Lord, R.G., 626

M

Maas, M., 10
MacArthur, Douglas, 525
MacKay, R.C., 346
Mackey, M.K.V., 357
Magee, J., 140
Magnet Hospital Recognition Program
    for Excellence in Nursing
    Services, 644
Magnet hospitals
  implications for a culturally sensitive
    workforce, 676–678
  staffing and scheduling, 350
Magnet Hospitals, the Attraction and
    Retention of Professional
    Nurses, 644
Magnetism, creating a culture of
  empirical quality outcomes
    outcomes, 660–661
    quality of care, 660
  evidence and outcomes, 644–645
  exemplary professional nursing
    practice, autonomous
    practice
    autonomy, 657–659
      evidenced-based practice, 658
      tools needed for clinical compe-
        tence, 658f
    consultations and resources, 659
  historical perspective
    eight essentials of magnetism, 644
    Magnet Hospitals, the Attraction
      and Retention of Professional
      Nurses, 644
    The Magnet Recognition Program,
      643–644
    Nursing Work Index, 644
    research and studies, 644
  introduction, 643
  knowledge, innovation, and im-
    provements, 659–660
  the Magnet Model
    five areas to be addressed, 646–647
    14 forces of magnetism, 647
  professional practice model, 654–655
  resource utilization and development
    community, 653
    image of nursing, 652
    organizational structure, 650
      implementing change, 650
      sustaining the change, 650–651
    policies and programs, 652–653
    professional development,
      651–652
  safe and ethical practice
    interdisciplinary relationships, 656
    nurses as teachers, 655–656
    quality of care (safe and ethical
      practice), 656–657
  self-assessment of the organization,
    645
  staff nurse self-assessment survey, 646f
  structural empowerment, leadership
    management style, 649–650
    quality of nursing leadership
      developing a vision, 647

developing commitment and
    trust, 648
  recognizing a need for change,
    647
  summary, 661
  transformational leadership, 647
Magnet Recognition Program, 21, 25,
    25f, 104, 147, 237, 350, 516,
    643, 676
Malcolm Baldridge National Quality
    Award, 512, 516
Malloch, K., 498, 634
Malpractice. *See* Medical malpractice
Management, historical perspective
  behavioral science and management,
    27
  definition of management, 26
  essential management practices,
    28–29
  evidenced-based management, 28
  Fayol's principle's of management,
    26–27, 27f
  human relations management, 27
  modern era, 26, 27
  post modern era, 26, 27
  premodern era, 26
  principle functions of managers, 27
Management and leadership
  differences between, 629
  similarities between, 630
Management by objectives (MBO)
  description of, 409–410
  process
    discussing the goals: first meeting,
      410
    learning the process, 410
    management by results, 411–412
    organizational development, 412
    problems with, 411–412
    taking action, 411
Management of attention, 628
Management of meaning, 628
Management of self, 629
Management of trust, 629
Managers, 161–162, 171–172
Managing a culturally diverse work-
    force
  characteristics that support reten-
    tion, 672–673
  cultural and diverse workforce issues
    guiding principle 1, 674, 675f
    population statistics, 675
    strategies for promoting cultural
      competence, 676f
  generational differences, 673–674
  introduction, 667–668
  Magnet Hospitals
    building healthy relationships,
      676–679
    evidenced-based practice, 677
    Magnet Recognition Program, 676
  outline of the nursing process, 668f
  recruitment issues
    creative collaboration, 669
    cultural sensitivity issues
      behavioral interviewing, 669,
        670f
      peer interviewing, 669–670
    culture described, 668
    devising individualized plans, 669

laws that impact the hiring process
  Age Discrimination in
    Employment Act (1967), 671
  Americans with Disabilities Act
    (1990), 671
  Civil Rights Act (1991), 671
  Equal Pay Act (1963), 671
  nurse retention factors, 668–669
  on-boarding: implications for cul-
    tural competence, 672
  strategies for, 671f
  summary, 678
MAPP mnemonic, 160–161
Marketing, strategies for, 264–265, 265f
Markham, J., 357
Martin, S.C., 8
Maslow, A. H.
  hierarchy of needs, 413–414,
    416–417
  holistic-dynamic theory, 415–416
  prerequisites to satisfying needs, 416
Mastal, M.F., 36
Mastorovich, M.J., 517
Matrix management model, 40
Matrix structure, 196, 196f
MBO. *See* Management by objectives
    (MBO)
McClelland, David, 414
McClure, M.L., 34, 643
McGrath, L.G., 277
McGregor, Douglas
  definition of leadership, 621
  Theory X and Theory Y, 418–419,
    623–624
McGuire, A., 421
McKay, P.S., 147
McKay-Dee education department
    (Ogden, UT), 358
Measures of Patient Safety Based on
    Hospital Administrative
    Data, 11
Measures of variability, 537
Medical Center of Central Georgia, 41
Medical malpractice
  definitions of, 472–473
  key areas for nursing negligence,
    473–474
  Monk v. Doctor's Hospital, 473
  National Practitioner Data Bank,
    2005 reports, 474f, 475f
  patient falls and medication errors,
    474
  statistics, 473
  strategies to reduce claims, 490f
  tort reform, 477
Medicare/Medicaid, 8, 458, 462–463
Medicus, 337
Meetings, 161
Meier, A.P., 310
Melnyk, B., 122
Mentoring, 672
Metamanagement
  definition of, 105
  principles of appreciative inquiry,
    106
  task-related actions for nurses,
    105–106
Metropolitan Medical Center, goals of,
    300f
Michigan Nurses Association, 91

Michigan studies of Likert, 624
Milio, N., 633
Mill, John Stuart, 76, 77
Milstead, J., 458
Mitchell, W.N., 630
Mitry, N.W., 633
Mittmann, N., 361
Mnemonics
  AIDA, 159
  DMAIC, 412
  MAPP, 160–161
  PREP, 159
Molloch, Kathy, 334
Monk v. Doctor's Hospital, 473
Morehead, S., 10
Morgan, Gareth, 6
Morgan, P., 156
Motivation
  enhancing
    building self-esteem, 420
    career planning, 419
    effective communication, 419
    encouraging self-actualization,
      420–421
    endorsing teamwork, 420
    other activities to stimulate moti-
      vation, 421
  theories
    content theories, 413–414
    described, 412–413
    Maslow, 413–414
      hierarchy of needs, 416–417
      holistic-dynamic theory, 415–416
      prerequisites to satisfying needs,
        416
    process theories
      arousal-activation theory, 414
      equity theory, 415
      expectancy-valence theory, 415
      intention-goal theory, 415
    questions to consider, 413
    usefulness to nurse managers, 417
Motorola, 558–559
Myers-Brigg type indicator, 145

N

Nagelkerk, J.M., 141
Naisbitt, John, 112
Nanus, B., 627
National Council Licensure
      Examination for Practical
      Nurses (NCLEX-PN), 465
National Council Licensure
      Examination for Registered
      Nurses (NCLEX-RN), 465
National Council of State Boards of
      Nursing (NCSBN), licensure
      of nurses, 464, 465
National Database of Nursing Quality
      Indicators (NDNQI), 10–11
National Healthcare Quality Report, 11
National Labor Relations Act (1947)
  definition of a professional em-
      ployee, 85–86
  termination of employees, 278
National League for Nursing, definition
      of residencies, 21
National Nursing Staff Development
      Organization, 594

National Patient Safety Goals (NPSGs),
      534, 535
National Practitioner Data Bank
  history of, 481
  reports, 474f, 475f
National Quality forum, 11
Natural Death Act (Texas), 82–83
Natural law, 77
Nave, J.L., 211
NCLEX-RN/NCLEX-PN, 465
NCSBN (National Council of State
      Boards of Nursing), 464, 465
NDNQI (National Database of Nursing
      Quality Indicators), 10–11
Needleman, J., 10
Negligence, 472
Negotiation
  introduction, 156–157
  principles of, 157
  steps in the process, 157
Nelson, E., 498
Newman's theory, 37
New York State Nurses Association, 92
Nightingale, Florence, 102, 620, 629
NMIS (nursing management informa-
      tion system), 336, 354–355
NMMDS (nursing management mini-
      mum data set), 443–444
Nominal group technique, 538
Nonmaleficence, 77, 80
Normative model, 139–140
Norton, D.P., 326, 327, 613
NPSGs (National Patient Safety Goals),
      534, 535
Nurse administrator
  certification, 26
  described, 23
  level of nursing administrative prac-
      tice
    nurse executive, 23–24
    nurse manager, 24
    standards of practice, 24–25
    standards of professional perfor-
      mance, 25
  magnet recognition program and
      scope and standards, 25, 25f
  qualifications of, 25–26
Nurse executive, 23–24
Nurse Executive Competencies (AONE),
      184–185, 186f, 187f
Nurse Leader-Patient Safety
      Competency Model,
      226–227f, 227f, 228f
Nurse manager, 24
Nurse Practice Acts, 464–465
Nurse recruiter, 264
*Nurse's Role in Promoting a Culture of
      Patient Safety,* 225–226
Nursing and leadership health care policy
  buffering, 633–634
  steps to prepare for, 633
Nursing Council Bylaws, 255–259
Nursing management
  management levels
    first-line nurses managers, 33–34
    nurse executive, 34–35
  role development, 32–33
Nursing Management Aging Workforce
      Survey, 262

Nursing management information sys-
      tem (NMIS), 336, 354–355
Nursing management minimum data
      set (NMMDS), 443–444
Nursing operating instructions, 507,
      508f, 509f
Nursing practice model of care, 238
Nursing rounds, 506–507, 507f
*Nursing's Agenda for the Future: A Call
      to the Nation,* 137
Nursing staff educator
  educator competencies, 595–596,
      596f
  educator roles
    change agent, 595
    consultant, 595
    continuing education responsibili-
      ties, 594
    definition of staff development,
      594
    facilitator, 594
    leader, 595
    researcher, 595
    structure and process changes, 594
  future planning for staff develop-
      ment, 605
    areas for insuring competency in,
      603–604
    coherence and trust, 604
    diversity of emotional competen-
      cies, 604
    focus on communication, 605
    other issues, 604–605
    strategies, 605
  introduction, 593
  organizational factors
    advisory groups, 597
    areas to be addressed, 596
    budgets, 597
    personnel, 597
  staff development evaluation,
      600–601
  staff development process
    case-based learning strategy, 599,
      599f
    characteristics of adult learners,
      598, 598f
    critical thinking, 599, 600f
    evidenced-based practice, 599, 600
    overview, 597
    principles and strategies of adult
      learners, 598
    simulation in, 600f
  summary, 605
  trends and issues in staff develop-
      ment
    legal and ethical, 601
    quality and safety: IOM compe-
      tencies, 602, 603f
    workforce diversity, 601–602
Nursing Work Index, 644
Nyberg, J., 353

O

Obligations, 77
O'Brien, M.A., 600
Occupational Safety and Health Act
      (OSHA) (1970)
  job termination and, 278

worker protection and considerations, 462f
Odiorne, G.S., 312, 409
Odomes v. Nucare, Inc., 462
Oermann, M.H., 603
Ohio State leadership studies, 625
Olivo, T., 645
Olney, Cynthia, 111
Olson, C.A., 579
Omnibus Budget Reconciliation Act (1990), 82
On-boarding: implications for cultural competence, 672
Open-door policy, 153
Operations management
  introduction, 496–497
  organizational transformation
    clinical microsystems, 498–499, 499f
    horizontal v. vertical hierarchy, 498
    quantum characteristics for organizational leaders, 498
Optimism, 57f, 58
Orem, D.E.
  definition of nursing, 292
  Orem's theory of self-care, 36, 536
Organizational awareness, 57f, 58
Organizational best practices
  employee attitude surveys, 171
  a good communication system, 171
  six critical factors, 170–171
Organizational climate, 228–229, 230f
Organizational culture
  culture of safety, 224–228
    competencies, 228f
    core patient safety technology competencies systems, 227f
    critical components relating to, 225
    Crossing the Quality Chasm, 224, 225f
    To Err is Human (IOM), 224, 224f
    Keeping Patients Safe (IOM), 224, 225f
    nurse executive's role, 226
    patient safety leadership competencies, 226–227f
    promoting, nurse's role in, 225–226
  introduction, 223–224, 223f
  summary, 246–248
Organizational publications, 168–169
Organizational structure and analysis.
    See also Restructuring nursing organizations
  AONE *Nurse Executive Competencies,* 184–185, 186f, 187f
  introduction, 184–185
  Nursing Council Bylaws, 255–259
  organizational climate, 228–229, 230f
  organizational culture (*See* Organizational culture)
  organizational theory (*See also* Team building)
    bureaucracy
      Hall's study of ten organizations, 189–190
      professsionalism and bureaucracy, 189f

strong points of bureaucratic organizations, 188
  term, 188
definitions of organizing, 186, 188
developing an organizational structure
  context, 192–193, 193f
  forms of
    decentralized structure, 196–197, 197f, 198f
    hierarchical structure, 194–196, 195f
    matrix structure, 196, 196f
  organization charts, 191–192, 192f
  overview, 191
introduction, 186
key organizational principles, 188f
organizational components, role theory: activities that reduce role conflict and ambiguity, 190–191, 190f
organizational development
  autonomy and accountability, 208–209
  introduction, 207–208
role of the nurse executive
  activities of nurses in participatory management, 205–205f, 205–206
  autonomy, 200–201
  commitment, 199–200
  communication and decentralization, 205
  communication and participation, 204–205
  conflict management, 200
  decentralization and, 197, 198f
  decentralization with participatory management, 203–204
  evidenced-based practice, 201–202, 204
  goals and objectives, 200
  good communication, 197–199
  participatory management, 197, 198f, 199f
  top management, 202
  training, 203
  trust, 199
  vertical *vs.* horizontal management, 202, 203f
shared governance, 206–207, 208f
  accountabilities for quality, 206
  accountabilities of management, 206–207
  accountabilities of practice, 206
  models of, 206
  preparing for, 207
  principles of, 206f, 207
organization of work, 229–231
summary, 246–248
Oryx, 558
Osborne, D, 383
OSHA. *See* Occupational Safety and Health Act (OSHA) (1970)
Outcome-based nursing practice, 41
Outcomes
  criteria/variables, process audits, 537
  empirical quality outcomes, 660–661
  quality of care, 660

evidence and outcomes, 644–645
expected, performance appraisal and, 575–576
measures, 500
potentially sensitive to nursing, 10

P

Pacini, C.M., 605
Pareto diagram, 542, 542f
Parish nursing, 235
Parissopoulos, S., 36
Participatory management, 197, 198f, 199f
  activities of nurses in, 205–205f, 205–206
  communication and, 204–205
  decentralization with, 203–204
Partnership clinical model of nursing practice, 236
Part-time nursing personnel, 342
Patient- and family-centered care model, 235–236
Patient classification systems (PCS), 350–351
  CASH system, 352
  components, 352
  computer models, 353
  desired characteristics, 351–352
  GRASP, 352, 361
  in-house *vs.* purchased, 353
  nursing models, 352–353
  problems, 354
  purposes, 351, 351f
Patient falls and medication errors, 474
Patient safety. *See also under* Organizational culture
  initiatives, 489f
  and the tort system, 477
Patient Self-Determination Act, 82
Patterson, K., 155
Paulanka, B.J., 675
Pavalko, R., 86
Pay
  equity, 206f
  merit pay increase
    award procedure, 582, 584f
    based on market value, 579–580
    budget, 580, 582, 583f, 584f
    measurement scales, 580, 583f
    performance standards, 580, 581–582f
    the process, 583, 585
  performance appraisal and designs, 579
    equity theory, 574
    expected outcomes, 575–576
    incentive-based programs, 575
Pay-for-performance process, elements of, 576–578
PCS. *See* Patient classification systems (PCS)
Pearson product-moment correlation, 537
Peer review, 88
  performance appraisal
    implementation of, 568–569
    Peer and Self-Evaluation System, 568
    phases of the review process, 569
    teaching peer review, 569

People v. Casa Blanca Convalescent Home, 480
Peplau's theory, 37–38
Performance appraisal
  as an uncomfortable task, 550–551
  developing and using performance standards
    based on core responsibilities, 554, 557
    for the clinical nurse, 554, 555–556f
    definition of standard, 554
    for the nurse executives/managers, 554
  evidenced-based practice, 551
  future of
    Deming's system, 573
    effective management of performance appraisals, 573–574
  group *vs.* individual plans
    competency model, 579
    group plans, 578–579
    individual plans, 579
  introduction, 549–550
    performance appraisal expectations
      required from employees, 550
      required from nurse executives, 550
  job analysis
    benefits of, 557
    downsizing, effects of, 558
    procedure, 557–558
    research on, 558
    steps to achieve statistical process control, 558–559
    uses of, 558
  job descriptions
    avoiding bias, 560
    bedside nurse (1887), 560
    as a contract, 559
    elements of, 560
    generalized clinical nurse (GCN), 562–563f
    that comply to legal, regulatory, and accrediting requirements, 560
    use of, 559
  literature, results from, 551
  merit pay increase
    award procedure, 582, 584f
    based on market value, 579–580
    budget, 580, 582, 583f, 584f
    measurement scales, 580, 583f
    performance standards, 580, 581–582f
    the process, 583, 585
  other rating methodologies
    Behavior-Anchored Rating Scales (BARS), 571
    task-oriented performance evaluation System (TOPES), 571
    team evaluation consensus (TEC), 571
  pay designs, 579
  pay for performance
    equity theory, 574
    expected outcomes, 575–576
    incentive-based programs, 575

peer ratings
  implementation of, 568–569
  Peer and Self-Evaluation System, 568
  phases of the review process, 569
  teaching peer review, 569
performance appraisals and job descriptions
  coaching, 565–566
  counseling
    directive approach, 567
    elective approach, 567
    importance of, 567
    interviews, 566
    nondirective approach, 567
  feedback, 565
  interviewing, 567–568
  job evaluation
    Hay Job Evaluation System, 561, 563
    work classification, 563–564
    as a tool, not a control mechanism, 560–561
    training, 564–565
    work redesign, 564
  problem areas in performance evaluation
    effectiveness, 571–572
    weaknesses, 572
  purposes
    motivation, 55
    other purposes, 553–554
    overview, 551–552
    salary problems
      equitable salary treatment, 552
      expectancy theory, 553
      explaining the basis for decisions, 552
      mixed-consequence system, 553
      relating rewards to job performance, 553
    the Xerox experience, 553
  self-rating
    effective, 570
    peer and supervisor ratings, 570
    questions to facilitate performance indicators, 569–570
    results of a two-part format to determine competence, 570
  summary, 585–586
  types of compensation programs, 576f
    pay-for-performance process, elements of, 576–578
Perry, D., 172
Personal digital assistants (PIAs), 443
Personal information manager (PIM), 443
Personalization, 205f
Persuasion, 110
Peter D. Hart Research Associates, 85
Peters, T., 162, 312, 496, 560
Pew Charitable Trusts, 54f
Pew Health Professions Commission study, 22
Phaneuf, Maria, process audit, 536
Phillips, J.S., 626
Phillips, P., 127
Physiological needs, 416, 417

PIAs (Personal digital assistants), 443
PIM (personal information manager), 443
Piper, L.R., 386
Planning. *See* Strategic planning and management
Plsek, P., 5, 6, 111, 614–615
Poetic principle, 106
Ponte, P.R., 604
Porter-O'Grady, Tim, 27, 197, 334, 498, 634
Portfolio, academic and clinical partnership
  designing markers of success, 614
  introduction, 609–610
  managing academic and clinical partners
    designated leader or champion, 614–615
    the synergy model as template, 615
  partnership performance issues, 612–614
  the portfolio, 610
  role of the academic partner
    benefits of partnership, 611
    evidenced-based practice, 611
    overview, 610–611
    using emotional intelligence, 611
  role of the clinical partner
    hospital-specific educational resources available, 613f
    hospital-specific resources available, 612f
    hospital-specific staffing data, 612f
  role of the liaisons and partnership committees, 611–612
  summary, 615
Positive principle, 106
Powell, John, 470
Powell, J.S., 348
Pozgar, G., 460
Preactivism, 305
Preceptorships and residencies, 21
Preferred provider organizations (PPOs), 400
Pregnancy Discrimination Act, 461f
PREP mnemonic, 159
Presence, 109
Price, E.M., 340–341
Price Waterhouse Coopers' Health Research Institute, nurse turnover rate, 271
Primary nursing, 205f
Principle of beneficence, 76
Principle of justice, 76
Principle of respect, 76
Principles of Nurse Staffing, 653
Prioritization matrix, 538–539, 538f
Process flowchart, 540, 540f
Process measures, 500
Process theories, 414–415
Product departmentation, 244
Productivity
  case study, 360
  definition, 355–356
  improving nursing productivity, 358–360
  measurement, 356–357

measuring
operational plan, 505–506f
overview, 504–506
model differences, 357–358
monitoring system for the recovery room, 357
problems in an operating room, 357
Professional nursing practice
autonomous practice
autonomy, 657–659
consultations and resources, 657–659
evidenced-based practice, 658
tools needed for clinical competence, 658f
differentiated nursing practice, 22
interdisciplinary collaboration
ANA, components of professional nursing practice environment, 22–23
characteristics of, 22
Pew Health Professions Commission study, 22
magnet recognition programs, 21
preceptorships and residencies, 21
professional practice model, 654–655
safe and ethical practice
interdisciplinary relationships, 656
nurses as teachers, 655–656
quality of care (safe and ethical practice), 656–657
Program evaluation and review technique (PERT), 510–511
Propaganda, 110
Provider-sponsored organizations, 401
Prudent buyer systems, 401
Publications, organizational, 168–169
Public speaking, techniques for, 163–164, 164–165f
Purnell, L.D., 675

Q

Quaker Oats, 579
Quality and safety: IOM competencies, 602, 603f
Quality awards
nursing excellence, 516, 517f
organizational excellence, 512, 516
Quality Interagency Coordination Task Force, 11
Quality management, 512
culture and climate, 530–531, 531f
customers, 530
data collection, nursing audits
process audits
evaluation, 536–537
Orem's categories of self-care requirements, 536
outcome criteria/variables, 537
Phaneuf audit, 536
Quality Patient-Care Scale, 536
structure of, 535
introduction
effective quality management, 53
JCAHO and IOM, 524
nursing QA programs, history of, 524
quality defined, 524

monitoring and feedback
customer satisfaction, 544
efficiency and effectiveness, 543–544
involvement of practicing nurses, 543
problem identification
evidence, 542
problem resolution, 542–543
program, components of
framework for continual improvement of health care, 533, 533f
list, 533
policies and procedures, 535
root cause analysis, adverse sentinel events, 534–535
standards for measuring quality of care, 534
statements of purpose, philosophy, and objectives, 534
quality as a philosophy, 530
quality circles/quality action teams, 532–533
research and, 544–545
summary, 545
tools
data analysis
brainstorming, 537–538
control charts, 539, 540f
Delphi method, 538
fishbone cause-and-effect diagram, 541
histogram or bar chart, 541, 541f
nominal group technique, 538
Pareto diagram, 542, 542f
prioritization matrix, 538–539, 538f
process flowchart, 540, 540f
run chart or trend chart, 539, 539f
quality improvement teams, 542
statistical techniques, 537
total quality management leaders, 529f
Donabedian model, 529–530
Joseph Juran, 527, 528f
Philip B. Crosby, 527–530
four absolutes of quality, 528f
Quality Management Maturity Grid, 529f
W. Edwards Deming, 524–527
application of Deming's theory, 525–526
Deming's 14 points, 525f
variation
causes, 526–527
concept, 526
Deming (Shewhart) APCD cycle, 526, 527f
Quality Patient-Care Scale, 346, 536
Quality processes
outcomes, 660–661
quality of care, 660

R

Rabin, J., 358
Rabkin, Mitchell, 64f
Rawls, A.C., 37

Reactivism, 304
Recruitment
assessment center process, 266, 268
interview, 265–266
candidates questions and interviewing tips, 266f
guide, 266f
illegal questions, 266f
responsibilities, nurse executive and candidate, 267f
marketing, 264–265, 265f
nurse recruiter, 264
recruiting nurses into employment
goal in recruiting, 262
opportunities for work-life balance, 264
providing up-to-date technology, 264
room for advancement, 264
strategic planning for, 263
recruiting students into nursing, 261–262, 263f
evidenced-based practice, 262
search committee, 269, 269f
Recruitment issues, in a culturally diverse workforce
creative collaboration, 669
cultural sensitivity issues
behavioral interviewing, 669, 670f
peer interviewing, 669–670
culture described, 668
devising individualized plans, 669
laws that impact the hiring process
Age Discrimination in Employment Act (1967), 671
Americans with Disabilities Act (1990), 671
Civil Rights Act (1991), 671
Equal Pay Act (1963), 671
nurse retention factors, 668–669
on-boarding: implications for cultural competence, 672
strategies for, 671f
Reddin, W.J.
theory of change, 113–114
three-dimensional theory of management, 627
Registered Nurse Ontario Association, 8
Regulatory issues. *See* Health policy, laws, and regulatory issues
Rehabilitation Act (1973), 461f
Reinkemeyer, M.H., 104
Relationship-based care model, 240–241
Relationship management, 57f, 59
Researcher role, 595
Residencies and preceptorships, 21
Resource acuity nurse, 348
Resource utilization and development
community, 653
image of nursing, 652
organizational structure, 650
implementing change, 650
sustaining the change, 650–651
policies and programs, 652–653
professional development, 651–652
Respondeat superior, 480–481
Restructuring nursing organizations
analyzing organizational structures, 241–242

Restructuring nursing organizations—
(*continued*)
departmentation, 244–245
standards for evaluation of, 243f
types of, 244
evaluating organizational function,
231–232f
consistency and inconsistency, 234
downsizing, 233–234
five steps of restructuring, 233, 233f
inhibitors to quick responses to
change, 234
mergers and acquisitions, 234
organizational analysis, 234.230f
synergies defined, 232
winning companies, 234
informal organization, 245
minimum requirements of an organizational structure, 242–243,
242f
models of nursing care delivery systems
collaborative patient management
model, 236
community-based nursing centers,
235
hospital at home, 236
key aspects of nursing practice
models, 235, 235f
parish nursing, 235
partnership clinical model, 236
patient- and family-centered care,
235–236
traditional model, 234
organizational effectiveness,
245–246, 245f
professional models of care
differential practice, 239–240, 240f
five subsystems, 237
group practice, 238–239
helper model, 239
Magnet Recognition Program, 237
nursing practice model, 238
relationship-based care model,
240–241
transforming care at the bedside,
238, 238f
professional nursing practice environment, 236–237f
challenges for, 236
evidenced-based practice, 237
summary, 246–248
symptoms of malorganization, 246
Retention of employees
ANA Bill of Rights for Registered
Nurses, 271f
introduction, 271
job expectations and satisfaction, 272
strategies
management education, 272
nurse retention coordinator, 272
retaining the older worker, 273
turnover, 271–272
Ridderheim, D.S., 209
Rigg, M., 569
Rights, 77
Rights-based ethics, 77–78
Risk management. *See also* Legal issues
documentation, 485–486, 487f

evidenced-based practice: genetic
screening, 491
incident/occurrence reporting
dos and don'ts of, 488f
preparation of, 488
use of, 487
nursing and, 489
patient safety initiatives, 489f
policies and procedures, 487–488
responsibilities
claims management, 485
competencies, 484f
compliance with regulatory and
accreditation agencies, 485
financial risk, 485
introduction, 483
loss and prevention reduction,
483–485
strategies to reduce malpractice
claims, 490f
summary, 491
Roberson v. Provident House, 478
Robert Wood Johnson Foundation, 63,
64f, 108, 238
Transforming Care at the Bedside
(TCAB), 8
Rogers, E.M., 614
Rogers, Martha, 37
Roger's theory of change, 115–116
*Role of the Nurse Executive in Patient
Safety: Guiding Principles
Toolkit,* 226
Roop, J.C., 603
Root cause analysis, 500–501, 501f
Rosener, J., 632
Rowland & Rowland, 307
Roy's theory, 36–37
Run chart or trend chart, 539, 539f
Russell, G., 10
Ryan, K., 172

S

Safety needs, 416, 417
Salary problems
equitable salary treatment, 552
expectancy theory, 553
explaining the basis for decisions,
552
mixed-consequence system, 553
relating rewards to job performance,
553
SBAR (situation, background, assessment, and recommendation),
605
Schlitzer v. University of Iowa Hospital,
460, 462
Schmalenberg, Claudia, 644, 651
Schwab, D.P., 579
Scoble, K., 10
*Scope and Standards for Nurse
Administrators,* 21–23, 25,
25f, 75–76, 209, 336, 458, 503,
516, 554, 643, 645, 654, 657
Scott, S., 156
Self-actualization
encouraging, 420–421
need, 416, 417
Self-care agency, 36
Self-control, emotional, 56, 57f

Self-esteem, 211, 420
Self-management, 56, 57f
Self-rating, performance appraisal
effective, 570
peer and supervisor ratings, 570
questions to facilitate performance
indicators, 569–570
results of a two-part format to determine competence, 570
Self-scheduling, staffing, 344f, 345–346
Senge, P., 499
Service departments, 195–196
Service orientation, 57f, 58
Shamian, J., 91
Shared governance, 205f, 206–207, 208f
accountabilities
of management, 206–207
of practice, 206
for quality, 206
models of, 206
preparing for, 207
principles of, 206f, 207
Shaw, George Bernard, 136
Sheats, P., 218–219f
Shortage of registered nurses by 2020,
261
Silber, J., 657
Silva, M.C., 36
Similar-to-me error, performance
appraisal, 572
Simmonds, T., 500
Situational awareness, 109
Sivell, S., 491
Six sigma strategies, 412, 413f
Skinner, B.F., 415
Sladek, R., 127
Slander, 478
Slippery slope argument, 77
Sloane, D.M., 657
Smith, H.L., 633
Smith, J.L., 357
Smith, T., 654
Sochalski, J., 657
Social awareness, 57f, 58
Social intelligence
Albrecht's model, 108–109
nourishing behavior, 108
principles of perception related to
change, 108
toxic behavior, 108
Society for Health Systems, 360–361
Software, general applications
communications, 440
database management, 440–441, 441f
personal digital assistants (PIAs), 443
personal information manager
(PIM), 443
spreadsheets, 442–443
word processing and desktop pub-
lishing, 441–442, 442f
Somera, Lorenza, 479
Somers, M.J., 570
Sorrell, J.M., 36
Span of control, 188f
Specialization, 188f
Speech making, techniques for,
163–164, 164–165f
Spradley's model for change, 117–118
Spreadsheets, 442–443

Stace, D.A., 118
Stacey, R.D., 4
Staff education and development. *See*
    Nursing staff educator
Staff function, 188f
Staffing and scheduling
    activities, 339–340
    decision making
        evidenced-based practices, 361
        mandated ratios, 360
        Society for Health Systems ap-
            proach, 360–361
    fixed-ratio staffing: The California
        experience, 354
    internship programs, 340
    introduction, 335–336
    magnet hospitals, 350
    models, 343, 344f, 345
        cross-training, 348
        cyclic scheduling, 343f, 345
        evidenced-based practice, 348
        flextime, 347–348
        modified work week
            10-hour shift, 346–347
            12-hour shift, 347
        resource acuity nurse, 348
        self-scheduling, 344f, 345–346
        temporary workers, 348–349
        weekend alternative, 347
    nursing management information
        system (NMIS), 336, 354–355
    orientation plan, 340, 341f
    patient classification systems (PCS),
        350–351
        CASH system, 352
        components, 352
        computer models, 353
        desired characteristics, 351–352
        GRASP, 352, 361
        in-house *vs.* purchased, 353
        nursing models, 352–353
        problems, 354
        purposes, 351, 351f
    policies, 340–341
    productivity
        case study, 360
        definition, 355–356
        improving nursing productivity,
            358–360
        measurement, 356–357
        model differences, 357–358
        monitoring system for the recov-
            ery room, 357
        problems in an operating room,
            357
    staffing philosophy, overview of, 336,
        336f
    strategic staffing, 349
    study
        data to be collected, 337–338
        forecasting staffing requirements,
            337, 338f
        planning for staffing, 338–339, 338f
        techniques, 337
    summary, 362
    transfer fair, 350
    travel nursing, 349
    unit staffing, 341–342
        complementary personnel, 342

        estimating a core staff per shift, 342f
        float personnel, 342
        full-time nursing personnel, 342
        part-time nursing personnel, 342
Staff nurse self-assessment survey, 646f
Standard of care, 511
    definition of, 474–475
    or "customary practice," 475–476
Standards of Clinical Nursing Practice,
    336, 503
Standards of practice, 24–25, 511–512
Standards of professional performance,
    25
Steffy, B.D., 29
Steinbeck, John, 552
Steinberg, D.L., 109
Stetler Model of evidenced-based prac-
    tice, 9
Stevens, D., 647
Stevens, Kathleen, 123
Stodgill's definition of leadership, 620
Stoltz, P.K., 533, 533f, 535
Strategic model, 141–142
Strategic planning and management
    evidenced-based strategic planning
        "balanced scorecard," 326–327
        evidenced-based practice, 327–328
        successful planning, 327
    introduction, 289, 290f
    mission, vision, and values
        mission or purpose, 290
        nursing mission or purpose, 291–294
            definition of nursing, 291–292
            focus on mission, 293
            mission statement of a division,
                293f
            mission statement of an organi-
                zation, 292f
            standards for the evaluation of
                mission statements, 294f
            statement of a unit, 293f
        values, 291
        vision, 291
    objectives
        areas of concentration, 297
        balanced objectives, 298f
        categorical areas for writing objec-
            tives, 298f
        described, 295–297
        of the division of nursing, 301f
        elements of objectives, 299f
        goals of the Metropolitan Medical
            Center, 300f
        long-term, 298
        of a nursing unit, 301f
        short-term, 298
        standards for evaluation of, 302f
    philosophy
        standards for evaluation of, 297f
        statement of a division, 296f
        statement of an organization,
            294–295, 295f
        statement of a unit, 296f
    planning
        Ackoff's four orientations to
            inactivism, 304–305
            interactivism, 305
            preactivism, 305
            reactivism, 304

        Ackoff's interactive planning-
            management model, 305,
            306f
        business planning, 319, 321
            key elements of, 319, 321–322
            operational plan-intensive care
                unit, 323–325f
        characteristics
            definitions of, 307
            examples of data for planning
                purposes, 308, 308f
            planning as the key element of
                nursing, 309
        choosing the best type of, 305–306
        divisional, 325
        elements
            assessment of strengths and
                weaknesses of the division,
                309
            good management, 310
            operational plans, 309
            premises, 309–310
            windows of opportunity,
                310–311
        factors relative to successful plan-
            ning, 304
        functional and operational plan-
            ning
            operational plan, 316f
            overview, 315–316
            participatory goal setting, 316,
                318
            standards for evaluation, 317f
            timetable for, 318f
        overview, 303–304
        planning new ventures, 319,
            320–321f
        practical planning actions, 322
        purposes, 306–307
        strategic planning
            benefits of, 314
            conclusions about the process,
                313f, 314–315
            crafting strategic plans, 312
            definition of, 311
            environmental scans, 311
            focus of, 312, 314
            implementation of, 314
            improving nursing management
                with, 312f
            phases of the process of, 313f
            seven areas of key results, 311
            use of, 311
        unit, 325–326, 326f
    strategy, 299–303
    summary, 328–329
Strauss, G., 86
Strengthening Hospital Nursing, 64f
Strong, A.G., 40
Structural empowerment, leadership
    management style, 649–650
    quality of nursing leadership
        developing a vision, 647
        developing commitment and
            trust, 648
        recognizing a need for change, 647
Structure standards, 511
Summer, C.E., 282
Swansburg, Russell, C., 140, 141f

Swanson, D.B., 600
"Swarmware," 5
Synergy
  defined, 232
  in managing academic and clinical
    partners, 615
  principle of, 210, 210f
System of policies, 188f
Systems thinking
  evaluation by root analysis, 500–501,
    501f
  introduction, 499–500
  management tools: measurement
    issues, 500
  management tools: performance
    issues
      approaches to controls, 502
      control functions, 502–503
      controlling mechanisms, 502
      elements of controls, 502
      self-control, 501–502
      task analysis and quality control,
        503

T

Talbott, C.M., 621
Task-oriented performance evaluation
  system (TOPES), 571
TCAB (Transforming Care at the
  Bedside), 8, 238, 238f
Team building
  committees
    evaluating meeting effectiveness,
      217f
    improving committee effective-
      ness, 216–217f
    organization of, 215–216, 215f
    purposes of committees, 215
    standards for evaluating, 214f
    types of, 214
  enhance self-esteem, 211
  group cohesiveness, 221
  group dynamics, 218–220
    functional roles of group mem-
      bers, 218–219f
  group leaders, 220
  Groupthink, 222–223, 222f
  phases of groups, 220–221
  principle of synergy, 210, 210f
  selected group techniques, 221–222f
  standards of practice and, 209–210
  steps to facilitate, 210–211, 211f
  summary, 246–248
  teams
    introduction, 211–212
    self-managed (self-directed) work
      team, 212–214, 213f
Team evaluation consensus (TEC), 565,
  571
Teamwork
  collaboration and, 57f, 60–61
  endorsing, motivation and, 420
Technology, 172
Temporary workers, 348–349
Tennessee Center for Nursing, 648
Termination phase, groups, 221
Termination report, example, 444f
Territorial departmentation, 244
Tests of significance, 537

*Theodore v. Department of Health and
  Human Services,* 460
Theory X and Theory Y, 418–419,
  623–624
The Sorry Works! coalition, 485
Third Wave, The, 429
Thomas, B., 211
Thomas, J., 40
Thompson, J.W., 172
Thompson, M.R., 265
Thoreau, Henry David, 184
Thorman, K., 348
Thriving on Chaos, 560
Time departmentation, 244
Tingey, S., 168
Tipping Point, 118
*To Err is Human: Building a Safer
  Health System* (1991), 7, 224,
  224f, 398
Toffler, A., 429
TOPES (task-oriented performance
  evaluation system), 571
Torts. *See under* Legal issues
Traditional model of nursing practice,
  234
Training, performance appraisals and
  job descriptions, 564–565
Training and education. *See also*
  Nursing staff educator
  for change
    anticipating potential failures,
      126–127
    communications, 125–126
    critical thinking, 125
    implementation science, 127
    organizational environment, 126
    rewards, 125
    using groups as change agents, 125
  continuing education online, 436
  management education, 272
  need for graduate-level education,
    9–10
  of nurse leaders, 631
  role of the nurse executive in, 203
Trait theory of leadership, 621–622
Transcendental systems, 32
Transfer fair, staffing and scheduling,
  350
Transformational leadership. *See*
  Leadership
Transformational Model for
  Professional Practice in
  Healthcare Organizations,
  648
Transforming Care at the Bedside
  (TCAB), 8, 238, 238f
Translation, ACE star model, 123
Transparency, 56, 57f, 58
Travel nursing, 349
Trends shaping nursing leadership
  complex adaptive systems (CAS)
    "clockware," 5
    how complexity science may im-
      prove organizations, 6–7
    macr-, micro-, and mesosystems
      as CAS, 6
    natural and human systems prop-
      erties, 6
    paradoxical questions, 5–6

placing your group at the edge of
  chaos, 5–6
principles, 5
"swarmware," 5
working in CAS, 7
creating healthy work environments,
  7–8
evidenced-based practice, 9, 10, 12
introduction, 3–4
nursing-sensitive indicators, safety
  standards, and quality indicators
    AHRQ quality indicators, 11
    IOM's Quality Initiative, 11
    National Database of Nursing
      Quality Indicators (NDNQI),
      10–11
    nursing-sensitive indicators, 10
    outcomes potentially sensitive to
      nursing, 10
    quality initiatives in public and
      private sectors, 11
organizational system: context for
  trends and change
    complex adaptive systems (CAS),
      4
    establishing informal groups, 4–5
    ordinary/extraordinary manage-
      ment, 4
    1980s approach to strategy, 4
professional organizations to improve care delivery, 8
safety, quality, and education
  integrating patient safety into
    nursing practice, 9
  need for graduate-level education,
    9–10
  nurse manager's role, 9
  skill sets and competencies for
    nurse executives, 10
summary, 12
websites, 17
Trinity Lutheran, performance improvement indicators for
  end-of-life care, 79
Trust, nurse executive role and, 199
Tuskegee experiment, 458

U

Ubiquitous computing, 446, 446f
Underwood, J., 466
Unintentional torts. *See under* Legal issues
Unit-based model of shared gover-
  nance, 206
Unity of command, 188f
U. of Iowa College of Nursing, 9, 41
U. of Kentucky Hospital model of case
  management, 39
U. of Pittsburgh Medical Center, 648
U. of Tennessee-Knoxville School of
  Nursing, 648
Upenieks, V., 677
Urwick, L., 186, 304, 495
U.S. Declaration of Independence, 76
Utilitarianism, 77

V

Valley Baptist Medical Center,
  Harlingen, TX, 238

Values, organizational culture, 223, 223f
Vega, K., 500
Veterans Administration medical system, 236
Veteran's Readjustment Assistance Act, 462f
Vik, A.G., 346
Virtual private networks, 435
Virtual reality (simulation), 446
Virtue-based ethics, 78
Vocational Rehabilitation Act, 278
Volunteer Hospitals of America Research Series, 657
Vroom, Victor, 415

W

Wah, S.S., 138
Walsh, M.B., 291
Wandelt, Mabel, 643
WANs (wide area networks), 434
Washington, Booker T., 522
Watson, Jean, Theory of Caring, 35
Webber, R.A., 282
Weber, Max, 188
Weekend work alternative, 347
Weeks, L., 266

Weihrich, H., 307, 496
Welty, Eudora, 50
West, M.E., 337
White, V., 29
WHO (World Health Organization), 457–458
Wide area networks (WANs), 434
Williams, E.G., 112
Wilson, C.K., 27
Wilson, R., 600, 601
Winitsky, M.L., 106
Wireless networks, 435
Witzel, P., 654
W.L. Gore Associates, 171–172
Wlody, G.S., 152
Wojcieszak, Doug, 485
Wolf, G., 235
Wolff, A.C., 606
Wolff, N., 353
Wong, C.L., 636
Woods, C., 237
Word processing, 441–442, 442f
Work, organization of, 229–231
Workforce diversity. *See also* Conflict management; Managing a culturally diverse workforce

staff development and, 601–602
Working or performing phase, groups, 221
Work redesign, performance appraisals and job descriptions, 564
Work week
    10-hour shift, 346–347
    12-hour shift, 347
World Health Organization (WHO), health policy process, 457–458

X

Xerox experience, 553

Y

Yura, H., 291

Z

Zaleznik, A., 629
Zander, K., 41
Zenger, T.R., 575
Zimmerman, B., 5, 6
Zurlage, C.L., 358